INTERNATIONAL HANDBOOK OF PANCREAS TRANSPLANTATION

DEVELOPMENTS IN SURGERY

INTERNATIONAL HANDBOOK OF PANCREAS TRANSPLANTATION

edited by

J.M. DUBERNARD

Edouard Herriot Hospital, Dept. of Urology and Transplantation Surgery, University of Lyon, Lyon, France

and

D.E.R. SUTHERLAND

University of Minnesota, Dept. of Surgery, Minneapolis, Minnesota, U.S.A.

SPRINGER-SCIENCE+BUSINESS MEDIA, B.V.

Library of Congress Cataloging in Publication Data

```
International handbook of pancreas transplantation / edited by J.M.
  Dubernard, D.E.R. Sutherland.
      p.   cm. -- (Developments in surgery)
    Includes index.

    1. Pancreas--Transplantation.   I. Dubernard, Jean-Michel.
  II. Sutherland, David E. R.   III. Series.
    [DNLM: 1. Pancreas--transplantation.   W1 DE998S / WI 800 I595]
  RD546.I55   1988
  617'.557--dc19
  DNLM/DLC
  for Library of Congress                                     88-13254
```

ISBN 978-94-010-6977-9   ISBN 978-94-009-1083-6 (eBook)
DOI 10.1007/978-94-009-1083-6

printed on acid free paper

Table of contents

List of first authors

Bartoš V. Institute for Clinical and Experimental Medicine, Vídeňská 800, P.O. Box 10, 140 00
  Prague 4, Czechoslovakia
  Co-author: I. Vaněk
Brekke I.B. National Hospital, Department of Surgery B, 0027 Oslo 1, Norway
Brons I.G.M. University of Cambridge Clinical School, Department of Surgery, Level 9,
  Addenbrooke's Hospital, Hills Road, Cambridge CB2 2QQ, United Kingdom
  Co-author: R.Y. Calne
Corry R.J. University of Iowa College of Medicine, Department of Surgery, Iowa City, IA
  52242, U.S.A.
  Co-authors: F.H. Wright, J.L. Smith
Dafoe D.C. University of Michigan Hospitals, Department of Surgery, D-2242 MPD, Ann
  Arbor, MI 48109, U.S.A.
  Co-authors: D.A. Campbell Jr, R.M. Merion, L. Rosenberg, L.L. Rocher, A.I. Vinik, J.G.
  Turcotte
Dubernard J.M. Edouard Herriot Hospital, Department of Urology and Transplantation
  Surgery, Pavillon V, Place d'Arsonval, F-69374 Lyon Cedex 08, France
  Co-authors: D.E.R. Sutherland, X. Martin, R. Sanseverino, A. Gelet, J. Traeger and N.
  Lefrançois, E. Herriot Hospital; E. La Rocca and M. Melandri, Clinica Medica VII, Istituto
  Scientifico S. Raffaele, Via Olgettina 60, 20090 Milano, Italy
Fernández-Cruz L. University of Barcelona, Department of Surgery, Villarroel 170, 08036
  Barcelona, Spain
  Co-authors: J.M. Gil-Vernet, J. Andreu, E. Esmatges, E.M. Targarona
Florack G. Technical University of Munich, Department of Surgery, Klinikum Rechts der Isar,
  D-8000 Munich 80, F.R.G.
Frisk B.A. Sahlgren's Hospital, Department of Surgery I, Transplant Unit, S-413 45 Göteborg,
  Sweden
  Co-authors: L.A. Hedman, H.A. Brynger
Garvin P.J. John Cochran Veterans Administration Medical Center and Department of
  Surgery, St. Louis University School of Medicine, St. Louis, MO 63104, U.S.A.
  Co-authors: M. Castaneda, K. Carney, D. Aridge, J. Hoff
Groth C.G. Huddinge Hospital, Department of Transplantation Surgery, 141 86 Huddinge,
  Sweden
  Co-authors: G. Tydén, J. Östman
Gunson B.K. Queen Elizabeth Hospital, Edgbaston, Birmingham B15 2TH, United Kingdom
  Co-author: P. McMaster

Land W. University of Munich, Division of Transplantatition Surgery, Klinikum Grosshadern, Marchionistrasse 15, D-8000 Munich 70, F.R.G.
Co-authors: R. Landgraf, W.D. Illner, D. Abendroth, A. Kampik, F.P. Lenhart, D. Burg, G. Hillebrand, L.A. Castro (‡), M.M.C. Landgraf-Leurs, M. Gokel, St. Schleibner, J. Nusser, M. Ulbig

Margreiter R. University Hospital, Division of Transplantation Surgery, Anichstrasse 35, Innsbruck, A-6020 Tirol, Austria
Co-authors: E. Steiner, A. Königsrainer, F. Aigner, M. Spielberger, C. Bösmüller

McMaster P. University of Birmingham, Queen Elizabeth Hospital, Edgbaston, Birmingham B15 2TM, United Kingdom

Michelsen B. Hagedorn Research Laboratory, Niels Steensensvej 6, DK-2820 Gentofte, Denmark
Co-authors: A. Grove, H. Vissing, H. Kofod, S. Baekkeskov, M. Cristie, M. Shak Pedersen, Å Lernmark

Monti L.D. Clinica Medica VII, Instituto Scientifico S. Raffaele, Via Olgettina 60, 20090 Milano, Italy
Co-authors: P.M. Piatti Clinica Medica VII; D. Long, Hospital Edouard Herriot, Department of Urology and Transplantation Surgery, Place d'Arsonval, F-69374 Lyon Cedex 08, France

Munda R. University of Cincinnati Medical Center, Department of Surgery, 231 Bethesda Avenue, Cincinnati, OH 45267-0558, U.S.A.
Co-author: J.W. Alexander

Pozza G. Clinica Medica, Istituto Scientifico San Raffaele, Via Olgettina 60, 20090 Milano, Italy
Co-authors: A. Secchi, E. La Rocca, M. Melandri

Scharp D.W. Washington University School of Medicine, Department of Surgery, 4939 Audubon Avenue, St. Louis, MO 63146, U.S.A.
Co-author: P.E. Lacy

Schilfgaarde R. van University Hospital Groningen, Department of Surgery, P.O. Box 30.001, 9600 RB Groningen, The Netherlands

Schlumpf R. University Hospital of Zurich, Department of Surgery, Rämistrasse 100, CH-8091 Zurich, Switzerland
Co-author: F. Largiadèr

Selam J.L. Lapeyronie hospital, Division of metabolic diseases, 34059 Montpellier, France, present address University of California at Irvine, College of Medicine, C-240, Medical Sciences 1, Irvine, CA 92717, U.S.A.

Sibley R.K. Stanford University Medical Center, Department of Pathology, 300 Pasteur Drive, Stanford, CA 94305, U.S.A.

Squifflet J.P. University of Louvain Medical School, Cliniques Saint-Luc, Department of Transplantation, 10 Avenue Hippocrate, 1200 Brussels, Belgium

Sutherland D.E.R. University of Minnesota Hospitals, Department of Surgery, 420 Delaware Street S.E., Box 280, Minneapolis, MN 55455, U.S.A.
Co-authors K.C. Moudry, F.C. Goetz, J.S. Najarian

Toledo-Pereyra L.H. Mount Carmel Mercy Hospital, Department of Surgery, Section of Transplantation, 6071 West Outer Drive, Detroit, MI 48235, U.S.A.
Co-authors: V.K. Mittal, D.A. Gordon

Traeger J. Edouard Herriot Hospital, Department of Nephrology and Metabolic Diseases, Place d'Arsonval, F-69374 Lyon Cedex 08, France
Co-authors: P.M. Piatti and L.D. Monti, Clinica Medica VII, Instituto-Scientifico S. Raffaele, University of Milan, Via Olgettina 60, 20090 Milano, Italy

Tydén G. Huddinge Hospital, Department of Transplantation Surgery, 141 86 Huddinge,
  Sweden
  Co-author: C.G. Groth
Tzakis A.G. University of Pittsburgh, Department of Surgery, 3601 Fifth Avenue, Falc Clinic
  4 West, Pittsburgh, PA 15213, U.S.A.
  Co-authors: P.B. Carroll, V. Kamp-Nielsen, T. Friberg, T.E. Starzl
Valente U. University of Genoa, Transplant Unit, Viale Benedetto XV 10, 16132 Genoa, Italy

Introduction and history of pancreatic transplantation

J.M. DUBERNARD and D.E.R. SUTHERLAND

Rationale for pancreas transplantation

In type I diabetes mellitus, insulin production by the pancreas progressively declines and ultimately disappears, as the Beta cells within the islets of Langerhans are destroyed by an autoimmune process resulting from a complex interplay between genetic and unknown environmental factors [1]. Searches for methods of total endocrine replacement therapy theoretically superior to simple exogenous insulin administration have taken three directions: 1) Connection to or implantation of an artificial (mechanical) pancreas, mimicking the betacell in its response to the need for and delivery of insulin; 2) transplantation of isolated islets as free grafts; and 3) solid organ, immediately vascularized pancreas transplantation. The first two approaches are currently impractical or ineffective in clinical practice, whereas the third has rapidly progressed during the past decade, to the point where its application is even becoming routine in a selected population of diabetic patients.

Pancreatic transplantation is performed to provide a self-regulated, endogenous source of insulin and other islet hormones, restoring normal metabolism, with the ultimate goals being prevention, stabilization or reversal of secondary degenerative complications of diabetes, complications that develop in spite of a well conducted exogenous insulin therapy because of the inherently imperfect nature of the therapy.

Diabetes mellitus is a world-wide health problem, with a high prevalence and a high incidence of microvascular complications. There are over 1 million insulin dependent type I diabetics in the United States and between 150,000 and 250,000 in France [2]. In Western countries, the incidence of type I diabetes mellitus is approximately 55 new cases per million population, all age groups being at risk, although the majority of the cases occurs in children [3]. Diabetes mellitus is the fourth leading cause of death by disease in occidental

Revised by Janet Sanders and Arnell Sandstrom.

1

J.M. Dubernard and D.E.R. Sutherland (eds.), International Handbook of Pancreas Transplantation, 1–11.

countries [4]. By the 20th year after onset of the disease, 50% of individuals with type I diabetes mellitus are either blind, in renal failure or have major sensory motor disturbances. Individuals with diabetes are 25 times more prone to blindness, 17 times more prone to renal failure, 5 times more likely to require an amputation and twice as likely to develop heart disease than the general population [5]. Improvements in treatment of the metabolic and degenerative complications of diabetes mellitus has led to an increase in the number of diabetic patients being treated for end stage renal failure, now representing 10 to 40% of the new patients admitted in dialysis centers [6]. This group of patients requires special therapeutic approaches because of the high rate of associated complications that occur while on dialysis as well as after renal transplantation. The desire to treat not only the manifestation of diabetic nephropathy but also its cause, is also apparent by the large number of simultaneous or successive renal and pancreatic transplants in patients with end stage diabetic nephropathy [7]. The majority of pancreas transplant recipients to date have been in this category of advanced disease.

Pancreatic transplantation has as its main purpose the prevention of secondary complications of diabetes, even though the factors influencing the development of microvascular and other lesions in the eyes, kidneys, nerves and other systems are not entirely understood [8]. The dysmetabolism of diabetes, as manifested by sustained or intermittent hyperglycemia, is known to play a dominant role in their genesis [9]. Normal beta cells are programmed to release insulin by demand to maintain plasma glucose and the concentrations of other metabolites at a constant level or within a very narrow range. Exogenous insulin administered by standard parenteral techniques, cannot reliably prevent wide excursions in plasma glucose levels [10]. Home glucose monitoring may improve diabetic control, but the instability of diabetes cannot be eliminated. Systems designed to administer insulin frequently or continuously, even with close monitoring of glucose plasma levels, do not mimic the precise control provided by functioning beta cells and carry the specific risk of hypoglycemia [11]. Insulin treatment regimens that induce 'near normoglycemia' have been applied in attempts to influence the late complications of diabetes, with some success [9]. Insulin pumps with intravenous injections have local infections problems [11]. Peritoneal infusion of insulin can improve glycemic control in some unstable diabetic patients, perhaps because of portal drainage of the intraperitoneal insulin. Even with these methods, however, non-physiological and predictible variations of glycemia occur. Most diabetic patients, therefore, are managed by exogenous insulin regimens that prevent or minimize the frequency of the extremes of either keto-acidosis or hypoglycemia.

Both the incidence and severity of degenerative complications are generally less in diabetic patients with a 'good' as opposed to a 'poor' control of hyperglycemia [9, 12]. Nephropathy and retinopathy can develop in patients who become diabetic as a result of total pancreatectomy or disease process that involves secondarly the islets [13, 14]. Lesions similar to those observed in diabetic patients also occur in the animal models of primary and secondary diabetes [15]. The lesions in animals can be prevented, arrested or reversed following restoration of normal metabolism by islets or pancreas transplantation [16, 17, 18]. Kidneys transplanted from normal donors to diabetic rats [19] or humans develop lesions of diabetic nephropathy [20]. Conversely, such lesions in kidneys taken from diabetic donors will regress following transplantation to non-diabetic rat [19] or human recipients [21].

Evidence that pancreas transplantation favorably influences the course of secondary complications in diabetic patients has slowly emerged [22, 23, 24, 25] and in some systems has been difficult to show because advanced lesions, often irreversible, were present at the time of transplantation [26]. However, kidneys transplanted to diabetic recipients simultaneously with a pancreas have not developed the lesions of diabetic nephropathy [22], that would otherwise be expected in a high proportion of grafts [20]. Regression of microscopic lesions of diabetic nephropathy has also been observed in the native kidneys of recipients of successful pancreas transplants alone [23]. An improvement in diabetic neuropathy following pancreas transplantation has also been reported [24]. Stabilization, and in some cases improvement of retinopathy, were observed in one series of diabetic recipient of simultaneous kidney and pancreas transplants [25], but not in another series of recipients of a pancreas transplant alone [26]. The extent to which pancreas transplantation can influence established complications is uncertain. The results of animal experiments suggest that the lesions should be in an early stage [16–18]. The observations have been an impetus for the clinical application of pancreas transplants alone in diabetic patients with degenerative complications just beginning to emerge, specifically those without renal failure [27].

Pancreas transplantation has the potential to have a significant impact on the health maintenance of two groups of diabetic patients, both grossly different according to the timing of the transplant: either at the end of evolution of disease in the kidney, in which case a renal graft is also required so kidney as well as pancreas function can be restored; or early in the cause of the disease, to replace pancreatic function alone in order to prevent degenerative complications.

It must be emphasized that finally, pancreas transplantation, unlike heart or liver transplantation, is not an immediate life saving measure. The objective of pancreas transplantation, is to improve the quality of life and to favorably influence the secondary complications of diabetes that would otherwise take their toll several years hence. Pancreas transplantation is akin to kidney transplantation, where if the kidney fails the patient can resume dialysis. Rejection, or other causes of pancreatic graft failure, should be followed by a return to exogenous insulin therapy and resumption of a life style no different than that achieved pretransplant.

History of pancreas transplantation

The discovery that the pancreas is an organ essential for carbohydrate metabolism was made by Von Mering and Minkowski, who in 1889, produced fatal diabetes in dogs by total pancreatectomy [28]. The first transplant of a pancreas was performed by Hedon, who in 1893 [29] reported that free grafting of a portion of a totally resected pancreas prevented the development of diabetes in a dog.

The impetus to pursue pancreas transplantation as a treatment for diabetes was diminished by the discovery of insulin by Banting and Best in 1922 [30]. Insulin was able to prevent the acute mortality from the metabolic derangements of diabetes and dramatically extended the life span of diabetic individuals. Before the discovery of insulin, the secondary complications of diabetes were rarely seen because most patients at risk did not survive sufficiently long for them to appear. After the discovery of insulin the secondary complications of diabetes became the major cause of diabetic morbidity and mortality [8]. The inability to achieve perfect metabolic control by exogenous insulin made prevention of complications difficult, and major efforts focused on treatment of secondary complications, culminating in the late 1960's and early 1970's with the application of kidney transplants for treatment of diabetic nephropathy [31] and laser and other procedures for diabetic retinopathy [32]. Such treatments, however, did not solve the basic problem, the dysmetabolism of diabetes, and a few individuals continued to pursue pancreas transplantation in the experimental setting.

The first successful transplants of immediately vascularized pancreatic grafts were made in dogs by Gayet and Guillaumie in 1927 [33], Houssay in 1929 [33] and Lexter in 1929 [34]. Brooks in the 1950's [36], Dejode and Howard in the early 1960's [37]. Lillehei and Largiarder and associates, from the mid 1960's to early 1970's [38, 39] worked out the techniques of pancreas transplantation in large animal models that lead to the first clinical attempts at pancreas transplantation and that formed the basis of current pancreas transplant research [40].

The first pancreas transplant in a human was performed by Kelly, Lillehei and associated at the University of Minnesota on December 17, 1966 [41]. A cadaver donor segmental (body and tail) pancreas graft, based on a vascular pedicle of the splenic artery in continuity with celiac axis and the splenic vein in continuity with the portal vein, was transplanted to the iliac fossa of an uremic diabetic woman. The duct of the graft was ligated. A kidney was transplanted to the opposite iliac fossa. The patient became normoglycemic and insulin-independent immediately, but she died two months posttransplant from a combination of rejection and sepsis. Lillehei and associates then went on to perform a series of 13 pancreas transplants between the end of 1966 and 1973, the first ten in uremic diabetic patients, of whom 9 also received kidney transplants, and the last three in nonuremic diabetic patients [39, 42]. The first 12 pancreas transplants were whole pancreaticoduodenal grafts anastomosed to a roux-en-Y loop of recipient jejunum, while the last one was a whole pancreas transplant in which the papilla of Vater was used for anastomosis to the recipient bowel [42]. Only one of the pancreas graft functioned for more than one year, while the others failed for a variety of reasons [43].

Lillehei had originally reasoned that for kidney transplants to succeed in uremic diabetic patients, the diabetic conditions would have to be corrected [39]. However, Najarian, Simmons, Kjellstrand and associates. in the early 1970's, showed that kidney transplantation could be performed with a success rate nearly as high in diabetic and nondiabetic recipients [44]. Thus, the rationale to perform pancreas transplants solely to promote kidney graft function became untenable and kidney transplantation alone became the treatment of choice in diabetic patients in most kidney transplant centers.

A few other groups also performed pancreas transplants in the 1960's and early 1970's, [45, 46, 47] but only one patient had long-term graft function, in the series of Gliedman et al. [48] transplanted at Montefiore Hospital in New-York. This patient died while on dialysis after rejection of the kidney with a functioning pancreas graft four and a half years after the transplant. Gliedman et al. [45] popularized the segmental pancreas transplant technique, that had been used by Kelly and Lillehei in their first case, but advocated exocrine drainage into a hollow organ, either the ureter or bowel [48].

Of the cases done in the late 1960's and early 1970's, approximately half were whole pancreas or pancreaticoduodenal grafts and half were segmental grafts. The success rate with either method was relatively low. The American College of Surgeons/National Institute of Health (ACS/NIH) maintained an organ transplant registry until June 30, 1977, and up to that time received information on 57 pancreas transplants in 55 diabetic recipients [49]. The one year pancreas graft function rate was only 3% and the one year patient survival rate was only 40% in these pioneering cases [50]. The first pancreas transplants were done, however, at a time when kidney transplantation was still in the early stages of development as the treatment for end stage renal disease and at a time when the clinical immunosuppressive protocols were just being formu-lated [39, 41, 45].

The incentive to perform pancreas transplants was low during these years, and in the 1970's a surge of interest developed in islet transplantation following the report by Ballinger and Lacy that islets from the rat pancreas could be transplanted as free grafts to ameliorate streptozotocin induced diabetes [51]. The development of islet isolation techniques in rodents, followed by their adaptation in the large animals, led many investigators to believe that islet transplantation would supercede pancreas transplantation for clinical application [52]. However, trials of islets transplantation in humans met with limited success, and an euglycemic state has not been induced in an islet transplant recipient [53, 54, 55, 56]. Isolation of a sufficient quantity of islets from the human pancreas has been a major difficulty but islet isolation and transplantation remains an area of active investigation in both animal [57] and humans [58].

The perception, or for some the ultimate realization, that development of islet transplantation into a clinical modality would take many years led to the resumption or expantion of pancreas transplantation in several centers in the late 70's and early 80's. The clinical application of the duct obstruction technique [59], a simple procedure was responsible for the renewed interest, but other innovations were also made [60] and a steady improvement in results has occurred [40]. Since 1978 a near doubling of pancreas transplant activity has occurred every other year [7].

The history of clinical pancreas transplantation largely revolves around development and application of various surgical techniques for grafting. As mentioned earlier, the first pancreas transplant was segmental with duct ligation [41]. Lillehei, however, favored the whole pancreas transplant technique with anastomosis of the graft duodenum or a button of the papilla of Vater to the recipient bowel [39, 42]. Gliedman et al. [45] introduced the novel technique of anastomosis of the duct of a segmental pancreas graft to the recipient ureter in uremic diabetic patients. A modification for urinary drainage was made by Sollinger et al. [61] at the University of Wisconsin in the early 1980's, in which the pancreatic duct of segmental grafts or a portion of the duodenum of whole pancreas grafts was anastomosed directly to the recipient bladder [65]. Groth et al. [46] at Huddinge Hospital in Stockholm, Sweden, applied segmental pancreas transplants with anastomosis to a Roux-en-Y loop of recipient bowel; this group has continued to use this basic technique with certain refinements into the 1980's [63, 64]. In 1978, Dubernard et al. [59], at Herriot Hospital in Lyon, France, reported on a new method of pancreas transplantation, in which the duct was injected with an synthetic polymer, reminiscent of the pancreatic duct obstruction experiment performed in dogs by Thiroloix in 1892 [65]. This technique completely avoided bacterial contamination, was safe, was soon adapted by several institutions, and has been used for more pancreas transplants than any other technique [7]. However, even this technique is not complication free, and fibrosis may be induced in the graft by duct injection [66, 67]. A return to the original method of Lillehei et al. [39, 42], in which a whole pancreas transplant was used with anastomosis of a patch or segment graft duodenum to the recipient bowel, also occurred in the 1980's [68, 69, 70, 71]. Today the three most popular techniques for management of the graft pancreatic duct are polymer injection, enteric drainage and bladder drainage [7]. The program with the largest number of cases (University of Minnesota) has used these three techniques, as well as some others, since resuming pancreas transplantation in 1978 [68, 71, 72]. The intraperitoneal duct open technique was initially tested [72]; even though it was ultimately abandoned, it was used in the patient with the longest pancreas graft survival (continous function since 1978). This group also has a large number of diabetic patients with a functioning renal graft from a living donor, and has expanded the living donor approach to pancreas transplants, both allografts and isografts [73, 74]. It was initially thought that transplants from living donors could be done with minimal or, in the case of twins, no immunosuppression, but when tried recurrence of disease with isletitis and/or selective beta cell destruction, occurred, without signs of rejection [75, 76], a key observation in the development of the hypothesis that Type I diabetes is an autoimmune disease [1]. Fortunately, recurrence of disease can be preserved by adequate immunosuppression, and the graft loss rate for immunological reasons is less for pancreas transplants from related than from cadaver donors [73], with a corresponding higher graft survival rate, justifying its continous application under rightly defined circumstances [77].

The development of pancreatic transplantation has been documented by the International Pancreas Transplant Registry [50]. The Registry was created at the First International Symposium on Pancreatic Transplantation, organized in Lyon in 1980 [78]. Since that time it has been maintained at the University of Minnesota [7], and has incorporated the data of the ACS/NIH registry that closed in 1977 [49]. The enthusiastic participation of virtually all pancreas transplant programs in the registry has allowed a comprehensive analysis of outcome to be performed, and has fostered close contact between the individuals involved in pancreas transplantation worldwide. Periodic workshops have also stimulated the development of and dissemination of information on pancreas transplants [60, 78].

Today, pancreatic transplantation is edging to the front of the stage in the management of the complicated diabetic patient. The time has come for a synthetic review of all the work performed during the past ten years, gathering experiences of the teams who have participated in the effort of promoting this method of endocrine replacement therapy. An aim of this book is also to show the magnitude of problems yet to be solved.

A technique of pancreatic transplantation with no negative and only positive features has not yet been described. Methods of diagnosis of rejection and prevention of rejection have to be improved before the procedure can be applied to the newly diagnosed diabetic patient. A fascinating challenge lies in

8

the extension of the indications and selection of patients, not only the Type I diabetic patients whose microangiopathy is clinically apparent and yet still potentially reversible, but also the group without such lesions but whose day-to-day living is handicaped by persistent or recurrent acute metabolic problems. As clinical results progress, pancreas transplantation will expand, and the foundation for this expansion, as well as for its current application, are described in this book.

References

1. Eisenbarth GS: Type I diabetes mellitus: A chronic autoimmune disease. New Engl J Med 314: 1360–1368, 1986.
2. LaPorte RE, Tajima N: Prevalence of insulin-dependent diabetes, diabetes in America (editors Harris MI and Hamman RF for national diabetes data group, NIADDK) NIH pub. no. 85-1468, U.S. dept health and human services, chapter V, pp 1–8, 1985.
3. LaPorte RE: Cruickshanks; Incidence and risk factors for insulin-dependent diabetes, diabetes in America (editors Harris MI and Hamman RF for national diabetes data group, NIADDK) NIH pub. no. 85-1468, U.S. dept health and human services, chapter III, pp 1–12, 1985.
4. Harris MI, Hanaman RF (eds): Diabetes in America NIH publication 85-1468, Bethesda, Maryland 1985.
5. Krolewski AS, Warram JH, Rand LI et al: Epidemiologic approach to the etiology of type I diabetes mellitus and its complications. N Engl J Med 317: 1390–1398, 1987.
6. Goetz FC, Elick B, Fryd D, Sutherland DER: Renal transplantation in diabetes. Clinics in Endocrinology and Metabolism 15: 807–821, 1986.
7. Sutherland DER, Moudry KC: Pancreas transplant registry: history and analysis of cases 1966 to October 1986. Pancreas 2: 473–488, 1987.
8. Tchobroutsky G: Relation of diabetes control to Development of microvascular complications. Diabetologia 15: 143–152, 1978.
9. Hanssen KF, Dahl-Jorgenson K, Lauritzen J et al: Diabetic control and microvascular complications: the near normoglycemic experience. Diabetologia 10: 677–684, 1986.
10. Service JS, Molnar GD, Rosevar JE, et al: Mean amplitude of glycemic excursions, a measure of diabetes instability. Diabetes 19: 644–655, 1970.
11. Ungar RH: Meticulous control of diabetes: Benefits, risks and precautions. Diabetes 31: 479, 1982.
12. Pirart J: Diabetes mellitus and its degenerative complications: A prospective study of 4,400 patients observed between 1947 and 1973. Diabetes Care 1: 168–188, 1978.
13. Passa P, Rousselie F, Gauville C, Canivet J: Retinopathy in idiopathic hemochromatosis with diabetes. Diabetes 26: 2: 113–120, 1977.
14. Doyle AP, Balcerzak SP, Jeffrey WL: Fatal diabetic glomerulosclerosis after total pancreatectomy. N Engl J Med 270: 623–624, 1964.
15. Salans LB, Graham BJ: Proceedings of a task force on animals appropriate for studying diabetes mellitus and its complications. Diabetes 31 (Supplement 1): 1–95, 1982.
16. Mauer SM, Sutherland DER, Steffes MW, et al: Pancreatic transplantation: Effects on the glomerular lesions of experimental diabetes in the rat. Diabetes 23: 748–753, 1974.
17. Orloff MJ, Yamanaka N, Greenleaf G, et al: Reversal of mesangial enlargement in rats with long-standing diabetes by whole pancreas transplantation. Diabetes 35: 347–354, 1986.

18. Orloff MJ, Maceto D, Greenleaf GE, et al: Effect of Pancreas transplantation of diabetic somatic neuropathy. Surgery 104: 437–444, 1988.

19. Lee CS, Mauer SM, Brown DM, Sutherland DER, Michael AF, Najarian JS: Renal transplantation in diabetes mellitus in rats. J Exp Med 139: 793–800, 1974.

20. Mauer SM, Steffes MW, Connett J, et al: Development of lesions in the glomerular basement membrane and mesangium after transplantation of normal kidneys to diabetic patients. Diabetes 32: 948–952, 1983.

21. Abouna GM, Al-Adnani MSA, Kremer GM, et al: Reversal of diabetic nephropathy in human cadaveric kidneys after transplantation into nondiabetic recipients. Lancet 2: 1274–1276, 1983.

22. Bohman SO, Tyden G, Wilezek A: Prevention of kidney graft diabetic nephropathy by pancreas transplantation in man. Diabetes 34: 306, 1985.

23. Bilous RW, Mauer SM, Sutherland DER, Steffes MW: Glomerular structure and function following successful pancreas transplantation for insulin-dependent diabetes mellitus. Diabetes 36: 43A, 1987. Nephropathy by Pancreas Transplantation in Man. Diabetes 34: 306, 1985.

24. van der Vliet JA, Navarro X, Kennedy WR, Goetz FC, Najarian JS, Najarian JS: The effect of pancreas transplantation on diabetic polyneuropathy. Transplantation 45: 368–370, 1988.

25. Ulbig M, Kampik A, Landgraf R, Land W: The influence of combined pancreatic and renal transplantation on advanced diabetic retinopathy. Transpl Proc 19: 3554–3556, 1987.

26. Ramsay RC, Goetz FC, Sutherland DER, Mauer SM, Robinson LL, Cantrill HL, Knobloch WH, Najarian JS: Progression of diabetic retinopathy after pancreas transplantation for insulin-dependent diabetes mellitus. H N Eng J Med 318: 208–214, 1988.

27. Sutherland DER, Kendall DM, Moudry KC, Navarro X, Kennedy WR, Ramsay RC, Steffes MW, Mauer SM, Goetz FC, Dunn DL, Najarian JS: Pancreas transplantation in nonuremic, type I diabetic recipients. Surgery 104: 453–464, 1988.

28. von Mering J, Minkowski O: Diabetes mellitus nach pancreas extirpation. Arch Exp Pathol Pharmakol 26: 371–379, 1889.

29. Hedon E. Sur la consommation du sucre ches le chien apres l'extirpation du pancreas. Arch Physiol Norm Pathol 5: 154–163, 1893.

30. Bliss M: The discovery of insulin. The univ. of Chicago press., 1982.

31. Najarian JS, Kjellstrand CM, Simmons RL et al: Renal transplantation for diabetic glomerulosclerosis. Ann Surg 178: 477–485, 1973.

32. Witkin SR, Klein R: Optholmologic care for people with diabetes. J Am Med Assoc 251–2534–37, 1984.

33. Gayet R, Guillaumie M: La regulation de la secretion interne pancreatique par un processus normalisateur demontree par des transplantations de pancreas. Cr Soc Biol 97: 1613–1627, 1877.

34. Houssay BA: Technique de la greffe pancreaticoduodenale an cou. C.R. Soc. Biol. (Paris) 100: 138–140, 1929.

35. Lexer E. Die freien transplantationen. Ferdinand Enke, Stuttgart 1919.

36. Brooks JR, Gifford GH: Pancreatic homotransplantation. Transplant Bull 6: 100–103, 1959.

37. DeJode LR, Howard JM: Studies in Pancreaticoduodenal homotransplantation. Surg Gyn Obst 114: 553–58, 1962.

38. Largiader F, Lyons GW, Hidalgo F, et al: orthotopic allotransplantation of the pancreas. Am J Surg 113: 70–76, 1967.

39. Lillehei RC, Simmons RL, Najarian JS, et al: Pancreatico-duodenal allotransplantation: Experimental and clinical experience. Ann Surg 172: 405–436, 1970.

40. Sutherland DER: Pancreas transplantation: an update. In Alberti KGMM, Krall LP (eds) Diabetes Annual/3; pp 159–188. Elsevier Science Publishers, Amsterdam, 1987.

41. Kelly, WD, Lillehei RC, Merkel FK, Idezuki Y, Goetz FC: Allotransplantation of the pancreas and duodenum along with the kidney in diabetic nephropathy. Surgery 61: 827, 1967.

42. Lillehei RC, Ruiz JO, Acquino C, Goetz FC: Transplantation of the pancreas. Acta Endocrinol 83 (Suppl 205): 303, 1976.

43. Sutherland DER, Goetz FC, Carpenter AM, Najarian JS, Lillehei RC: Pancreaticoduodenal grafts: clinical and pathological observations in uremic versus nonuremic recipients. In: Touraine JL, Traeger J, Betuel H, Brochier J, Dubernard JM, Revillard JP, Triau R (eds): Transplantation and clinical immunology; vol X, pp 190–195. Excerpta Medica, Amsterdam-Oxford, 1979.

44. Najarian JS, Sutherland DER, Simmons RL, Howard RJ, Kjellstrand CM, Ramsay RC, Goetz FC, Fryd DS, Sommer BG: A ten year experience in kidney transplantation in juvenile onset insulin dependent diabetics. Ann Surg 190: 487–500, 1979.

45. Gliedman ML, Gold M, Whittaker J, Rifkin H, Soberman R, Freed S, Tellis V, Veith FJ: Clinical segmental pancreatic transplantation with ureter–pancreatic duct anastomosis for exocrine drainage. Surgery 74: 171–180, 1973.

46. Groth CG, Lundgren G, Arner P, Cellste H, Hardstedt C, Lewander R, Ostman J: Rejection of isolated pancreatic allografts in patients with diabetes. Surg Gynecol & Obstet 143: 933–940, 1976.

47. Largiader F, Uhlschmid G, Binswanger U, et al: Pancreas rejection in combined pancreaticoduodenal and renal allotransplantation in man. Transplantation 19: 185–187, 1975.

48. Gliedman ML, Tellis VA, Soberman R, et al: Long-term effects on pancreatic transplant function in patients with advanced juvenile onset diabetes. Diabetes Care 1: 1–9, 1978.

49. American college of surgeons/national institute of health: organ transplant registry: first scientific report. JAMA 217: 1520–1529, 1971.

50. Sutherland DER: International Human pancreas and islet transplant registry. Transpl Proc 12 (No. 4, Suppl 2): 229–236, 1980.

51. Ballinger WF, Lacy PE: Transplantation of intact pancreatic islets in rats. Surgery 72: 175, 1972.

52. Sutherland DER: pancreas and islet transplantation. I. Experimental studies. Diabetologia 20: 161–85, 1981.

53. Sutherland DER: Pancreas and islet transplantation. II. Clinical results. Diabetologia 20: 435–50, 1981.

54. Sutherland DER, Matas AJ, Najarian JS: Pancreatic islet cell transplantation. Surg Clinics of No Amer 58: 365–382, 1978.

55. Sutherland DER, Matas AJ, Goetz FC, Najarian JS: Transplantation of dispersed pancreatic islet tissue in humans: Autografts and allografts. Diabetes 29 (suppl 1): 31–44, 1980.

56. Scharp DW, Lacy PE: Human islet isolation and transplantation. Diabetes 34 (suppl 1): 5A, 1985.

57. Lacy PE: Islet transplantation. In: Alberti KGMM, Krall LP (eds) The diabetes annual/3; pp 189–200. Elsevier Science Publishers, Amsterdam, 1987.

58. Scharp DW, Lacy PE, Finke E, et al: Low temperature culture of human islets isolated by the distention method and purified with ficoll or percoll gradients. Surgery. 102: 869–879, 1987.

59. Dubernard JM, Traeger J, Neyra P, Touraine JL, Tranchant D, Blanc-Brunat N: A new method of preparation of segmental pancreatic grafts for transplantation: trials in dogs and in man. Surgery 84: 633–640, 1978.

60. Land W, Landgraff R: clinical pancreas transplantation, the world experience: Proceedings of the second international workshop on clinical pancreas transplantation. Transp Proc 19 (Suppl 4): 1–45, 1987.

61. Sollinger HW, Cook K, Kamps D, Glass NR, Belzer FO: Clinical and experimental experi-

ence with pancreaticocystostomy for exocrine pancreatic drainage in pancreas transplantation. Transpl Proc 16: 749–531, 1984.

62. Sollinger H, Kalayoglu M, Hoffman RM et al: Experience with whole pancreas transplantation and pancreaticoduodenocystostomy. Transpl proc 18: 1759–1761, 1986.

63. Groth CG, Collste H, Lundgren G et al: Successful outcome of segmental human pancreatic transplantation with enteric exocrine diversion after modifications in technique. Lancet 2: 522–524, 1982

64. Tyden G, Reinholt G, Brattstrom C et al: Diagnosis of rejection in recipients of pancreatic grafts with enteric exocrine diversion by monitoring pancreatic juice cytology and amylase excretion. Transpl Proc 19: 3892–3894, 1987.

65. Thiroloix J., Le diabete pancreatique masson ed, Paris 1892.

66. Blanc-Brunat N, Dubernard JM, Touraine JL, et al: Pathology of the pancreas after intraductal neoprene injection in dogs and diabetic patients treated by pancreatic transplantation. Diabetologia 25: 97, 1983.

67. Sibley RK, Sutherland DER: Pancreas transplantation: An immunohistological and histopathologic examination of 100 grafts. Am J Pathol 128: 151–170, 1987.

68. Sutherland DER, Goetz FC, Najarian JS: One hundred pancreas transplants at a single institution. Ann Surg 200: 414–440, 1984.

69. Starzl TE, Hakali TR, Shaw BW et al: A flexible procedure for multiple cadaveric organ procurement. Surg Gynecol Obstet 158: 223–230, 1984.

70. Corry RJ, Nghiem DD, Schulak JA, Beutell WD, Gonwa TA: Surgical treatment of diabetic nephropathy with simultaneous pancreatic duodenal and renal transplantation. Surg Gyn Obstet 162: 547–555, 1986.

71. Prieto M, Sutherland DER, Goetz FC et al: Pancreas transplant results according to technique of duct management: Bladder versus enteric drainage. Surgery 102: 680–691, 1987.

72. Sutherland DER, Goetz FC, Najarian JS: Intraperitoneal transplantation of immediately vascularized segmental pancreatic grafts without duct ligation: A clinical trial. Transplantation 28: 485–491, 1979.

73. Sutherland DER, Goetz FC, Najarian JS: Pancreas transplants from related donors. Transplantation 38: 625–633, 1984.

74. Sutherland DER, Sibley R, Zu X-Z, Michael A, Srikanta S, Taub F, Najarian J, Goetz FC: Twin-to-twin pancreas transplantation: Reversal and reenactment of the pathogenesis of type I diabetes. Trans Assoc Amer Phys XCVII: 80–87, 1984.

75. Sutherland DER, Goetz FC, Elick BA, Najarian JS: Experience with 49 segmental pancreas transplants in 45 diabetic patients. Transplantation 34: 330–338, 1982.

76. Sibley RK, Sutherland DER, Goetz, FC, Michael AF: Recurrent diabetes mellitus in the pancreas iso- and allograft. A light and electron microscopic and immunohistochemical analysis of four cases. Laboratory investigation. 53: 132–144, 1985.

77. Sutherland DER, Goetz FG, Moudry KC, Najarian JS: Pancreatic transplantation – a single institution's experience. Diabetes, Nutrition and Metabolism 1: 57–66, 1988.

78. Dubernard JM, Traeger J: Transplantation of the pancreas. Transplant proc 12 (suppl 2): 1, 1980.

1. Modern concepts of diabetes and its pathogenesis

B. MICHELSEN, A. GROVE, H. VISSING, H. KOFOD,
S. BAEKKESKOV, M. CHRISTIE, M.S. PEDERSEN and
Å. LERNMARK

Introduction

Diabetes mellitus affects a large number of individuals and represents a syndrome which is characterized by chronic hyperglycemia. Since blood glucose is controlled by a number of mechanisms, several abnormalities of different etiology and pathogenesis may cause hyperglycemia. The major types of diabetes are non-insulin dependent (Type 2) diabetes (NIDDM) and insulin-dependent (Type 1) diabetes (IDDM). NIDDM can affect as much as 3–4 percent of the population in Western Europe and North America and is probably a heterogeneous disease with multiple etiologies. Obesity is one of the suspected factors. Insulin receptor defects and mutant insulin molecules are etiological factors for only a few IDDM patients. In the majority of patients, onset starts after the age of 40, and about 60–90 percent of the patients are obese. Since most of the problems discussed in this book are less relevant to NIDDM, the modern concepts of diabetes and its pathogenesis that will be discussed in this chapter will refer to insulin-dependent (Type 1) diabetes mellitus (IDDM).

A patient with IDDM is dependent on injections of insulin to prevent ketosis and to preserve life. The disease is characterized by insulinopenia and onset is usually found in young people, but may occur at any age. The major features of IDDM are the association with certain HLA types, autoimmunity, including also autoreactivity against the islet B cells and an etiology which may involve environmental factor(s) including chemicals, microorganisms or virus. IDDM appears to develop after a prodrome of autoimmunity directed towards the islet B cells to include islet cell antibodies [1, 2], insulin autoantibodies [3] or antibodies against a human islet M_r 64000 (64K) protein [4]. At the time of clinical diagnosis, a major portion of the B cells has been lost [5, 6] and islets of Langerhans with inflammatory cells are often found [7, 8]. While the islet B cells are greatly diminished in number, the other endocrine cell types remain and the islets of Langerhans now consist of A, D, and PP cells. It is possible

13

J.M. Dubernard and D.E.R. Sutherland (eds.), International Handbook of Pancreas Transplantation, 13–24.
© *1989 by Kluwer Academic Publishers.*

that the autoimmune reactions involve mechanisms which specifically remove the B cells.

The pathogenesis of the loss of B cells remains obscure. However, the fact that both humoral [9, 10] and cellular [11] anti-B-cell immune activities have been demonstrated raises the possibility that the immune response, which normally is protective to an individual, may be involved in causing the disease. Although B-cell specific cytotoxic T lymphocytes have yet to be demonstrated, earlier studies have shown evidence of cellular hypersensitivity to islet cell antigens in migration inhibition tests [12]. Cells armed with antibodies against surface-expressed islet cell antigens may mediate antibody-dependent cellular cytotoxicity [13]. Cells stationary or able to home in on the islets and produce Interleukin-1 (IL-1) are potentially harmful, since the latter has been found to be highly cytotoxic to islet cells [14].

Antibodies detecting B-cell specific, cell-surface expressed antigen(s) may be cytotoxic either by mediating complement-dependent cytotoxicity [9, 10] or by inhibiting the B-cell function [15] or replication [16]. Whatever may be the mechanisms, the specific removal of the B cells would seem to require one or several B cell specific molecules which are recognized by the different arms, cellular or humoral, of the immune response (Figure 1).

The immune response is controlled by several important elements. First, a foreign antigen or as we assume, an autoantigen as well, is processed by an antigen-presenting cell. Macrophages, dendritic cells or monocytes are all cells capable of processing and presenting antigens. The processing apparently allows fragments of the antigen to appear on the cell surface in close association with, and perhaps even bound to, an HLA-D region Class II molecule. Second, a specific T helper lymphocyte receptor will recognize the presented antigen in the context of the Class II molecule. Third, the T helper lymphocyte responds to the antigen-Class II molecule complex by rapid proliferation and elaboration of IL-2, a T-cell growth factor. Fourth, B lymphocytes carrying membrane-bound antibodies for the antigen are activated to proliferate, differentiate and to produce antibodies. Fifth, T cytolytic lymphocytes (CTL) are activated by the T helpers, as well. By having their receptors recognize the antigen shown on the target cell surface, CTL's are able to kill target cells, provided these and the CTL's share the same Class I antigen specificity.

There are two features of the immune response towards the pancreatic islet cells which are of particular interest. First, many IDDM patients, at clinical onset, also have other organ-specific autoantibodies apart from those directed against islet cell antigens. The background of this increased level of autoimmunity is not understood, but it has been noted that healthy family members to IDDM patients also have an increased prevalence of a variety of autoantibodies [17–19]. Second, more than 93 percent of all IDDM individuals are HLA-DR3 and/or DR4 positive [20, 21]. The association to these Class II

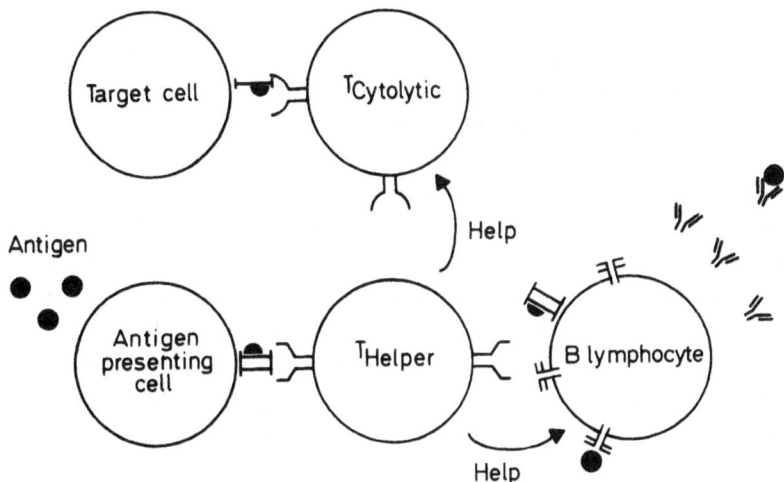

Figure 1. Schematic representation of different components of the immune system, the molecular biology of which is thought to be involved in the pathogenesis of insulin-dependent diabetes mellitus (IDDM).

specificities may signify that either these molecules are involved in the pathogenesis of IDDM or that they mark genes in linkage disequilibrium with a hypothetical diabetogenic gene located on chromosome 6. Recent approaches directed towards analyzing the IDDM susceptibility genes with cloned HLA Class II gene probes to determine restriction fragment length polymorphism (RFLP) have shown that HLA-DR identical control and IDDM patients may be different [22]. This observation suggests that RFLP analysis with a cloned HLA-DQ β-chain gene may better define a susceptibility to develop IDDM. The Class II molecules belong to a family of polymorphic molecules which also include the Class I transplantation antigens, the T lymphocyte receptor subunits and membrane-bound antibodies. Common to these molecules are their structural polymorphism and ability to bind molecules. Recently, Class II molecules have been shown to be able to bind antigens, or rather, fragments thereof. It will therefore be important to determine the structure and function of those HLA-D region encoded proteins which provide susceptibility to develop IDDM. Although the information in man is fragmentary, extensive studies in the mouse have shown the Class II β-chain amino acid sequence capable of determining the degree by which a mouse is able to respond to certain antigens.

The rationale to understanding the pathogenesis of IDDM should therefore include attempts to identify firstly; specific islet cell autoantigens detected by autoreactive immune effectors including autoantibodies and T lymphocytes, and secondly; the HLA Class II molecules which are able to present an antigen which initiates an immune response against a B cell specific determinant. Methods of molecular analysis, that allow cloning and sequencing of genes which encode proteins that may represent autoantigens, are an important approach to the understanding of the molecular biology of autoimmunity.

In this respect, molecular cloning of both the T cell receptor and the HLA Class II molecules offers a novel way of determining the mechanisms by which an antigenic epitope is able to initiate an immune response. Our approach is to use antibodies against synthetic peptides, whose sequence has been derived from the nucleotide sequence of cloned HLA Class II molecule genes. The antibodies are raised to determine the extent by which Class II molecules are expressed on the surface of immune competent cells. In future attempts, such antibodies may be useful in controlling or influencing the immune response to certain antigens.

Detection of islet cell autoantigens

Numerous investigations suggest that patients with IDDM of short duration have a variety of autoantibodies (Table 1). The disappearence of the islet B cells need to be explained against this background of autoimmunity. The question to be asked is, therefore, whether the islet B cells possibly express

Table 1. Autoantibodies found at an increased frequency among IDDM patients.

Type	Antibody
1. Organ-specific	
Pancreatic islet	ICA (Cytoplasmic)
	ICSA (Cell surface)
	C'AMC (Cytotoxic)
	IAA (Insulin autoantibody)
	64K (M_r 64000 autoantigen)
Thyroid	Thyroid microsomal
Stomach	Gastric-parietal cell
	Intrinsic factor
Adrenals	Adrenal cell
Pituitary	Pituitary cell
2. Non-organ specific	
Peripheral lymphocytes	Lymphocytotoxic
Nucleic acids	Single-stranded DNA
	Double-stranded RNA
Cell constituents	Tubulin
	Insulin receptor

cell-specific antigens that allow antibodies and/or immune effector cells to be directed towards them. At least three antigens of possible importance have been identified: 1. *Insulin*. Using sensitive radioimmunoassay [3] or ELISA [31] tests, autoantibodies against insulin have been described among 30–40 percent of newly diagnosed IDDM patients that have not yet been treated with insulin. 2. $M_r 64000$ *(64K) autoantigen*. The detection of islet cell autoantigens by immunoprecipitation of detergent-solubilized human islets labelled metabolically by ^{35}S-methionine is outlined elsewhere [30]. Serum samples, from IDDM patients [4] or individuals followed for several years before developing IDDM [3, 32], have been positive for autoantibodies against 64K protein. More than 80 percent of newly diagnosed IDDM patients were found positive compared to only 1/22 healthy controls (Table 2). 3. $M_r 38000$–40000 *(40K) autoantigen*. Immunoprecipitation as described above with both human [4, 32] and polyclonal islet cell antisera [33, 34] showed the presence of a 40K autoantigen in islet cells. This protein could be islet B-cell specific and represent a plasma membrane anchored glycoprotein [34]. In IDDM patients, as well as in the individuals followed from 4 months and up to 8 years before the clinical onset of IDDM, this component, so far, has only been detected in HLA-DR3 positive human islet cell preparations [4, 32]. Studies are in progress to isolate the 64K and 40K islet cell autoantigens to determine their structure, function and ability to initiate an immune response.

Analysis of HLA-D region genes

HLA-D region Class II genes are analyzed by RFLP [22, 23]. Initially, an HLA-DQ β-chain cDNA probe [24] was used to analyze HLA-DR identical IDDM patients and control individuals [22]. Using BamHI restriction enzyme digestion of blood leukocyte DNA, electrophoretic separation in agarose gels and transfer of DNA fragments to nitrocellulose paper by the method of Southern [25], it was found that the HLA-DQ β-chain cDNA probe detected a 3.7 kb fragment (Table 3) more often among controls than in IDDM patients [22]. A BamHI 3.7 kb fragment from an HLA-DR4-containing chromosome

Table 2. Prevalence of autoantibodies against the human islet M_r 64000 autoantigen.

Individuals tested	n	Positive reaction	%
Healthy controls	22	1	4%
Newly diagnosed IDDM patients	32	28	88%
Appearance before the clinical onset	12	9	75%

was cloned and sequenced [26, 27]. The fragment was found to be confined to the HLA-DQ β-chain gene; the BamHI sites being located in the first and third intervening sequences, respectively. A probe representing part of the first intervening sequence was prepared [27] and used to dissect further the RFLP between IDDM patients and healthy controls (Table 3).

Refinement of the HLA-DQ β-chain gene Restriction Fragment Length Polymorphism (RFLP)

The second generation HLA-DQ β-chain gene probe representing the first intervening sequence (IVS1) of an HLA-DQ β-chain gene, revealed a simplified restriction fragment pattern (Table 3). It was possible to demonstrate that those HLA-DR 3/4-positive IDDM patients who were negative for the BamHI 3.7 kb fragment had a 12 kb fragment. IDDM, therefore, is most likely to occur more often in HLA-DR 3- and/or 4-positive individuals who have a 12 kb BamHI-fragment than in those who have a 3.7 kb fragment.

Analysis of a large population sample with the IVS1-probe showed 7 fragments which varied between individuals (Table 3). IDDM was significantly associated with the presence of 12 kb and/or 4 kb fragments, while fragments of 7.5 kb, 3.7 kb and 3.0 kb decreased in frequency. The demonstration that the RFLP observed between IDDM and controls, particularly in those individuals having an identical HLA-DR specificity, suggests that the susceptibility to develop IDDM might be closer to the HLA-DQ locus than to HLA-DR. Since only three specificities for HLA-DQ serological typing is currently available, the present approach to define IDDM susceptibility by molecular cloning of individual fragments should permit a final identification of HLA-D region sequences showing the greatest degree of association with IDDM.

Table 3. Restriction fragments detected with HLA-DQ β-chain gene probes following BamH1 endonuclease digestion.

DNA fragment size (kb)	cDNA probe		DNA fragment size (kb)	Intervening sequence probe	
	IDDM n = 29	Controls n = 25		IDDM n = 117	Controls n = 177
6.2	10%	40%	12	63%	37%
5.8	79%	40%	7.5	19%	50%
3.7	0%	40%	4.0	63%	36%
3.2	10%	60%	3.7	2%	29%
			3.0	7%	37%

The prevalence (%) is shown for 25–177 individuals and only when the statistical test (Fischer's exact test with corrected p-values) showed p_c <0.05.

Antibodies against synthetic peptides

Sequence determination of cloned genes permits the expected amino acid sequence to be derived based on the genetic code. Peptides are synthetized and following coupling to a carrier, peptide antibodies are prepared either as a polyclonal antiserum or as monoclonal antibodies. Antibodies prepared against the peptides are usually coupled covalently to a carrier protein before immunization [28]. Enzyme-linked immunoassay (ELISA) is used to analyse the specificity of the peptide antibody. Western blotting allows an analysis of the ability of the antibody to detect denatured antigen transferred into nitrocellulose. Indirect immunofluorescence analysis on living cells by the Fluorescence-activated Cell Sorter (FACS IV) makes it possible to determine whether the peptide antibody is able to bind to native Class II molecules on the surface of immune-competent cells.

Antiserum against synthetic peptides detect HLA-D region molecules on immune cells

The possibility that certain HLA-DQ Class II molecules may confer a risk of developing IDDM makes it important to evolve means by which these molecules can be detected on cells and thereby determine their function. The preparation of antibodies against synthetic peptides, the sequence of which has been derived from the nucleotide sequence of the gene, offers a way to study a cell surface molecule even if the protein itself has never been isolated to determine its structure.

The N-terminal end of the HLA-DQ and HLA-DR β-chains differs in 6 out of 8 amino acids (Table 4). Several rabbit antisera were raised against the peptides coupled to thyroglobulin as a carrier [29]. It was demonstrated by ELISA that the antisera specifically detected the peptide used for immunization. The DQ1–8 antiserum did not cross-react with the DR1–8 peptide and

Table 4. HLA-DQ and -DR N-terminal nucleotide and predicted amino acid sequences used to prepare synthetic peptide antibodies.

	Sequences							
Position in polypeptide:	1	2	3	4	5	6	7	8......
DR 1–8	Gly	Asp	Thr	Arg	Pro	Arg	Phe	Leu....
	GGG	GAC	ACC	CGA	CCA	CGT	TTC	TCC...
	AGA	GAC	TCT	CCC	GAG	GAT	TTC	GTC...
DQ 1–8	Arg	Asp	Ser	Pro	Glu	Asp	Phe	Val....

vice versa. A plasma membrane enriched fraction from AL-34 cells, a lympho-blastoid cell line, was subjected to gel electrophoresis during denaturing conditions and the separated proteins electrophoretically transferred to nitro-cellulose filters. Strips of the nitrocellulose filters were incubated with anti-serum and antibodies which bind to the antigen demonstrated with a second antibody labelled with peroxidase. It was found that the DQ1–8 as well as the DR1–8 antiserum detected a M_r 29000 component which is the expected size of an HLA-D region β-chain peptide [29]. It was concluded therefore that the two antisera detected molecules of similar size despite their amino acid se-quences being different. (Table 4). The question remained whether the anti-sera would be able to detect the native molecules. The HLA-region Class II molecules are heterodimeric proteins composed of an α-chain and a β-chain. The protein complex has yet to be crystallized to determine its three-dimen-sional structure. Therefore, it was not possible to predict whether the N-terminal ends of the β-chain would be accessible for antibodies to bind or not.

Suspensions of cells from either lymphoblastoid cell lines or blood mononu-clear cells were incubated with the antisera and bound antibodies detected by indirect immunofluorescence analysis. It was found that both antisera induced a cell surface immunofluorescence reaction on the cell lines and on peripheral blood cells. However, it is well-known that Class II antigens are restricted in their expression. In general, the antigens are primarily confined to B lympho-cytes and monocytes, while T lymphocytes are negative. We used the Fluores-cence-activated Cell Sorter (Figure 2) to distinguish monocytes from lympho-cytes by low angle forward light scatter.

In the mononuclear blood cells from a healthy individual (Figure 2), it was demonstrated by indirect immunofluorescence that neither the DQ1–8 nor the DR1–8 antiserum bound to the lymphocytes. In contrast, both antisera bound to the monocyte population. We therefore conclude, that locus-specific anti-sera may be used to distinguish between HLA-DR and -DQ β-chains. These antisera are currently being used to determine the expression of these Class II molecules on mononuclear blood cells from healthy individuals and for com-parison with IDDM patients that are being treated with Cyclosporin A or a placebo in a double-blind, controlled trial.

Conclusion and future studies

The pancreatic islet B cells seem to be the specific target in an autoimmune process which leads to the development of IDDM, and this process appears to be initiated before the clinical onset of the disease. The initiating event and the development of an autoimmune response against specific islet B-cell autoanti-gens are not understood at all. In addition to insulin as a possible autoantigen,

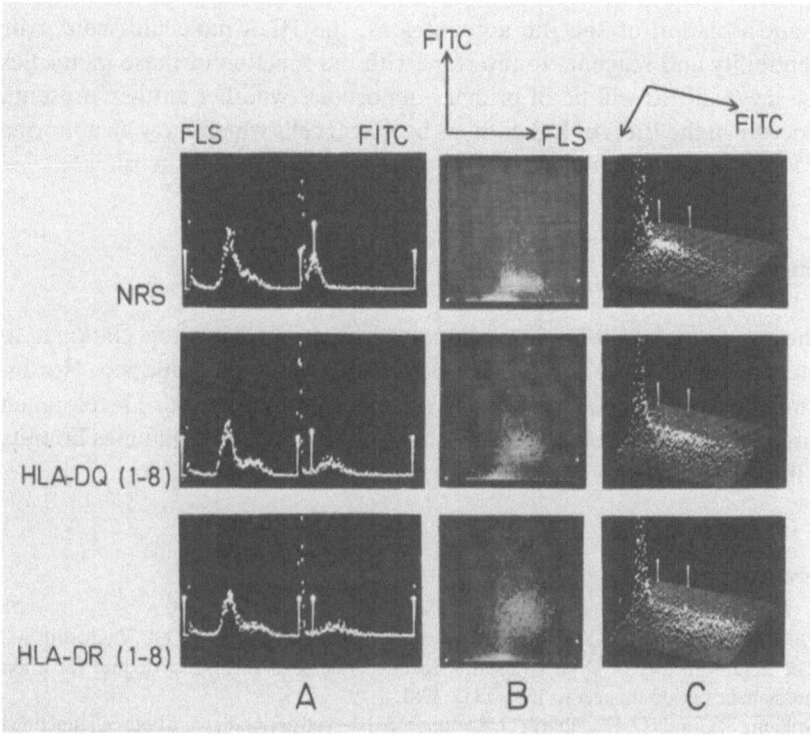

Figure 2. Analysis of cell surface binding of synthetic peptide rabbit antisera against the N-terminal sequences of the β-chains of HLA-DR (DR1–8) and -DQ (DQ1–8). Panels A, B, and C demonstrate 3 different modes of analysing the results obtained in the Fluorescence-activated Cell Sorter. NRS is normal rabbit serum. FLS is forward low angle scatter, and FITC is fluorescine isothiocyanate-induced fluorescence due to antibody binding.

the 40K and the 64K proteins need to be characterized fully. Molecular cloning of polymorphic genomic DNA fragments detected by RFLP analysis with HLA-D region gene probes allows for an effective analysis of IDDM susceptibility genes. Current results indicate that genes encoded in the HLA-DQ locus are more closely associated to the development of IDDM than those encoded in HLA-DR. These gene products are instrumental in antigen presentation and they may provide elements of risk in an autoimmune process. Attempts, therefore, are being made to develop reagents that permit the detection and functional analysis of HLA Class II molecules. The production of antibodies against the N-terminal sequences of Class II β-chain polypeptides has shown, that locusspecific immunological reagents can be prepared to distinguish between HLA-DR and -DQ. The aim of future studies is to test, whether an antigen-specific immunosuppression in IDDM-susceptible individuals will prevent the loss of pancreatic B cells. Such experiments require the identifica-

22

tion and isolation of specific autoantigens, the HLA-molecules conferring susceptibility and reagents to interfere with the function of these molecules. These mechanisms will be of primary importance whether antigen presentation occurs in the islets of Langerhans by islet B cells which show an abnormal expression of Class II molecules [35] or at a site away from the islets.

Acknowledgement

Studies at our laboratory were supported by grants from the National Institutes of Health (AM 26120, AM 33873) and from the foundation, Nordisk Insulinlaboratorium. S. Baekkeskov is supported by a Career Development Award and B. Michelsen by a fellowship from the Juvenile Diabetes Foundation International.

References

1. Gorsuch AN, Spencer KM, Lister J, McNally JM, Dean BM, Bottazzo GF, Cudworth AG: The natural history of Type I (insulin-dependent) diabetes mellitus: evidence for a long prediabetic period. Lancet ii: 1363–1365, 1981.
2. Srikanta S, Gunda O, Eisenbarth G, Soeldner JS: Islet cell antibodies and beta cell function in monozygetic triplets and twins initially discordant for Type I diabetes mellitus. N Engl J Med 308: 322–325, 1983.
3. Palmer JP, Asplin CM, Clemons P, Lyen K, Tatpati O, Raghu PK, Paquette TL: Insulin-dependent diabetics before insulin treatment. Science 222: 1337–1339, 1983.
4. Baekkeskov S, Nielsen JH, Marner B, Bilde T, Ludvigsson J, Lernmark Å: Autoantibodies in newly diagnosed diabetic children immunoprecipitate specific human pancreatic islet cell protein. Nature 298: 167–169, 1982.
5. Rahier J, Goebbels RM, Henquin JC: Cellular composition of the human diabetic pancreas. Diabetologia 24: 366–371, 1983.
6. Foulis AK, Stewart JA: The pancreas in recent-onset Type 1 (insulin-dependent) diabetes mellitus: insulin content of islets, insulitis and associated changes in the exocrine acinar tissue. Diabetologia 26: 456–461, 1984.
7. Gepts W: Pathologic anatomy of the pancreas in juvenile diabetes mellitus. Diabetes 14: 619–633, 1965.
8. Bottazzo GF, Dean BM, McNally JM, MacKay EH, Swift PGF, Gamble R: In situ characterization of autoimmune phenomena and expression of HLA molecules in the pancreas in diabetic insulitis. N Engl J Med 313: 353–360, 1985.
9. Dobersen MJ, Scharff JE, Ginsberg-Fellner F, Notkins AL: Cytotoxic autoantibodies to beta-cells in the serum of patients with insulin-dependent diabetes mellitus. N Eng J Med 303: 1493–1498, 1980.
10. Marner B, Lernmark A, Ludvigsson J, MacKay P, Matsuba I, Nerup J, Rabinovitch A: Islet cell antibodies in insulin-dependent (Type 1) diabetic children treated with plasmaphoresis. Diabetes Res 2: 231–236, 1985.
11. Lernmark Å: Cell-mediated immunity in Type 1 (insulin-dependent) diabetes: Update 1984.

23

In: Andreani D, di Mario U, Federlin KF, Heding LG (eds) Immunology of Diabetes; pp 121–131. Kimpton Medical Publications, London, 1984.

12. Nerup J, Andersen OO, Bendixen G, Egeberg J, Poulsen JE: Antipancreatic cellular hypersensitivity in diabetes mellitus. Diabetes 20: 424–427, 1971.

13. Maruyama T, Takei I, Matsuba I, Tsuruoka A, Taniyama M, Ideda Y, Kataoka K, Abe M, Matsuki S: Cell-mediated cytotoxic islet cell surface antibodies to human pancreatic beta cells. Diabetologia 26: 30–33, 1984.

14. Mandrup-Poulsen T, Bendtzen K, Nielsen JH, Bendixen G, Nerup J: Cytokines cause functional and structural damage to isolated islets of Langerhans. Allergy 40: 424–429, 1985.

15. Kanatsuna T, Baekkeskov S, Lernmark A, Ludvigsson J: Immunoglobulin from isulin-dependent diabetic children inhibits glucose-induced insulin release. Diabetes 32: 520–524, 1983.

16. Lernmark A, Kanatsuna T, Rubenstein AH, Steiner DF: Detection and possible functional influence ofantibodies directed against the pancreatic islet cell surface. Adv Exp Med Biol 119: 157–163, 1979.

17. Bottazzo GF, Mann JIl, Thorogood M, Baum JD, Doniach D: Autoimmunity in juvenile diabetes and their familes. Br Med J i: 165–168, 1978.

18. MacLaren NK, Riley WJ: Throid, gastric, and adrenal autoimmunities associated with insulin-dependent diabetes mellitus. Diabetes Care 8, 1: 1–109, 1985.

19. Hägglöf B, Rabinovitch A, MacKay P, Huen A, Rubenstein AH, Marner B, Nerup J, Lernmark Å: Islet cell and other organ specific autoantibodies are increased among healthy first-degree relatives to insulin-dependent diabetic children. Acta Paediatr. Scand (in press).

20. Platz P, Jakobsen BK, Morling M,, Ryder LP, Svejgaard A, Thomsen M, Christy M, Kroman H, Benn J, Nerup J, Green A, Hauge M: HLA-D and DR-antigens in genetic analysis of insulin-dependent diabetes mellitus. Diabetologia 21: 108–115, 1981.

21. Wolf E, Spences KM, Cudworth, AG: The genetic susceptibility to Type 1 (insulin-dependent) diabetes: analysis of the HLA-DR association. Diabetologia 24: 224–230, 1983.

22. Owerbach D, Lernmark A, Platz P, Ryder LP, Rask L, Peterson PA, Ludvigsson J: HLA-D region β-chain DNA endonuclease fragments differ between HLA-DR identical healthy and insulin-dependent diabetic individuals. Nature 303: 815–817, 1983.

23. Owerbach D, Lernmark Å, Rask L, Peterson PA, Platz P, Svejgaard A: Detection of HLA-D/DR-related DNA polymorphism in HLA-D homozygous typing cells. Proc Natl Acad Sci USA 80: 3758–3761, 1983.

24. Larhammar D, Schenning HLA, Gustafsson K, Wiman K, Claesson L, Rask L: Complete amino acid sequence of an HLA-DR antigen-like β chain as predicted from the nucleotide sequence: Similarities with immunoglobulins and HLA-A, -B, and -C antigens. Proc Natl Acad Sci USA 79: 3687–3691, 1982.

25. Southern EM: Detection of specific sequences among DNA fragments separated by gel electrophoresis. J Med Biol 98: 503–517, 1975.

26. Michelsen B, Kastern W, Lernmark Å, Owerbach D: Identification of an HLA-DC β-chain related genomic sequence associated with insulin-dependent diabetes. Biomed Biochim Acta 44, 1: 33–36, 1985.

27. Michelsen B, Lernmark Å: Molecular cloning of a polymorphic DNA endonuclease fragment associates insulin-dependent diabetes with HLA-DQ. J Clin Invest 79: 1144–1152, 1987.

28. Tager HS: Coupling of peptides to albumin with dinitrofluorobenzene. Anal Biochem 71: 367–375, 1976.

29. Deufel T, Grove A, Kofod H, Lernmark Å: Locus-specific detection of HLA-DQ and -DR antigens by antibodies against synthetic N-terminal octapeptides of the β-chain. Febs Letters 189, 2: 329–337, 1985.

30. Baekkeskov S: Radiolabelling and immunoprecipitation of islet cell antigens. In: J. Larner

and S.L. Pohl (eds.) Methods in diabetes research, vol. I: Laboratory methods, Part A, John Wiley and Sons, New York, pp. 129–140, 1984.

31. Wilkin T, Armitage M, Casey C, Pyke DA, Hoskins PJ, Rodier M, Diaz JL, Leslie RDG: Value of insulin autoantibodies as serum markers for insulin-dependent diabetes mellitus. Lancet 2: 480–481, 1985.

32. Baekkeskov S, Kristensen JK, Srikanta S, Bruining, GJ, Mandrup-Poulsen T, Beaufort C, Soeldner JS, Eisenbarth G, Lindgren F, Lernmark Å: Antibodies to a M_r 64000 human islet cell antigen precede the clinical onset of insulin-dependent diabetes. Submitted for publication.

33. Dyrberg T, Baekkeskov S, Lernmark Å: Specific pancreatic β-cell surface antigens recognized by a xenogenic antiserum. J Cell Biol 94: 472–477, 1982.

34. Baekkeskov S, Lernmark Å: A β-cell glycoprotein of M_r 40000 is the major immunogen following xenogenic immunization. Diabetologia 27: 70–73, 1984.

35. Hanafusa T, Pujoll-Borrel R, Chlovata L, Russell RCG, Doniach D, Bottazzo GF: Aberrant expression of HLA-Dr antigen on thyrocytes in Graves' disease: relevance for autoimmunity. Lancet ii: 1111–1115, 1983.

2. Experimental pancreas transplantation: a survey of relevant issues

R. VAN SCHILFGAARDE

Introduction

The aim of pancreas transplantation is to provide for a source of endogenous insulin production in type 1 diabetics. The concept is that by this means normoglycemia will be maintained in a more physiologic fashion than by means of administration of exogenous insulin. This would ameliorate the quality of life not only by deleting the obligatory insulin injections and dietary restrictions, but also by yielding the best chance for the prevention or reduction of late complications such as retinopathy, nephropathy, neuropathy, and vascular disease.

Transplantation of the pancreas differs from transplantation of other organs in two aspects. First, there is a very realistic alternative for pancreas transplantation. Exogenous insulin treatment is the conventional approach in diabetics, and long-term treatment during several decades is normal practice. The alternative for kidney transplantation is dialysis, but throughout the years it has been well established that, in general, kidney transplantation should be favoured over dialysis. Alternatives for heart or liver transplantation are not available. Second, unlike other organ transplants, only part and not all of the transplanted pancreas is meant to serve its purpose, since the pancreas is composed for less than 5 percent of endocrine and for more than 95 percent of exocrine tissue. Exocrine replacement is not the purpose of pancreas transplantation, and this consideration is of specific interest if one realizes that it is the 95 percent of exocrine tissue which should to a large extent be held responsible for many of the surgical complications associated with pancreas transplantation.

Obviously, therefore, research has concentrated on two approaches. One is to find clinically applicable and effective methods of transplanting the endocrine but not the exocrine tissue. Islet transplantation has made significant progress in the animal setting during the last few years but, in contrast to pancreas transplantation, results of clinical application are still disappointing.

J.M. Dubernard and D.E.R. Sutherland (eds.), International Handbook of Pancreas Transplantation, 25–47.
© *1989 by Kluwer Academic Publishers.*

The other approach is to concentrate on methods for the prevention of complications associated with exocrine secretion.

Experimental pancreas transplantation has, throughout the years, yielded substantial information in regard to the feasibility of different methods for managing exocrine secretions. In addition, it has been applied for refining other aspects of the surgical technique, such as evaluating the methods of vascular anastomoses in order to prevent thrombosis. Methods of preservation are of utmost importance in regard to clinical applicability and they, too, have been studied experimentally. Experimental pancreas transplantation appears to have occupied itself predominantly with surgical techniques and methods of preservation rather than with questions regarding the wide field of methods of preventing, detecting and treating rejection, since the number of studies in this latter category is relatively small. The major part of experimental work has been done in large animals and mainly in dogs.

General aspects

Early research regarding pancreas transplantation has mainly occupied itself with developing an adequate model. Interestingly, however, the first application of experimental pancreas transplantation did not intend to determine the eventual feasibility of clinical application, but was rather designed to investigate the source and action of insulin [1]. Nevertheless, these early experiments in dogs could later be interpreted as an important contribution to the basic concept of clinical pancreas transplantation, since they clearly showed that a pancreatic allograft is capable of maintaining normoglycemia in totally pancreatectomized dogs.

Approximately three decades later, pancreas transplantation started to be investigated from the point of view of finding new means of treating diabetics. Initial efforts restricted themselves to the transplantation of non-vascularized pancreatic fragments, and the first to study not only the transplantation of non-vascularized fragments but also the transplantation of the vascularized organ systematically were Brooks and Gifford [2]. Although none of their pancreatic transplants were successful, their study yielded two pertinent pieces of information. First, it indicated that, in principle, pancreas transplantation should be taken to be technically feasible, since after declamping the graft was always seen to become pink, pulsate, and appear to be viable. Second, it indicated that causes of failure were always deducible to either vascular thrombosis or complications from the side of exocrine secretions, or to a combination of both.

Obviously, subsequent efforts for developing adequate models of pancreas transplantation have concentrated on these two aspects. Initially, several investigators have used vascular anastomoses between the donor celiac trunk and portal vein and the recipient femoral artery and vein, respectively, while placing the pancreas graft subcutaneously in the groin of the recipient dog. DeJode and Howard [3] have used this vascular technique for transplanting partial pancreaticoduodenal grafts of which the duodenum was fashioned into a conduit brought out through the skin, from which the exocrine secretions drained externally. Reemtsma et al. [4] have used the same vascular technique for transplanting the left pancreatic segment of which the exocrine secretion was abolished by means of ductligation. Then, Bergan et al. [5] used the whole pancreas and placed it intraperitoneally by connecting the celiac axis and portal vein to the recipient's aorta and caval vein, respectively. They, too, used ductligation for abolishing exocrine secretion. The first to aim at maintaining not only endocrine but also exocrine integrity of the pancreas graft without external drainage was Lillehei's group in Minneapolis [6]. They used the complete pancreas and duodenum of the donor for allotransplantation into completely pancreaticoduodenectomized recipient dogs. Vascular anastomes were made onto the recipient's aorta and caval vein, the donor duodenum was interposed between the recipient's stomach and distal duodenum, and bile drainage was re-established by means of cysto-enterostomy.

Although technical problems continued to be substantial and failure rates were high, the studies in these early years of experimental pancreas transplantation share two general conclusions. One is that they certainly proved a technically successful pancreas graft to be capable of maintaining normoglycemia in pancreatectomized dogs. The other is that these allograft models offered the opportunity for short-term but not long-term interpretation of various surgical modalities, since rejection interfered with long-term graft survival.

Consequently, the introduction of a model for segmental pancreatic autotransplantation by Mitchell et al. [7] was an important contribution to further research into the technical aspects. They used the left lobe of the pancreas with the splenic artery and vein, which were connected to the iliac vessels. Thus, the celiac trunk with the hepatic artery could be left intact. After removal of the right lobe of the pancreas, the dogs could be tested for evaluation of the endocrine function of the autografted left lobe. Several modifications have been described, and a schematic drawing of the modified technique as applied in our experiments is presented in Figure 1. Obviously, this model can not only be used for testing pancreas transplants in the absence of immunological rejection, but it can also be applied as an allograft model for investigating immunological factors. In addition, it can be readily modified in various fashions such as to address the surgical issues of main importance, i.e. the management of exocrine secretion, the vascular technique, and preservation of the pancreas (Table 1).

28

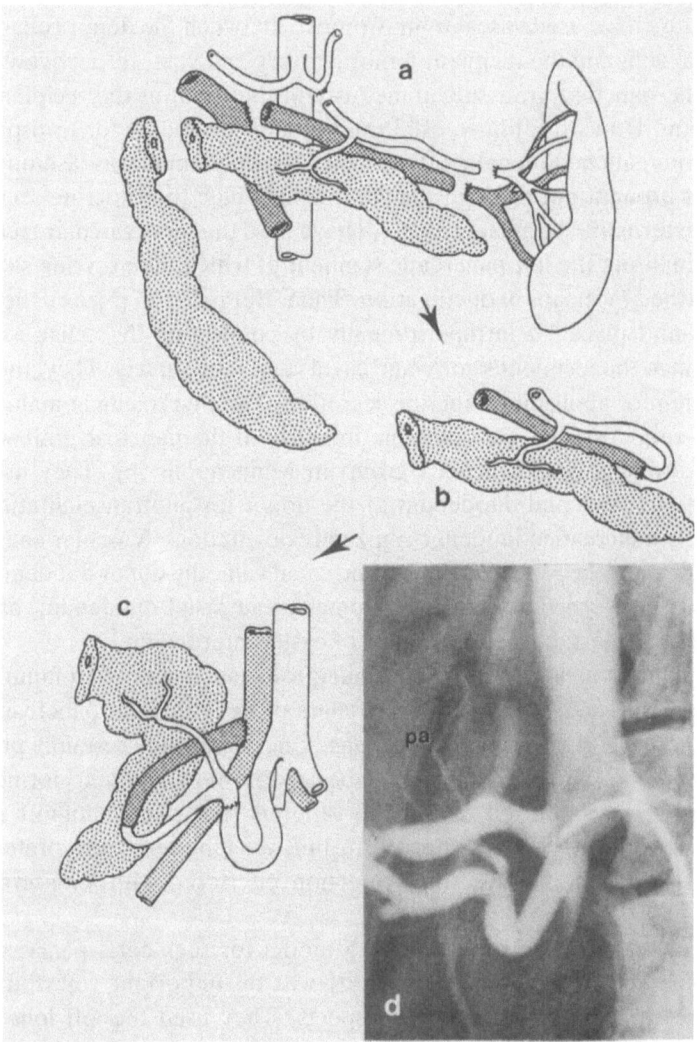

Figure 1. Schematic drawing of the surgical procedure for segmental pancreas autotransplantation in dogs. a) Isolation of the left pancreatic lobe. b) Construction of an arteriovenous fistula. c) Implantation of the graft. d) Postoperative angiogram showing the pancreatic artery (pa) and the arteriovenous fistula. Reproduced by courtesy of Surgery [28].

Management of exocrine secretion

There are, in principle, three options for managing the exocrine secretion. One is to take measures for its maintenance, the second is to do nothing while leaving the pancreatic juice freely draining into the peritoneal cavity, and the third is to take measures for its abrogation (Table 1).

Maintenance of exocrine secretion

Maintenance of exocrine secretion requires the pancreatic juice to be capable of continuously flowing out of the main pancreatic duct without any impediment and without causing peripancreatic or other unwanted inflammatory reactions. Theoretically, this can be accomplished by way of external drainage, for instance through a duodenal conduit attached to the skin. However, this is a highly unpractical solution with many obvious disadvantages. The more appropriate method is internal drainage, which can be accomplished by anastomosing the ductal system to either the intestinal tract (stomach or small bowel) or the urinary tract (pyelum, ureter, or bladder). Various technical approaches and modifications have been described during the late sixties [8] and early seventies [9, 10] both for allografts and autografts. Apparently, whole rather than segmental pancreas grafts offer the best opportunity for long-term unimpeded outflow of the pancreatic juice. With whole grafts the duodenum [8] or the papilla with only a duodenal patch [9] can be used for connecting the ductal system to the intestine. But with segmental grafts (i.e. a transsected pancreas and main duct) it is difficult to fashion the anastomosis between the ductal system and the intestine or urinary tract with reasonable certainty of long-term patency of the main duct, which is a prerequisite for long-term maintenance of exocrine secretion. Techniques for long-term maintenance of exocrine secretion always require extended operations with an increased chance for surgical complications, which is the draw-back they have in common.

Table 1. Surgical issues of main importance in pancreas transplantation.

Management of exocrine secretion	
– Maintenance	– external drainage
	– internal drainage
– Free drainage	
– Abrogation	– duct ligation
	– duct obliteration
Vascular technique	
– Prevention of thrombosis	– arterial interposition
	– arteriovenous fistula
	– surgical technique
– Venous anastomosis	– caval vein
	– portal vein
Preservation	– machine perfusion
	– cold storage

Free drainage

Free drainage of pancreatic juice is the least cumbersome technique, since it requires no specific measures but to place the graft intraperitoneally. In dogs, the technique is safe since, unlike man, the canine exocrine secretion from freely draining grafts tends to decrease gradually and eventually to cease completely. Long-term endocrine function of freely draining grafts has been reported excellent in dogs [11] which may imply that this technique is useful for investigating immunological factors. Its pertinence for studying technical aspects remains doubtful, however, since free drainage in the clinical situation has disappointingly proved to be associated with many complications and technical failures [12].

Abrogation of exocrine secretion

Abrogation of exocrine secretion can be accomplished in two fashions. Ligation of the pancreatic duct is simple and often effective. It has, however, two major disadvantages. First, it has been well established that long-term effects of otherwise successful ductligation include not only the exocrine but also the endocrine tissue. Ductligated canine pancreases not only develop atrophy of the exocrine tissue and severe fibrosis, but also endocrine insufficiency in the majority of cases [13]. The second disadvantage of ductligation is that its acute effect on the exocrine tissue is highly unpredictable, and there is a substantial risk of inducing acute pancreatitis with autolysis and peripancreatic abcesses. Although this risk is relatively low in dogs, it is conspicuous in man. Therefore, ductligation has become obsolete in clinical pancreas transplantation and, consequently, of marginal relevance as an experimental technique.

The other method for abrogating exocrine secretion is ductobliteration or ductinjection. The basic principle is that the ductal system is filled with a fluid substance which solidifies within several minutes. The effect is that the exocrine secretion is completely abolished. The method was introduced by Dubernard et al. in 1978 [14], who showed it to be safe and very effective both in dogs and in man. Understandably, the availability of this new and safe procedure had a very stimulating influence on clinical pancreas transplantation which, until that time, had been associated with highly disappointing results and many technical complications [15]. However, the initial enthousiasm was tempered by the observation that initially succesful, ductobliterated grafts spontaneously ceased to function several months after transplantation [12]. The extensive fibrosis induced by ductobliteration was generally taken as the cause of such late failures, although it remained unclear to what extent rejection may have contributed in individual cases [12, 16]. The obvious dilemma was whether the safety of the procedure or the chance for long-term endocrine function should prevail. The first option would favour ductobliteration, while accepting the risk of endocrine failure. The second option would favour maintenance of exocrine secretion, while accepting an increased risk of serious surgical complications. The relevance of this dilemma is obvious since diabetics, on the one hand, represent an increased risk for surgery in general and for organ transplantation in particular while, on the other hand, the purpose of pancreas transplantation is to provide for long-term endocrine sufficiency in order to reduce the late complications of the diabetic disease itself. However, insufficient data appeared to be available for choosing either of both options. For that reason, our group has tried to analyze the effects of ductobliteration in some detail, for which purpose we have used beagles. A summary of the results is presented below.

The effects of pancreatic ductobliteration

The main findings of our work in regard to the effect of ductinjection are threefold. They relate to changes in endocrine function, to histologic changes, and to pancreatic blood flow.

When the right lobe of the pancreas was removed and the left lobe was injected with approximately 0.2 ml of ductobliterant while leaving it otherwise untouched, K-values with intravenous glucosetolerance testing (IVGTT) were reduced to about half of normal as of one month [17] and even two weeks [18] after operation, and a similar reduction was observed with the quantitative insulin response to IVGTT [19]. In spite of this reduced glucosetolerance and insulin response, normoglycemia was maintained up to at least two and even three years postoperatively, during which time period no significant further deterioration of either K-values or insulin responses was observed. These findings did not appear to depend conspicuously upon the type of ductobliterant used, since similar results were obtained with neoprene, polyisoprene, and prolamine [17].

The information concerning the endocrine function as obtained by sampling peripheral venous blood should be taken as not more than an indirect assessment of actual beta-cell performance. Since we were interested in determining the loss of beta-cell performance as induced by ductobliteration more accurately, a model was developed for directly measuring the insulin output by the left pancreatic lobe [18]. The model is schematically presented in Figure 2. By inserting a silastic cannula into the distal splenic vein and re-introducing the cannula into the portal vein, the undiluted pancreatic venous blood can be completely and continuously diverted through this cannula when the splenic vein is clamped more proximally. Through a three-way stopcock not only blood samples can be drawn but also the pancreatic blood flow can be measured in a direct fashion by using a stopwatch while collecting blood during a

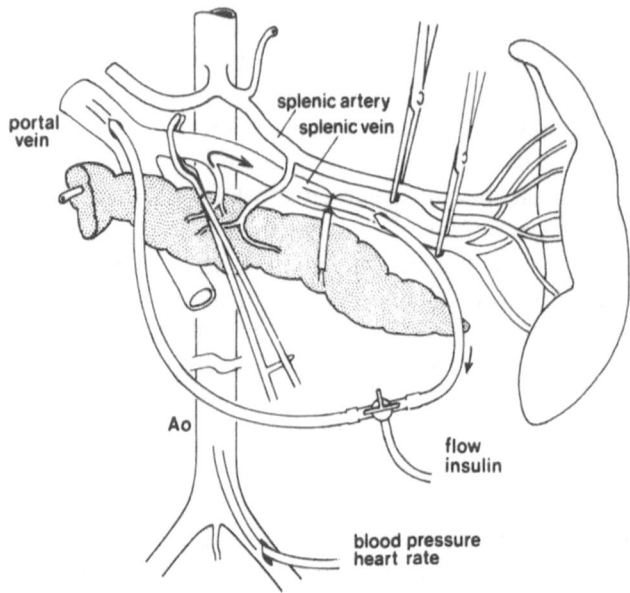

Figure 2. Schematic drawing of the model for the direct determination of insulin output by the left lobe of the canine pancreas. Reproduced by courtesy of H.G. Gooszen [18].

fixed time interval. The actual insulin secretion expressed in microunits of insulin per minute can now be calculated as the product of the insulin concentration in each sample (μU/ml) and the blood flow while taking that sample (ml/min). Samples were taken at standard intervals after intravenous infusion of glucose, identical to the intervals applied with regular IVGTT's. Obviously, this model is applicable not only with left pancreatic segments kept in situ, but also with heterotopically autografted segments by cannulating the common iliac and inferior caval vein [18]. We have used this model to test unmodified left pancreatic segments and left pancreatic segments at 6 weeks and 18–24 months after ductobliteration. Results are graphically presented in Figure 3. The mean insulin secretion in each group during the whole test period of sixty minutes decreased from approximately 9,700 μU/min to approximately 3,100 μU/min at 6 weeks and 3,000 μU/min at 18–24 months after ductobliteration [18]. These findings clearly demonstrate that, within six weeks postoperatively, ductobliteration induces a reduction in insulin secretory capacity to about thirty percent of normal, and that no further reduction is apparent during at least 18–24 months postoperatively.

The second topic of our investigations into the effects of ductobliteration regards histologic changes. They were studied qualitatively by means of standard tissue staining and by means of immunohistochemical staining techniques using an indirect peroxidase labeled antibody method for the detection of

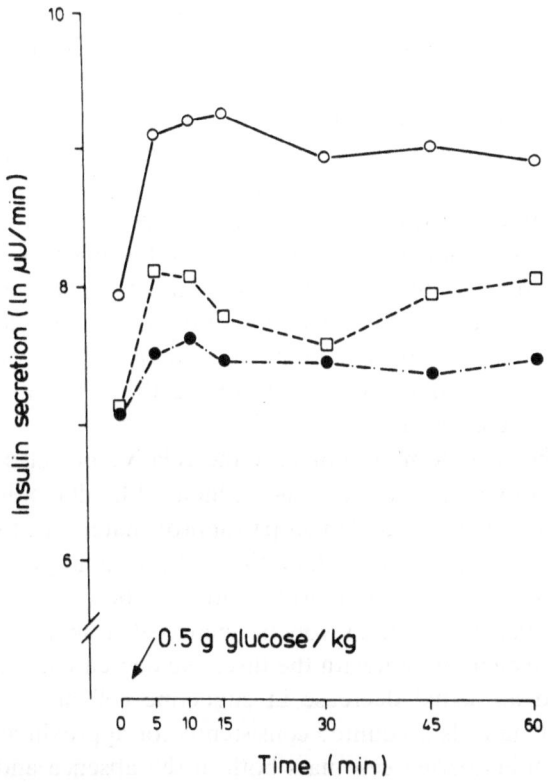

Figure 3. Insulin output by the left lobe of the canine pancreas as determined directly in the unmodified situation (O——O, n = 8), at 6 weeks (□---□, n = 5) and at 18–24 months (●---●, n = 7) after ductobliteration and autotransplantation. Reproduced by courtesy of H.G. Gooszen [18].

insulin, glucagon, somatostatin, and pancreatic polypeptide. The same staining techniques were used for quantitative studies.

When studied qualitatively, the most conspicuous histologic changes were twofold. First, already at one month after ductobliteration only remnants of exocrine acini were detectable. The exocrine tissue had for the major part been replaced by loose fibrous tissue becoming more dense in the following months, during which the initial inflammatory reaction gradually subsided. Evidently, the pancreases had always considerably shrunken with gross examination. Second, ductobliteration was invariably associated with a severe disturbance of the architecture of the islets, and endocrine cells were found dispersed throughout fibrous tissue as of one month postoperatively. In some instances, the endocrine cells tended to re-arrange in islet-like clusters which failed, however, to display the intrinsic topographical relationship of different endocrine cell-types as in normal islets [17].

For quantitative studies the relative amounts of exocrine and endocrine tissue were morphometrically assessed in biopsies taken from normal pancreases and at one, three, and twelve months after ductobliteration. Irrespective of the type of ductobliterant applied, the exocrine tissue was found to have decreased from more than ninety-five percent in unmodified pancreases to less than ten percent of pancreatic tissue already at one month after ductobliteration. As of three months, it had completely disappeared. The relative amounts of different endocrine cell-types within the endocrine compartment were also morphometrically assessed. Only insignificant changes were observed since, at twelve months after ductobliteration, the relative contribution of beta-, alpha-, delta-, and pancreatic polypeptide producing cells to the endocrine cell mass was similar to the composition of the endocrine compartment of unmodified pancreases [17].

We have tried to determine not only the relative but also the absolute changes in quantity of endocrine tissue as induced by ductobliteration [18]. The pancreatic weight was found to drop to approximately one third of normal within a few months after ductobliteration. The volume percentage of endocrine tissue was determined morphometrically both in unmodified and ductobliterated pancreases. This volume increased from 1.4 to 2.5 percent which finding, in combination with the threefold decrease in whole pancreas weight, implied an actual decrease in endocrine cell mass of about fifty percent. Since beta-cells accounted consistently for approximately sixty percent of the total endocrine cell mass both in the absence and presence of ductobliteration, it should be concluded that ductobliteration is associated with a reduction of the total beta-cell mass to about half of normal.

The third topic of our investigations into the effects of ductobliteration regards eventual changes in pancreatic blood flow. We used an electromagnetic device with perivascular probes placed around the splenic artery, which was temporarily clamped distally to the origin of the pancreatic artery for measuring flow. By this means, the blood flow was determined both in unmodified and in ductobliterated left pancreatic lobes at different time intervals up to eight [20] and twelve months [18] after ductobliteration. The basal pancreatic blood flow through unmodified segments was found to be in the order of 8 ml/min when determined electromagnetically. This value was quite similar to the basal flow levels as observed with the direct method for measuring flow as described above in the context of directly assessing the actual insulin secreting capacity, since with that technique we found a basal pancreatic blood flow of about 6 ml/min [18]. Basal flow levels remained similar at all intervals after ductobliteration, indicating that neither ductobliteration as such nor the conspicuous fibrosis as induced by ductobliteration appear to exert a detrimental effect on basal pancreatic blood flow.

Next, we have looked into pancreatic blood flow not only under basal conditions but also after stimulation. To this end, we first used papaverine as a direct vasodilator. Intra-arterial injection of papaverine was found to be associated with an approximately threefold increase of blood flow through unmodified as well as ductinjected left lobes up to six [21] and twelve months [18] after ductobliteration. This observation showed that the severe fibrosis and shrinkage as induced by ductobliteration did not prevent the pancreatic vasculature to dilate in response to a direct but metabolically aspecific stimulus. The next step was to determine the effect of a more physiologic stimulus on pancreatic blood flow, for which purpose we could use the repeated assessments during sixty minutes after intravenous glucose injection as performed by the direct, instead of electromagnetic, method while determining the actual insulin secreting capacity as described above. Here, too, we found the blood flow to increase significantly. The peak was reached within five to ten minutes after glucose injection, and the blood flow had always returned to its basal level at fortyfive or sixty minutes after glucose injection. This observation was made in unmodified pancreases and also at six weeks after ductobliteration. However, when tested at 18 to 24 months after ductobliteration, the blood flow was found not to increase any more in response to intravenous glucose loading [18]. The absence of this response could not be explained by an inability of the pancreas to react with vasodilation because of a mechanical impediment from the side of the interstitial fibrosis, since direct stimulation with papaverine was followed by an increase in blood flow [21]. Therefore, these findings were interpreted as an inability of the pancreas to respond to a specific metabolic stimulus, which inability was explained by the observed distortion of islet architecture as induced by ductobliteration. Conceivably, this distorted architecture could be held responsible for a decreased or absent capability for adequately being triggered by a specific metabolic stimulus.

Together, the findings regarding the effects of ductobliteration as reviewed above lend themselves for the following interpretation. It appears that ductobliteration induces an acute inflammatory reaction which not only causes the acinar tissue to atrophy and disappear and to be replaced by fibrous tissue, but also interferes with the integrity of the islets. This interference includes the destruction of both the subtle islet architecture and about half of the endocrine cell mass itself. This acute inflammatory reaction is at its height already within the first two weeks after ductobliteration, and gradually fades out during the first two to three months. From then on a stable situation is maintained with clusters of endocrine cells and fragments of endocrine tissue in a quantity of about half of normal lying scattered throughout dense fibrous tissue. These features are not associated with changes in pancreatic blood flow. In terms of functional performance these features are associated with a reduction to less than half of normal and actually to about one third of normal. This is explained by the fact that not only quantitative but also qualitative changes of endocrine tissue derive from ductobliteration. This latter notion is clearly illustrated by comparing insulin responses to intravenous glucosetolerance testing under different circumstances [19]. Insulin response curves obtained with ductobliterated but otherwise untouched left pancreatic segments displayed not only a far lesser response (quantitative) but also a flattened curve (qualitative) when compared to unmodified segments. When such ductobliaterated segments had been autografted onto the iliac vessels, i.e. onto the systemic circulation and thus bypassing the liver, the quantitative insulin response as expressed in area-under-the-curve was similar to that with unmodified segments, but the slope of the curve remained similar to that observed with ductobliterated but non-transplanted segments (Figure 4). Obviously, the severely reduced insulin secreting capacity of ductobliterated segments is apparent both quantitatively and qualitatively with portal venous drainage, whereas with systemic venous drainage the quantitative defect is artificially masked as a consequence of bypassing the liver while the qualitative defect continues to be similarly apparent.

Consequences for clinical applicability

The main conclusion emerging from the foregoing paragraphs is that normal endocrine performance cannot be maintained in the absence of normal pancreatic histology and integrity of both the exocrine and endocrine tissue. Our work clearly shows that such integrity is abolished by ductobliteration. Others have demonstrated similar effects to occur after ductligation [13] which knowledge, interestingly, was already available from much earlier work directed to investigate exocrine physiology rather than surgical techniques regarding pancreas transplantation [22].

It should be recognized that the findings as reviewed above relate to the canine, and not the human, pancreas. However, there is no basic consideration to assume that eventual differences in the response to abrogation of exocrine secretion between the canine and the human pancreas are of a fundamental nature. With this proviso, the dilemma as presented in the paragraph 'Abrogation of exocrine secretion' tends to discredit not only ductligation, but also ductobliteration in spite of its well-recognized safety. Transplanting less than half of the endocrine cell mass actually available within the donor pancreas should be taken to jeopardize eventual chances for long-term endocrine function on an adequate level, not only because of the reduced endocrine cell mass as such, but also because this reduced mass can be taken to be quite easily destructed by eventual rejection episodes. Therefore, it seems that maintenance of exocrine secretion should be favoured as the surgical modality to be applied with clinical pancreas transplantation. Gladly, clinical experience with intestinal drainage has proved to be associated with a decreas-

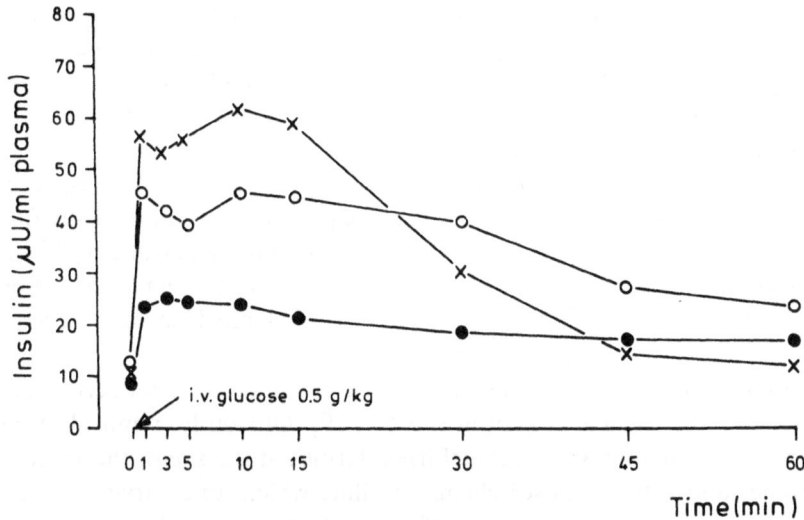

Figure 4. Insulin response curves after intravenous glucose injection in unmodified dogs (X——X, n = 6), at 6 months after removal of the right lobe and autotransplantation of the ductobliterated left lobe (O——O, n = 6), and at 6 months after removal of the right lobe and in situ ductobliteration of the left lobe (●——●, n = 6). Reproduced by courtesy of Diabetes [19].

ing complication rate during the last few years [23]. In addition, drainage into the urinary tract, i.e. more specifically into the bladder, has proved to be a reliable technique for maintaining exocrine secretion not only in dogs [24] but also in man [25].

Vascular technique

The first item relating to the vascular technique with pancreas transplantation regards the prevention of vascular thrombosis. The second item regards the site of the venous anastomosis, i.e. whether it should be onto the systemic or portal venous circulation (Table 1).

The prevention of thrombosis

Thrombosis and subsequent ischemic graft necrosis are the complications that have substantially contributed to the extremely high failure rate of early experimental pancreas transplantation, and they are frequently observed with clinical pancreas transplantation. It should be acknowledged, though, that not every occurrence of ischemic graft necrosis can be attributed to thrombosis. Many are the anatomical variations of the arterial and venous pancreatic vessels [26, 27] and, in dogs, the pancreatic artery derives not always from the splenic artery but in about twenty percent of cases it comes from the cranial mesenteric artery [28]. Ischemic grafts necrosis is inevitable should the arterial anastomosis in these instances be made with only the splenic artery and without additional surgical adaptations.

The high incidence of thrombotic complications with pancreas transplantation is commonly explained by the fact that the pancreas is a so-called low-flow organ. It takes about ten percent of the celiac blood flow at maximum [29] and not much more than approximately twenty percent of the splenic blood flow [20]. Therefore, the splenic vessels have a relatively large diameter in relation to the volume of the isolated left segment.

Thrombotic complications as seen after transplantation do not occur when the isolated left segment is kept in situ [17, 19]. Obviously, removal of the spleen in combination with eventual irregularities at the site of the vascular anastomes and with the post-ischemic swelling which, to a varying degree, always follows ex situ preservation of the graft, may easily be sufficient to reduce the flow just sufficiently so as to facilitate the occurrence of thrombosis.

Thrombotic complications have been tried to overcome by interposing the splenic artery of the graft between the cut ends of the recipient artery, since it was felt that the abrupt decrease in diameter from splenic into pancreatic artery was adding to the risk of thrombosis [26]. This technique of double arterial anastomosis has subsequently been tested by several others and at various implantation sites, but its effectiveness could not be conclusively confirmed. This is not surprising, since the high chance for thrombosis comes from the venous rather than the arterial pole. Predictably, therefore, an arteriovenous fistula between the distal splenic vessels as introduced by Calne et al. [29] has a better chance for preventing thrombosis since it induces a more than twofold increase of blood flow through the splenic vessels [20]. We have used such a fistula routinely in our experimental setting [28]. Since these fistulas tend to occlude within a few weeks postoperatively while the vasculature of the graft remains patent, we feel that the fistula serves it purpose especially during the early postoperative period when chances for thrombosis are increased because of post-ischemic swelling of the pancreatic tissue. However, it should be recognized that the actual merit of an arteriovenous fistula has never been confirmed in any controlled trial, and that many groups achieve excellent surgical results by merely anastomosing the donor splenic vessels onto the recipient circulation while not using a fistula or any other specific modification of the standard surgical technique. Such a specific modification has been applied by transplanting the pancreas together with the spleen, in order to maintain normal flow relations through the splenic vessels and their pancreatic branches. Although this technique undoubtedly yields an optimal hemodynamic situation, it should preferably be restricted to autografts since a combined pancreatico-splenic allograft carries the risk of inducing fatal graft-versus-host disease [25].

It appears, therefore, that the most important factor in securing successful transplantation is a meticulous surgical technique. This includes the recognition of eventuel anatomical variations of the pancreatic vessels, and extremely careful handling of the graft during dissection in order to minimize the chance for postoperative pancreatitis and post-ischemic swelling. The latter factor, of course, is closely related to the method and duration of preservation of the graft. However, the factor of main importance is a very subtle and precise vascular technique in order to avoid irregularities of suture lines and kinking of the vessels [27]. In addition to these surgical aspects one can consider medical treatment by means of anticoagulant prophylaxis such as coumadin derivates, or anti-platelet agents such as dipyridamol and salicylates. Their clinical application is associated with some risk, however, which many groups do not wish to take.

The site of the venous anastomosis

The commonly applied technique is to anastomose the donor vein, i.e. the portal or splenic vein, to the caval or iliac vein of the recipient. However, this does not mimick the physiologic situation since, in normal individuals, the pancreatic venous blood is delivered directly to the liver through the portal vein.

Systemic instead of portal venous drainage may have consequences which are clinically pertinent. Conceptually, permanently low concentrations of insulin in the portal venous blood may, in the long run, exert a detrimental effect on the liver since, under physiologic conditions, the liver is used to be exposed to varying and intermittently very high concentrations of insulin in the portal blood. Systemic instead of portal venous drainage not only deprives the liver from physiologic concentrations of insulin in the portal blood, but this bypass of the liver also prevents that forty to fifty percent of the insulin secreted by the pancreas is cleared by the liver prior to being delivered to the peripheral systemic circulation, which is one of the normal processes taking place within the liver under physiologic conditions. Consequently, systemic instead of portal venous drainage may be associated with a relative hyperinsulinemia in the systemic circulation, which may account for the conspicuous hypoglycemia which is frequently observed during the early postoperative period after pancreas transplantation [5, 6, 30]. It may also account for the fact that normal or nearly normal glucosetolerance has been reported after transplantation of ductobliterated left pancreatic segments [12, 31], in spite of the fact that such segments exhibit a clearly reduced insulin secreting capacity. As was already mentioned in the paragraph 'The effects of pancreatic ductobliteration' and also illustrated in Figure 4, the seemingly normal glucosetolerance with such segments should not be equated with normal beta-cell performance but rather be interpreted as artificially normal by virtue of systemic as opposed to portal venous drainage, since portally draining but otherwise identical segments are associated with severely reduced glucosetolerance [19]. Finally, systemic instead of portal venous drainage may have consequences for the graft itself, since preliminary but suggestive evidence is available in dogs that, in the long run, systemic but not portal drainage exerts a detrimental effect on the endocrine performance of the graft [32].

The answer to the question if the venous anastomosis should be made onto the systemic or portal circulation should ultimately come from clinical work. In the majority of clinical cases, the vein has been anastomosed onto the systemic circulation. The theoretically more physiologic method of anastomosing the vein onto the portal circulation is currently being tested in humans [33]. The long-term results of both approaches should be meticuously compared over the years to come.

Preservation of the pancreas

Reliable preservation of the graft is an important logistic prerequisite of clinical organ transplantation. Therefore, experiments investigating methods of preserving the pancreas were initiated as soon as pancreas transplantation was taking shape as a clinical feasibility. Not only the first clinical pancreas transplant but also the first systematic preservation studies were performed in Minneapolis. Idezuki et al. used canine pancreaticoduodenal grafts which, after flush perfusion with dextran in balanced salt solution, were subjected to hypothermic storage in a hyperbaric oxygen chamber. When tested in vitro by perfusion with oxygenated diluted blood to which glucose had been added, these grafts were shown to sustain a preservation period of 24 hours but not longer, as judged by the amount of insulin released in response to glucose stimulation [34]. This finding was subsequently confirmed in vivo by allotransplantation of pancreaticoduodenal grafts preserved in this fashion, since preservation up to 24 hours was associated with viable grafts but a longer preservation period was not [35]. Later, De Gruyl et al. have compared simple flush perfusion and cold storage (Collin's solution) with pulsatile machine perfusion (cryoprecipitated plasma) of canine pancreatic allografts [36]. They found both preservation methods to be equally effective both in terms of graft function and graft histology. Collin's solution for simple flush perfusion and cold storage of canine pancreatic grafts was later compared to silica gel filtered dog plasma (SGF) by Florack et al. [37]. They found that preservation up to 24 and even 48 hours was feasible with both methods, but that SGF was more reliable in terms of long-term graft function to be expected when preservation had been extended to 48 hours. This preservation study is of significance since it was the first to use autografts instead of allografts, thus excluding eventual interference of immunologic phenomena with the interpretation of results. Subsequently, the same authors compared these results of simple flush perfusion and cold storage with pulsatile machine perfusion [38]. In spite of careful monitoring the flow rate which was kept on a mean level well below 10 ml/min, results of machine preservation were found to be inferior when expressed in failure rates of autotransplantation after 24 and 48 hours of preservation. Interestingly, mean flow rates during preservation were higher in failed than in successful machine preserved grafts, and post-transplantation mean peak serum amylase levels were lower after machine preservation than after cold storage. These findings seem to indicate that higher flow rates are detrimental to the graft, and that pulsatile machine perfusion may be associated with inferior preservation of the exocrine tissue as evidenced by its inadequate capability for producing or secreting amylase. This consideration appears relevant in view of the fact that, under certain circumstances, the capability of producing and secreting amylase may well be interpreted as a reliable monitor of graft function (see paragraph 'Prevention and detection of rejection').

Although these experimental findings in dogs seem very encouraging in regard to eventual clinical applicability, preservation of the human pancreas is still associated with somewhat unpredictable results. Several cases of successful long-term preservation have been described by some [12], but others reported human pancreatic transplants to function well when the cold ischemic period had been shorter than 10 hours, but inadequately or not at all when it had been longer [39]. It appears that the human pancreas responds unlike the human kidney to preservation, in spite of the fact that the canine pancreas can be readily subjected to similar preservation techniques as the canine kidney. There may well be a species specific angle to the matter since porcine, unlike canine, pancreatico-duodenal grafts have recently been reported to be detrimentally affected by cold storage during more than 4 hours [40].

Prevention and detection of rejection

Prevention of rejection of pancreatic allografts, similar to other organ transplants, can be pursued by way of two narrowly related options; one is by choosing the optimal histocompatibility match, and the other by using the most effective immunosuppressive medication.

That matching may prolong pancreas allograft survival has experimentally been demonstrated in DLA-typed beagles both in regard to a minimal number of haplotype mismatches [41] and MLC-identity [42]. In both studies, immunosuppressive therapy was shown to further increase pancreas allograft survival. Questions regarding the influence of histocompatibility matching on pancreas allograft survival have further been investigated in rodents. Unlike other vascularized organ transplants, pancreas allografts in the rat have been found to be not only rejected in the presence of major histocompatibility complex (MHC) disparity, but also and with similar vehemence with non-MHC incompatibility even in the presence of MHC-identity [43]. Although this suggests that not only MHC-alloantigens but also non-MHC-alloantigens may contribute to eliciting the rejection of pancreas allografts, it remains unclear whether these alloantigens are located within the exocrine or endocrine compartment of the pancreas, or both.

It should be noted that rejection is not the only immunologic phenomenon which may occur within the endocrine tissue of the allografted pancreas. Since type 1 diabetes should be interpreted as an autoimmune disease of the beta-cells, the endocrine tissue of the transplanted pancreas is at risk for destruction by recurrence. The clinical reality of this risk was clearly demonstrated in recipients of pancreas transplants procured from identical twin donors [12], and it was recently reinforced experimentally in a model of islet allotransplantation in spontaneously diabetic BB rats [44].

Evidently, questions regarding the place of histocompatibility matching in pancreas transplantation address the type and location of alloantigens within the exocrine and endocrine compartment of the pancreas, as well as the biological interrelationship of rejection and recurrent autoimmune disease of the endocrine tissue. Some answers may derive from clinical experience [12], but systematic work in the experimental setting of vascularized pancreas as well as islet grafts appears indispensable.

In regard to the optimal choice of immunosuppressive medication for the prevention of pancreas allograft rejection, a detailed coverage of the numerous studies investigating the efficacy of different immunosuppressive regimens in rats, pigs, dogs and primates, would take us beyond the scope of this overview. Results may be summarized by stating that conventional immunosuppression with azathioprine and corticosteroids appears to be less effective with experimental pancreas as compared to other experimental organ allografts such as heart or kidney. In addition, cyclosporine and especially cyclospirine in high doses can induce long-term experimental pancreas allograft survival. These findings, however, appear of limited relevance for the current practice with clinical pancreas transplantation, since most centers choose their immunosuppressive regimens for clinical application on the basis of their own or other center's previous clinical experience rather than data derived from experimental work. This, of course, is the obvious consequence not only of the ever present difficulty with interpreting animal work for its clinical applicability, but also of the comfortable circumstance that the number of clinical pancreas recipients is rapidly growing, thus offering an increasingly reliable and relevant source of information for deciding upon the optimal choice of immunosuppressive medication. This consideration implies that experimental work with immunosuppressants may prove to have its value predominantly in association with unraveling the relationship between rejection and recurrent autoimmune disease of the endocrine tissue, rather than with finding optimal regimens of immunosuppressive therapy for clinical application.

An issue of main importance regards the timely detection of rejection. It is well known that the blood glucose level is a poor indicator, since elevated levels are almost always associated with irreversible damage to the betacells. That early treatment is of utmost importance has recently been confirmed in rats [45] and in dogs [46]. Simultaneous kidney transplantation may partly serve the purpose of immunological monitoring [47], but more pertinent methods focus on the pancreas graft itself. Fine needle aspiration cytology has yielded disappointing results in the dog [48]. Infusion of indium-labeled platelets with subsequent and repeated scanning has been tested with some success in dogs [49] and also in man [50]. There is strong evidence that the surgical technique with which exocrine secretion is preserved by drainage into the bladder is currently the best option for the early detection of eventual rejection, since a decrease in urinary amylase content is invariably an early indicator. This was recently confirmed experimentally in dogs [46], which supports the favourable clinical experience [25].

The issue of treating rejection has not been systematically investigated in the experimental setting. Information concerning this topic is mainly derived from clinical experience [12]. In view of the difficulty of detecting eventual rejection in due time, it is not surprising that the available information is sparse and largely anecdotal. Experimental pancreas transplantation may well prove worthwhile for obtaining some pertinent insights.

Concluding considerations

This overview does not attempt to cover each aspect of experimental pancreas transplantation as it has developed during the past few decades. It rather tries to focus on those selected topics which appear of direct relevance to the current status of clinical pancreas transplantation and the differing views in which its clinical execution may be held. Therefore, many excellent studies regarding certain topics in this wide field, be it technical, metabolic, or immunologic in nature, have not been mentioned; their inclusion would have served the purpose of completeness but not the purpose of a more conceptual (and, admittedly, sometimes defective) approach.

44

Finally, it should be suggested that experimental pancreas transplantation in the years to come may prove to be a substantial asset not only for answering some questions relevant to clinical pancreas transplantation, but also (and perhaps: especially) for elucidating more basic questions regarding the etiology and treatment or prevention of diabetes. The latter proposition requires a sound cooperation between experimental pancreas and islet transplantation.

References

1. Gayet R, Guillaume M: La régulation de la sécrétion interne pancréatique par un processus humoral, démontrée par des transplantations de pancréas. Expériences sur des animaux dépancréatés. C R Soc Biol 97: 1615–1618, 1927.
2. Brooks JR, Gifford GH: Pancreatic homotransplantation. Transplant Bull 6: 100–103, 1959.
3. DeJode LR, Howard JM: Studies in pancreaticoduodenal homotransplantation. Surg Gynec Obstet 114: 553–558, 1962.
4. Reemtsma K, Lucas JF, Rogers RE, Schmidt FE, Davis FH: Islet cell function of the transplanted canine pancreas. Ann Surg 158: 645–654, 1963.
5. Bergan JJ, Hoehn JG, Porter N, Dry L: Total pancreatic allografts in pancreatectomized dogs. Arch Surg 90: 521–526, 1965.
6. Largiader F, Lyons GW, Hidalgo F, Dietzman RH, Lillehei RC: orthotopic allotransplantation of the pancreas. Am J Surg 113: 70–76, 1967.
7. Mitchell RI, Rappaport AM, Davidson JK: Autotransplantation of the pancreas. Can J Surg 9: 192–198, 1966.
8. Idezuki Y, Feemster JA, Dietzman RH, Lillehei RC: Experimental pancreaticoduodenal preservation and transplantation. Surg Gynec Obstet 126: 1002–1014, 1968.
9. Aquino C, Ruiz JO, Schultz LS, Lillehei RC: Pancreatic transplantation without duodenum in the dog. Am J Surg 125: 240–244, 1973.
10. Toledo-Pereyra LH, Castellanos J, Lampe EW, Lillehei RC, Najarian JS: Comparative evaluation of pancreas transplantation techniques. Ann Surg 182: 567–571, 1975.
11. Cutfield RG, Kyriakides GK, Olson L, Condie RM, Mintz DH, Miller J: Late observations of canine segmental pancreatic autografts. Transplant Proc 16: 762–763, 1984.
12. Sutherland DER, Goetz FC, Najarian JS: One hundred pancreas transplants at a single institution. Ann Surg 200: 414–440, 1984
13. Idezuki Y, Goetz FC, Lillehei RC: Late effect of pancreatic duct ligation on beta cell function. Am J Surg 117: 33–39, 1969.
14. Dubernard JM, Traeger J, Neyra P, Touraine JL, Tranchant D, Blanc-Brunat N: A new method of preparation of segmental pancreatic grafts for transplantation: trials in dogs and in man. Surgery 84: 633–639, 1978.
15. Sutherland DER: Pancreas and islet transplant registry statistics. Transplant Proc 16: 593–598, 1984.
16. Van Schilfgaarde R, Lemkes HHPJ, Paul LC, Gooszen HG, Terpstra JL: Pancreas transplantation in The Netherlands: report of the first case. Neth J Surg 39: 29–31, 1987.
17. Gooszen HG, Bosman FT, Van Schilfgaarde R: The effect of duct obliteration on the histology and endocrine function of the canine pancreas. Transplantation 38: 13–17, 1984.
18. Gooszen HG: Canine segmental pancreatic autotransplantation. An analysis of the effects of duct obliteration. Thesis, Leiden University. Pasmans, 's-Gravenhage, 1984. (ISBN 90-9000830-6).

19. Gooszen HG, Van Schilfgaarde R, Frölich M, Van der Burg MPM: The effects of duct obliteration and of autotransplantation on the endocrine function of canine pancreatic segments. Diabetes 34: 1008–1013, 1985.
20. Gooszen HG, Van Schilfgaarde R, Terpstra JL: Arterial blood supply of the left lobe of the canine pancreas. II. Electromagnetic flow measurements. Surgery 93: 549–553, 1983.
21. Van Schilfgaarde R, Gooszen HG: The persisting capability for vasodilatation in duct-occluded canine pancreatic segments. Horm Metab Res Suppl 13: 12–15, 1983.
22. Dragstedt LR: Some physiologic problems in surgery of the pancreas. Ann Surg 118: 576–593, 1943.
23. Tydén G, Brattström C, Lundgren G, Ost L, Gunnarsson R, Ostman J, Groth CG: Pancreas transplantation in type 1 diabetes mellitus. Transplant Proc 18: 1753–1754, 1986.
24. Sollinger HW, Cook K, Kamps D, Glass NR, Belzer FO: Clinical and experimental experience with pancreaticocystostomy for exocrine pancreatic drainage in pancreas transplantation. Transplant Proc 16: 749–751, 1984.
25. Sollinger HW, Kalayoglu M, Hoffman RM, Deierhoi MH, Belzer FO: Quadruple immunosuppressive therapy in whole pancreas transplantation. Transplant Proc 19: 2297–2299, 1987.
26. Collin J: Current state of transplantation of the pancreas. Ann Roy Coll Surg 60: 21–27, 1978.
27. Florack G, Sutherland DER, Cavallini M, Najarian JS: Technical aspects of segmental pancreatic autotransplantation in dogs. Am J Surg 146: 565–574, 1983.
28. Van Schilfgaarde R, Gooszen HG, Overbosch EH, Terpstra JL: The arterial blood supply of the left lobe of the canine pancreas. I. Anatomical variations relevant to segmental transplantation. Surgery 93: 545–548, 1983.
29. Calne RY, McMaster P, Rolles K, Duffy TJ: Technical observations in segmental pancreas allografting: observations on pancreatic blood flow. Transplant Proc 12 (suppl 2): 51–57, 1980.
30. Bewick M, Mundy AR, Eaton B, Watson F: Endocrine function of the heterotopic pancreatic allotransplant in dogs. III. The cause of hyperinsulinemia. Transplantation 31: 23–25, 1981.
31. Pozza G, Traeger J, Dubernard JM, Secchi A, Pontiroli AE, Bosi E, Malik MC, Ruiton A, Blanc-Brunat N: Endocrine responses of type 1 (insulin-dependent) diabetic patients following successful pancreas transplantation. Diabetologia 24: 244–248, 1983.
32. Van Goor Hm, Slooff MJH, Sluiter WJ, Wijffels RTM: Changes in beta-cell response after segmental pancreatic autotransplantation. Transplant Proc 18: 1790–1791, 1986.
33. Brons IGM, Calne RY, Rolles K, Lobo A, Evans DB: Paratopic segmental pancreas with simultaneous kidney transplantation in diabetics. Transplant Proc 18: 1757–1758, 1986.
34. Idezuki Y, Goetz FC, Kaufman SE, Lillehei RC: In vitro insulin productivity of the preserved pancreas: a simple test to assess the viability of pancreatic allografts. Surgery 64: 940–947, 1968.
35. Idezuki Y, Goetz FC, Lillehei RC: Experimental allotransplantation of the preserved pancreas and duodenum. Surgery 65: 485–493, 1969.
36. De Gruyl J, Westbroek DL, MacDicken I, Ridderhoff E, Verschoor L, Van Strik R: Cryoprecipitated plasma perfusion preservation and cold storage preservation of duct-ligated pancreatic allografts. Br J Surg 64: 490–493, 1977.
37. Florack G, Sutherland DER, Heil J, Zweber B, Najarian JS: Long-term preservation of segmental pancreas autografts. Surgery 92: 260–269, 1982.
38. Florack G, Sutherland DER, Heil J, Squifflet JP, Najarian JS: Preservation of canine segmental pancreatic autografts: cold storage versus pulsatile machine perfusion. J Surg Res 34: 493–504, 1983.
39. Largiader F, Baumgartner D, Uhlschmid G: Ischemia tolerance of human pancreatic transplants. Transplant Proc 16: 1285–1286, 1984.
40. Dafoe DC, Campbell DA, Marks WH, Borgstrom A, Marion RM, Berlin RE, Turcotte JG:

Detrimental effects of four hours of cold storage on porcine pancreaticoduodenal transplantation. Surgery 99: 170–177, 1986.

41. De Gruyl J, Westbroek DL, Dijkhuis CM, Vriesendorp HM, MacDicken I, Elion-Gerritsen W, Verschoor L, Hulsmans HAM, Hörchner P: Influence of DLA-matching, ALS, and 24-hour preservation on isolated pancreas allograft survival. Transplant Proc 5: 755–759, 1973.

42. Kyriakides GK, Rabinovitch A, Mintz D, Olson L, Rappaport FT, Miller J: Long-term study of vascularized free-draining intraperitoneal pancreatic segmental allografts in beagle dogs. J Clin Invest 67: 292–303, 1981.

43. Klempnauer J, Hoins L, Steiniger B, Günther E, Wonigeit K, Pichlmayr R: Evidence for a differential importance of MHC and non-MHC alloantigens in pancreas and heart transplantation in the rat. Transplant Proc 16: 778–780, 1984.

44. Woehrle M, Markman JF, Silvers WK, Barker CF, Naji A: Effect of temperature of pretransplant culture on islet allografts in BB rats. Transplant Proc 18: 1845–1847, 1986.

45. Schulk JA, Drevyanko TF: Experimental pancreas allograft rejection: correlation between histologic and functional rejection and the efficacy of antirejection therapy. Surgery 98: 330–337, 1985.

46. Prieto M, Sutherland DER, Fernandez-Cruz L, Heil J, Najarian JS: Early diagnosis and treatment of rejection in pancreas transplantation. Transplant Proc 18: 1805–1806, 1986.

47. Severyn W, Olson L, Miller J, Kyriakides G, Rabinovitch A, Flaa C, Mintz D: Studies on the survival of simultaneous canine renal and segmental pancreatic allografts. Transplantation 33: 606–612, 1982.

48. Steiner E, Hammer C, Land W, Gruner P, Schneeberger H, Stangl M, Steimer W: Fine needle biopsy of canine pancreas graft: an attempt at cytologic diagnosis in graft rejection. Transplant Proc 16: 789–790, 1984.

49. Sollinger HW, Lieberman LM, Kamps D, Warner T, Cook K: Diagnosis of early pancreas allograft rejection with indium-111-oxine-labeled platelets. Transplant Proc 16: 785–788, 1984.

50. Jurewicz WA, Buckels JAC, Dykes JGA, Gunson BK, Hawker RJ, Chandler ST, McCollum CN, McMaster P: Indium-111 labeled platelets in monitoring pancreatic transplants in humans. Transplant Proc 16: 720–723, 1984.

Commentary

Without the aforementioned efforts of the various researchers in the field of pancreas transplantation, clinical pancreas transplantation as it is known today, would not be possible. Early experimental work provided us with an understanding of the pancreas and its functions, and much of it was geared toward obtaining meticulous surgical technique. This proved to be necessary in the laboratory setting, since vascular thrombosis was a frequent cause of graft failure among the early transplants. However, clinically, this was not seen. Instead, the main obstacle which prevented success of these grafts, was the inadequate management of the exocrine secretions. Since it had already been clearly demonstrated that pancreatic allografts were indeed capable of maintaining normoglycemia in totally pancreatectomized dogs, subsequent experiments were therefore focused on various techniques which provided for optimal duct management. Nevertheless, progress in this area has been slow, especially since an 'ideal' experimental model has yet to be developed.

To date, there is only a small number of animal models with naturally occurring diabetes mellitus. As a result, the majority of the experimental work has been done in the surgically induced, diabetic canine (recipient) model that is free of secondary diabetic complications; whose graft has been harvested from a healthy, anesthetized donor dog. Hence, it is easy to see why a fair percentage of the experimental data is often not applicable in the clinical setting. What is needed, therefore, is an experimental model which closely mirrors the entire clinical pancreas transplant scenario. In retrospect, however, some of the experimental studies have failed to incorporate all of the pathophysiological changes occurring along with brain death, into their animal models; and have not been able to successfully report on a test for determining the viability of the donor pancreas prior to transplantation.

It is apparent, in reading this chapter, that we are still searching for ways to improve pancreatic graft function, especially from the viewpoint of procurement and preservation. Recent experimental studies seem to indicate that the viability of the donor organ following transplantation, can be dictated, by the type of care given to the donor prior to and during harvesting of the pancreas; by the formulation of the preservation solution(s) used to flush out and preserve the pancreas; and by the method of preservation used. Nevertheless, we are able at the present time, to successfully preserve canine pancreases for as long as 72 hours in the laboratory setting, which is way beyond the limits that were thought to be impossible only a decade ago.

As discussed by Van Schilfgaarde, the prevention and detection of pancreas rejection remains as the final obstacle to long-term success. Although a considerable amount of studies have assessed various combinations of immunosuppression for pancreas transplantation, including graft and/or donor pretreatment with various potential immunomodulators, few centers have altered their immunosuppressive regimens based on this experimental work. Development of an optimal regimen for immunosuppressive therapy would contribute to a reduction in morbidity and mortality, and reduce the length of postoperative hospitalization.

It is obvious, that future research in experimental pancreas transplantation is still needed, if we are to eliminate or stabilize the secondary complications associated with diabetes.

Luis H. Toledo-Pereyra
Chief, Transplantation
Director, Research
Mount Carmel Mercy Hospital
Detroit, Michigan USA

3. Indication for combined pancreas and kidney transplantation**

J. TRAEGER*, P.M. PIATTI and L.D. MONTI

Introduction

The discovery of insulin in 1921 radically changed the outlook for diabetic patients. The acute complications, as hyperosmolar or ketoacidotic coma, were no longer the main cause of death and life expectancy progressively improved, leading to an increase in micro- and macroangiopathic complications.

In the last years many efforts have been done to optimize insulin therapy in order to restore diabetic patients in a condition of normoglycemia with a normal life [1, 2]. For this, many approaches were employed as multiple insulin injections, continuous subcutaneous insulin infusion and intraperitoneal or intravenous insulin infusions. However, even the more sophisticated insulin treatment cannot prevent development of micro and macroangiopathic complications of diabetes mellitus at the present time. The National Commission on Diabetes in the United States has reported that patients with insulin-dependent diabetes are 25 times more prone to blindness, 17 times more prone to kidney disease, 5 times more often afflicted with gangrene, and twice as often afflicted with heart disease than are non-diabetic individuals. Furthermore, one of the most important complications of diabetes mellitus remains renal microangiopathy.

End stage renal disease (ESRD) in patients with diabetes mellitus currently comprises 20% to 30% of the population referred for dialysis or transplantation. It was calculated that the cumulative incidence of diabetic nephropathy was 45% after 40 years of diabetes. Recent statistics have shown that ESRD is the primary cause of death in type I diabetic patients, and is responsible for one third of all cases of renal failure [3].

Initial changes in renal function are elevated glomerular filtration rate (GFR), renal hypertrophy and increased renal plasma flow. Some years after

* Aural, 10 Impasse Lindberg, Lyon 69003, France.
** This review was sent to the editor in June 1986.

49

J.M. Dubernard and D.E.R. Sutherland (eds.), International Handbook of Pancreas Transplantation, 49–57.
© 1989 by Kluwer Academic Publishers.

the appearance of these functional renal changes, structural lesions begin to appear [4, 5]. In this period it is possible to demonstrate the appearance, on a clinical level, of proteinuria followed by progressive deterioration of GFR. Clinical proteinuria is defined as urinary excretion in excess of 0.5 g/24 hr in at least four consecutive 24 hr urine specimens [6]. The transition phase between microalbuminuria with negative Albustix and clinical proteinuria often lasts five to ten years. After this period, diabetic nephropathy rapidly progresses to ESRD that requires dialysis, kidney transplantation or simultaneous kidney plus pancreas transplantation.

Dialysis of kidney transplantation in diabetic patients

In the past, uremic patients with diabetes were usually excluded from dialysis and transplantation because of a general fear that their basic disease and its complications will make either dialysis or transplantation unable to give a satisfactory life expectancy. Patient and graft survival rates after renal transplantation are 10 to 20 per cent lower in diabetic patients then in non-diabetic patients [7, 8]. The most recent innovation in standard hemodialysis and CAPD has actually improved the prognosis for diabetic patients on dialysis. However, dialysis of the uremic diabetic patient is still with greater morbidity and mortality than the same therapy for the non-diabetic patients, and progressively more centers have opted for early, even pre-dialysis, transplantation of diabetic patients [9]. It is reported that 38% of diabetic patients treated by dialysis will live for 3 years, while 82% of patients and 59% of grafts survive 3 years following living donor renal transplantation [10]. In a report of Rohrer [11] the patient and graft survival rates of 144 kidney grafts performed in diabetic patients do not differ significantly from 120 kidney grafts performed in non diabetic patients, even if patient survival is higher in non-diabetic patients. The overall one year patient and graft survival rates for primary cadaver grafts was 89.4% and 74.5% with all therapeutical approaches.

The improvement of patient and graft survival in the last years has increased the risks of recurrence of diabetic nephropathy in transplanted kidney. In fact, the kidney graft, exposed to a diabetic environment, has proved to be susceptible to microscopic recurrence of diabetic nephropathy within the first four post-operative years [12]. Other data have demonstrated that two patients who became uremic more than ten years post-transplant, had histologic lesions of advanced diabetic nephropathy in the graft without evidence of rejection [13]. Thus, kidney transplantations in diabetic patients has provided one of the most important bits of evidence that the complications of diabetes mellitus in the various organ systems are secondary to dysmetabolism and are not an independent disease process.

Mauer [14] has demonstrated that recurrence of diabetic nephropathy occurs in the transplanted kidney within two years after transplantation, also in presence of a good metabolic control with exogenous insulin. Studies performed by Abouna [15] showed the possibility of regression of diabetic renal lesions when normal glycemic levels are achieved. His team transplanted in two uremic patients kidneys from a diabetic cadaver donor with slight proteinuria but normal creatinine. They observed a complete histological regression of diabetic renal disease after 7 months of functioning graft.

Evolution of micro and macrovascular complication in renal transplanted patients is another important problem. Progression of diabetic complications does not seem to change after kidney transplantation. Even if dialysis seems to determine a deterioration of retinopathy (probably due to metabolic disturbance, hypertension and heparinization for hemodialysis treatment [16–18]) after renal transplantation a stabilization and often a deterioration of retinopathy is seen. This is probably due to metabolic disturbance which is not satisfactorily corrected by exogenous insulin administration [19, 20].

Simultaneous kidney plus pancreas transplantation

Indications for simultaneous kidney plus pancreas transplantation

Transplantation of insulin-producing tissue for the achievement of insulin independence is now feasible in humans by means of pancreas transplantation. With the association of a pancreas graft to a kidney graft it is possible to resolve many problems of renal transplantation in diabetic patients, such as recurrence of nephropathy in the transplanted kidney, difficulty of diagnosis of pancreatic rejection and reversal or halt of degenerative complications of diabetes mellitus.

In patients who are candidates for major surgical intervention (kidney transplantation) and immunosuppression, the addition of a pancreatic graft appears to be a logical attempt to treat diabetes mellitus and renal failure at the same time [21]. First of all, pancreas transplantation seems not to add surgical risks to kidney transplantation. In our experience no patients died for technical problems related to pancreas transplantation as pancreatitis or infection of the pancreatic graft. Furthermore, in patients treated with immunosuppressive drugs for kidney transplantation, the same immunosuppressive schedule is also used for pancreas transplantation. In our opinion, the side effects of immunosuppression are too hard to perform a pancreas transplantation alone in which graft survival is relatively low. This is especially true in patients at a relatively early stage of diabetic disease with possibility of a long period of life free of complications of diabetes mellitus. One of the most important problems, in diabetic patients treated with kidney transplantation, is the recurrence of diabetic nephropathy. Although it is still unclear to what extent the recurrence of diabetic nephropathy will affect graft survival, it is hoped that a pancreas graft performed simultaneously with a kidney graft will prevent recurrence of diabetic nephropathy in the transplanted kidney.

In rodents with functioning kidney, it has been shown by several investigators that when pancreas grafts are performed immediately after induction of diabetes, the typical glomerular lesions do not occur [22–26]. If simultaneous pancreas and kidney transplantation is carried out in diabetic patients, no renal lesions are seen after several years of successful grafts [22–26].

Diagnosis and treatment of rejection as early as possible are the most important problems related to the outcome of pancreas and kidney transplantation. In patients who receive pancreatic and renal grafts from the same donor, the kidney serves as an excellent marker of rejection [27], in fact deterioration of kidney function may be the only sign of rejection, without rise in blood glucose level. Studies of Severyn [28] demonstrated that in animals submitted to kidney plus pancreas transplantation, an increase of serum creatinine as expression of renal rejection occurred 6 to 22 days before the onset of hyperglycemia. Renal allograft biopsies revealed generalized mononuclear infiltration, but islets of Langerhans appeared to be spared of immunological infiltrate. This is in accordance with experimental findings of Kyriakides et al. [29], who showed in a canine model of kidney plus pancreas transplantation that mononuclear infiltration of the pancreas is confined to exocrine tissue when serum creatinine first begins to rise. Changes in renal function are the first and most reliable indicators of rejection of both organs while changes in the pancreatic function occur late in the course of rejection. Hyperglycemia is too late a sign of rejection, because the fasting blood glucose level does not rise until 90% to 95% of the islet mass has been eliminated. Moreover, hyperglycemia, in patients treated with steroids, looses its original importance as a primary sign of rejection because it is difficult to distinguish between associated pancreatic rejection and functional changes due to steroid therapy [30]. On the other hand, the treatment of renal rejection could completely prevent pancreatic rejection.

The early kidney rejection diagnosis after pancreas plus kidney transplantation reduces the percentage of subsequent pancreas rejection. Only 50% of the irreversible kidney graft rejections were associated with pancreatic graft rejection detected by serum c-peptide reduction. Furthermore, there was a very low percentage of isolated pancreas rejection with undamaged kidney graft. Immunosuppressive therapy also seems play an important role. In fact, with triple therapy (cyclosporin, azathioprin and low doses of steroids), we have no isolated rejection of pancreas graft in comparison with 22.2% shown during conventional therapy (Table I). Many reports showed an amelioration of degenerative complications with kidney plus pancreas transplantation. Land [31] reported an improvement of visual acuity in a group of diabetic patients submitted to simultaneous kidney plus pancreas transplantation and Black [32] demonstrated a regression of prolipherative retinopathy with amelioration of visual acuity. In our experience an amelioration of visual acuity is seen in most of the patients, 50% of cases presented an amelioration of exudative retinopathy, and in almost all cases no progression of proliferative retinopathy is seen. These results are encouraging in performing simultaneous kidney and pancreas transplantation in diabetic patients with ESRD.

Patient selection and risk factors

The clinical conditions of the patients are relatively poor at the time of transplantation because of moderately severe peripheral vascular disease with a large percentage of amputation of the lower limb. If a major stenosis is present in a large vessel of the lower limb, this may represent a strict indication for a single renal transplantation on the side opposite to the stenosis, because of a possibility of gangrene of lower limb due to insufficient blood flow. Atherosclerotic coronary artery disease and cardiomyopathy occur commonly and are accelerated with chronic hemodialysis. Cardiovascular complications are the major cause of mortality in type I diabetic patients [33], and in our experience cardiovascular complications represent the major cause of death in a group of 69 patients submitted to kidney plus pancreas transplantation (30%). These data are not different from those reported in the literature for kidney transplantation (38.5%) [11]. Pancreas transplantation does not seem to add risks in patients with cardiovascular problems.

Table 1. Pancreatic and kidney graft outcome in 54 simultaneous pancreas and kidney transplantations.

	n	Pancreas alone[a]	Pancreas and kidney[a]	Kidney alone[a]
Ster. + AZA	9	2 (22%)	3 (33%)	1 (11%)
CsA + ster.	31	4 (13%)	2 (6%)	5 (16%)
triple th.	14	0 (0%)	1 (7%)	0 (0%)
		Pancreas[b]	Kidney[b]	
Ster. + AZA		12,5%	37,5%	
CsA + ster.		39,3%	49,5%	
triple th.		50,0%	58,0%	

[a] = Pancreatic and/or kidney graft losses for rejection according to the different immunosuppressive therapies; [b] = Pancreatic and kidney graft survivals at 15 months, according to different immunosuppressive therapies.

It is important to perform a detailed cardiac assessment, with coronary arteriography, in order to identify the patients at higher risks for cardiac complications, but also the patients eligible for a pre-transplant surgical correction of the coronary disease. Toledo-Pereyra suggests that patients with a left ventricular ejection fraction of less than 45%, and right ventricular ejection fraction of less than 35%, are at increased risk and should not be considered for transplantation (pancreas or kidney) [34].

Besides specific indications for surgical interventions, the prevention of progression of cardiac and vascular complications must be pursued in order to achieve better pre-transplant clinical conditions. This can be done by means of diabetes control, dietary measures, maintenance of satisfactory nutritional conditions and agressive treatment of hypertension.

Patient and pancreatic graft survival

Since 1979, the results of transplantation in diabetic patients, at least during the first two years of follow-up have been mainly the same as in non-diabetic renal allograft recipients. In an analysis [35] performed without regard to the timing of kidney transplantation, pancreas graft survival was significantly higher in recipients with ESRD (38% at 1 year) than in those without ESRD (24% at 1 year). On the contrary, patient survival rate was significantly higher in recipients without (84% at 1 year) than in those with ESRD (74% at 1 year). Our experience (in 69 pancreatic grafts performed from 1968 to June 1986) evidences that no pancreas was functioning at 1 year, while pancreas survival rate at the same time after simultaneous kidney and pancreas transplantation was 35%. In the case of patients treated with triple therapy (cyclosporin, azathiprin, steroids) pancreatic graft survival was 50% at 1 year (Figs 1, 2).

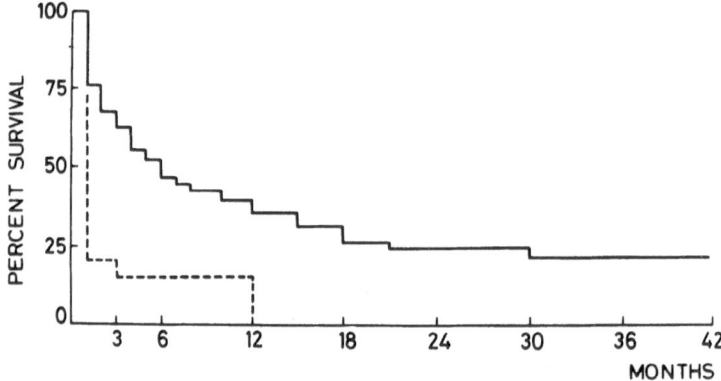

Figure 1. Pancreatic-graft survival in 15 diabetic patients with transplanted pancreas alone (---) and in 54 diabetic patients with simultaneous kidney and pancreas grafts (---) performed in Lyon.

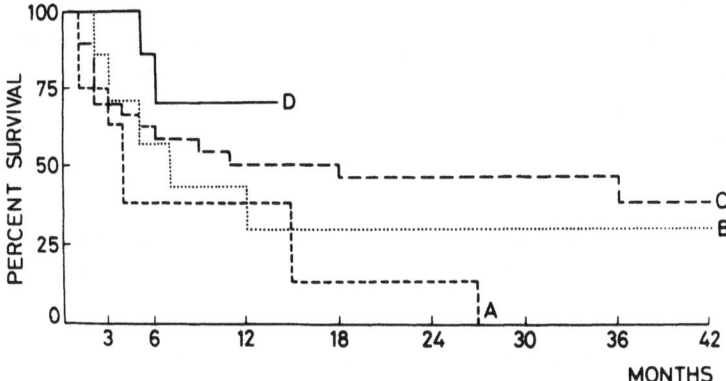

Figure 2. Pancreatic-graft survival in 54 diabetic patients submitted to simultaneous pancreas and kidney transplantation according to different immunosuppressive therapies: A = conventional therapy, B = CsA from the beginning, C = CsA after conventional therapy, D = triple therapy (CsA, Aza, low doses of steroid).

Kidney graft survival ranged from 50% to 70% at 1 year in observations reported by several groups [31, 36].

Conclusion

Pancreas graft in diabetic renal transplant patients is the only method that can truly provide endocrine replacement therapy. The objective of such treatment is to prevent or halt the progression of complications of diabetes in the eyes, kidney, nervous or other systems. In diabetic patients without renal failure, pancreas transplantation could be performed but one of the most important problems is the difficulty in the detection of early rejection. Classical parameters of glucose homeostasis (glycemia, insulinemia and c-peptide) are not adequate, since important modifications of each parameter might depend on multiple factors (steroid administration, post-surgical complications, etc.) even in the absence of an episode of rejection.

In simultaneous pancreas and kidney transplanted patients both the uremic problems and the diabetic syndrome should be alleviated and the impact on the morale of the patient should not be underestimated. The diabetic patients experience an improvement in their sense of well-being, they are able to eat normally and avoid insulin injections for the first time in perhaps 20 or 30 years. In conclusion, we prefer to perform a simultaneous kidney and pancreas transplantation, because pancreas transplantation is a 'life enriching' rather than a 'life sustaining' procedure and many problems as rejection, technical failure, side effects of immunosuppression are to be solved before to perform pancreas transplantation alone.

56

Pancreas transplantation can be performed only in selected diabetic patients, who require kidney transplantation with immunosuppressive therapy, provided their secondary complications of diabetes are more serious than the potential side effects of anti-rejection therapy.

References

1. Pozza G, Spotti D, Micossi P, Cristallo M, Melandri M, Piatti PM, Monti LD, Pontiroli AE: Long term continuous intraperitoneal insulin treatment in brittle diabetes. Brit Med J 286: 255–257, 1983.
2. Shade DS, Eaton RP, Warhol RM, Gregory JA, Dorbernek RC: Subcutaneous peritoneal access device for type I diabetic patients nonresponsive to subcutaneous insulin. Diabetes 31: 470–473, 1982.
3. Christiansen JS, Andersen AR, Andersen JK, Deckert T: The natural history of diabetic nephropathy. Diabetic Nephropathy 4: 104–106, 1985.
4. Ditzel J, Junker K: Abnormal glomerular filtration rate, renal plasma flow and renal protein excretion in recent and short term diabetes. Brit Med J 2: 13–19,1972.
5. Christiansen JS, Gammelgaard J, Frandsen M, Parving HM: Increased kidney size, glomerular filtration rate, and renal plasma flow in short-term insulin-dependent diabetics. Diabetologia 20: 451–456, 1981.
6. Andersen AR, Christiansen JS, Andersen JK, Kreiner S, Deckert T: Diabetic nephropathy in type I (insulin dependent) diabetes: an epidemiological study. Diabetologia 25: 496–501, 1983.
7. Belzer FO, Glass N, Sollinger H, Miller D: Functional survival of juvenile diabetic patients after renal transplantation. In: Friedman EA, L'Esperance SA (eds) Diabetic renal retinal syndrome, prevention and management; 2nd edition. Grune and Stratton, New York, 1982.
8. Standards committee of the American society of transplant surgeons: Current results and expectations of renal transplantation. JAMA 246: 1330–1334, 1983.
9. Sutherland DER, Morrow CE, Fryd DS, Ferguson R, Simmons RL, Najarian JS: Improved patient and primary renal allograft survival in uremic diabetic recipients. Transplantation 34: 319–323, 1982.
10. Friedman EA: Comprehensive care essential to success in diabetic nephropathy. Transplant Proc 16: 569–572, 1984.
11. Rohrer RJ, Madras PN, Sahyoun AI, Monaco AP: Renal transplantation in the diabetic. World J Surg 10: 397–403, 1986.
12. Bohman SO, Tyden G, Wilczek H, Lundgern G, Jarenko G, Gunnarson R, Ostman J, Groth CG: Prevention of kidney graft diabetic nephropathy by pancreas transplantation in man. Diabetes 34: 306–308, 1985.
13. Sutherland DER, Morrow CE, Fryd DS, Ferguson R, Simmons RL, Najarian JS: Improved patient and primary renal allograft survival in uremic diabetic recipients. Transplantation 34: 319–325, 1982.
14. Mauer SM, Steffes MW, Connett J, Najarian JS, Sutherland DER, Barbosa J: The development of lesions in the glomerular basement membrane and mesangium after transplantation of normal kidneys to diabetic patients. Diabetes 32: 948–952, 1983.
15. Abouna GM, Kremer GD, Dadah SK, Al-Aduani MS, Kemar SA, Kusma G: Reversal of diabetic nephropathy in human cadaveric kidneys after transplantation into non-diabetic recipients. Lancet ii: 1274–1276, 1983.
16. White N, Snowden SA, Parsons V, Sheldon J, Bewick M: The management of terminal renal failure in diabetic patients by regular dialysis therapy. Nephron 11: 261–275, 1973.

17. Blagg CR: Visual and vascular problems in dialysed diabetic patients. Kidney Int 6 (suppl 1): 527–531, 1974.
18. Amair P, Khanna R, Letbel B, Pierratos A, Vas S, Meema E, Blair G, Chisol ML, Vas M, Zingg W, Digenis G, Oreopulos D: Continuous ambulatory peritoneal dialysis in diabetics with end stage renal disease. N Engl J Med 306: 625–630, 1982.
19. Ramsay RC, Knobloch WH, Barbosa JJ, Sutherland DER, Kjellstrand CM, Najarian JS, Goetz FC: The visual status of diabetic patients after renal transplantation. Am J Ophthal 87: 305–310, 1979.
20. Mitchell JC: End stage renal failure in juvenile diabetes mellitus: a 5 year follow-up of treatment. Mayo Clin Proc 52: 281–288, 1977.
21. Hattler BG Jr, Miller J, Johnson MC: Cellular and humoral factors governing canine mixed lymphocyte culture after renal transplantation. II Cellular. Transplantation 14: 47–50, 1972.
22. Mauer SM, Sutherland DER, Steffes MW, Leonard RJ, Najarian JS, Michael AF, Brown DM: Pancreatic islet transplantation: effects on the glomerular lesions of experimental diabetes in the rat. Diabetes 23: 748–753, 1974.
23. Weil R III, Nozawa M, Koss M, Weber C, Reemtsma K, McIntosh RM: Pancreatic transplantation in diabetic rats: renal function, morphology, ultrastructure, and immunohistology. Surgery 78: 142–148, 1975.
24. Orloff MJ, Lee S, Charters C III, Grambort DE, Storck LG, Knox D: Long term studies of pancreas transplantation in experimental diabetes mellitus. Ann Surg 182: 198–206, 1975.
25. Federlin K, Bretzel RG, Schmidtchen U: Islet transplantation in experimental diabetes of the rat. V. Regression of glomerular lesions in diabetic rats after intraportal transplantation of isogeneic islets: preliminary results. Horm Metab Res 8: 404–406, 1976.
26. Gray BN, Watkins E Jr: Isolated islet transplantation in experimental diabetes. Aust J Exp Biol Med Sci 54: 57–70, 1976.
27. Tyden G, Lundgren G, Gunnarsson R, Ostman J, Groth CG: Laboratory findings during rejection of segmental pancreatic allografts. Transplant Proc 16: 715–717, 1984.
28. Severyn W, Olson L, Miller J, Kyriakides G, Rabinovitch A, Flaa C, Mintz D: Studies on the survival of simultaneous canine renal and segmental pancreatic allografts. Transplantation 33: 606–612, 1982.
29. Kyriakides G, Olson L, Severyn W, Flaa C, Rabinovitch A, Mintz D, Miller J: Early detection of pancreatic allograft rejection in dogs: Immunologic and physiologic monitoring in simultaneous kidney and pancreas transplantation and response in immunosuppression. World J Surg 5: 430, 1981.
30. Dubernard JM, Traeger J, Touraine JL, Betuel H, Malik MC: Rejection of human pancreatic allografts. Transplant Proc 12: 103–106, 1980.
31. Land W, Langraf R, Illner WD, Jensen U, Gokel M, Castro LA, Fornara P, Burg D, Kampi K: Improved results in segmental pancreatic and renal transplantation in diabetic patients under cyclosporine therapy. Transplant Proc 17: 317–324, 1985.
32. Black PD: Visual status of diabetic patients after pancreatic and other organ transplantation. Trans Ophtal Soc U K 101: 100–104, 1981.
33. Braun WE, Phillips D, Vidt D, Novick AC, Nakamoto S, Popowniak K, Magnusson M, Pohl M, Paganini E, Steinmuller D, Protiva D, Buszta C: The course of coronary artery disease in diabetics with and without renal allografts. Transplant Proc 15: 1114–1119, 1983.
34. Toledo-Pereyra LH: The importance of myocardial imaging as a selection criterion of patients prior to pancreas transplantation. Transplant Proc 16: 671–674, 1984.
35. Sutherland DER, Moudry K: Pancreas transplant registry report. Transplant Proc 1986 (in press).
36. Traeger J, Dubernard JM, Piatti PM, Bosi E, El Yafi S, Lefrancois N, Cantarovich D, Secchi A, Gelet A, Kamel G, Monti LD, Touraine JL, Pozza G: Cyclosporine in double simultaneous pancreas plus kidney transplantation. Transplant Proc 17: 336–339, 1985.

4. Indication for pancreas transplantation alone

D.E.R. SUTHERLAND

Introduction and general considerations

Ideally, pancreas transplants should be performed in diabetic patients who do not yet have, but are destined to develop, secondary lesions of diabetes more serious than the potential side effects of antirejection therapy. Currently, there is no way to predict which patients will develop secondary complications before the earliest lesions appear. Thus, pancreas transplants have largely been restricted to patients who already have clinical manifestations of diabetic retinopathy, neuropathy or nephropathy.

Even though the potential for benefit is greatest in patients without terminal manifestations of the complications, most pancreas transplants have been performed simultaneous with a kidney transplant in uremic patients with end stage diabetic nephropathy [1]. Kidney transplantation is the best treatment for diabetic patients with renal failure [2], and the addition of a pancreas entails only the surgical risks, since immunosuppression is already obligatory. Diabetic patients who meet the criteria for kidney transplantation, and who do not have a contraindication to an extended surgical procedure, are appropriate candidates for a simultaneous pancreas transplant. Indeed, most uremic diabetic patients should be candidates for the combined operation, as outlined in the preceeding chapter.

Of the 1077 recipients of primary pancreas grafts reported to the Pancreas Transplant Registry through April of 1987, more than two thirds (685, or 64%) received simultaneous kidney transplant [1]. The remaining patients received a pancreas transplant alone; of these, nearly hàlf (183, or 17% of the total number of pancreas transplant recipients), had received a previous kidney transplant. Again, in recipients of a pancreas after a kidney, only the surgical risks needed to be considered, since immunosuppression is obligatory. In kidney transplant recipients, a pancreas transplant is justified simply to avoid the need for exogenous insulin therapy, with the improvement of lifestyle that ensues, even if secondary complications are advanced. This is not to say that a

J.M. Dubernard and D.E.R. Sutherland (eds.), International Handbook of Pancreas Transplantation, 59–70.
© *1989 by Kluwer Academic Publishers.*

beneficial effect on secondary complications will not occur, but any negative effect that immunosuppression may have on these complications has already been accepted, unlike the situation in a nonuremic nonkidney transplant patients. Thus, for patients who already have a kidney graft, a pancreas transplant can be considered, unless they are in a high operative risk category (e.g., previous myocardial infarct, or presence of specific uncorrectable lesions on coronary arteriogram). For patients who have have had or need a kidney transplant, even such pre-existing conditions as blindness would not be a contraindication to a pancreas transplant. The management of diabetes by such patients is more difficult than the management of immunosuppression, and the latter treatment is necessary anyway for the kidney transplant.

The selection process must be much more rigorous for the nonuremic, nonkidney transplant patients who do not have end stage diabetic nephropathy. In such candidates, both the surgical and the immunosuppressive risks must be balanced against the benefits of pancreas transplantation. Only one-fifth (184 or 18%) of the recipients of primary pancreas transplants reported to the Registry as of April, 1987, were in this category [1]. The potential for benefit is greater in this than in any other group of diabetic patients. Except for the rare patient with such severe lability that the diabetes itself is incapacitating, secondary complications should be present in recipients of pancreas transplants alone, but at a stage where reversal or stabilization is possible. However, the lesions should also be at a stage where progression to a level more serious than the potential side effects of antirejection treatment would occur if diabetes were not corrected. In other words, the risks of immunosuppression, as well as the surgical risks of transplantation, should be less than the risks of remaining diabetic.

The surgical risks of pancreas transplantation are now low. Because cyclosporin is a relatively new drug, the long-term risks of its use are not completely known [3], but it must be used in such a fashion as to minimize its nephrotoxic effect [4].

Precisely determining the risks of remaining diabetic can also be difficult for some patients, since no absolutely reliable markers indicate which cases are prone to develop secondary complications before the earliest lesions appear. Markers have been proposed, such as stiff joints in childhood [5] or high plasma levels of inactive renin [6] indicating patients at high risk for microvascular complications, or high insulin like growth factor I levels identifying patients in which the course of retinopathy is accelerated [7]. However, not everyone with these markers follows a predictable course, and in some the complications are present before the markers become positive.

Once lesions are present, however, there are markers to predict progression, including retinopathy [8] and neuropathy [9]. Another example is proteinuria [10]. Even microalbuminuria identifies patients in which diabetic nephropathy who will inevitably progress to end stage renal disease [11], at least if they remain diabetic [12]. The central question is whether a pancreas transplant could halt the progression of this process. This question leads to the additional question of whether cyclosporin nephrotoxicity, superimposed on pre-existing diabetic nephropathy, would actually accelerate or augment the process. Evidence to date suggests that this is not the case in the most recipients [13], but certainly such a risk has to be considered [14].

There is also the subgroup of patients who have extreme difficulty with diabetic control on a day to day basis [15]. There are tests to predict which patients are at high risk for hypoglycemic episodes on intensified insulin therapy regimens, such as the epinepherine response to stress [16]. If such a patient also has early secondary complications, there is no doubt that the risks of remaining diabetic outweigh the risks of immunosuppression.

On the other hand, a pancreas transplant in a diabetic individual with no evidence of secondary complications places the patients at risk for complications of immunosuppression, without sure knowledge of benefit other than the ability to obviate the need for exogenous insulin. Thus, the selection of patients without any evidence of secondary complications must be extremely rigorous, with clear evidence that insulin treatment is so difficult a pancreas transplant is warranted. If completely innocuous antirejection methods were available, recipient selection criteria for pancreas transplantation could be very liberal, but current methods of immunosuppression dictate the need to restrict its application to the type of patient described in the following section.

There is abundant evidence to support the concept that the complications of diabetes are secondary due to disordered metabolism [17]. Whether lesions once present can be influenced is another question, but pancreas transplantation establishes a euglycemic state [18], a goal that is nearly impossible to achieve by exogenous insulin [19]. In addition, there is evidence, presented in a separate chapter, that the progression of established lesions in the eyes, nerves and kidneys [13, 20, 21] can be prevented, and that some lesions can regress [14, 20, 21].

Criteria for pancreas transplants alone

In general, nonuremic diabetic candidates for pancreas transplantation should have at least early diabetic nephropathy, with proteinuria or lesions on biopsy predicting progression. Even without a pancreas transplant, immunosuppression would eventually be necessary since progression to end stage disease without a pancreas transplant would be inevitable. A pancreas transplant mainly entails assuming the risk of immunosuppression early rather than late in the course of the disease, with the need for kidney transplant either obviated or unaltered, except perhaps for the timing. These patients need to be studied to determine if a detrimental effect of chronic cyclosporin nephrotoxicity is offset by a beneficial amelioration of diabetic renal lesions.

Some nonuremic diabetic patients, without or with minimal renal disease, in whom the potential for development of progressive nephropathy is uncertain, but in whom other problems exist that could be relieved by a pancreas transplant, such as extreme difficulty with metabolic control, or progressively severe neuropathy, may also be candidates. With current immunosuppressive regimens, the number of recipients in this category is small since the problems of diabetes must be more serious than the potential side effect of chronic immunosuppression. The criteria used for selection of candidates for pancreas transplant alone at the University of Minnesota are summarized in Table 1, and are more fully discussed in the following section.

Justification for pancreas transplants alone according to past and current results

In considering whether to perform pancreas transplantation alone in nonuremic nonkidney transplant patients, it is important to know current graft survival rates. It is also important to know what the effects have been on secondary complications in patients who have maintained functioning grafts. Only a small number of patients in this category have been transplanted, but preliminary studies of the effect on secondary complications show:

1. Microscopic lesions of early diabetic nephropathy regress [13], but creatinine clearance is decreased because of cyclosporin [22].

2. Retinopathy may progress during the first year, but thereafter the process seems to stabilize [20]. Most recipients had advanced eye disease, and were not in the category of background retinopathy thought to be ideal according to the criteria outlined in Table 1. In the patients studied, progression has been seen in approximately 30% of recipients during three years; thereafter retinopathy has remained stable in patients with functioning grafts, while continous deterioration has been seen in those with failed grafts [20].

3. Neuropathy appears to improve, in patients with functioning grafts [14, 21, 23]. Subjective improvement in pereperhial sensory deficitis has been described [23]. Objective, electrophysiological tests, show that nerve convection velocities increase, and deterioration of evoked muscle action potentials ceases [21]. In contrast, neurological deterioration has continued to progress in patients whose grafts have failed [14].

The details of the studies are summarized in a separate chapter on secondary complications. In essences, the studies show that patients with functioning grafts achieve the benefits desired from pancreas transplant, but at the expense of cyclosporin nephrotoxicity and the need for life-long immunosuppression.

Even though a benefit can be shown, the success rate also has to be sufficiently high to justify the procedure. In the Pancreas Transplant Registry, pancreas graft survival rates have been lowest in recipients of pancreas transplants alone [11], but patient survival rates have been the highest in this category (see Registry chapter). Patient survival rates are higher than in the patients with end stage diabetic nephropathy, because the recipients of pan-

Table 1. Criteria for pancreas transplantation alone in nonuremic, nonkidney transplant diabetic patients.

A. Nephropathy (pre-uremic or non end-stage)
   1. Albuminuria[a]
   2. Mesangium <30% of glomerular volume on renal biopsy (<20% normal; >30% severe disease)
   3. Creatinine clearance >50 ml/min[b]
B. Retinopathy
   1. Preferable to be in background or nonproliferative stage where early stabilization, or even regression, is theoretically possible [8].
   2. Pre-proliferative or proliferative stage is acceptable; probability of progression unchanged during first year but long-term stabilization may occur if diabetic state is corrected [18].
C. Neuropathy
   1. Sensory loss, pain or motor dysfunction[c]
   2. Severe autonomic dysfunction[d]
   Stage at which various lesions or manifestations of neuropathy are inevitably progressive or are potentially reversible have not been defined.
D. Severe dysmetabolism (hyperlabile diabetes)
   Frequent episodes of hypoglycemia and ketoacidosis in face of diligent efforts by patient and physician to control diabetes with exogenous insulin (functionally incapacitated by diabetes).

Early nephropathy (A) in combination with one of the other lesions (B, C, or D) indicates a favorable risk: benefit ratio. The risk of pancreas transplantation and immunosuppression is no greater than the risk of remaining diabetic, and there is potential for benefit. The isolated presence of B or C without other lesions does not necessarily indicate a risk of diabetes greater than that of pancreas transplantation and immunosuppression, and transplants in such patients should be preformed in an investigational setting. D by itself can be an indication for transplantation; D in combination with any of the other criteria clearly defines a risk of diabetes greater or equal to that of pancreas transplantation and immunosuppression, and a successful transplant solves the rare diabetic management problem.

[a] Progression to uremia (end-stage disease) is inevitable if diabetic state continues, but regression or stabilization is possible if diabetes is corrected [13].
[b] Renal function is good enough to tolerate cyclosporin, although the long-term effect is unknown [3].
[c] Subjective improvement in sensation [23], objective improvement in nerve conduction velocities [21] and stabilization of evoked muscle action potentials [12] have occurred after successful pancreas transplants.
[d] No data on autonomic studies after pancreas transplants alone has been published.

creas transplants alone have less advanced complications, and less coronary artery disease; thus a higher survival rate is expected (90% at one year in the Registry). Graft survival rates may be lower because of difficulty in diagnosing and treating rejection in the absense of the kidney from the same donor [24]. In recipients of simultaneous pancreas and kidney transplants, the physiological manifestation of rejection may occur earlier in the kidney than in the pancreas, but the kidney mirrors events ongoing the pancreas. Treatment of kidney rejection is automatically associated with earlier treatment of pancreatic rejection than when a recipient of a pancreas transplant alone is treated based on a rise in plasma glucose. With the advent of the bladder drainage technique [25] the situation has improved [26], and in the Registry figures, recipients of pancreas transplants alone managed by bladder drainage have graft survival rates equilivent to that in patients with end stage diabetic nephropathy who receive simultaneous pancreas and kidney transplants [1].

The largest experience with pancreas transplantation alone is at the University of Minnesota, where 111 such procedures were performed between 1980 and January of 1988 [14]. The results in these cases will be summarized here as an example of what can be achieved and to give some historical perspective to the application of pancreas transplants alone. Results have improved as advances in immunosuppression and surgical technique have been made [27].

Of the 111 Minnesota pancreas transplants alone performed since 1980, the surgical techniques for duct management was open intraperitoneal in 3, polymer injection in 13, enteric drainage in 65 and bladder drainage in 30. The first two techniques are no longer used. In addition, the enteric drainage technique in no longer used for recipients of cadaver grafts, but is still applied to related donor transplants. With related donor transplants, rejection is most likely to occur, compensating for the inability to monitor a parameter independent of glucose for rejection. All bladder drained pancreas transplants alone have been from cadaver donors, and rejection has been monitored by urine amylase as well as by plasma glucose levels [26]. The difference that these approaches make is apparent from the results. In the overall series of 111 pancreas transplants alone, one year patient and graft survival rates were 90% and 39%; for the 81 technically successful cases, the 1 year graft survival rate was 53%. Before November 1984, the recipients were immunosuppressed with two drugs only (either azathioprine and prednisone or cyclosporin and prednisone). Since November 1984, the recipients have been immunosuppressed with cyclosporin, azathioprine and prednisone in combination (triple therapy). Comparing the results in Era 2 versus Era 1, 1 year patient survival rates were 93% versus 86%; graft survival rates were 48% versus 29% for all cases, and 63% (n = 47) versus 41% (n = 34) for technically successful cases. The results by technique and donor source of pancreas transplants alone since

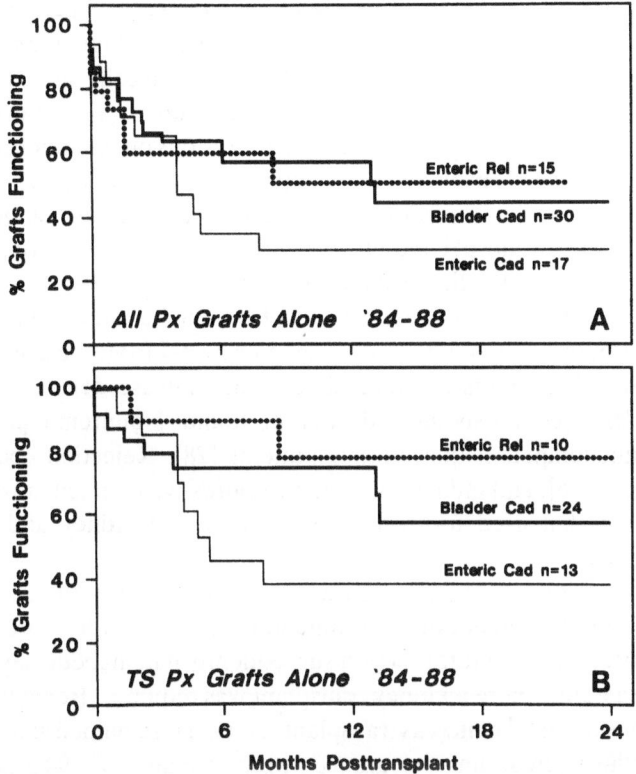

Figure 1. Graft functional survival rates for (A) all and for (B) technically successful pancreas transplants alone, performed at the University of Minnesota from October 1984 to January 1988, in nonuremic, nonkidney transplant recipients, according to donor course and duct management technique. Enteric drained (ED) grafts from cadaver donors had the lowest long-term success rate, primarily because of the inability to diagnose and treat rejection early, while bladder drained (BD) grafts from cadaver and enteric drained grafts from related (REL) donors had a relatively high success rate because of the ability to diagnose and treat rejection episodes early based on urine amylase monitoring in the BD and because of the low incidence of rejection in the REL category. Currently only BD is used for cadaver donor transplants while both ED and BD are used for related donor pancreas transplants alone. From Sutherland et al, Surgery 104: in press, 1988 [14].

November 1984 are illustrated in Figure 1. The one year graft survival rates for bladder drained cadaver (n = 30), related donor enteric (n = 15) and cadaver donor enteric (n = 17) pancreas transplants alone cases were 58%, 51%, and 21%, and for technically successful cases were 75% (n = 24), 77% (n = 10), and 38% (n = 13). Thus, with bladder drainage from cadaver donors and enteric drainage from related donors, a high success rate is achieved; with enteric drainage from cadaver donors the success rate has been low because of the inability to diagnosis and treat rejection early and we have abandoned this approach. Using the current approach with cadaver bladder and related enteric drainage, the overall one year patient and graft survival rate for 45 pancreas transplants alone cases were 95% and 56%; for technically successful cases, the 1 year graft survival rate was 76%. These results were achieved with a protocol that includes preoperative blood transfusions on immunosuppression (to reduce sensitation), triple immunosuppressive therapy posttransplant and diligent monitoring for rejection episodes, with daily home blood glucose monitoring, daily urine pH monitoring, and urine amylase levels checked three times a week for the first two months and weekly thereafter. A decline in urine amylase activity (units/hour) by 50% from the baseline prompts admission for treatment of rejection. A decline in urine pH from the usual baseline of 7 to 9 to <7 prompts an immediate urine amylase determination and admission for rejection should a decline be found. Nonuremic patients are more immunocompetent than uremic patients [28]. Rejection episodes are more frequent [26], and induction immunosuppressive regimen must be more vigorous than that used for recipients of combined kidney and pancreas transplants [4].

In the analysis of the 111 pancreas transplant alone cases at the University of Minnesota, serial assement of renal function has been made. Three patients who have lost pancreas graft function subsequently had diabetic nephropathy progress to a point where a kidney transplant was required. Renal function in recipients of successful pancreas transplants alone has remained stable after an initial decline (creatinine clearance pretransplant of 94 ± 30 versus 52 ± 19 ml/min by one year). However, two cyclosporin patients with pretransplant creatinine clearances of 55 and 70 ml/min had exceptional courses, with a decline during the first year post transplant to <25 ml/min. Both underwent successful kidney transplants at that time. In the recipients of pancreas transplants alone who have had serial studies of visual acuity and retinopathy, visual acuity has remained stable in 79%, improved in 5% and worsened in 15%. Retinopathy has remained stable in 59%, but progressed in 41% over the first year; thereafter, retinopathy has remained stable in almost all patients, with a deterioration between the first and the second year occurring in only 4% [14].

The neurological changes in recipients of pancreas transplants alone, are given in detail in the chapter on secondary complications. In patients with functioning grafts studied at one and two years, motor and sensory nerve connection parameters improved and evoked muscle amplitude potentials remained stable [14]. Recipients with failed grafts continued to have progressive deterioration in evoked muscle amplitude potentials is usually the course in diabetic patients.

Summary and conclusions

Prospective recipients for pancreas transplants alone who meet the criteria listed in Table 1 will have secondary complications involving either the eyes, nerves, or kidneys, or difficulty with diabetic control so great that it is justified to substitute management by immunosuppression (transplant) for management by exogenous insulin. Except for the exceptional patients who meet the criteria of hyperlabile diabetes, early lesions of nephropathy must generally by present for a diabetic individual to be considered for a pancreas transplant. The lesions should be at the stage predicting a high probability of end stage disease should conventional diabetic management continue to be used. Creatinine levels should be $<2\,mg/dl$ and a creatinine clearance $>50\,ml/min$. Otherwise the cyclosporin required to prevent rejection will not be tolerated. It is unlikely the disease process in a patient with a creatinine clearance $<50\,ml/min$ would be stabilized or reversed. For some patients with a creatinine clearance between 50 and 70, the disease process may continue to progress, but in such patients even if end stage diabetic nephropathy occurs secondary to cyclosporin, the recipient is no worse off (regarding the kidney) than if the transplant had not been done. If end stage disease from either diabetes or cyclosporin does not occur the patient will have benefited.

Patients with a creatinine clearance of between 20 and 50 ml present a dilemma. Progression to uremia after a solitary pancreas transplant may be accelerated because of the nephrotoxic effect of cyclosporin superimposed on severe diabetic nephropathy. In such patients consideration can be given to performing an early kidney transplant in combination with the pancreas. Otherwise the pancreas transplant should be deferred until a kidney transplant is necessary to treat uremia.

Patients with no evidence of nephropathy who undergo a pancreas transplant must accept the potential risk of progressive cyclosporin nephrotoxicity, without knowing whether they are at risk for end stage diabetic nephropathy had they remained diabetic. These patients must be clearly at risk for other complications of their diabetes, with either neuropathy or backround diabetic retinopathy, or must have such difficulty with diabetic control that they are nearly incapacited. When immunosuppression without nephrotoxicity or other side effects is available, the pool of nonuremic diabetic patients considered for pancreas transplantation will broaden, and even children could be considered.

Pancreas transplant recipient should thoroughly understand the risks and uncertainties associated with the procedure. For kidney transplant recipients, the additional risks of a pancreas transplant are minimal, but for the nonuremic nonkidney transplantation, the immunosuppressive risks are not fully known. Nevertheless, diabetic patients who are faced with the prospect of progressive deterioration of bodily functions, and who find it difficult to accept established therapy even when the alternative contains known as well as unknown risks, are appropriate candidates. Prospective recipients should be given written information on all aspects of pancreas transplantation, including immunosuppression, results and possible complications, and should participate in frank and open discussion with physicians and other personel involved with the program.

It is also mandatory that physicians preforming the transplants in nonuremic nonkidney recipients, study the recipients diligently. Serial examinations of eye, nerve and kidney function are needed to document the degree of baseline disability and to assess the effect of transplantation on the subsequent course of secondary complications.

In the United States, pancreas transplantation is not funded by government programs and the patients have to have insurance coverage or pay out-of-pocket. Thus, financial considerations also limit the application of pancreas transplantation. Several insurance companies provide coverage for pancreas transplants, and indeed it is responsible to do so since the procedure is cost-effective if serious secondary complications of diabetes are ameloriated. Some companies specify such coverage in the policies they write, while others have provided coverage with prior authorization obtained on a case-by-case basis.

The criteria nonuremic, nonkidney transplant diabetic patients should meet in order to receive a pancreas are being continuously redefined as results improve and more effective, less toxic immunosuppressive protocols are devised. Thus, the criteria outlined above for recipient selection should be considered only a guideline, to be modified according to individual circumstances and future changes in the approaches to endocrine replacement therapy for diabetes.

References

1. Sutherland DER, Moudry KC: Pancreas transplant registry. Pancreas 2: 473–388, 1987.
2. Sutherland DER, Canafax DM, Goetz FC et al: Renal transplantation in diabetic patients, the treatment of choice. In: Mogensen CE (ed) The kidney and hypertension of diabetes mellitus; pp 341–348. Martinus Nijhoff Publishers Company, Boston, 1988.
3. Humes HJD, Jackson NM, O'Connor RP, Nunt DA, White MD: Pathogenic mechanisms and insights into cyclosporin toxicity. Transpl Proc 17: 51–51, 1985.
4. Sutherland DER, Goetz FC, Najarian JS: Improved pancreas graft survival rates by use of multiple drug combination immunotherapy. Transpl Proc 18: 1770–1773, 1986.
5. Rosenbloom AL, Sliverstein JH, Lezote DC et al: Limited joint mobility in childhood diabetes mellitus indicates increased risk for microvascular disease. N Engl J Med 305: 191, 1981.
6. Luetscher JA, Kraemer FS, Wilson DM et al: Increased plasma inactive renin: a marker to

microvascular disease. N Engl J Med 312: 1412, 1985.

7. Merimee TJ, Zapf J, Froesch ER: Insulin-like growth factors. Studies in diabetes with and without retinopathy. N Engl J Med 390: 527, 1983.
8. West KM, Erderich LJ, Stover JA: A detailed study of risk factors for retinopathy in diabetes. Diabetes 29: 501–508, 1980.
9. Young RJ, Mac Intyre CC, Martyn CN, Prescott RJ, Ewing DJ, Smith AF, Viberti GC, Clark BF: Progression of a subclinical polyneuropathy in young patients with type 1 (insulin-dependent) diabetes: associations with glycaemic control and microangiopathy (microvascular complications). Diabetologia 29: 156–161, 1986.
10. Mogenson CE, Christiansen CK: Predicting diabetes nephropathy in insulin-dependent diabetic patients. N Engl J Med 311: 89–93, 1984.
11. Viberti GC, Hill RD, Jarre HRJ et al: Microalbuminuria as a predictor of clinical diabetic nephropathy. Lancet 1: 1430–1432, 1982.
12. Anderson AR, Christiansen JS, Anderson JK et al: Diabetic nephropathy in type I insulin dependent diabetes. Diabetologia 25: 496–501, 1983.
13. Bilous RW, Mauer SM, Sutherland DER et al: Glomeural structural function following treatment by pancreas transplantation for insulin dependent diabetes mellitus. Diabetes 36: 43A, 1987.
14. Sutherland DER, Kendall DM, Moudry KC et al: Pancreas transplantation in nonuremic type I diabetic recipients. Surgery 104: 453–464, 1988.
15. Malone JI, Hellrrunj JM, Melphrusew et al: Good diabetic control: A study in mastilousion. J Peds 88: 943–947, 1976.
16. White N, Skor DA, Cryer PE et al: Identification for type I diabetic patients at increased risk of hypoglycemia during intensive therapy. N Engl J Med 308: 485, 1983.
17. Tchobroutsky G: Relation of diabetes control to development of microvascular complications. Diabetologia 15: 143, 1978.
18. Sutherland DER, Najarian JS, Greenberg BZ et al: Hormonal and metabolic effects of an endocrine graft. Vascularized segmental transplantation on the pancreas in insulin-independent patients. Ann intern Med 5: 537, 1981.
19. Unger RH: Meticulous control of diabetes: Benefits, risks and precautions. Diabetes 31: 479, 1982.
20. Ramsey RC, Goetz FC, Sutherland DER et al: Progression of diabetic retinopathy after pancreas transplant regimen patient for insulin dependent diabetes mellitus. N Engl J Med 318: 208–214, 1988.
21. van der Vliet JA, Navarro X, Kennedy WR et al: The effect of pancreas transplantation in diabetic polyneuropathy. Transplantation 45: 368–379, 1988.
22. DeFransisco AM, Mauer SM, Steffes MW et al: The effect of cyclosporin in native renal function in nonuremic diabetic recipients of pancreas transplants. J Diabetic Complications 1: 128–131, 1987.
23. Sutherland DER, Goetz FC, Hesse UJ, Kennedy WR, Ramsay RC, Mauer SM, Steffes MW, Kendall DM, Najarian JS: Effect of multiple variables on outcome in pancreas transplant recipients at the university of Minnesota and preliminary observations on the course of pre-existing secondary complications of diabetes. In: Friedman EW, L'Esperance FA (eds) Diabetic renal retinal syndrome 3: therapy; pp 481–499. Grune and Stratton Inc, New York, 1986.
24. Dubernard JM, Traeger J, Touraine L et al: Patterns of renal and pancreatic rejection in double-grafted patients. Transpl Proc 13: 305, 1981.
25. Sollinger HW, Cook K, Kamps D et al: Clinical and experimental experience with pancreaticocystostomy for exocrine pancreatic drainage in pancreas transplantation. Transpl Proc 16: 749, 1984.

26. Prieto M, Sutherland DER, Goetz FC, Najarian JS: Pancreas transplant results according to technique of duct management: Bladder versus enteric drainage. Surgery 102: 680–691, 1987.
27. Sutherland DER, Goetz FC, Moudry KC, Najarian JS: Pancreatic transplantation: a single institution's experience. Diab Nutr Metabol 1: 57–66, 1988.
28. Lawrence HS: Uremia: Nature's immunosuppressive device. Ann Intem Med 2: 166–8, 1965.

5. Surgical techniques and complications

J.M. DUBERNARD, X. MARTIN, R. SANSEVERINO and A. GELET

Introduction

There is no optimal technique for pancreatic transplantation. Of the various techniques that have been described, one or the other may be the most appropriate depending on the indication for transplantation and the character-istics of the recipient. Ideally, the surgical approach should be adapted to the specific circumstances of each case.

Historically, the first pancreas transplantation was segmental with ligation of pancreatic duct [1]. Pancreaticoduodenal transplants with enteric drainage [2] and segmental transplants with urinary drainage [3] were also used in many of the early cases. Although these cases demonstrated that diabetes could be cured by pancreatic transplantation, most failed from technical complications and the surgical techniques used were largely abandoned.

In 1976 we applied the technique of duct obstruction using neoprene for human pancreas transplantation [4]. This simple and safe technique was rapidly adopted by several centers and was a stimulus for further development of clinical pancreatic transplantation. This technique has been used in more than half of pancreas transplants performed world-wide during the last 10 years [5]. Various substances other than neoprene (Silicone, Prolamine, Polyi-soprene, etc . . .) have been used, all with similar results.

Other techniques have also been used. Duct open with free intraperitoneal drainage had some success, but the complication rate in humans was higher than in animal experiments and is no longer used [6]. Enteric drainage of a segmental pancreas was used in some early cases [7], but the results were not satisfactory until relatively recently [8].

Cyclosporin has been available in most institutions since 1982, and its use has been associated with a reduction in steroid dose for transplant recipients.

Syntactically Revised by Dr. David Sutherland and retyped by Arnell Sandstrom and Janet Sanders. Illustrations by Martin Finch.

J.M. Dubernard and D.E.R. Sutherland (eds.), International Handbook of Pancreas Transplantation, 71-130.

Concomitantly, old techniques have been resurrected and new techniques developed, including use of a segment for bladder drainage [9]; the whole pancreas without duodenum for polymer injection [10], or with a small patch of duodenum for pancreatico-duct-enterostomy [10], or pancreatico-duct-cystostomy [11]; or the whole pancreas with a segment of duodenum for pancreatico-duodeno-enterostomy [12, 13] or pancreatico-duodeno-cystosto-my [13, 14]. The management of exocrine secretions, the mass of pancreatic tissue required, and the physiological character of the technique have to be considered when analyzing surgical strategy in pancreatic transplantation. None of the techniques have been demonstrated to be superior to the others in terms of graft survival rates [5].

Leaving the pancreatic duct open in the abdominal cavity was successful in dogs and some early human cases, but the incidence of complications (ascitis, peritonitis) was high [6], and the technique has been abandoned for clinical use. Duct obstruction produces extensive fibrosis of exocrine tissue, and theoretically may affect endocrine function long term. However, our experimental data did not confirm this hypothesis [15], and a detrimental effect of exocrine parenchyma fibrosis on endocrine function has not been well documented [16]. Diversion of pancreatic juice into intestinal tract is more physiological than the others, but results in bacterial contamination.

Pancreatic juice can be diverted in the urinary tract by anastomosis of the duct to the ureter [17] or directly to the bladder [9]. The theoretical advantage of this technique relates mainly to the ability to diagnose rejection early, by a drop in urinary amylase. Theoretically, the maximum islet mass should be transplanted and whole pancreas grafts should be prefered to segmental grafts. However there is no clear demonstration of the superiority of whole over segmental transplants in terms of graft survival or metabolic function.

The most physiological approach is paratopic transplantation with diversion of the pancreatic juice into the upper intestinal tract and drainage of the graft venous effluent into the portal system so that the secreted insulin makes a first passage through the liver [18].

The details of the various surgical steps and approaches are described in the following sections. The relative advantages and disadvantages of alternative methods are also discussed.

Pancreas harvesting

Cadaver donor selection

The general criteria for selection of cadaver pancreas donors, are similar to those for liver, kidney or heart donors, but for the pancreas a history of diabetes is a contraindication. Hyperglycemia occurring after brain death is not a contraindication to pancreas harvesting, and is often a consequence of intravenous glucose infusions given to the donor. If there is any suspicion of diabetes, the glycosolated hemoglobin level is a means to assess the average glucose levels during the previous weeks. Amylase levels are not very helpful since head injury patients often become hyperamylasemic. Surgical exploration is often the best or only way to check pancreas integrity.

Donor operation

The donor should be placed on the surgery table with a rigid support between the scapulae. This position superficializes the pancreas and facilitates its dissection. The incision can be altered depending on which organs are to be retrived from cadaver donors. (Figure 1). If only the pancreas and kidneys are removed, a bilateral subcostal incision is adequate, and may be combined with a midline incision. When the heart is also harvested a sternotomy plus a xyphopubic incision is performed. When combined with liver procurement, a bilateral subcostal incision combined with a xyphopubic incision and a sternotomy should be done.

Segmental pancreas procurement from cadaver donors

The gastrocolic ligament is divided from the pylorus to the splenic flexure of the colon (Figure 2). The branches of the gastroepiploic vessels are ligated or clipped before division. The dissection is facilitated by upward retraction of

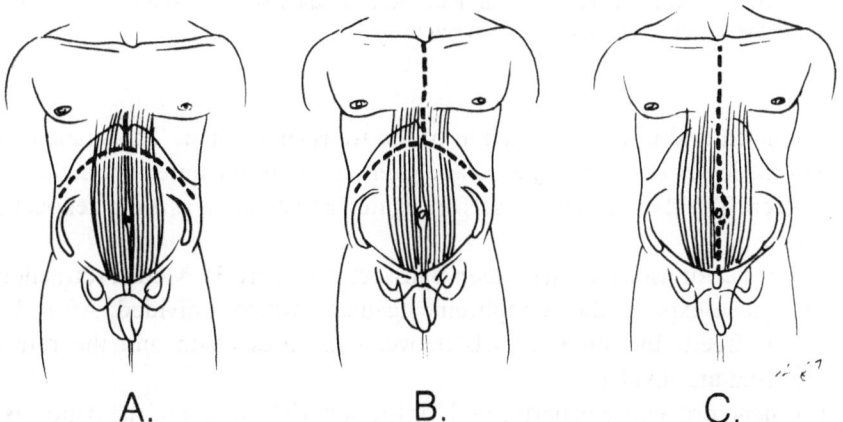

A.   **B.**   **C.**

Figure 1. Surgical access: A) Bilateral subcostal incision for pancreas and kidney removal B) Bilateral subcostal and sternotomy incision for pancreas, kidney, liver and heart removal C) Xyphopubic and sternotomy incision for pancreas and kidney and heart.

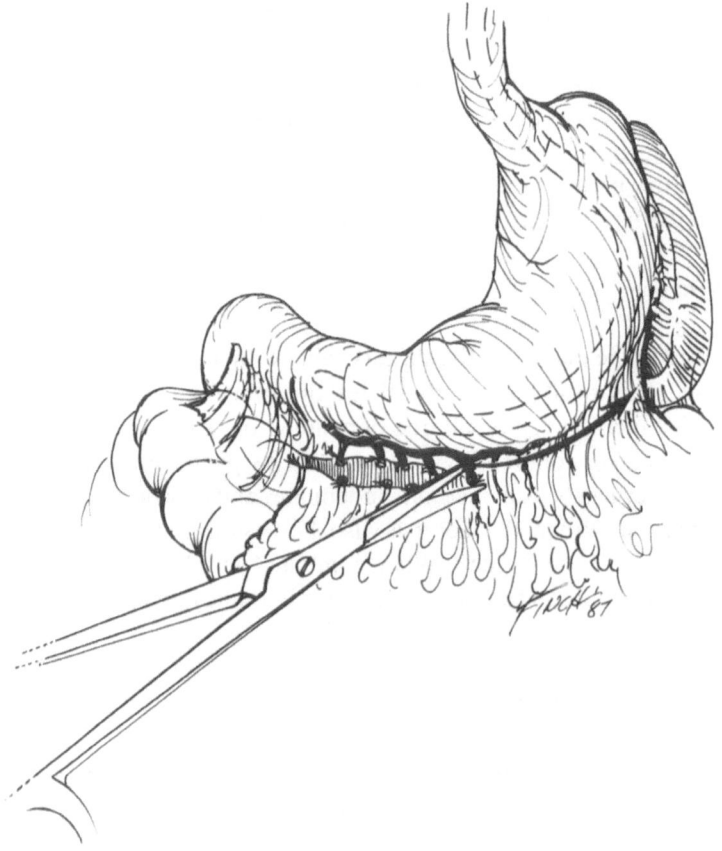

*Figure 2.*Transection of the gastrocolic ligament to enter the lesser sac. The branches of the gastroepiploic vessels are ligated or clipped before division.

the stomach and inferior retraction of the transverse colon. This maneuver allows the lesser sac to be entered and gains access to the anterior portion of the spleen. The short gastric vessels are ligated and divided, as is the lienocolic ligament.

The posterior aspect of the spleen is dissected (Figure 3). Medial retraction of the spleen exposes the lienophrenic ligament, which is divided. After the spleen is freed, the small vessels between the mesocolon and the retro-peritoneum are divided.

The same procedure is performed for the superior margin of the pancreas, taking care not to jeopardize the splenic artery in its course on the upper border of the gland. Using the spleen as a handle the distal pancreas is retracted medially; the posterior surface of the gland is exposed with the

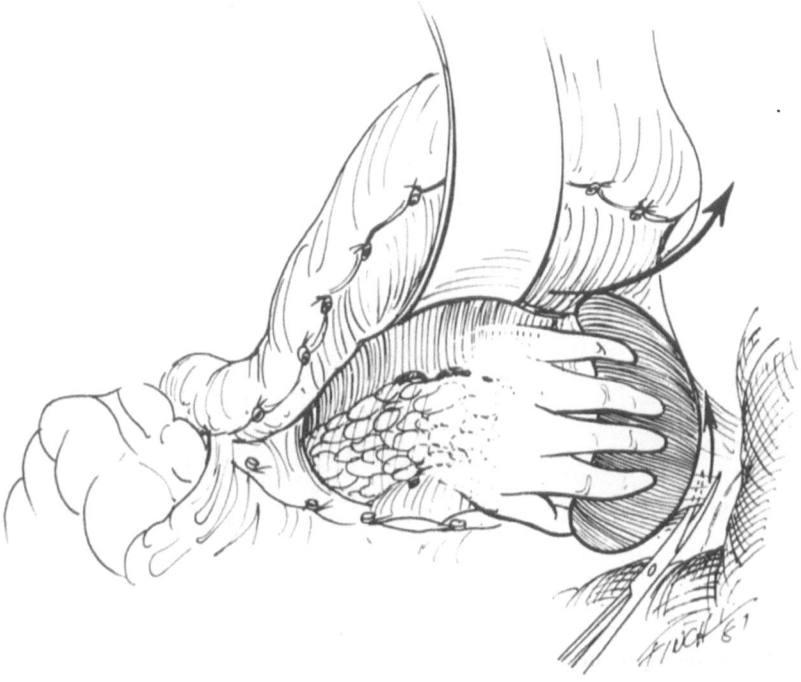

Figure 3. Dissection of the spleen. After division of the gastroepiploic vessels the spleen is freed from its posterior peritoneal attachments.

splenic vein running through the midportion. The inferior mesenteric vein is identified and divided at its confluence with the splenic vein, allowing a further medial mobilization of the body of the pancreas (Figure 4).

The celiac axis is now approached, if necessary by tracing the splenic artery to its origin (Figure 5). The spleen and distal pancreas are retracted to the left as the dissection of the celiac axis is started. In our early cases, the common hepatic artery was freed from its origin to its bifurcation in an antegrade way. Currently, we use the gastroduodenal artery as a guide to the common hepatic artery, proceeding retrograde to the celiac axis (Figure 6).

The gastroduodenal artery is identified at the superior margin of the head of the pancreas and freed to the bifurcation of the common hepatic artery. The common hepatic and hepatic artery proper are encircled by loops, but are not ligated and divided until the end of the procedure to minimize coagulation disturbances due to hepatic ischemia. The left gastric artery is identified, ligated and divided, completing the dissection of the celiac axis. The crura of the diaphragm are incised, and a loop is placed around the abdominal aorta, above the celiac axis.

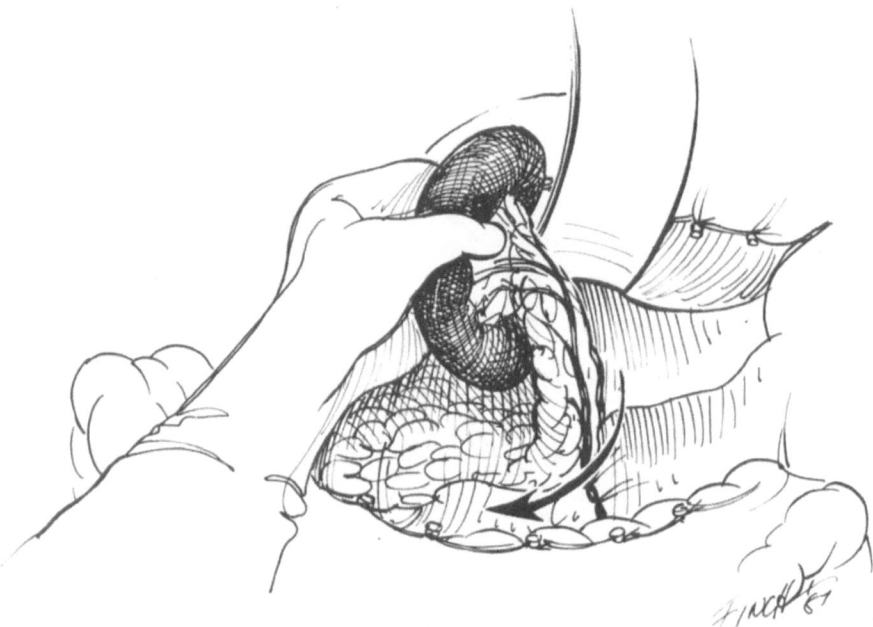

Figure 4. Mobilization of the distal pancreas (inferior margin). The spleen and tail of the pancreas are retracted medially, and the inferior mesenteric vein is ligated and divided.

The superior mesenteric vessels are identified and dissected close to the inferior border of the pancreatic gland. The superior mesenteric vein is traced to its confluence with the splenic vein, originating the portal vein. The tips of a scissor are passed behind the neck of the pancreas, in the avascular plane between the gland and the anterior surface of the portal vein (Figure 7). This maneuver identifies the site of section to separate the body and the tail from the head of the pancreas. The portal vein is dissected for 2 or 3 cm into the porta hepatis, and looped by a tape. The remaining attachments between the neck of the gland and aorta are ligated and divided.

The gland is now ready for removal. Cooling may be performed at this point by inserting a canula in the distal splenic artery in the splenic hilum, and flushing the pancreas by a retrograde infusion of cold preservation solution after having placed a 'bull dog' clamp at the origin of the splenic artery (Figure 8). This method allows the quality of the graft arterial vascularization to be assessed from the immediate change in color of the pancreatic parenchyma.

With evolution of multiorgan harvesting, at present cooling is usually performed via a cannula placed in the lower abdominal aorta; this technique permits simultaneous perfusion of the kidneys, pancreas and liver.

After the dissection is completed, the superior mesenteric vein is ligated and

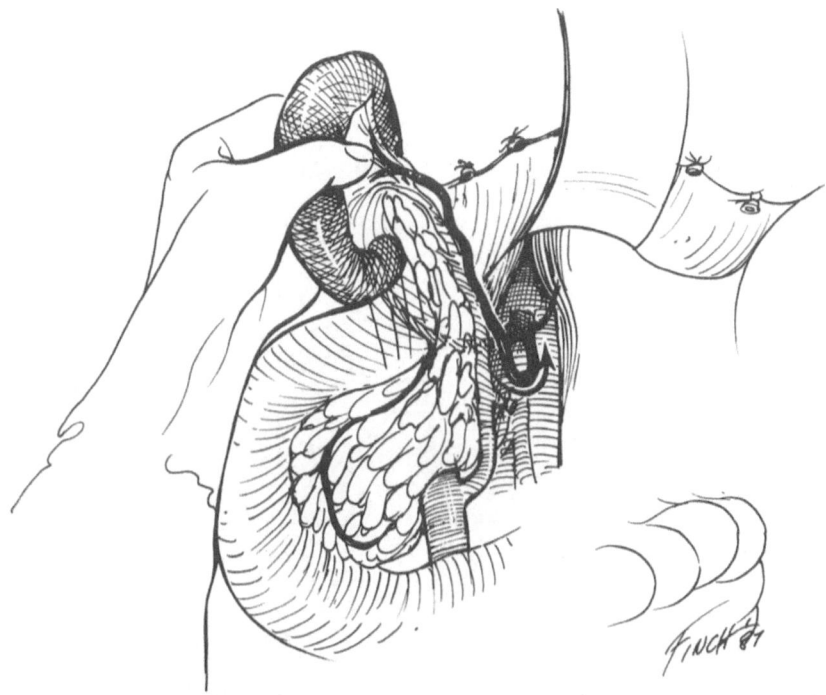

Figure 5. Retrograde dissection of the splenic artery, toward the celiac axis. The branches of the celiac axis – hepatic, left gastric and splenic arteries – are identified. The left gastric artery is ligated and divided.

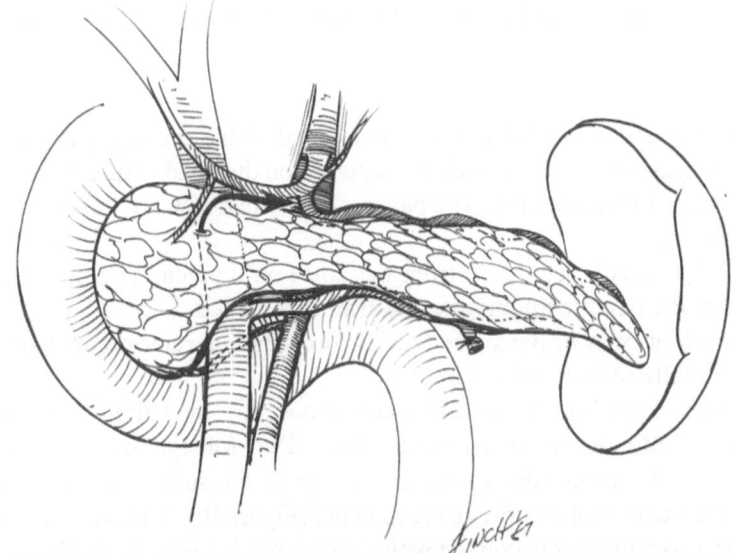

Figure 6. Retrograde dissection of the common hepatic artery and celiac axis, starting from gastroduodenal artery at the superior border of the pancreatic gland.

78

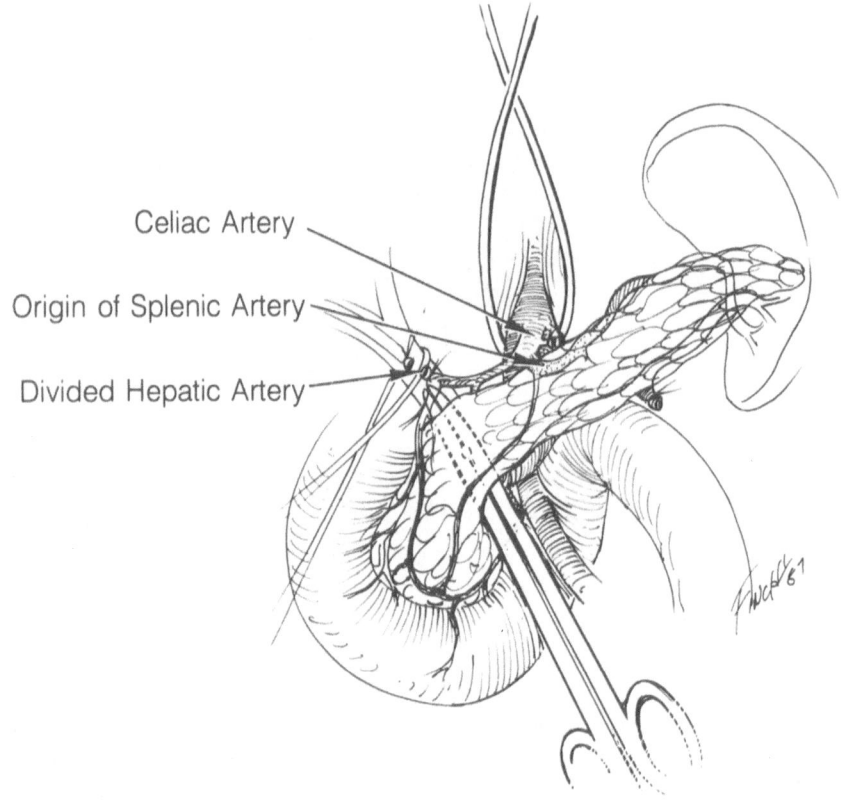

Celiac Artery

Origin of Splenic Artery

Divided Hepatic Artery

Figure 7. The pancreatic neck is freed from the portal vein by blunt dissection with passage of a scissor.

divided; the abdominal aorta is cross-clamped above the celiac axis and the arterial perfusion is started. A clamp is placed on the head of the gland as close as possible to the duodenum. The pancreas is divided distal to the clamp with a knife (Figure 9).

The celiac axis is separated from the aorta on a patch. The portal vein is divided in the hepatic hilum, and the graft is removed.

Splenectomy may be performed just before pancreas removal or ex situ. The graft is usually reflushed ex situ.

When the duct obstruction technique is choosen, a small blunt-tip catheter is introduced into the main pancreatic duct. Two forceps are placed at the extremities of the cut edge of the graft, a no. 2 silk suture is placed around them, and 3 to 6 ml of Neoprene are injected (Figure 10). The synthetic rubber progressively solidifies in contact with the pancreatic juice. When the catheter is removed the duct is ligated with a 4/0 Prolene suture. The parenchyma of the pancreatic neck is ligated with multiple no. 2 silk sutures to prevent Neoprene extravasation.

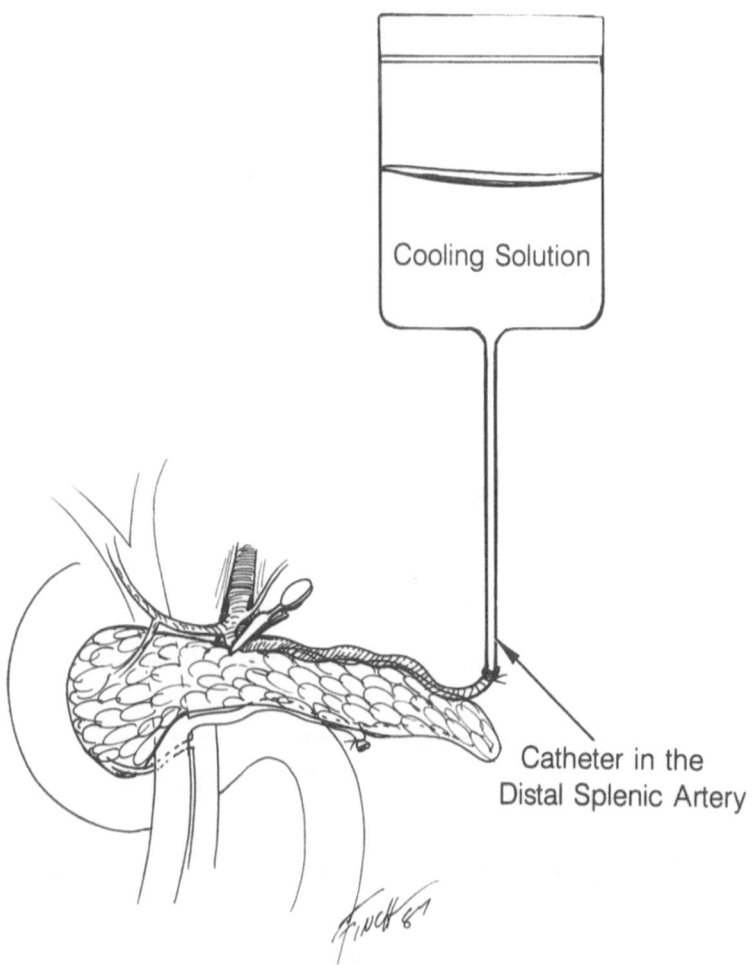

Cooling Solution

Catheter in the
Distal Splenic Artery

Figure 8. Cooling of the pancreas by retrograde perfusion via a catheter in the distal splenic artery. This technique was used in our early cases to check pancreatic arterial vascularization.

The kidneys are usually harvested with the pancreas. In our early experience two different surgical options were used, depending on the kidney arterial supply. When each kidney was vascularized by only one artery, the renal pedicles were dissected first; the suprarenal abdominal aorta and vena cava were clamped and the kidneys were removed and flushed ex situ. The pancreatic dissection was then performed.

In donors with multiple renal arteries, the pancreatic dissection was performed first and after removal flushed ex situ. The kidneys were then dissected and removed.

Our present strategy is to remove the kidneys 'en bloc' with the vena cava

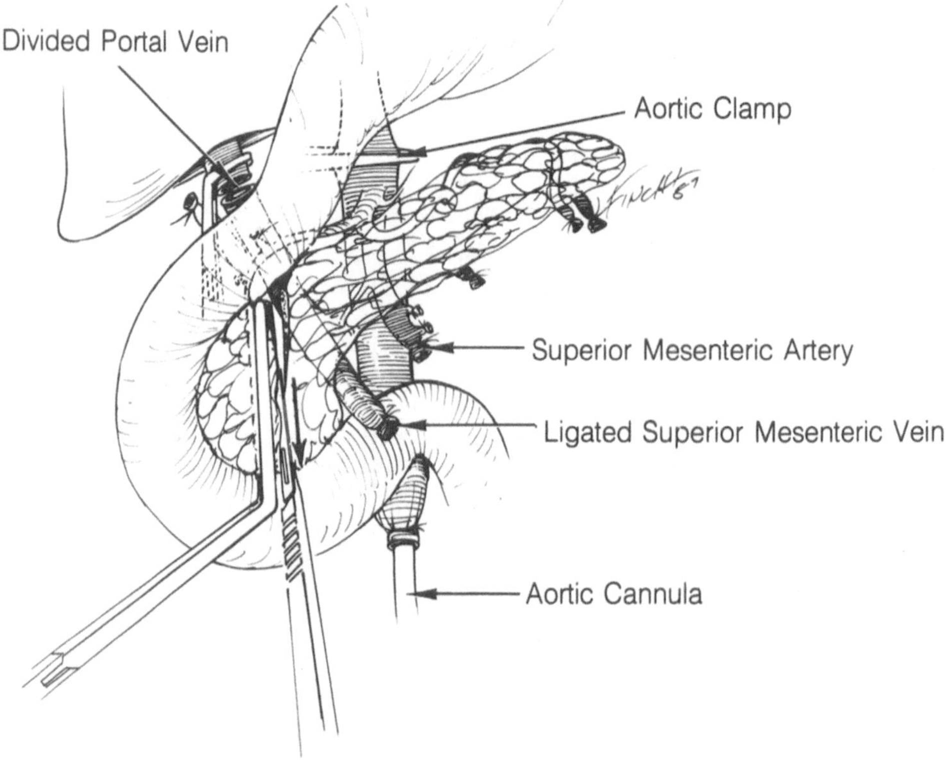

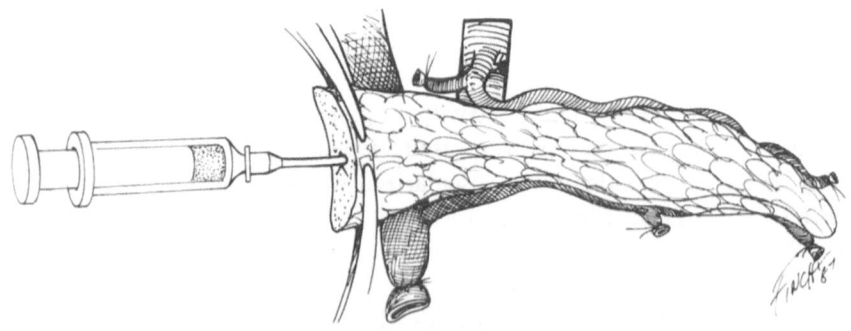

Divided Portal Vein

Aortic Clamp

Superior Mesenteric Artery

Ligated Superior Mesenteric Vein

Aortic Cannula

Figure 9. Section of head of the pancreas, after cooling by an aortic flush, followed by removal of the distal segment as the graft.

Figure 10. Neoprene injection of a segmental graft. This maneuver is usually performed ex situ via a small catheter introduced in the duct of Wirsung.

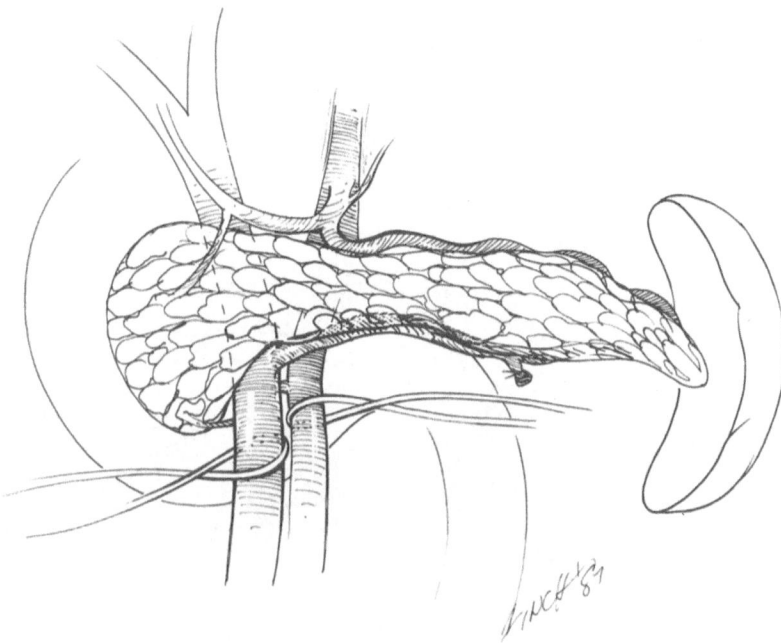

Figure 11. Whole pancreas harvesting: Dissection of superior mesenteric vessels. The loop on the superior mesenteric artery is distal to the origin of the inferior pancreatico-duodenal artery.

and corresponding segment of aorta, and the pancreas with the portal vein and aortic segment encompasing the celiac axis and in some cases the superior mesenteric artery. This technique is described in detail in the section on multiorgan procurement.

Whole pancreas procurement

When a whole pancreas is harvested the surgical procedure is exactly the same concerning dissection of the spleen and distal pancreas. The superior mesenteric vessels are identified at the inferior margin of the pancreas and a loop is passed around the vein proximal to the mesocolic branches and around the artery distal to the inferior pancreatico-duodenal artery (Figure 11). The celiac axis is dissected as previously described, but the common hepatic and gastroduodenal artery is conserved to preserve the vascularity to the proximal pancreas and duodenum. A Kocher maneuver is performed to free the duodenum from its retroperitoneal attachments. The hepatic artery proper is ligated and divided distal to gastroduodenal artery; the common bile duct is ligated and divided; and a loop is passed around the portal vein (Figure 12).

When a whole pancreatic graft is harvested alone without duodenum, a

82

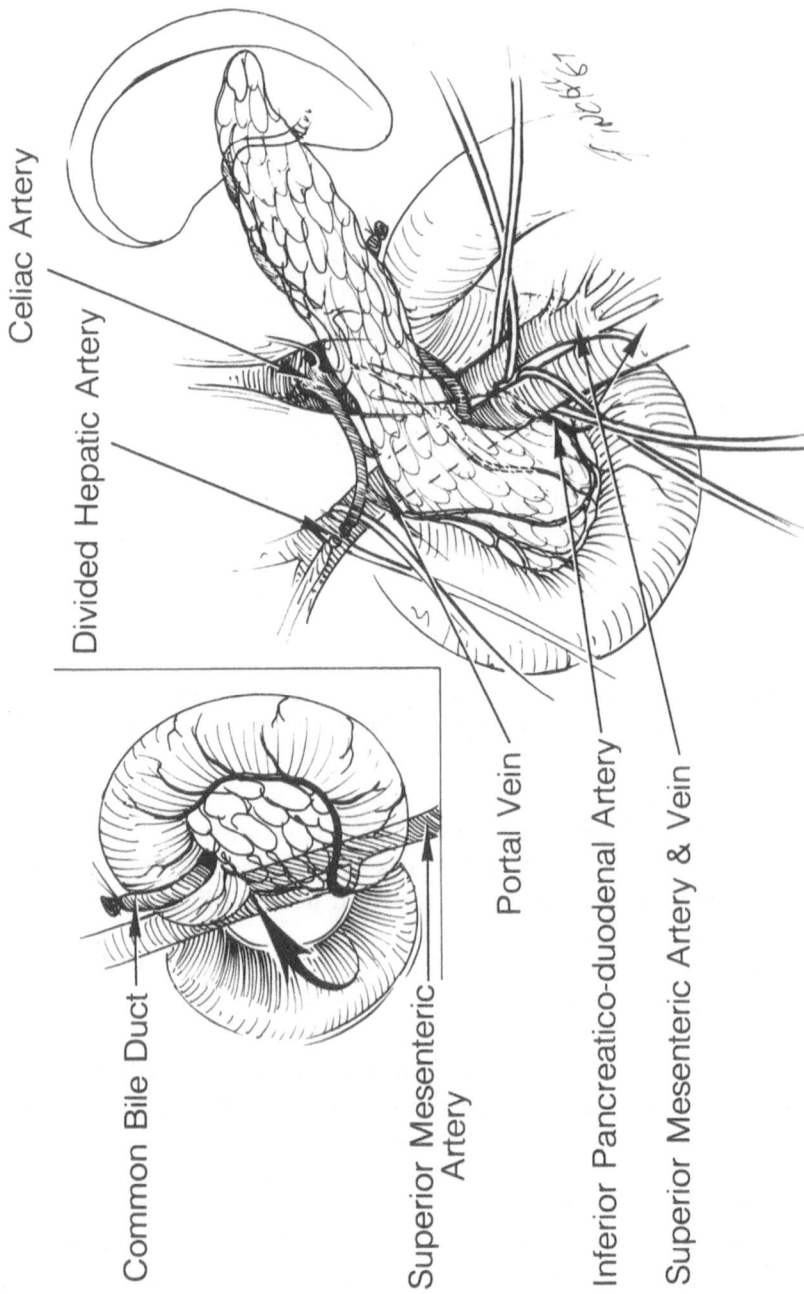

Celiac Artery

Divided Hepatic Artery

Common Bile Duct

Superior Mesenteric
Artery

Portal Vein

Inferior Pancreatico-duodenal Artery

Superior Mesenteric Artery & Vein

Figure 12. A Kocher maneuver is followed by dissection of the porta hepatis for whole pancreas harvesting.

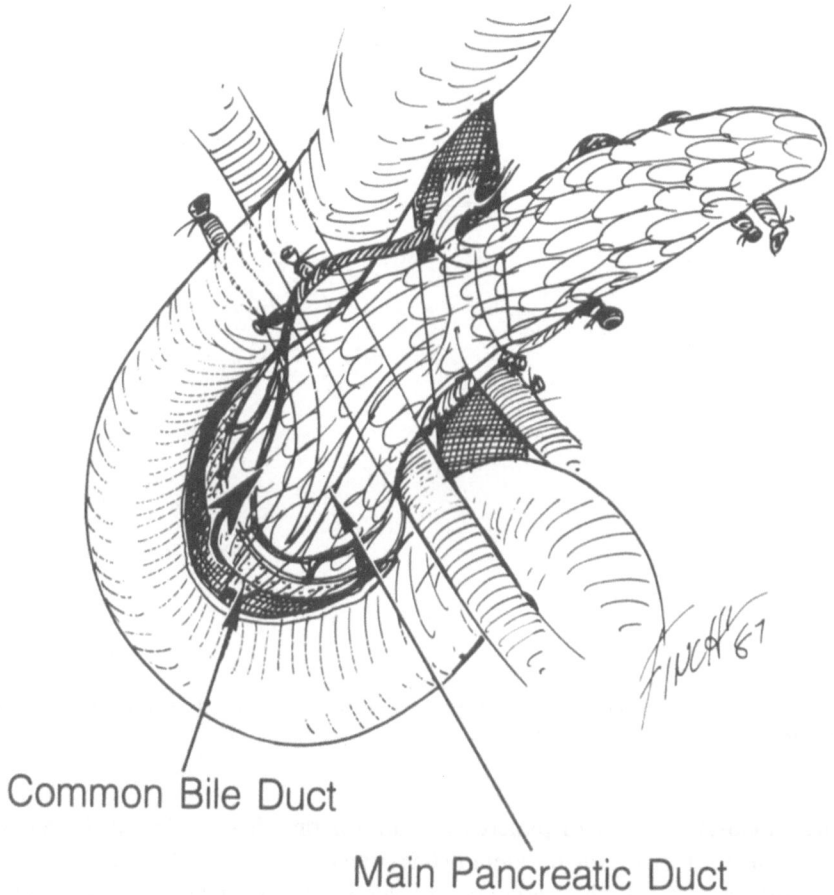

Common Bile Duct

Main Pancreatic Duct

Figure 13. The pancreatic head is separated from the duodenum when a whole pancreas alone is procured.

careful dissection is performed to separate the pancreatic head and duodenum, dividing the small vessels entering the duodenum from the pancreaticoduodenal arcades. This is a meticulous and time consuming procedure necessitating ligation and/or coagulation of numerous small vessels (Figure 13). Futhermore if duct injection is intended, difficulties might occur due to poor injection of the pancreatic segment drained by the accessory duct (Figure 14).

In the case of a pancreatico-duodenal graft, the segment of duodenum corresponding to the head of the pancreas is transected using a G.I.A. automatic stapling device (Figure 15). In order to reduce the risks of bacterial contamination, antibiotic solutions can be injected in the duodenal segment.

An alternative approach consists of excising the duodenum except for a patch surrounding the ampulla of Vater. This technique is used when a

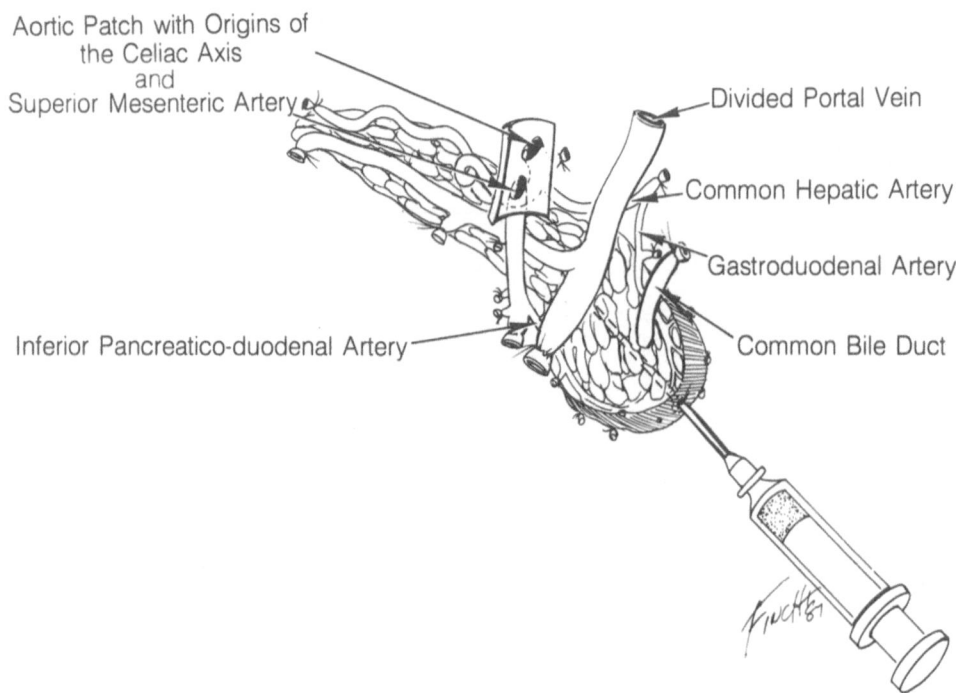

Aortic Patch with Origins of
the Celiac Axis
and
Superior Mesenteric Artery

Divided Portal Vein

Common Hepatic Artery

Gastroduodenal Artery

Inferior Pancreatico-duodenal Artery

Common Bile Duct

Figure 14. Ex vivo duct injection of a whole pancreas after separation of the pancreatic head and duodenum.

pancreatico-cystostomy or pancreatico-enterostomy is intended in the recipient (Figure 16). After the duodenum has been isolated with or separated from the pancreatic head, the vascular pedicles of the graft are prepared. The superior mesenteric vessels are ligated and divided at the inferior margin of the pancreatic neck. The abdominal aorta is cross-clamped above the celiac axis, and in situ perfusion is started via a cannula placed in the lower abdominal aorta. The portal vein is divided as high as possible in the porta hepatis; the aorta is transected and a vascular patch is prepared to include the origins of celiac and superior mesenteric arteries. After pancreas removal the graft is reflushed ex situ and stored at 4° C in preservation solution. The spleen can be separated from the pancreas at the time. When we harvest a whole pancreas, we use the 'en bloc' technique for rapid procurement of the kidneys.

Segmental pancreas procurement from living related donors

The Minnesota group has described a technique for distal pancreas harvesting from living related donors [19]. This approach is justified by the shortage of cadaver donors, and the improved functional survival of living related grafts because of the reduced risks of rejection. The selection of living related

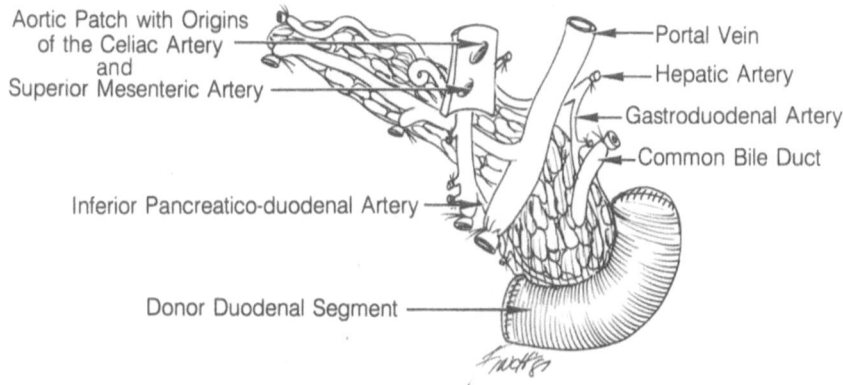

Aortic Patch with Origins
of the Celiac Artery
and
Superior Mesenteric Artery

Portal Vein
Hepatic Artery
Gastroduodenal Artery
Common Bile Duct

Inferior Pancreatico-duodenal Artery

Donor Duodenal Segment

Figure 15. Appearance of whole pancreatico-duodenal graft after removal from donor.

pancreas donors requires that many conditions be fulfilled. Some have previously donated a kidney to the recipient. The donor must be healthy enough to undergo a major surgical procedure. Metabolic studies including oral and intravenous glucose tolerance test results must be normal. If pancreatic function is normal, half a pancreas should maintain a non-diabetic state in both the donor and recipient (for potential surgical complications and risk of occurrence of diabetes see commentary).

A bilateral subcostal or midline incision is performed. The peritoneal cavity is opened and the gastrocolic ligament divided to enter the lesser sac. The ligatures must be close to the transverse colon to preserve the gastroepiploic artery supplying the greater curvature of the stomach and the spleen. Care must be taken not to devascularize other abdominal organs supplied by the celiac axis, particularly the spleen.

Dissection is restricted to the inferior and medial borders of the spleen, but without dividing the lienocolic ligament. The short gastric vessels are preserved. The lienophrenic ligament is not interrupted and the spleen is not mobilized (Figure 17). The stomach, decompressed by a nasogastric tube, is retracted upward. The posterior peritoneum is incised over the tail of the pancreas and distal splenic vessels are ligated into the splenic hilum. The artery is ligated before the vein to avoid venous congestion of the spleen.

After careful dissection of superior and inferior margin of the gland, distal pancreas is retracted medially and the inferior mesenteric vein is divided if it joins the splenic vein (Figure 18). The splenic artery is isolated at its origin from the celiac axis. The pancreatic neck is dissected by passing a finger along the portal vein in the avascular space between posterior surface of the gland and anterior surface of the portal vein (Figure 19). The pancreatic neck is divided and the small vessels on the two cut surfaces are ligated with 5/0

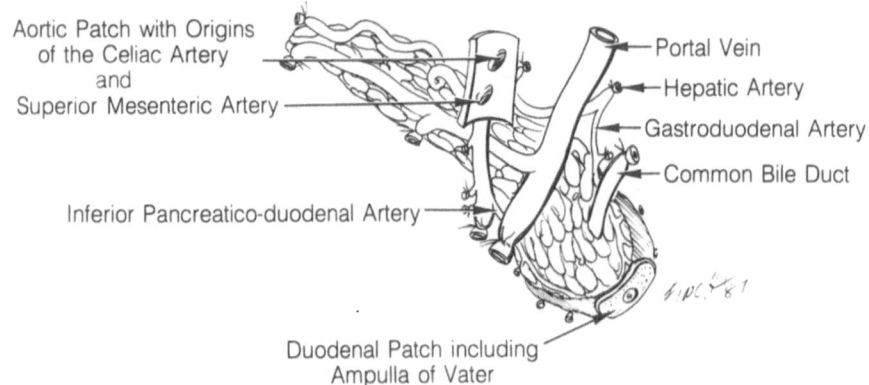

Aortic Patch with Origins of the Celiac Artery and Superior Mesenteric Artery

Portal Vein

Hepatic Artery

Gastroduodenal Artery

Common Bile Duct

Inferior Pancreatico-duodenal Artery

Duodenal Patch including Ampulla of Vater

Figure 16. Whole pancreas with a duodenal patch.

prolene sutures. A blunt tip catheter is introduced into the main duct of distal pancreas for drainage or obstruction. The cut edge of the proximal pancreas is sutured with 4/0 Prolene sutures to prevent any postoperative fluid leakage from small ducts (Figure 20).

Systemic heparinization of the patient is now performed (70 U/kg). A vascular clamp is placed on the origin of the splenic artery from the celiac axis and at the confluence of splenic vein into the portal vein. The vessels are divided and the graft is removed and flushed with cold electrolyte solution. Prolamine sulfate is used to reverse the effect of heparine.

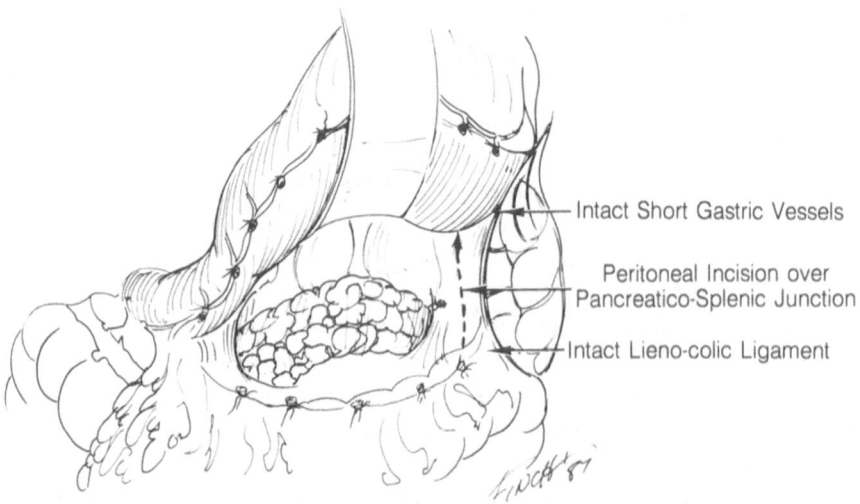

Intact Short Gastric Vessels

Peritoneal Incision over Pancreatico-Splenic Junction

Intact Lieno-colic Ligament

Figure 17. Removal of distal pancreas segment from a living related donor: The pancreas is dissected without mobilizing the spleen.

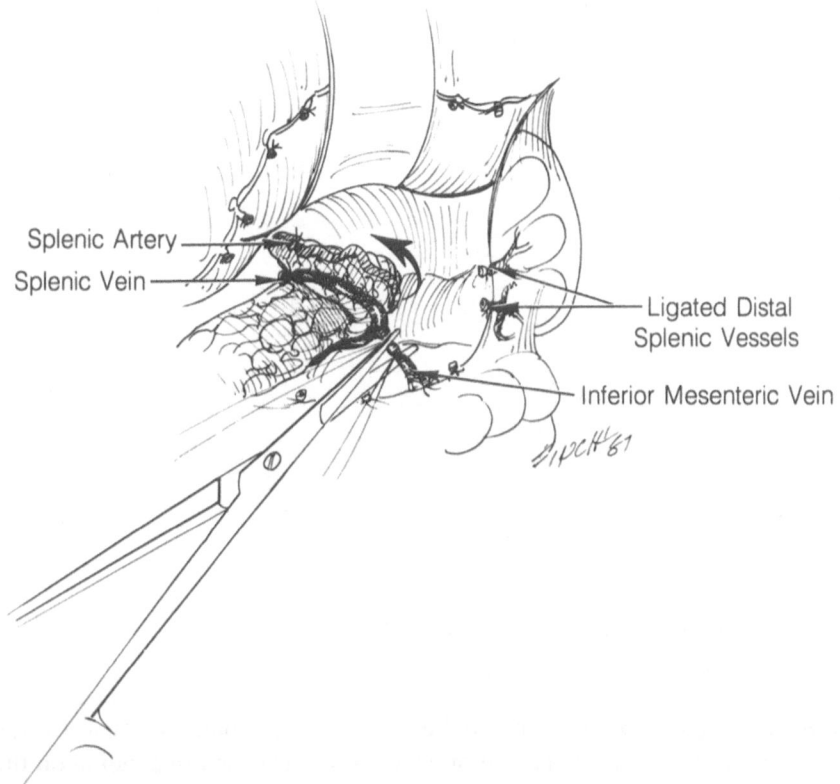

Splenic Artery

Splenic Vein

Ligated Distal Splenic Vessels

Inferior Mesenteric Vein

Figure 18. Medial mobilization of the tail of the pancreas and ligation and division of the inferior meseneric vein (not always necessary) in a living donor.

The stumps of the splenic artery and vein in the donor are oversewn with 5/0 Prolene running sutures. Hemostasis and spleen viability are assured and the abdominal wall is closed without drainage.

Multiple organ procurement

Multiple organ harvesting is now widely used because of the development of heart and liver transplantation programs. All organs can be harvested together with a pancreas.

At our institution kidneys are always removed; the heart is removed when the donor is young and in good general condition. Liver and pancreas harvesting from the same donor requires a specific surgical approach, which is always possible when a segmental pancreatic graft is harvested. It is also possible to remove both a liver and a pancreatico-duodenal graft under precise anatomical conditions.

88

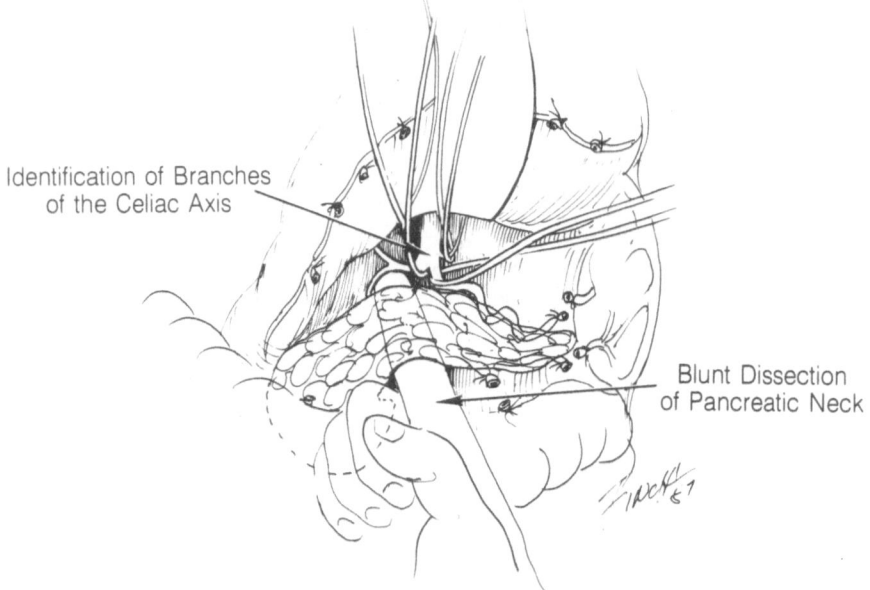

Identification of Branches
of the Celiac Axis

Blunt Dissection
of Pancreatic Neck

Figure 19. Isolation of pancreatic neck and proximal splenic artery.

Kidneys and pancreas. In our initial experience we separately removed the pancreas and kidneys, the choice of which to remove first depending on the renal arterial supply as previously described. Our present strategy is to remove the kidneys and pancreas 'en bloc'.

A large subcostal incision is performed (Figure 1), and the inferior lip is retracted downward and fixed to the abdominal wall. The retroperitoneal space is entered by mobilizing the ascending colon and small bowel upward and medially (Figure 21). The distal aorta and venous cava are mobilized just proximal to their bifurcation and looped with no. 1 silk (Figure 22).

The left retroperitoneal space is exposed by dividing the inferior mesenteric artery and upward retraction of the descending colon. After the pancreas dissection is completed, the kidneys are further mobilized. The distal ureters are divided and the posterior surfaces of kidneys are freed from their retroperitoneal attachments. If a segmental pancreas is to be harvested, the superior mesenteric artery is ligated at its origin so the flushing solution is not dispersed into the small bowel.

The distal great vessels are now ligated with the no. 1 silks. The aortic wall is incised and the cannula for in situ cooling is introduced and secured with the proximal no. 1 silk loop. The vena cava is also incised and a large cannula is introduced to drain by gravity blood and the cooling solution. The cannula is secured with the proximal no. 1 silk loop (Figure 23). The abdominal aorta is

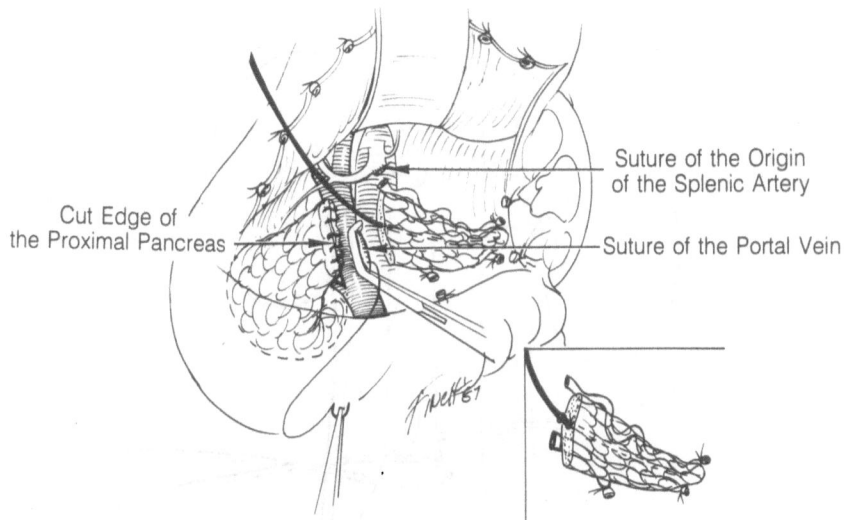

Figure 20. Completion of segmental pancreatectomy in a living donor.

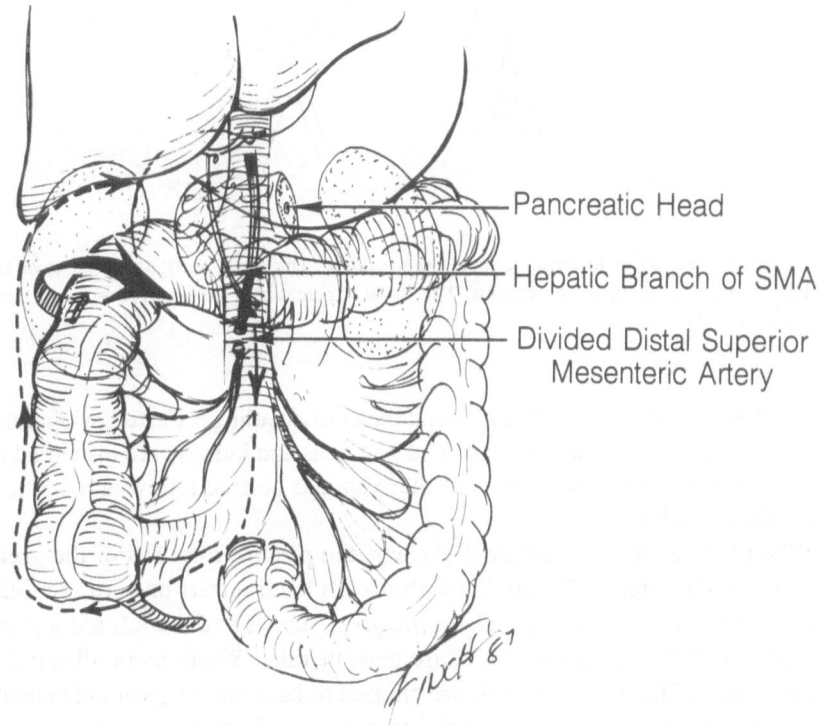

Figure 21. Access to retroperitoneal space for multiple organ harvesting. Medial mobilization of the ascending colon and small bowel is facilitated by division of the distal superior mesenteric artery.

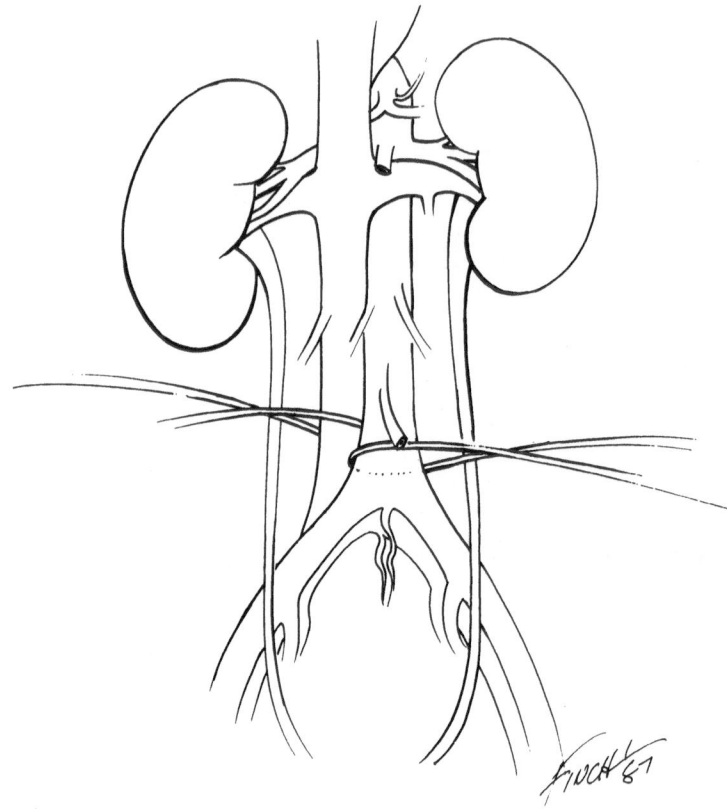

Figure 22. Dissection of lower abdominal great vessels. The distal aorta and vena cava are mobilized proximal to their bifurcations. The distal pancreas may be removed prior to these maneuvers.

cross-clamped above the celiac axis and the in situ cooling is started by opening the aortic and vena cava cannulae. The pancreas and kidneys are inspected to ensure they are pale and cool, and there should be free inflow and outflow from the cannules.

When the venous fluid effluent is clear, the posterior aspects of the great vessels are dissected. The surgeon with his left hand retract upward the right kidney. The ureters and cannulae in the great vessels and the left kidney are retracted upward by an assistant. Care must be taken not to jeopardize polar renal vessels. The lumbar vessels are clipped to keep the surgical field clean. When dissection is complete the in situ cooling is stopped, the aorta is transected above and below celiac axis and below renal vessels, the vena cava is transected above the renal veins, the portal vein is divided at the hepatic hilum, and the pancreas and kidneys are removed en bloc and later divided ex situ (Figure 24).

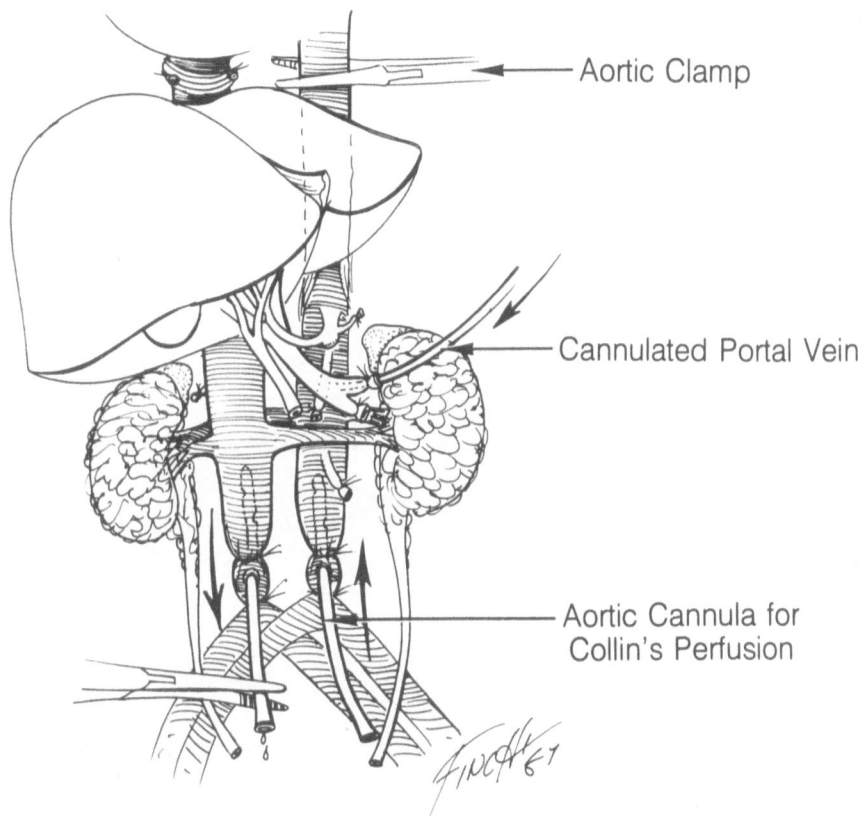

Figure 23. Cannulation of distal great vessels and cooling of the kidneys and liver.

Pancreas and kidneys and heart. When the heart along with the pancreas and kidneys are procured, the procedures in the previous sections are carried out as described. Before aortic cross clamping, the cardiac surgeon dissects the heart.

The donor is systematically heparinized (3 mg/kg). Cardioplegic solution is infused into the heart. The aorta is cross-clamped, and the distal aorta is perfused with cold preservation to cool the abdominal organs. After cardiectomy, the dissection of the kidneys and pancreas are completed, as previously described.

Liver and pancreas and kidneys and heart. Removal of liver and pancreas from the same donor can be performed so both organs can be adequately revascularized in the recipient.

i) *Distal pancreas donation with liver harvesting*
Two different surgical options are possible when a segmental pancreas graft is procured with a liver: 1. Transection of the splenic artery at its origin from

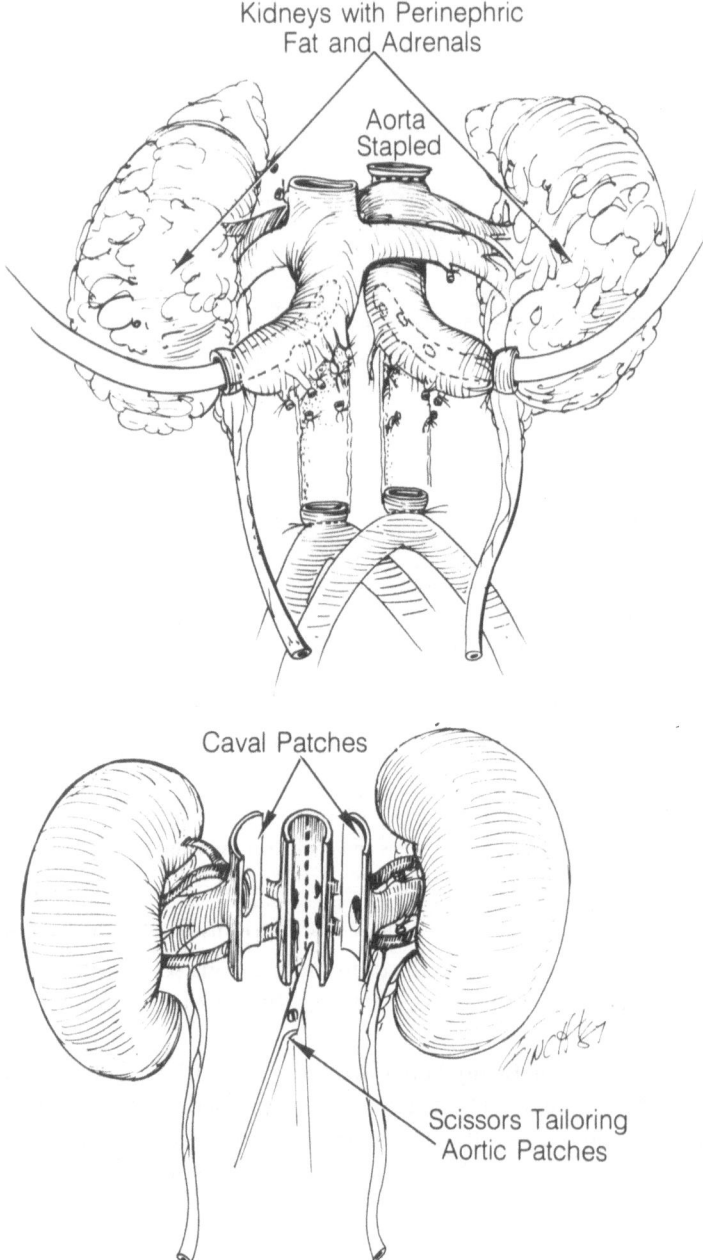

Figure 24. Dissection of posterior aspect of the great vessels in situ, and separation of the kidneys ex situ.

celiac axis (this technique can be utilised in all donors); 2. Retention of the celiac axis with an aortic patch (This technique cannot be utilized in presence of a left hepatic artery originating from the left gastric artery).

I Distal pancreas with splenic artery without patch

Dissection of the distal pancreas is performed first when the graft arterial supply is to be based on the splenic artery without a patch. The porta hepatis is dissected in the following sequence:

- The common bile duct is ligated and divided as distal as possible.
- The hepatic artery is isolated and looped distal to the origin of the right gastric and gastroduodenal arteries, and both of the latter ligated and divided.
- The portal vein is isolated behind the hepatic artery and looped.

Scissors are passed in the avascular plane between the portal vein and the pancreatic gland, isolating the pancreatic neck (Figure 7).

A cannula is introduced into the portal vein through a transverse venotomy in the first branch of the superior mesenteric vein, and advanced to the porta hepatis. Two ligatures previously placed around either the first branch of the superior mesenteric vein or the portal vein (1–2 cm below its bifurcation into the porta hepatis) are tied (Figure 25). The liver is pre-cooled in situ by perfusion with Ringer's lactate at 4° C. The perfusion rate is adjusted according to the central body temperature and the central venous pressure (less than one litre is infused before clamping).

The distal aorta and inferior vena cava are cannulated as previously described. The abdominal aorta is isolated and looped above celiac axis.

Cardioplegia is now induced and a clamp is placed across the diaphragmatic aorta. Cold preservation solution is infused via the catheter previously placed in lower abdominal aorta. Ringer's lactate is infused into the portal system. The superior mesenteric artery is ligated at its origin to avoid dispersion of the cooling solution into the small bowel. The heart is removed as these maneuvers are performed.

The neck of the pancreas is now divided at the level of the portal vein (Figure 9). The splenic artery is divided at its origin from celiac axis and the stump is oversewn with a 5/0 prolene running suture (Figure 26). The portal vein is incised longitudinally on its right side between the two ligatures previously placed and maintained on the portal vein and on the first branch of superior mesenteric veins, allowing the splenic vein to be removed and stored. If neoprene or another substances is to be injected, it now can be performed as previously described (Figure 10).

When the iliac vessels of the recipient are not diseased, the splenic artery can be easily sutured, either end-to-end to the internal or end-to-side to the external iliac artery. However, the iliac vessels of diabetic recipients often are atherosclerotic and the anastomosis is facilitated by an extension arterial graft.

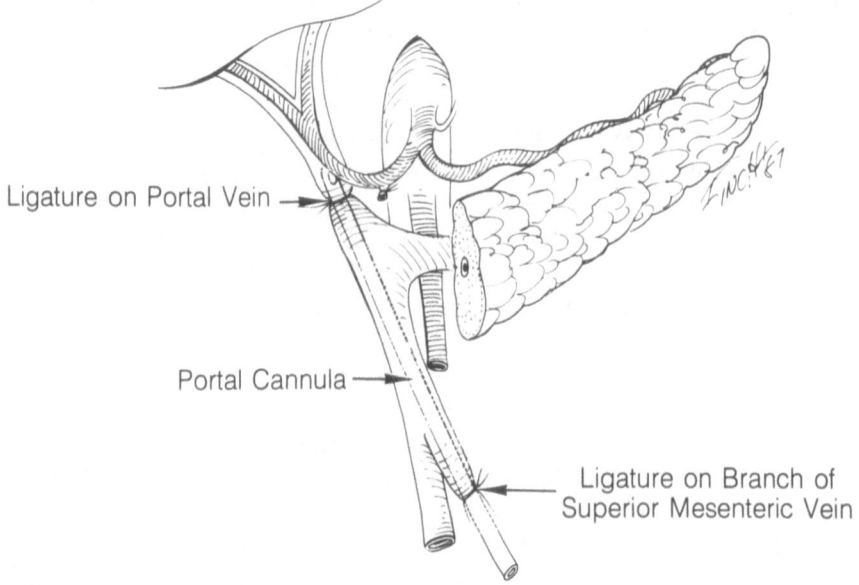

Figure 25. Simultaneous segmental pancreas and liver harvesting: the portal vein is cannulated via the first branch of superior mesenteric vein.

Thus, we always procure the donor's iliac vessels in order to have this option. In this case the donor external iliac artery is anastomosed end-to-end to the donor splenic artery, and a patch, fashioned at the site of bifurcation of common iliac artery, is used for anastomosis and for graft revascularization in the recipient (Figure 27).

It is preferable to leave the hepatic portion of the portal vein as long as possible when the liver is donated. In this case, the splenic vein is transected at its confluence with the portal vein. Removal of an iliac vein segment from the donor can be used as an extension graft to lenghten the short segment of splenic or portal vein on the pancreas (Figure 27).

After completion of the distal pancreatectomy, the liver and kidneys are removed as previously described.

II Retention of the celiac axis on an aortic patch

This technique of retaining the celiac axis with the pancreas can be used if there is normal hepatic vascular anatomy and if there is a right hepatic artery originating from superior mesenteric artery (20% of cases), but not if the left hepatic artery originates from the left gastric artery (17% of cases).

When the celiac axis is retained, the distal pancreas is dissected as previously described, with one difference. The common hepatic artery is divided at its origin from the celiac axis (Figure 28). The left gastric artery is divided at its

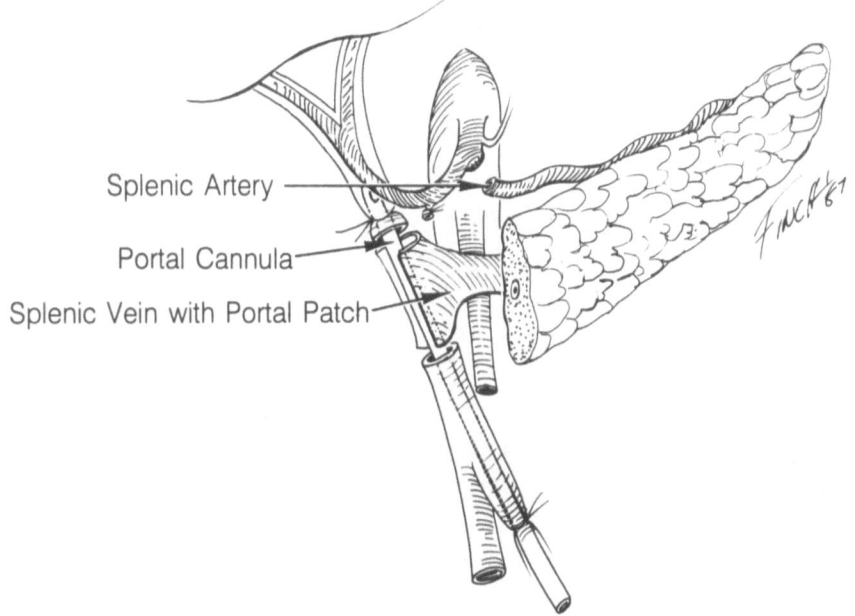

Figure 26. Simultaneous segmental pancreas and liver harvesting: Division of splenic artery and portal vein.

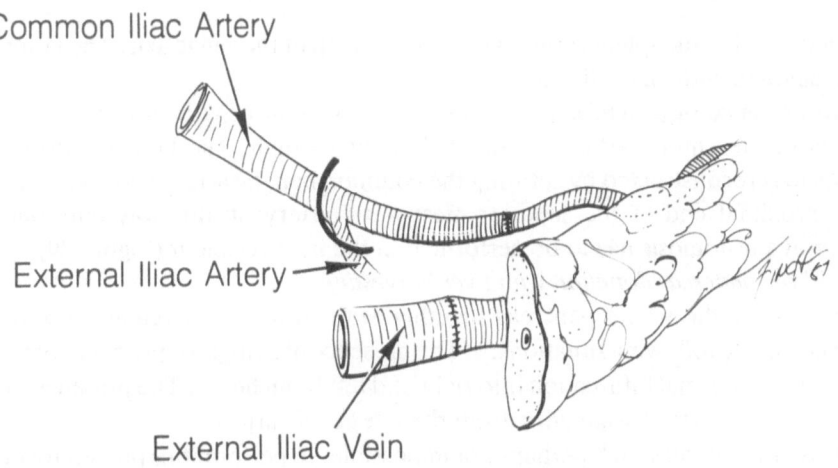

Figure 27. Iliac vessel extension grafts can facilitate transplantation of segmental pancreas grafts removed from donors.

96

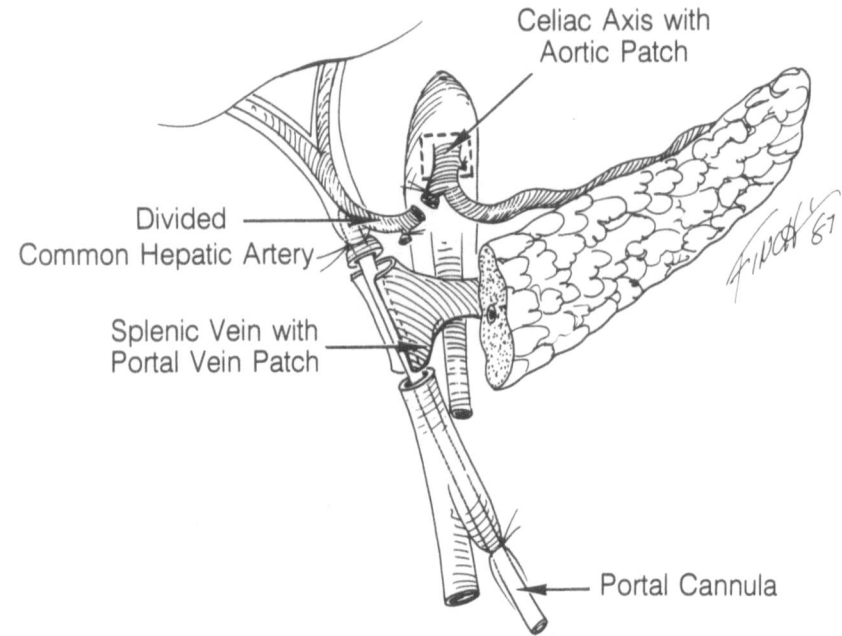

Figure 28. Procurement of segmental pancreas vascularized by celiac axis with an aortic patch and a portal vein patch, while retaining vascularity to the liver.

origin, leaving the splenic artery alone as a branch of the celiac axis. The latter is fashioned with an aortic patch.

In presence of a right hepatic artery, the common hepatic artery and the superior mesenteric artery are divided at their origin. The hepatic arterial pedicle is reconstructed by suturing the common hepatic artery end-to-end to the proximal end of the superior mesenteric artery; in this way only one arterial anastomosis has to be performed in the liver recipient (Figure 29).

ii) *Whole pancreas donation with liver harvesting*
Removal of the whole pancreas together with liver can be readily accomplished in the following situations: 1. The presence of a single or proper hepatic artery with normal bifurcation into right and left branches; 2. The presence of a left hepatic artery originating from the left gastric artery.

It is difficult, although perhaps not impossible, to perform this procedure in presence of a right hepatic artery originating from the superior mesenteric artery.

1. In cases of *normal hepatic vascularization* (single hepatic artery), the whole pancreas is dissected as previously described. Various options are existing to prepare vascular pedicles for graft revascularization, but certain basic maneuvers must be carried out.

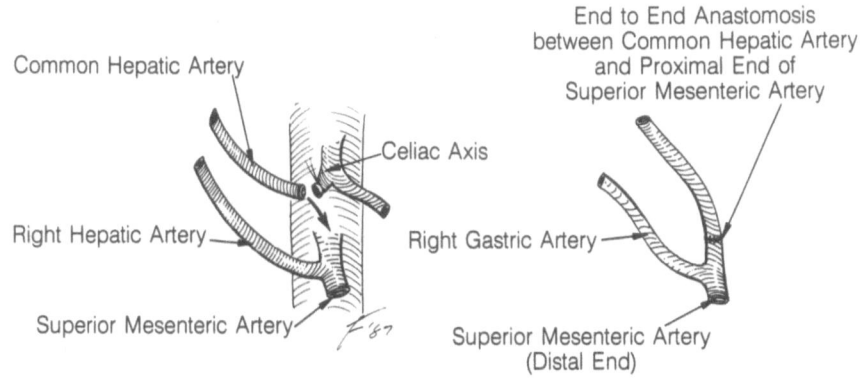

Figure 29. Hepatic revascularization after pancreas harvesting in presence of a right hepatic artery.

The gastro-duodenal artery is ligated as close as possible to its origin from the common hepatic artery, in order to avoid damage to the pancreatico-duodenal superior branches. A cannula is inserted into the first branch of the superior mesenteric vein and advanced into the portal vein. The ligature previously placed around the first branch of superior mesenteric vein is secured to fix the catheter within the portal vein lumen. A purse string is placed around the portal vein distal to the site of transection but not tied. Ringer's and Collins' or other appropriate solutions are now perfused as previously described.

At the time of pancreas removal, the common hepatic artery is divided at its origin from the celiac axis. The arterial supply to the pancreatic graft is ensured by retaining the celiac axis and superior mesenteric artery on an aortic patch (Figure 30). The portal vein is divided at the superior margin of the pancreatic gland, Care must be taken not to section the cannual which is totally removed with the pancreas (Figure 31a).

After pancreas removal, the liver is reperfused through another cannula introduced into the portal vein stump. The purse string, previously placed around the portal vein, is now tightened around the new perfusion cannula (Figure 31b).

2. *In donors with an anomalous origin of the left hepatic artery,* the procedure differs from above. The splenic artery is divided at its origin, leaving the celiac axis in continuity with the common hepatic artery and the left gastric artery with its aberrant left hepatic branch (Figure 32a). The superior mesenteric artery is retained with an aortic patch for pancreas revascularization.

The splenic and superior mesenteric artery can be connected by an external iliac artery extension graft, anastomosed end-to-end to the proximal end of splenic artery and the distal end of superior mesenteric artery. Arterial graft

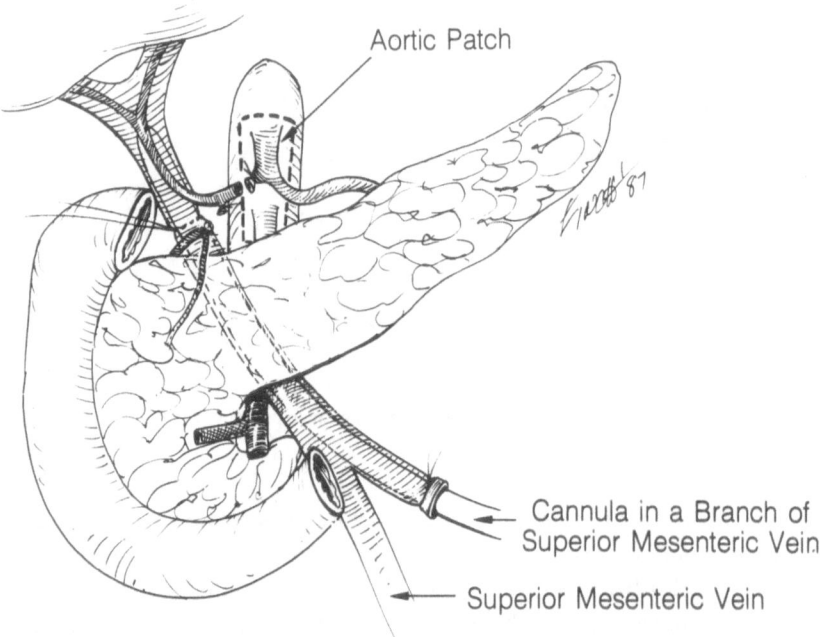

Figure 30. Simultaneous harvesting of a whole pancreas and liver.

revascularization is acomplished with only one anastomosis via the superior mesenteric artery with its aortic patch (Figure 32b).

3. When an *aberrant right hepatic artery* originates from the superior mesenteric artery, it is not advisable to procure the whole pancreas with the liver. The inferior pancreatico-duodenal artery also originates from the superior mesenteric artery, and is as necessary to revascularize the pancreas as the right hepatic artery is for the liver. Since division of the gastro-duodenal artery is mandatory in case of liver harvesting, the arterial supply of the head of the pancreas and duodenum is provided only in a retrograde fashion from the collaterals between the inferior pancreatico-duodenal artery and the superior pancreatico-duodenal artery. In the other situations described, the inferior pancreatico-duodenal artery can be preserved, but with an aberrant right hepatic artery this is most likely not possible.

Organ preservation

Preservation will be extensively discussed in another chapter. Cold storage at 4°C is considered the best way to preserve a pancreatic graft. If Collins solution is used, the cold ischemia should not exceed 6 hours; beyond this limit transplant results are less good (see chapter on International Pancreas Trans-

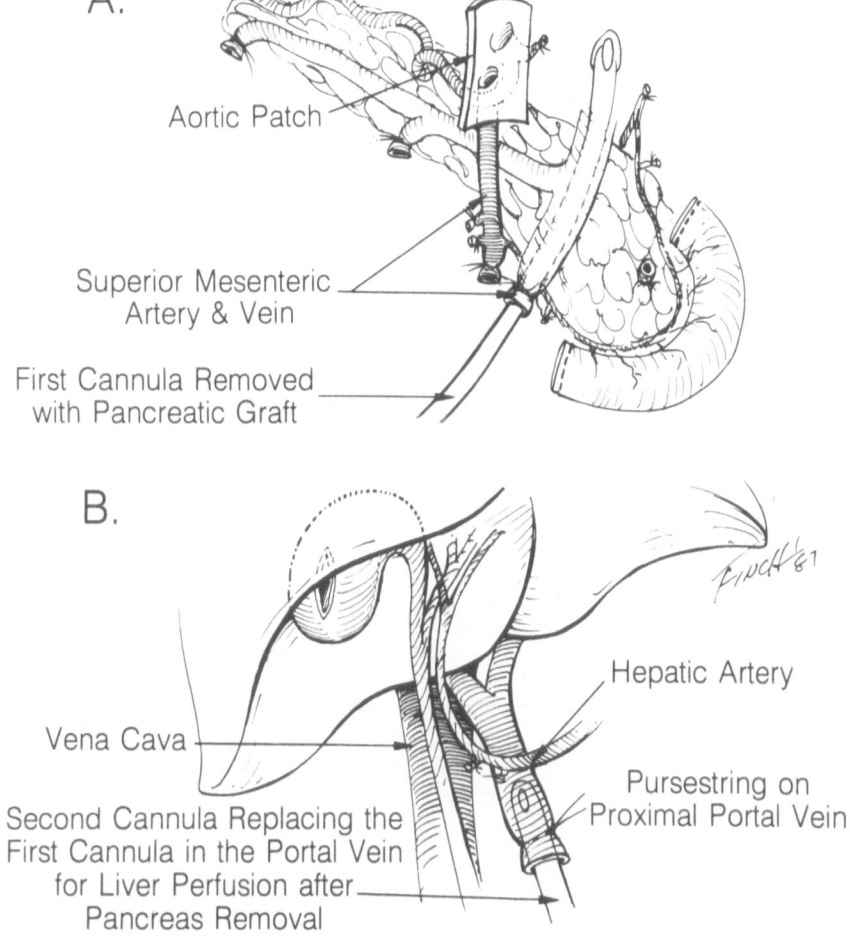

A.

Aortic Patch

Superior Mesenteric
Artery & Vein

First Cannula Removed
with Pancreatic Graft

B.

Vena Cava

Second Cannula Replacing the
First Cannula in the Portal Vein
for Liver Perfusion after
Pancreas Removal

Hepatic Artery

Pursestring on
Proximal Portal Vein

Figure 31. A) Whole pancreas removed with first portal cannula B) Liver perfused by second portal cannula after pancreas removal.

plant Registry). However, new preservation solutions have been developed, and new guidelines for the duration of preservation are being developed.

Pancreatic transplantation

Several different approaches have been described for pancreas transplantation. Various options exist for the graft position in the abdominal cavity, the site of implantation, the mass of pancreatic tissue grafted (whole versus segmental gland), and the handling of the exocrine secretion.

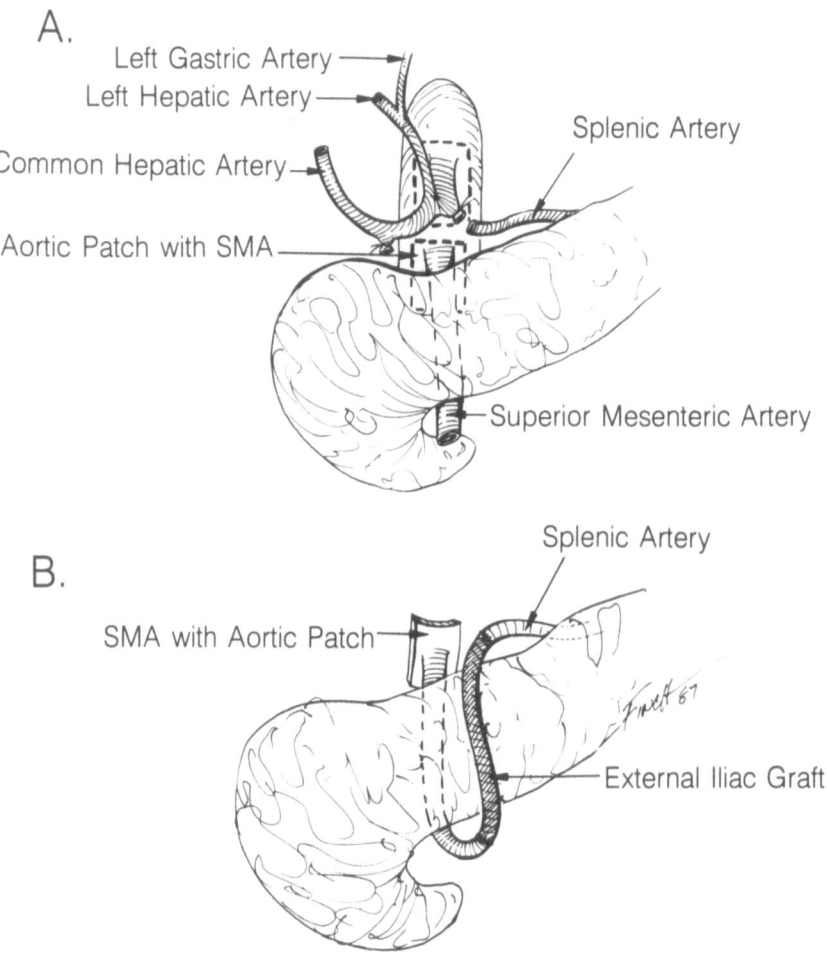

A.

Left Gastric Artery

Left Hepatic Artery

Common Hepatic Artery

Aortic Patch with SMA

Splenic Artery

Superior Mesenteric Artery

B.

Splenic Artery

SMA with Aortic Patch

External Iliac Graft

Figure 32. A) Whole pancreas removal in presence of a left hepatic artery B) Splenic and superior mesenteric artery of pancreas are joined with an iliac artery interposition graft.

Incision and position of the graft

We have used various sites for graft placement in the abdominal cavity. In our early cases [14], we placed pancreatic graft extraperitoneally in the left or right iliac fossa through a J-shaped iliac incision, similar to that used for kidney transplantation (Figure 33). Frequent perigraft collections and local wound infection were observed, and we next tested an 'intra-extraperitoneal' placement of the graft. The same extraperitoneal access was used as described above, but a 4 cm peritoneal incision was performed after graft revascularization. The omentum was advanced through the peritoneal window and

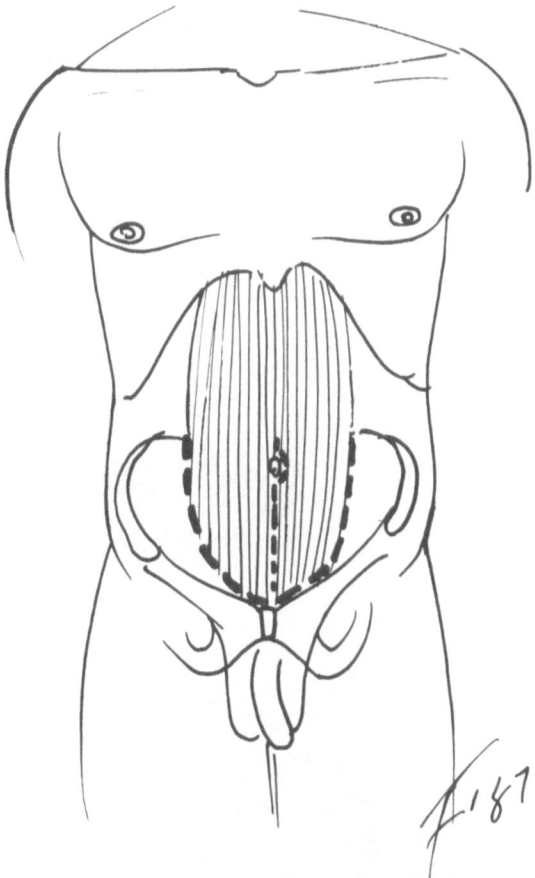

Figure 33. Double J shaped skin incisions for simultaneous kidney and pancreas transplantation by the retroperitoneal approach used in our early cases midline incision.

wrapped around the pancreas [17], facilitating, if necessary, absorption of perigraft leakage (Figure 34).

Currently, we place the pancreas graft entirely in the peritoneal cavity [20]. A lower midline incision from just above the umbilicus to the pubis is used (Figure 33). The peritoneal cavity is opened, and the small bowel retracted upward. This approach is used for either segmental or whole pancreas transplantation. It facilitates peritoneal drainage of pancreatic leakage, should it occur. In addition, a single incision can be used for double kidney and pancreas transplantation.

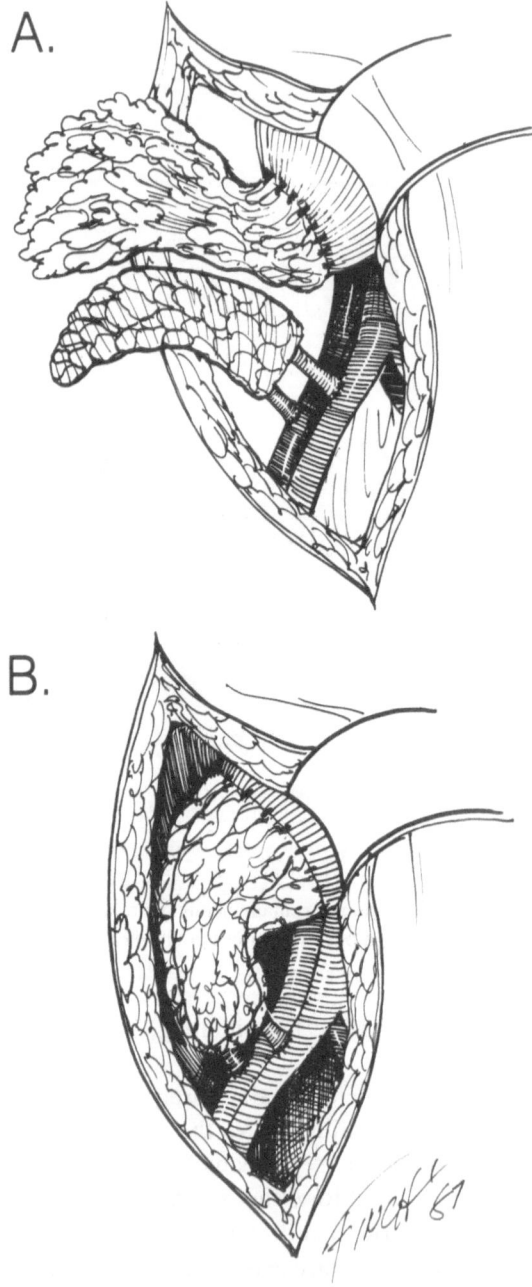

Figure 34. Intra-extraperitoneal placement of the graft with omentoplasty: after the graft is revascularized the omentum is brought through a peritoneal incision (A), wrapped around the graft and sutured to the peritoneum (B).

Preparation of the site and graft revascularization

General considerations

The common or external iliac vessels are usually used for vascular anastomoses. Either the left or right side can be choosen. The left side is usually preferred for the pancreas when a double kidney and pancreas transplantation is scheduled or when a previous kidney graft has been placed on the right side. If a retroperitoneal approach is used, the iliac vessels are exposed by retracting the sigmoid colon medially on the left side. The ureter is displaced laterally and the iliac artery and vein are isolated and looped by tapes.

At present, we prefer a midline incision with trans-mesocolic approach to the left iliac vessels. This approach facilitates intra-abdominal placement of the pancreatic graft, makes it easier to avoid kinking or twisting of the graft vein, and reduces the risk of early postoperative venous thrombosis (Figure 35).

After the vessels are prepared, the pancreas graft is removed from its container and arterial and venous patches are tailored to fit the iliac vessels. The common iliac vein is clamped and a venotomy is performed; a small part of the venous wall is excised to ensure a patuous anastomosis and promote venous outflow from the graft. An end-to-side anastomosis is performed between the vein of the graft and the iliac vein with a 5/0 prolene running suture. When the venous anastomosis has been completed a 'bull-dog' clamp is placed on the graft vein to avoid venous reflux and the iliac vein clamps are released. The common iliac artery is now clamped. The site of iliac arteriotomy is carefully choosen to correspond to the graft artery. An end-to-side anastomosis is performed with a 6/0 or 5/0 prolene running suture. The venous 'bull-dog' clamp is first released, followed by release of the arterial clamps. The graft should rapidly regain a normal color and consistency.

Strong pulsations of the graft splenic artery are usually observed; oedema of the pancreatic gland sometimes occurs, but usually lasts only a short time after the vascular clamps have been released, unless the preservation time has been excessive.

Surgical strategy differences for segmental versus whole pancreas transplants

Segmental graft revascularization. When a segmental graft is performed several options exist for graft revascularization. In grafts from living related donors, the graft splenic vein must be used for end to side anastomosis with recipient iliac vein (Figure 36), and either end-to-side anastomosis of the splenic artery to iliac artery or end-to-end to the hypogastric artery are realized.

When the distal pancreas is harvested from a cadaver, three technical

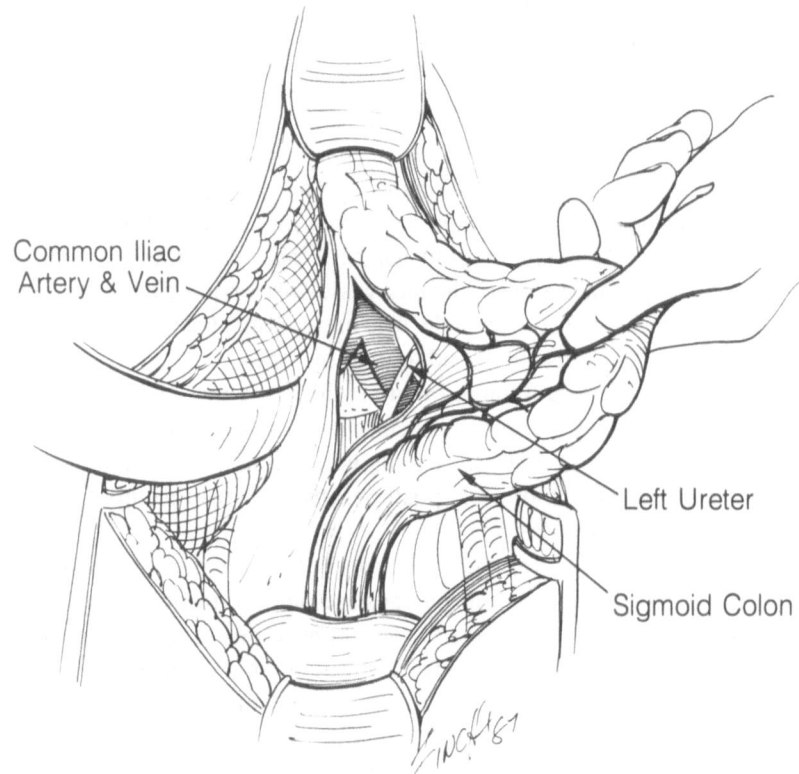

Common Iliac
Artery & Vein

Left Ureter

Sigmoid Colon

Figure 35. Transmesocolic approach to the left common iliac vessels of the recipient.

options exist for arterial revascularization. A patch of donor celiac axis and common hepatic artery can be fashioned to facilitate anastomosis of the graft splenic artery to the recipient common iliac artery. In case of severe atheroma, it is sometimes advantageous to use the celiac axis with or without an aortic patch, after ligation of common hepatic and left gastric arteries (Figure 37).

In our earlier cases [4], the venous anastomosis was performed using a patch of donor portal and superior mesenteric vein (Figure 38a). The anastomosis was difficult to perform because the proximity of the cut edge of the gland to the iliac vessels. Our present strategy is the remove the donor pancreas with a segment of portal vein, after ligation of superior mesenteric vein (Figure 38b). Care has to be taken to adjust the length of portal vein in order to avoid any kinking or twisting. A flexible approach is required, and the graft tail may be projected upward or downward in the abdominal cavity. Separate sutures between the body or the pancreas and the abdominal wall can help maintain the graft in the best position [4].

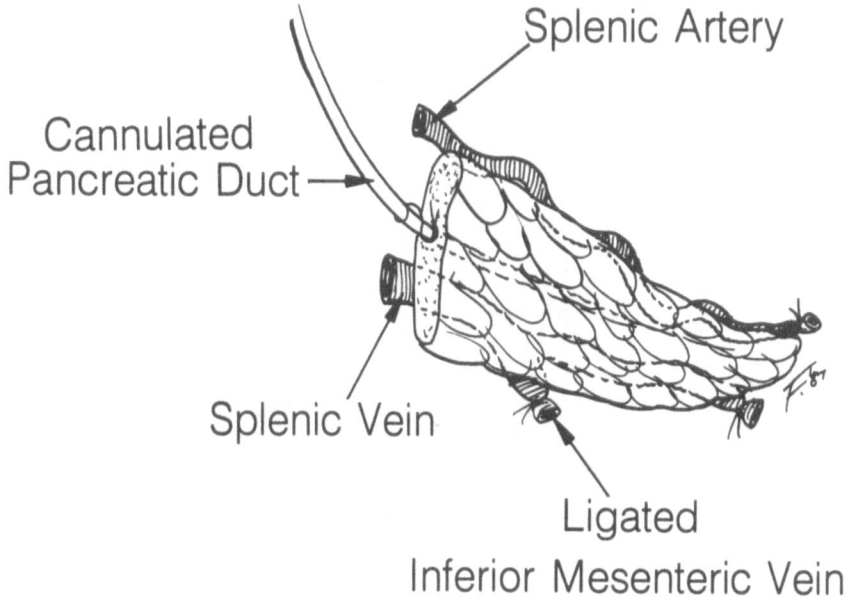

Figure 36. Segmental graft from living related donor after preparation for transplantation.

Whole pancreas revascularization. For whole pancreas transplants, the portal vein and an aortic patch including the celiac axis and superior mesenteric artery are usually sutured end to side to iliac vein and artery respectively (Figure 39). In cases of whole pancreas grafts procured from cadaver liver

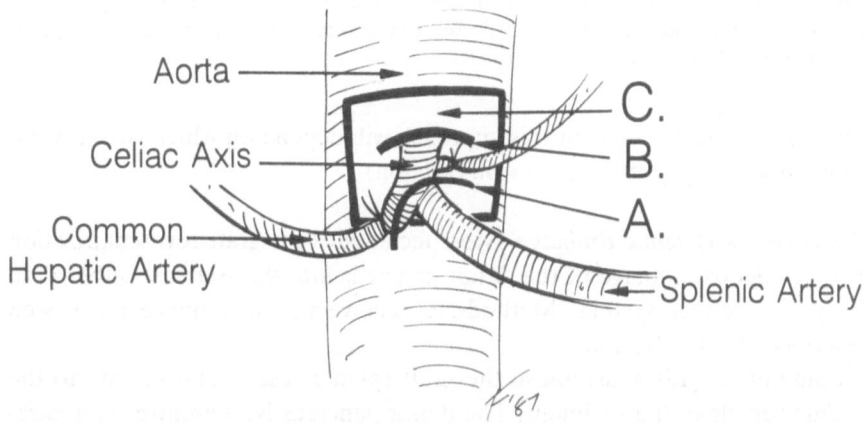

Figure 37. Alternative methods for arterial revascularization of a segmental pancreatic graft depending on the circumstances of the donor operation: A: Splenic artery with a patch of celiac axis and common hepatic artery B: Celiac axis C: Celiac axis with aortic patch.

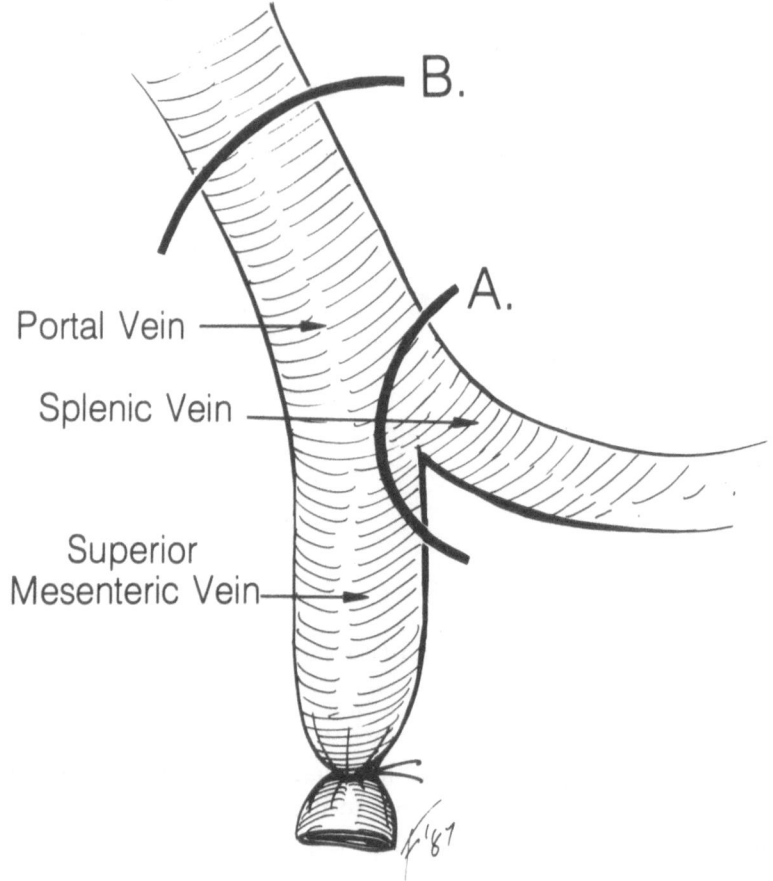

Figure 38. Alternative methods for venous drainage of a segmental pancreatic graft depending on the circumstances of the donor operation: A: Splenic vein with a patch of portal vein and superior mesenteric vein B: Portal vein.

donors, the arterial anastomosis approach will depend on which vessels were retained with the graft (see previous section).

Portal versus systemic drainage. Most techniques for graft revascularization involve venous drainage of the donor pancreas into the systemic rather than the portal venous system. Methods to achieve portal drainage have been described [17, 18, 21, 22].

Calne et al. [18] anastomose the graft splenic vessels end to side to the splenic vessels of the recipient. The donor pancreas is, therefore, in a paratopic position, close to the patient's own pancreas (Figure 40). The approach is difficult, and is performed through a left subcostal incision. Alternatives are to use the recipient's mesenteric vessels, either the inferior [21] or superior [22],

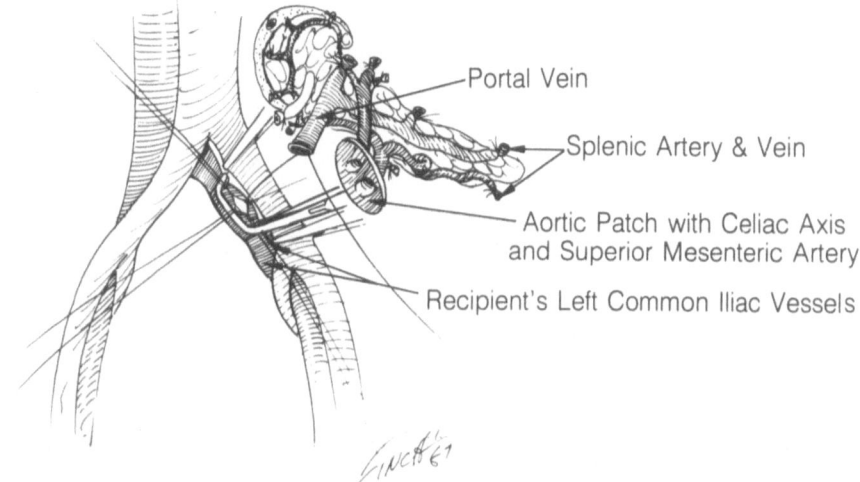

Figure 39. Revascularization of a whole pancreas transplant.

for the anastomosis to the graft vessels. Although there are only a few cases, the use of the inferior mesenteric vessels [21] has been associated with a higher success rate than the use of the superior vessels [22]. However, a clear metabolic advantage of portal over systemic drainage has not been shown [22].

Management of graft endocrine secretion

Management of the exocrine secretion is a central problem in pancreas transplantation. The approaches may differ with the type of transplant, segmental or whole pancreas.

Segmental pancreas

Several techniques have been described for the management of exocrine secretion of a segmental pancreatic graft.

Duct obstruction (Figure 10). This technique was first applied in humans in 1976, and entails injection of the main pancreatic duct with a synthetic polymer [4, 23–25]. Since 1976 we have used Neoprene for duct obstruction [4]. This liquid synthetic polymer flocculates with changes in pH. It is liquid at its commercial pH of 12 to 14. The pH of the pancreatic juice is 8 to 9. The polymer solidifies when injected into the pancreatic duct; 3 ml are usually sufficient for injection of a segmental graft. Neoprene extravasation should be avoided. The pancreatic duct is sutured with a 4/0 prolene and the pancreatic neck totally ligated with a purse-string 2–0 silk.

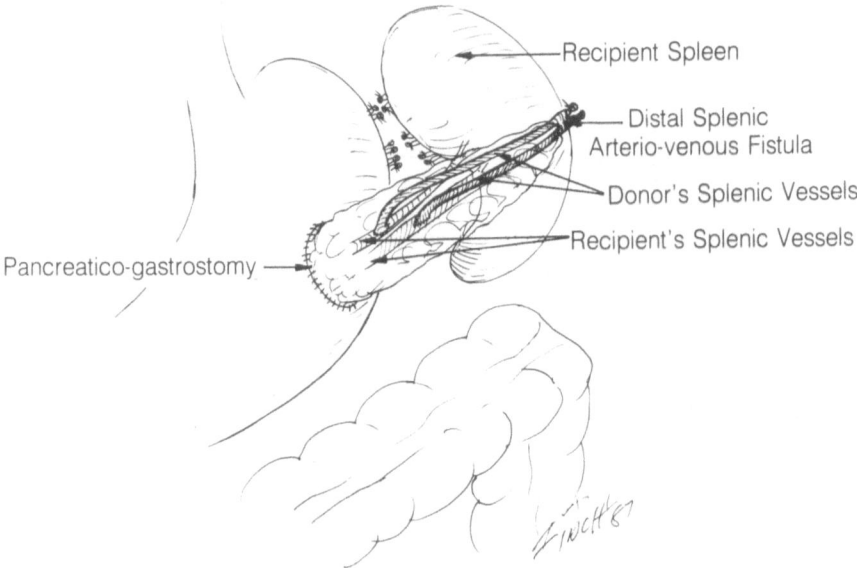

108

Figure 40. Segmental pancreas transplanted in the paratopic position; the splenic vessels of the graft are sutured end-to-side to splenic vessels of the recipient and the graft duct is anastomosed to the splenic vessels of the recipient.

Other substances have been used including prolamine [23], polyisoprene [24] and silicone [25]. Silicone theoretically might not adhere to the duct wall, a possible disadvantage. Prolamine is a slowly resorbable substance and might not be as 'obstructive' as Neoprene, accounting for the apparently higher complication rate observed by the group using the substance [23]. Neoprene is very easy to inject, it adheres very well to duct walls, and is not reabsorbed. We believe it is the best available substance for duct obstruction.

After the graft has been harvested and splenectomy performed, the duct of Wirsung is cannulated with a small blunt-tip catheter. The polymer is injected and the neck of the pancreas is ligated. When a duct-obstructed segmental pancreas is transplanted, graft revascularization is the only major surgical maneuver necessary in the recipient.

Recently, some groups have placed a catheter in the duct and brought it out externally, delaying injection until several weeks post-transplant [21, 27]. This technique allows exocrine function to be monitored in the early post-transplant period, but an advantage of this approach over immediate injection has not been demonstrated.

Intestinal drainage (Figure 41). Intestinal drainage of segmental grafts is usually performed into a Roux-en-Y loop of jejunum [7]. The small bowel is

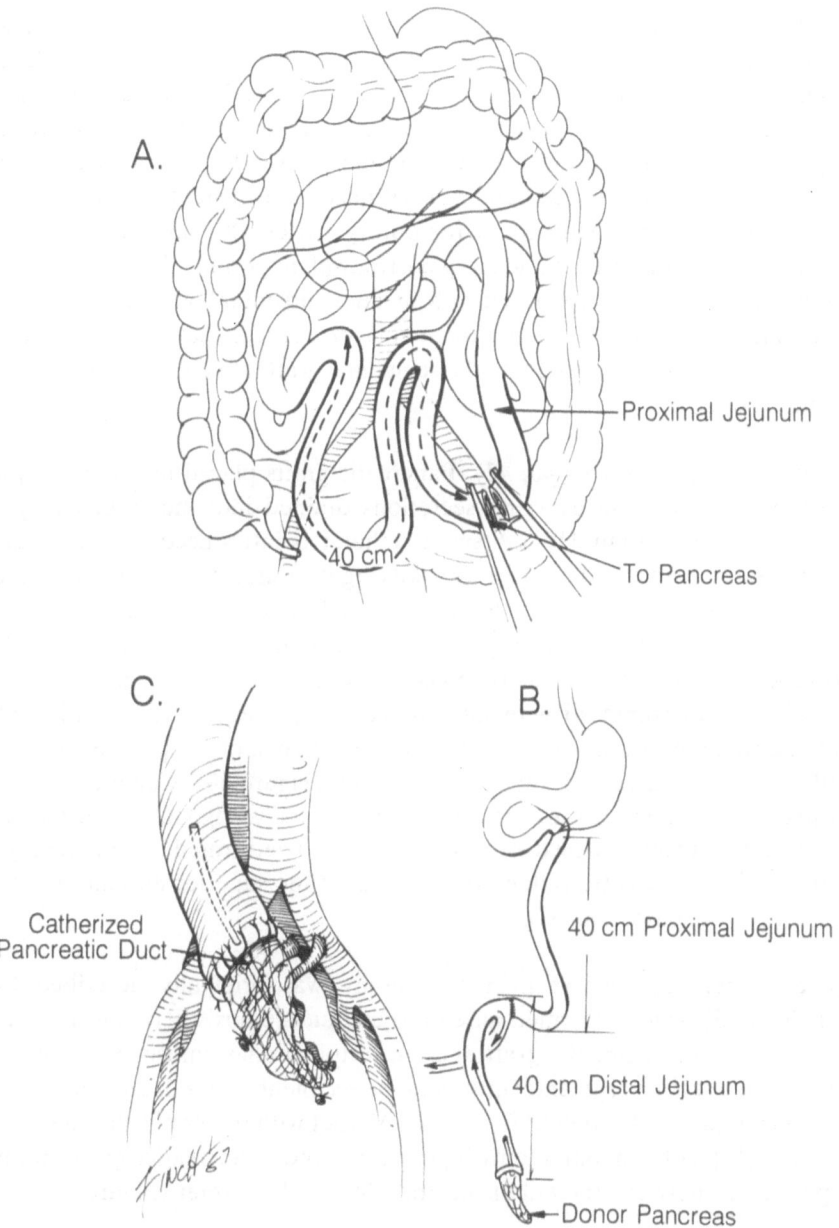

Figure 41. Enteric drainage of a segmental graft into a Roux-en-Y loop. A) Isolation of recipient jejunum B) Entero-enteric and pancreatico-enteric anastomoses C) Completed pancreatico-jejunostomy by two layers, intussusception technique.

divided between intestinal clamps approximately 40 cm distal to Treitz ligament (Figure 41a). An end to side jejuno-jenunostomy is performed at least 40 cm distal to pancreatico-jejunostomy to ensure an adequate defunctionalized limb for drainage of pancreatic secretion (Figure 41b). Different techniques can be used for the pancreatico-jejunostomy. The pancreatic duct can be intubated with a small cathether or left unstented. If stented, the catheter can be brought externally for a temporary period [8], allowing exocrine function to be monitored in the early posttransplant period. The pancreatico-jejunostomy is usually performed with an inner and outer layer. A nonabsorbable continuous suture is used for the first layer. A second layer of 3/0 prolene sutures is then used to invaginate the segmental graft into the intestinal lumen (Figure 41c).

Gastric drainage (Figures 40, 42). Pancreatic grafts placed in the paratopic position have had the exocrine secretions drained into the stomach by a pancreaticogastrostomy [18]. A small catheter is introduced into the main pancreatic duct and held in place by a 4/0 catgut suture. It is inserted into and back out the stomach and brought out through the abdominal wall and fixed to the skin with a suture, allowing external pancreatic drainage for the early postoperative period. The gastric mucosa and the wall of the pancreatic duct are directly anastomosed with interrupted 7–0 prolene sutures, and a 5/0 prolene running suture is used to secure the cut edge of the pancreatic graft within the seromuscular layer of the stomach (Figure 40). Calne et al. [18] wrap the pancreatic graft in omentum, and place a drainage tube near the tail of the graft. Pancreaticogastrostomy has also been performed in some cases of heterotopic pancreas transplantation [28] using the superior mesenteric vessels for revascularization (Figure 42).

Ureteral drainage. Pancreaticoureterostomy was originally described by Gliedman [3], who performed an end to end anastomosis between the pancreatic duct of a segmental graft and the recipient anastomosis between the pancreatic duct of a segmental graft and the recipient ureter in the iliac fossa. This technique has been modified by Gil-Vernet with paratopic placement of the graft [17]. A left nephrectomy is performed and a pancreatico-pyelostomy is performed between the tail of the graft and the left ureter (Figure 43).

Bladder drainage (Figures 44, 45). Pancreaticocystostomy was first described for segmental grafts [9]. A segmental pancreas is harvested by the standard techniques described previously. Vascular anastomoses are accomplished to external iliac vessels. The pancreaticocystostomy has been performed in two different fashions. In the first method (Figure 44), the pancreatic duct is cannulated and sutured to the bladder mucosa, and the cut edge of the

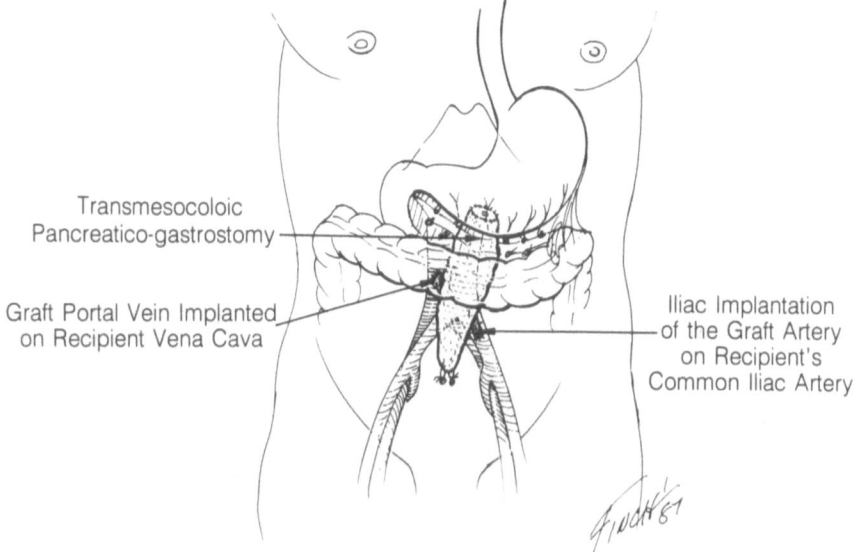

Transmesocoloic
Pancreatico-gastrostomy

Graft Portal Vein Implanted
on Recipient Vena Cava

Iliac Implantation
of the Graft Artery
on Recipient's
Common Iliac Artery

Figure 42. Transmesocolic pancreatico-gastrostomy after heterotopic transplantation of a segmental pancreatic allograft. Graft vessels are anastomosed to the caval vein and the common iliac artery (Figure) or to the superior mesenteric artery and vein.

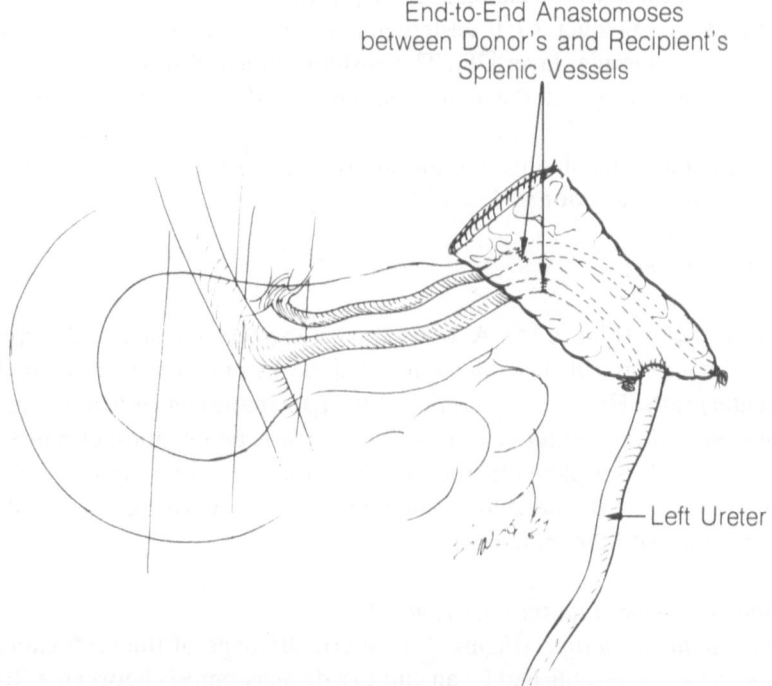

End-to-End Anastomoses
between Donor's and Recipient's
Splenic Vessels

Left Ureter

Figure 43. Pancreaticopyelostomy technique for segmental grafts.

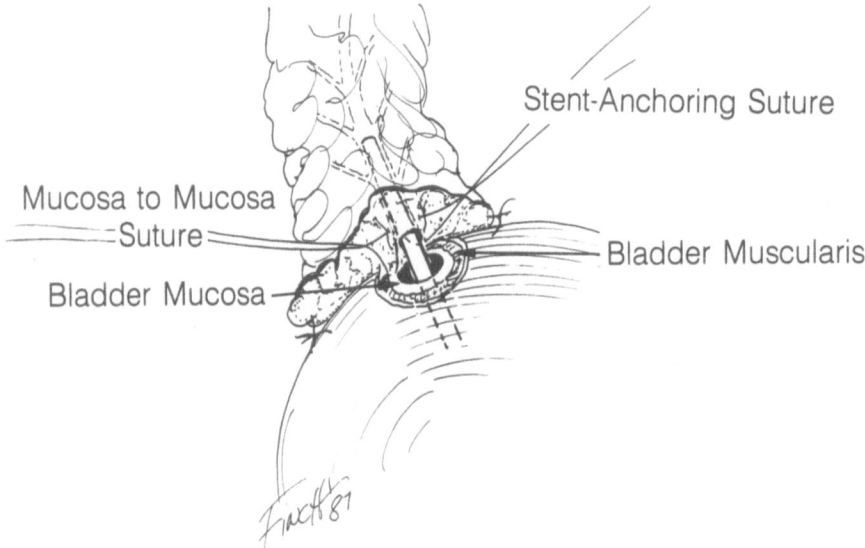

Figure 44. Pancreaticocystostomy for segmental grafts with duct cannulation and one layer anastomosis.

pancreas is sutured to the bladder serosa [9]. In the second technique (Figure 45), the pancreatic duct is left unstented and the bladder mucosa is dissected free from the muscular layer [28]. The posterior mucosal surface is sutured to the posterior surface of the pancreas. The periductal pancreatic tissue is anastomosed to a small opening in the bladder mucosa. The pancreatic neck is intusscepted into the bladder and the anterior lip of the seromuscular incision is sutured to the anterior surface of the graft [29].

Whole pancreas

Duct obstruction (Figure 14). A total pancreas can be harvested and prepared with duct injection [10]. The injection technique is similar to that described for segmental grafts. However separation of the pancreatic head is a time consuming procedure necessitating meticulous hemostasis and ligation of numerous small vessels. A complete obstruction of the duct might be more difficult to achieve because of the need to cannulate the accessory pancreatic duct if it is not confluent with the main duct.

Intestinal drainage (Figures 46, 47, 48, 49).
i) *Whole pancreas alone.* (Figure 46) Enteric drainage of the graft exocrine secretions can be established by an end to side anastomosis between a Roux-in-Y intestinal loop and a small patch of duodenum encompassing the pan-

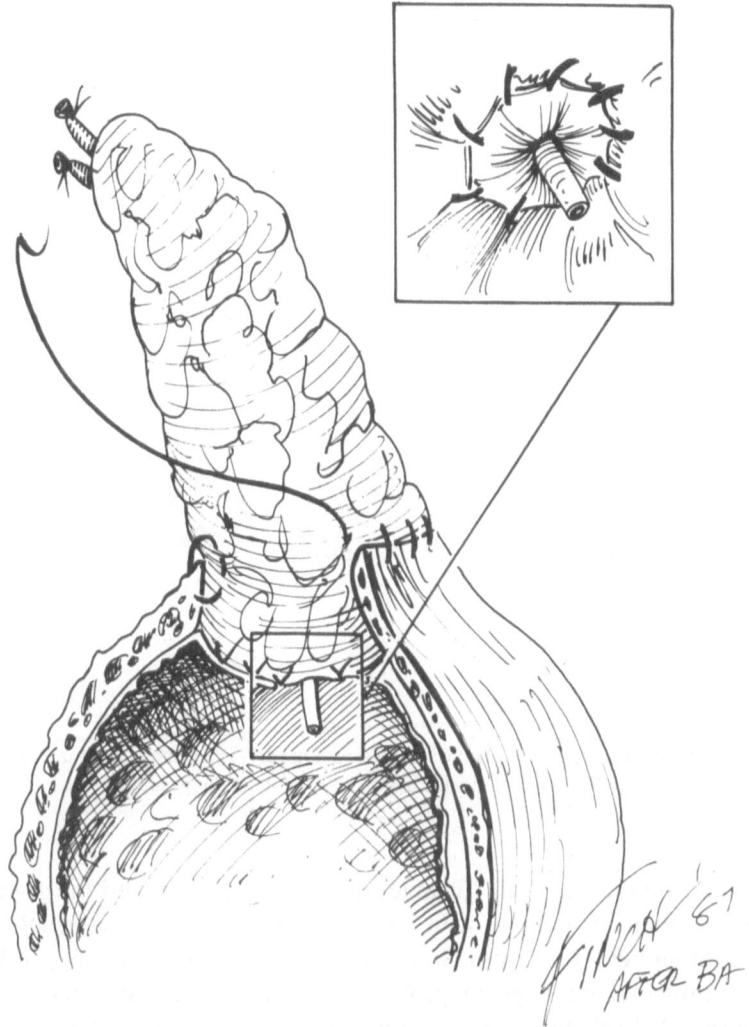

Figure 45. Pancreaticocystostomy of a segmental pancreatic graft in two layers with duct left unstented.

creatic ducts [10]. In either case, a small incision is made in the antimesenteric wall of the jejunum and the pancreatic duct or duodenal patch is anastomosed with 5/0 Prolene separate stitches (Figure 46a). The sutures include the full thickness of the intestinal wall and the small duodenal patch surrounding the papilla of Vater. A second layer invaginates the donor pancreatic duct into the intestinal lumen (Figures 46b). The head of the donor pancreas is secured to the jejunal wall by separate 4/0 prolene separate stitches.

ii) *Pancreaticoduodenal graft* (Figure 47, 48, 49). Intestinal drainage of a

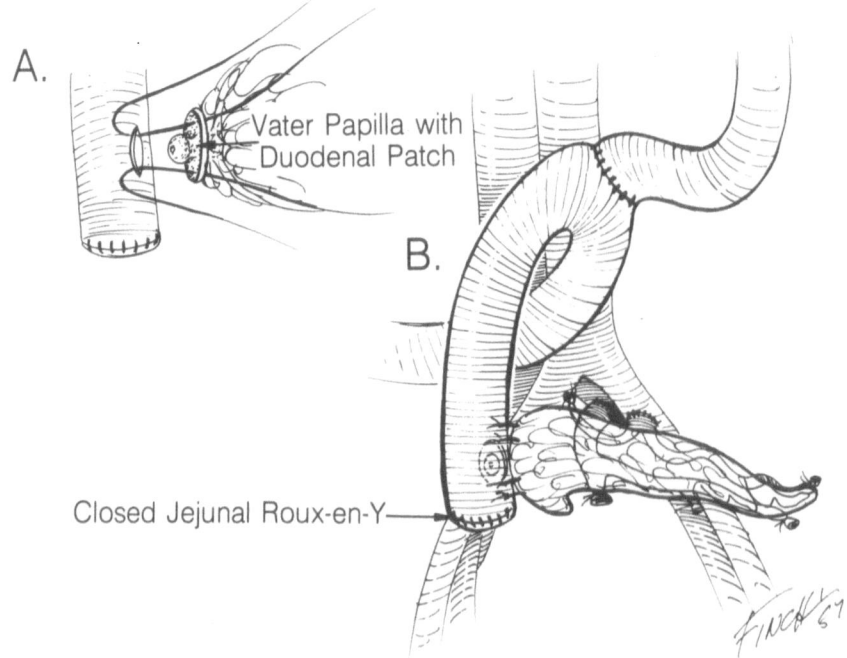

Figure 46. Whole pancreas transplant with enteric drainage: A) Placement of sutures for pancreatic duct-jejunostomy B) Completed anastomosis to Roux-en-Y loops in intestine.

pancreaticoduodenal graft (includes the whole pancreas and the segment of donor duodenum intimate with pancreatic head) is easily accomplished by standard surgical techniques. Starzl et al. [12] and Corry et al. [30] performed the anastomosis to a single loop. We used this approach in one of our patients (Figure 47). Prolonged postoperative leakage of the intestinal anastomosis convinced us to anastomose the donor duodenum to a defunctionalized Roux-en-Y intestinal limb in subsequent cases (Figure 48), an approach also used by others [13].

The Roux-en-Y intestinal loop is fashioned as previously described. The distal end of the defunctionalized limb is closed in two layers with a non-absorbable suture. After revascularization, the proximal and distal end of donor duodenum, resected during the donor operation by using an automatic suture device type GIA, are invaginated with a 4/0 prolene running suture. A small incision is made in the antimesenteric wall of recipient jejunum and in the wall of donor duodenum. The GIA automatic suture device is introduced into the recipient jejunal and in the donor duodenal lumens, and a side to side anastomosis is accomplished. Alternatively, the anastomosis may be hand sewn.

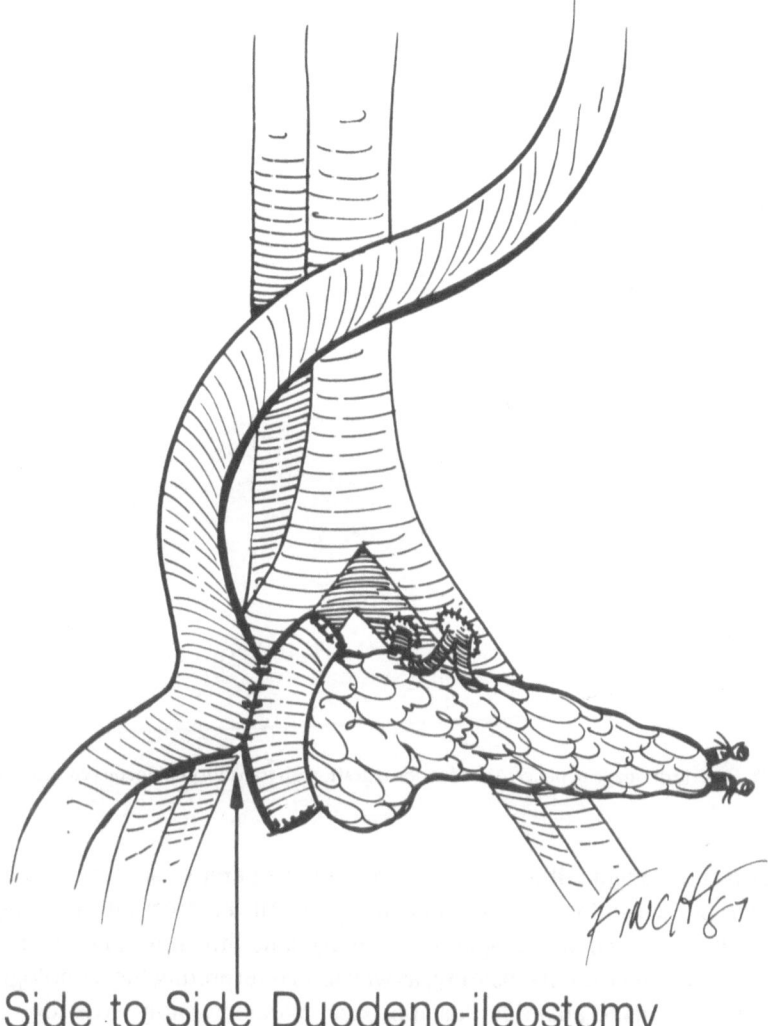

Side to Side Duodeno-ileostomy

Figure 47. Enteric drainage of whole pancreaduodo-duodenal transplant by side-to-side duodeno-enterotostomy to a free loop of bowel.

When the duodenojejunal anastomosis is delayed, for example in double pancreas and kidney transplantation, and the renal graft is revascularized before performing the enteric drainage in order to minimize renal ischemia care must be taken when opening the segment of donor duodenum which becomes distended by pancreatic and duodenal secretions which begin to form immediately after pancreatic revascularization. This problem can be avoided by performing the enteric anastomosis before revascularization of the kidney.

In our first few pancreatico-duodenal transplants, a cutaneous enterostomy

116

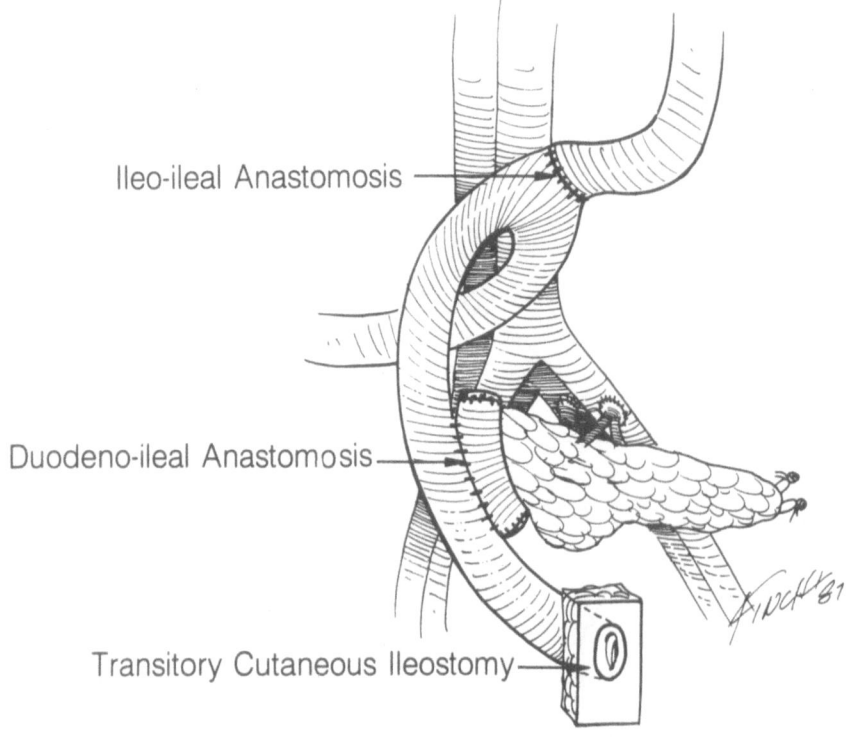

Ileo-ileal Anastomosis

Duodeno-ileal Anastomosis

Transitory Cutaneous Ileostomy

Figure 48. Enteric drainage of pancreaticoduodenal graft, with transitory cutaneous enterostomy.

was performed (Figure 48). In order to drain postoperative secretions and to perform repeated endoscopic duodenal biopsies. The enterostomy was closed at 3 months. Absence of postoperative leakage and difficulties in performing endoscopy through the enterostomy, as well as in interpreting the pathological data, convinced us to abandon this approach. We now simply close terminal end (in two layers) of the defunctionalized Roux-en-Y limb (Figure 49).

Bladder drainage (Figures 50, 51). Bladder drainage of the exocrine secretion of the whole pancreas transplant can be accomplished by several variations [11, 13, 14, 31]. Either a duodenal patch [11, 31] or a duodenal segment [13, 14] can be anastomosed to the bladder. The first technique is similar to that described for pancreatico-jejunostomy. A small patch of the donor duodenum, surrounding the ampulla of Vater, is sutured to the bladder mucosa of a posterior cystostomy with interrupted absorbable stitches (Figure 50). The sutures can be placed in the inside of the bladder through an anterior cystostomy (Figure 50a). Alternatively [31], the duodenal patch can be anastomosed to the bladder through a single posterior incision (Figure 50b). For

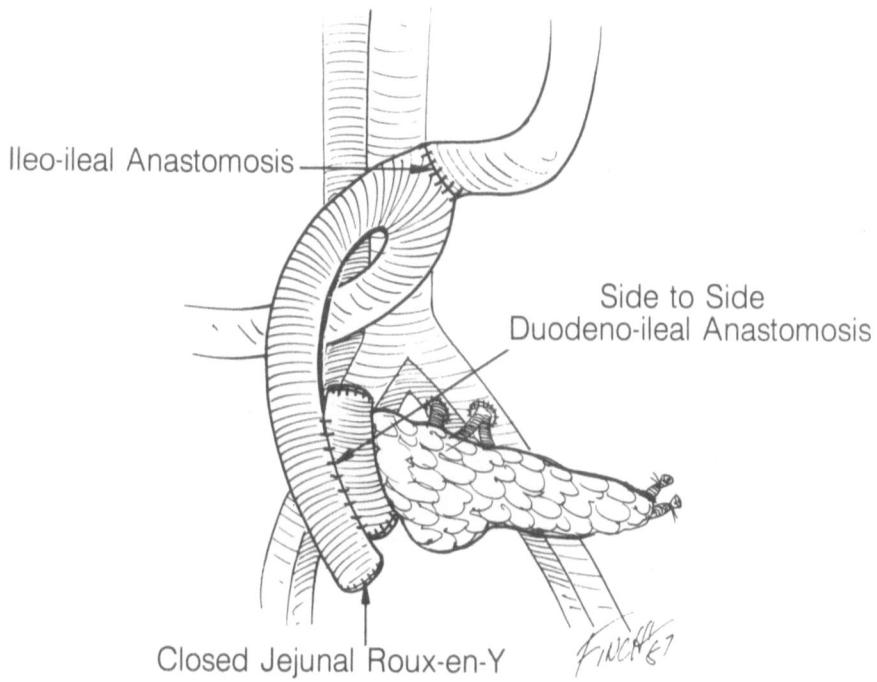

Ileo-ileal Anastomosis

Side to Side
Duodeno-ileal Anastomosis

Closed Jejunal Roux-en-Y

Figure 49. Enteric drainage of pancreaticoduodenal graft to a Roux-en-Y loop with strict internal drainage.

pancreaticoduodenal grafts a two layer duodenocystostomy is performed by making a lateral incision in the duodenum for anastomosis to a corresponding incision in the posterior aspect of the dome of the bladder (Figure 51). With all of these techniques, a catheter is left in the bladder for 1 or 2 weeks.

Surgical complications

Various surgical complications can occur after pancreas transplantation. Some are specific and some non-specific for the pancreas.

Non-specific complications

Postoperative bleeding is a risk for all operations. Anastomotic bleeding is rare, but the poor quality of the vessels in some diabetic patients predisposes to this complication. Graft hemorrhage may occur because of poor hemostasis during graft harvesting, and laxity in this regard is more likely to occur with whole organ grafts. During multiorgan harvesting the surgeon is under pressure to proceed rapidly, and a careful graft hemostasis is not always obtained.

118

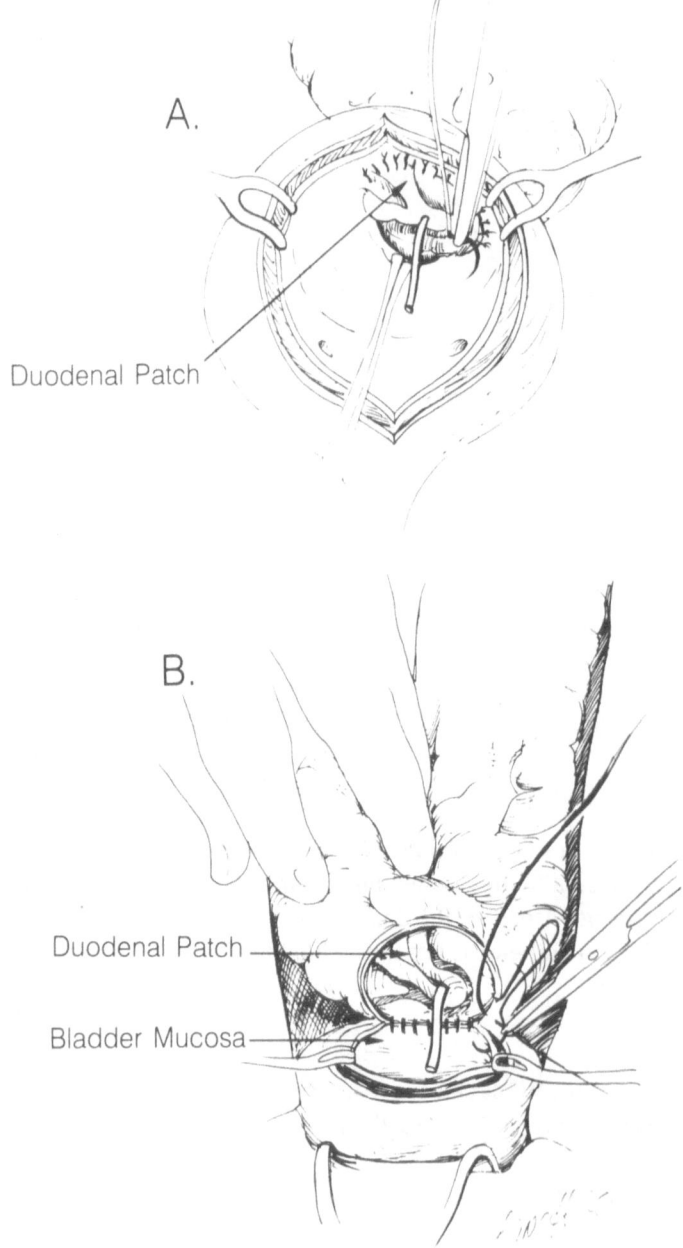

A.

Duodenal Patch

B.

Duodenal Patch

Bladder Mucosa

Figure 50. Whole pancreas transplant with bladder drainage: A) Pancreatico-cystostomy by implantation of a duodenal button through an anterior cystostomy B) Direct implantation of the of duodenal button into a posterior cystostomy. The inferior row of sutures is placed first.

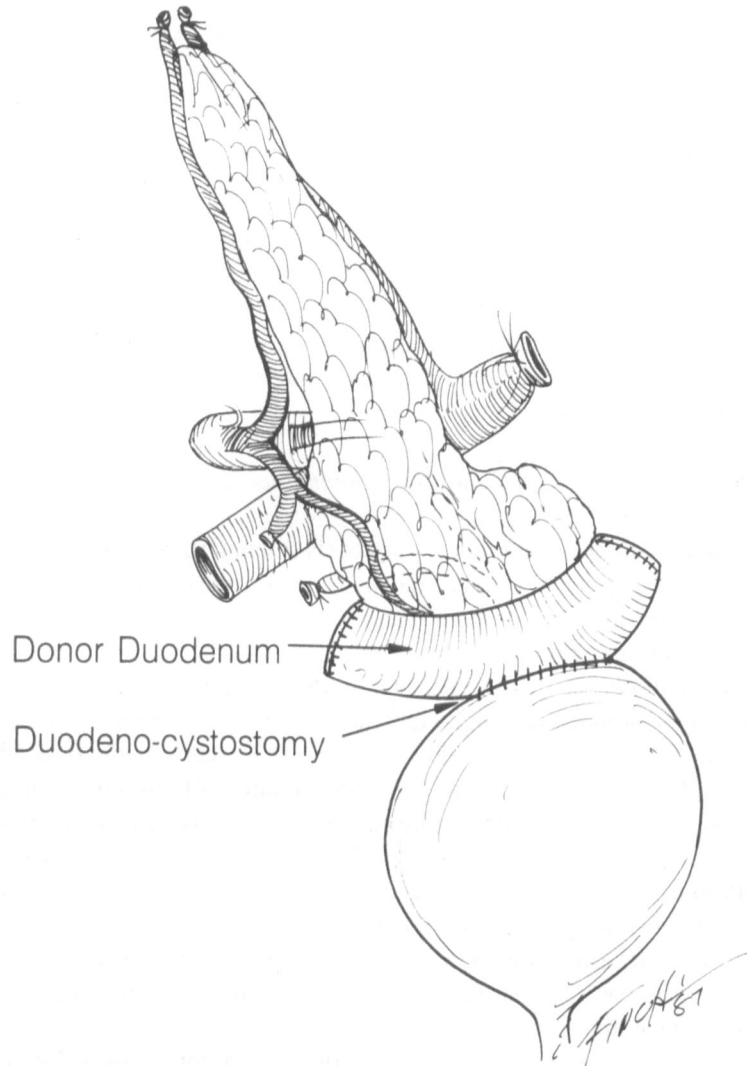

Donor Duodenum

Duodeno-cystostomy

Figure 51. Whole pancreaticoduodenal transplantation by bladder drainage through a side-to-side pancreaticoduodeno-cystostomy.

Therefore, meticulous attention to graft hemostasis must be made after pancreas revascularization in the recipient.

Intra-abdominal complications such as ileus or small bowel obstruction due to adhesions are also common to all types of abdominal surgery. In our series the incidence has been highest in the group with enteric drained whole pancreas grafts [32].

Leakage of intestinal anastomoses occurred in the earliest series of pancreas transplant [1, 2]. Improvement in the surgical techniques and, the use of lower doses of steroids have made enteric drainage reliable and reduced the frequency of the complication [13].

Wound infections occur in all types of surgery. Transplant patients are immunosuppressed and are at high risk for septic complications. In pancreas transplant recipients, collections of pancreatic juice can lead to abscess or fistula formation and even wound dehiscence. In our experience, intraperitoneal placement of the pancreatic graft has significantly reduced the frequency of such complications, perhaps because the peritoneal cavity can absorb peripancreatic collections [20].

Complications specific to pancreas transplantation

One of the major causes of pancreatic graft loss is vascular thrombosis. Several hypothesis have been proposed as to mechanisms of this complication.

Arterial thrombosis is less frequent than venous thrombosis. Atherosclerotic recipient vessels may predispose to its occurrence.

Venous thrombosis usually occurs in the early postoperative period and is not entirely understood. Hemodynamic changes due to donor splenectomy could explain the high incidence of this complication by reducing the flow rate in the large splenic vessels. Interruption of the collaterals between the distal and proximal pancreas in segmental grafts has also been considered as favoring venous thrombosis. However the complication also occurs in whole pancreas transplantation. Some groups give heparin or low molecular weight dextran to the patient in the early postoperative period in an attempt to prevent graft thrombosis. Long term anticoagulant drugs are also sometimes given. There is no evidence, however, that anticoagulation is helpful, and the treatment predisposes to bleeding.

Two main surgical options have been proposed to compensate for the hemodynamic disturbances: distal arterio-venous fistula of the splenic vessels and pancreatico-splenic transplantation. A distal arteriovenous fistula, first used by Calne et al. [33] in segmental grafts, theoretically reduces blood pressure in the splenic artery, increases blood pressure in the splenic vein, and increases blood flow in both vessels. Its efficacy in reducing the incidence of thrombosis has not been proved. Moreover, the hemodynamic consequences of venous hyperpressure are not known, and in baboons hemodynamic pancreatitis has been described [34].

Pancreatico-splenic transplantation, initially proposed by Starzl et al. [12] is a logical technical approach because the pancreas and spleen share the same vascular supply. Unfortunately, major immuno-hematologic complications, specifically graft versus host disease [35, 36] have occurred, and splenic rupture and hemorrhage have also occurred [12]. Irradiation of the graft spleen may obviate graft versus host disease [37], but there is no evidence that inclusion of the spleen reduces the incidence of thrombosis.

Occurrence of ascitis was frequent in case of intraperitoneal open free duct grafts [6]. Fluid collections (pseudocysts) occur with all types of grafts. The major hazard of intraabdominal fluid collection is secondary infection, which usually leads to graft loss. In our experience, the incidence of this complication was lower with the duct obstruction than with the enteric drainage technique [32].

Conclusions

Many different surgical techniques have been described for pancreas transplantation. The increased pancreatic mass of whole vs segmental pancreas graft has not been demonstrated to provide metabolic control superior to that achieved with segmental grafts. The technical failures rates (including vascular thrombosis), has also been no different for whole and segmental grafts. Duct obstruction is the simplest and safest technique for handling of the exocrine secretions. Graft fibrosis might have a deleterious effect on the endocrine tissue at long term, although this has not occurred in our experimental and clinical experience. Pancreatico-duodenal transplantation with enteric diversion is more physiological, but in our experience has been more complicated and time consuming, and with no difference in outcome.

In the Transplant Registry, the results with the commonly used techniques are reported to be the same [13]. Bladder drainage, enteric drainage and duct obstruction all have similar long term graft survival rates. However, the advantage of diagnosing graft rejection by measuring changes in urinary amylases or pH may give bladder drainage an advantage in nonuremic, non-kidney transplant recipients [11]. Comparative studies under standard conditions (same surgical team, comparable criteria for patients selection, same immunosuppression, etc.) are needed in order to determine the technique of choice for pancreas transplantation. The optimal technique may differ for different categories of patients, and studies in which the recipients are appropriately stratified could help in this determination. Meanwhile, the results with all techniques continue to improve, and multiple options exist for the pancreas transplant surgeon.

References

1. Kelly WD, Lillehei RC, Merkel FK et al: Allotransplantation of the pancreas and duodenum along with a kidney in diabetic nephropathy. Surgery 61: 827–837, 1967.
2. Lillehei RC, Simmons RL, Najarian JS et al: Pancreaticoduodenal allotransplantation: experimental and clinical experience. Ann Surg 172: 405–436, 1970.
3. Gliedman ML, Gold M, Whitker J et al: Pancreatic duct to ureter anastomosis in pancreatic transplantation. Am J Surg 125: 245–252, 1973.
4. Dubernard JM, Traeger J, Neyra P et al: A new method of preparation of segmental pancreatic grafts for transplantation: trials in dogs and in man. Surgery 84: 633–639, 1978.
5. Sutherland DER, Moudry KC: Pancreas transplant registry: history and analysis of cases 1966 to october 1986. Pancreas 2: 473–488, 1987.
6. Sutherland DER, Baumgartner D, Najarian JS: Free intraperitoneal drainage of segmental pancreas grafts: clinical and experimental observations on technical aspects. Transpl Proc 12 (Suppl 2): 26–32, 1980.
7. Groth CG, Lundgren G, Gunnarson R, Hardstedt C, Ostman J: Segmental pancreatic transplantation with special reference to the use of ileal exocrine diversion and to the hemodynamics of the graft. Transpl Proc 12 (Suppl 2): 62–67, 1980.
8. Groth CG, Collste H, Lundgren G et al: Successful outcome of segmental human pancreatic transplantation with enteric exocrine diversion after modifications in technique. Lancet 2: 522–524, 1982.
9. Cook K, Sollinger HW, Warner T, Kamps D, Belzer FO: Pancreaticocystostomy: an alternative method for exocrine drainage of segmental pancreatic allografts. Transpl 35: 634, 1983.
10. Sutherland DER, Goetz FC, Najarian JS: One hundred pancreas transplants at a single institution. Ann Surg, 200 (No 4): 414–440, 1984.
11. Sollinger H, Kalayoglu M, Hoffman RM et al: Experience with whole pancreas transplantation and pancreaticoduodenocystostomy. Transpl Proc 18: 1759–1761, 1986.
12. Starzl TE, Iwatsuki S, Shaw BW Jr, Green DA, van Thiel DH, Nalesnik MA, Nusbacher J, Diliz-Pere H, Hakala TR: Pancreaticoduodenal transplantation in humans. Surg Gynecol Obstet 159: 265–272, 1984.
13. Prieto M, Sutherland DER, Goetz FC, Najarian JS: Pancreas transplant results according to technique of duct management: Bladder versus enteric drainage. Surgery 102: 680–691, 1987.
14. Nghiem DD, Corry RJ: Technique of simultaneous pancreaticoduodenal transplantation with urinary drainage of pancreatic secretions. Am J Surg 153: 405–406, 1987.
15. Dubernard JM, Martin X, Faure JL et al: Effect of intraductal injection of Neoprene on the canine pancreas. Transpl Proc 12 (Suppl 2): 123, 1980.
16. Dubernard JM, Traeger J, Devonec M, Touraine JL: Pancreatic transplantation in man: Surgical technique and complications. Transpl Proc 12 (Suppl 2): 40, 1980.
17. Gil-Vernet JM, Fernandez-Cruz L, Andren J et al: Clinical experience with pancreaticopyelostomy for exocrine pancreatic drainage and portal venous drainage in pancreas transplantation. Transpl Proc 17 (No 1): 342–345, 1985.
18. Calne RY: Paratopic segmental pancreas grafting: A technique with portal venous drainage. The Lancet, March 17, 595–597, 1984.
19. Sutherland DER, Goetz FC, Najarian JS: Living related donor segmental pancreatectomy for transplantation. Transpl Proc 12 (Suppl 2): 19–23, 1980.
20. Dubernard JM, Traeger J, Bosi E, Gelet A et al: Transplantation for the treatment of insulin-dependent diabetes: Clinical experience with polymer-obstructed pancreatic grafts using neoprene. World J Surg 8, 262–266, 1984.
21. Sutherland DER, Goetz FC, Abouna GM et al: Use of recipient mesenteric vessels for revascularization of segmental pancreas transplants. Transpl Proc 19: 2300–2304, 1987.

22. Wilczek H, Gunnarsson R, Felig P et al: Normalization of hepatic glucose regulation following heterotopic pancreatic transplantation in humans. Transpl. Proc 17: 315–316, 1985.
23. Land W, Liebe W, Kuhlmann H, Eberhard E: Stimultaneous kidney and pancreas transplantation using prolamine for duct obstruction. Transpl Proc 12 (Suppl 2): 76–77, 1980.
24. McMaster P, Gibby OM, Evans DB, Calne RY: Human pancreatic transplantation with polyisoprene and cyclosporin A immunosuppression. Proc. 1980 EASD satellite symposium islet-pancreas transplantation and artificial pancreas. Horm Metab Res 22, 151–156, 1981.
25. Sutherland DER, Goetz FC, Elick BA et al: Experience with 49 segmental pancreas transplants in 45 diabetic patients. Transplantation 34: 330–336, 1982.
26. Steiner E, Klima J, Niederwieser D et al: Monitoring of the pancreatic allograft by analysis of exocrine secretion. Transpl Proc 19: 2336–2338, 1987.
27. Baumgartner D, Bruhlmann W, Largiader F: Technique and timing of pancreatic duct occlusion with prolamine in recipients of simultaneous renal and segmental pancreas allotransplants. Transpl Proc 16: 1134–1135, 1986.
28. Tyden G, Wilezek H, Lundgren G, Osteman J et al: Experience with 21 intraperitoneal segmental pancreatic transplants with enteric drainage or gastric exocrine diversions in humans. Transpl Proc 17 (No 1): 331–335, 1985.
29. Frisk BA, Hedman LA, Brynger HA: Segmental pancreas transplantation with exocrine drainage into the bladder in man-technique outcome. Transplantation (in press).
30. Corry RJ, Nghiem DD, Schulark JA et al: Surgical treatment of diabetic nehropathy with stimultaneous pancreatico-duodenal and renal transplantation. Surg Gynecol Obstet 162: 547–555, 1986.
31. Sollinger HW: Transplantation of the intact pancreas organ: Urinary drainage for pancreas transplantation. Transplantation and Immunology Letter 3 (No 1): 1–10, 1986.
32. Dubernard JM, La Rocca E, Gelet A, Faure JL, Long D, Martin X, Lefracois N, Blanc N, Monti L, Touraine JL, Traeger J: Simultaneous pancreas and kidney transplantation long-term results and comparison of two surgical techniques. Transpl Proc 19: 2285–2287, 1987.
33. Calne RY, McMaster P, Rolles K et al: Technical observations in segmental pancreas transplantation: Observations on blood flow. Transpl Proc 12 (Suppl 2): 51–57, 1980.
34. Du Toit DF, Heyrenrych JJ, Smit B, Louw G, Zuurmond T, Laker L, Els D, Weideman A, Wolfe-Coote S, van der Merwe EA, Gorenewald WA: Segmental pancreatic allograft survival in baboons treated with combined irradiation and cyclosporin: a preliminary report. Surgery 97 (No 4): 447–453.
35. Deierhoi MH, Sollinger HW, Bozdech MJ, Belzer FO: Lethal graft versus host disease in a recipient of a pancreas-spleen transplant. Transpl 41: 544–546, 1986.
36. DaFoe DC, Campbell DA, Marks WH et al: Karyotypic chimerism and rejection in a pancreaticoduodenal splenic transplant. Transplantation 40: 572–574, 1985.
37. Koostra G, van Hooff JP, Jorning PJG, Leunissen KML, van der Linden CJ, Beukers E, Buurman WA: A new variant for whole pancreas grafting. Transpl Proc 19: 2314–2318, 1987.

Commentary I

The Chapter by Dubernard on Pancreas Transplants and Surgical Techniques describs in detail the necessary surgical maneuvers in both the donors and recipients, including techniques now rarely used but of historical interest, as well as those in common use today. The approaches at the University of

Minnesota differ in some details with those described by Dubernard, and in this commentary these differences are stressed.

In regard to cadaveric donors, there is no reason to use a limited incision, even when only a kidney and pancreas are harvested. Thus, we make a (cruciate bilateral subcostal and xyphopubic) incision in all cadaver donors, and add a sternotomy when the liver and heart are also harvested (most donors). There is no need to achieve less than perfect hemostasis, even when procuring a whole pancreas in conjunction with the liver and other organs, and we perform a complete dissection of the pancreas, ligating all lymphatics, and only the vascular attachments remain at the end of the dissection. The pancreas is then removed along with other organs, with or without in situ flushing.

In the situation in which the whole pancreas and liver are procured, the options Dubernard describes for division of the vascular supply between the pancreas and liver are logical. One can retain the celiac axis with either the pancreas or the liver. When it is retained with the liver, only the superior mesenteric artery and the splenic artery go with the pancreas, and we have used a different arterial reconstruction technique than that described by Dubernard. Either we have directly anastomosed the end of the proximal splenic artery to the side of the proximal superior mesenteric artery, or we have used an iliac artery bifurcation grafts, anastomosing the hypogastric to the splenic and the external to the superior mesenteric artery, with the common iliac stump as the conduit for anastomosis in the recipient.

In regard to living related pancreas donation, Dubernard has described the surgical maneuvers precisely and concisely. The largest experience with living donation has been at the University of Minnesota, where over 60 such procurements have been carried out. The rationale for the use of living related donors has been the shortage of cadaver donors and the immunological advantage, with a decreased propensity for rejection. However, since pancreas transplantation is not a life saving measure, we largely restrict living related donations to specific situations, such as for individuals who have a high percentage of antibodies to the panel and in whom matching with a cadaver donor is unlikely, but a suitable living related donor exists to whom the recipient has a negative crossmatch. We have also used a living related donor in the situation where the donor has previously given a kidney, rejection has not occurred, and the pancreas can be transplanted with assurance that rejection is also unlikely. In such cases, we have yet to see loss of either a pancreas or a kidney graft from rejection. The surgical complications have occurred in 8 of 63 donors (12%), and include splenectomy in 2, reoperation for religation of pancreas duct in one, and percutaneous drainage of fluid collections in 5, 3 sterile and 2 infected. Oral glucose tolerance test (OGTT) results have remained normal in two-thirds and have become abnormal in one-third of the donors after distal pancreatectomy. Two donors developed a type II diabetes. The changes in glucose tolerance tests are similar magnitude to those in creatinine clearance following uninephrectomy for living related kidney donation. In a retrospective analysis of test results, all with an adnormal OGTT result postoperatively had a low first phase insulin release during a preoperative intravenous glucose tolerance testing. While not all with a low first phase insulin release developed an abnormal OGTT result, all those with normal first phase insulin release had normal postoperative OGTT results. Thus, we now select donors from volunteers who have a high first phase insulin release on IVGTT, and exclude those that do not.

In regard to the recipient operation, of the techniques described by Dubernard, only three are in common use today, duct injection, enteric drainage, and bladder drainage. At the University of Minnesota we now use bladder drainage nearly exclusively for cadaver donor transplants, because of the advantage of using urinary amylase for early diagnosis of rejection, the only marker other than plasma glucose in nonuremic, nonkidney transplant recipients of pancreas grafts. For living related transplants we still use enteric drainage because of the ease with which segmental grafts may be enteric drained, but we have also used bladder drainage in this group. Until new markers for early diagnosis of rejection are available, we will continue to use the bladder drainage technique.

In regard to the site of graft placement, we differ with Dubernard and prefer the right side for the pancreas graft. The right iliac vessels are easily approached without the need to reflect the colon no matter which drainage technique. Bladder drainage is particularly facilitated by use of the right side, whether pancreatic-ducto-cystostomy for segmental or pancreatic-duodeno-cystostomy for whole organ grafts. However, if the right side has been used for previous kidney transplant, the left side is perfectly acceptable using the transmesocolic approach described by Dubernard in which the pancreas graft is easily placed intraperitoneally. For simultaneous transplantation of pancreas and kidney grafts, we place the pancreas on the right side and the kidney on the left side, but the kidney is placed lateral to the sigmoid colon rather than transmesocolic. We use the transmesocolic approach only when it is the pancreas that is placed on the left side.

As noted by Dubernard, several options are available for the pancreas transplant surgeon, and the choice of technique may depend on the individual situation. For example, a recipient with pancreatic exocrine deficiency, might benefit from enteric drainage for relief of this problem, and we have done so in two cases. Otherwise, bladder drainage is preferred because of the provision of a marker (urine amylase) for early diagnosis and treatment of rejection. Dubernard and his colleagues are to be congratulated for carrying out a prospective study comparing two techniques, enteric drainage and duct injection, in uremic recipients of simultaneous pancreas and kidney transplants.

As Dubernard indicates, other techniques should also be compared in prospective studies, stratified according to the category of recipient, in order to determine which is the best approach in a given situation.

D.E.R. Sutherland
Department of Surgery
Medical School
University of Minnesota
Minneapolis, Minnesota 55455

Commentary II

For the development of a successful method in pancreatic transplantation four different techniques were used consecutively in Zurich. The initial approach with extraperitoneal pancreas organ transplantation and enteric drainage [1] as well as the second attempt with intrasplenic or intraportal transplantation of pancreatic microfragments [2] gave an unsatisfactory result (see Experience of the University Hospital of Zurich, chapter 13). In a third step since 1980, the program was continued with the technique of intraperitoneal segmental pancreatic transplantation with Prolamin duct obliteration and hence more encouraging results [3]. However, recurrent pancreatic fistulae, caused by premature degradation of the occlusive material, led to a last modification of the procedure in 1983. Since then the technique of delayed percutaneous duct obliteration with Prolamin remained our method of choice. Thereupon the incidence of early loss of graft function, exocrine fistulae and the number of subsequent reoperations was markedly reduced, whereas the one-year graft survival rate improved close to 50% average [4].

Surgical technique

This has been described previously in detail [5]. Briefly, pancreatic segments based on the splenic vessels were transplanted intraperitoneally to the left iliac vessels through a lower midline incision, the graft being placed in the pouch of Douglas. A silicon rubber catheter was inserted into the pancreatic duct and brought out through a stab would in the abdominal wall, temporarily diverting the exocrine juice to the exterior. Four to eight weeks later occlusion of the pancreatic duct was performed by fluoroscopically controlled Prolamin injection through the catheter which was withdrawn afterwards.

Discussion

In spite of a definite progress during the recent years, the worldwide one-year pancreas allograft survival rate is still well under the results of other solid organ transplants. The reasons for this are mainly technical complications, primarily due to exocrine secretion and graft thrombosis. Numerous methods have been employed to overcome these delicate obstacles, however, the uniform results [6] do not indicate at present a preferable surgical procedure. On the contrary, even the optimal transplant size and the implantation site resumed to be a subject of discussion. But the real issue remains the question whether drainage of the superfluous exocrine secretion into a hollow viscus or sealing of the exocrine tissue by the duct occlusion technique is the method of choice.

The distinct disadvantage of the *drainage procedures* is the increased risk for complications due to extended surgical manipulations in the immunocompromised host. In the case of enteric drainage, opening of the small intestine contaminates the field, causing frequent wound sepsis. Moreover, activation of the drained pancreatic enzymes due to enteric and microbial contamination often led to anastomotic breakdown and consequent infectious complications. This became somewhat better with the introduction of a pancreatic duct diversion catheter, preserving the pancreaticoenteric anastomosis temporarily from digestive enzymes [7, 8]. The bladder drainage on the other hand seemed to offer a relative simple technique with minimal bacterial contamination at the time of transplantation as well as the possibility of monitoring urinary amylase and pH. The latter promised to be valid markers of rejection, particularly interesting in isolated pancreas transplantation, but their usefulness is still controversial [9, 10]. Furthermore, the pancreaticocystostomy procedure also was subject to complications in that serious metabolic acidosis may occur, sometimes requiring intravenous bicarbonate infusion, whereas casual enzyme activation may cause autodigestional erosions of bladder mucosa and severe urethritis [11].

In regard to these considerable problems and the fact that the latest pancreas transplant registry report [6] revealed no distinct advantage of any drainage procedure, it seems reasonable to us to continue with the *duct obliteration method*. Complications with this technique – mainly exocrine fistulae –, formerly not less frequent but anyhow less dangerous for the patient, have been further reduced since the postponement of duct occlusion. Prolamin appears the most suitable occlusive material due to its property of being reabsorbed and radiopaque. The latter is an essential prerequisite for the delayed injection technique. The argument that occlusion-induced fibrosis of the pancreatic transplant may lead to gradual deterioration of endocrine function has yet to be proven. Our patient with the longest functioning graft survival is actually $6^{1}/_{2}$ years from transplantation and presents consistently a normal glucose metabolism.

The question of whether *a whole organ or a segmental graft* should be used depends in part upon the employed technique for exocrine management. The supporters of the whole organ technique argue at least, that the utilization of a donor duodenal portion for cystostomy or jejunostomy would better prevent exocrine drainage complications [12, 13]. However, when duct occlusion is established a pancreatic segment is preferable, the exocrine tissue amount to be sealed and becoming fibrotic desirably being as small as possible. Futhermore, the donor operation to harvest a segment is easier compared to the removal and meticulous ex vivo preparation of a whole pancreatico-duodenal graft and may therefore be less traumatic, this possibly being important as a prophylaxis against pancreatitis and thrombosis. Finally, the technique of pancreatic segment retrieval is more easily compatible to liver procurement from the same donor and allows even living-related pancreas graft donation, the latter not suitable in our clinic.

The *intraperitoneal positioning* as optimal site for pancreas transplantation has been long since widely accepted. The resorptive capacity of the peritoneum prevents peritransplant fluid collections and consequent abscess formation. Thereby tube drainage of the transplantation site, frequently starting point for infection or chronic fistulae, becomes unnecessary or of very short duration. For this reason duct-occluded pancreatic segments with inevitable transcapsular exsudation and secretion of exocrine juice from the cut end should be placed intraperitoneally. Whenever extraperitoneal implantation of a whole or segmental transplant with exocrine drainage is performed, large windows are usually created by widely opening of the peritoneum. This precaution is necessary due to lymphatic fluid secretion from the pancreas surface. Furthermore, specific and unspecific defense mechanisms of the peritoneum decrease the risk of secondary bacterial contamination [14].

Compared to all these advantages, it is of minor importance whether an untouched peritoneal cavity might be beneficial in patients on CAPD, as argued by one of the few groups that resumed total extraperitoneal pancreas transplantation [15]. *Pancreatic graft thrombosis* on the contrary, originating mainly from the abnormal hemodynamic situation in the transplant, still represents a major drawback. The pancreas originally takes only a small percentage of the celiac blood flow, thus after removal of the spleen a poor blood flow results in the feeding and draining transplant vessels. Moreover, coagulation abnormalities and poor quality of the arteriae wall in the diabetic recipient increase the risk for venous and arterial thrombosis. With the aim of increasing graft vessels blood flow, creation of an av-fistula between the distal splenic vessels [16] as well as interposition of the splenic artery [17] have been tried, a distinct advantage not being clearly evident. For the same purpose inclusion of the donor spleen with the transplanted pancreas was attempted but later generally abandoned due to the risk for GVHR. In any case, the following preventive measures seem advisable. Meticulous surgical technique during the donor operation to prevent trauma to the pancreas, as well as during the recipient operation to avoid any kinking, twisting or tensing of the graft vessels. Anticoagulation prophylaxis, at least for the first postoperative period. Finally, through patient selection criteria to eliminate inappropriate candidates having severe macroangiopathic lesions.

In *conclusion*, our current technique of intraperitoneal segmental pancreas transplantation with delayed Prolamin duct occlusion is based on the following well-established technical principles: 1 the use of a segment enables a simple donor operation and is easily compatible to multi organ harvesting from the same donor. 2 the duct occlusion method allows an uncomplicated and safe surgical procedure in the recipient as it saves a risky accompanying drainage operation. 3 the postponement of duct obliteration facilitates early graft function monitoring and reduces incidence of fistulae. 4 Prolamin provides a convenient occlusive material since it is radiopaque and reabsorbable. 5 the intraperitoneal positioning takes advantage of the indispensable resorptive and defensive qualities of the peritoneal cavity. 6 no-touch technique for the donor pancreatectomy and meticulous anastomosis installation in the recipient together with an anticoagulation prophylaxis are reliable means to prevent graft thrombosis.

References

1. Largiadèr F: Clinical cases of pancreatic organ allotransplantation. Transplant Proc 12: 81–82, 1980.
2. Kolb E, Largiadèr F: Clinical islet transplantation. Transplant Proc 12: 205–207, 1980.
3. Baumgartner D, Largiadèr F: Simultaneous renal and intraperitoneal segmental pancreatic transplantation: the Zurich experience. World J Surg 8: 267–269, 1984.
4. Decurtins M, Schlumpf R, Baumgartner D, Largiadèr F: Three years experience with delayed duct occlusion in intraperitoneal pancreas transplantation. Transplant Proc 19: 3939–3940, 1987.
5. Schlumpf R, Largiadèr F, Decurtins M: Experience in clinical pancreas transplantation – university of Zurich. Transplant Proc 19 (Suppl 4): 92–95, 1987.
6. Sutherland DER, Moudry KC: Pancreas transplant registry report – 1986. Clin Transplantation 1: 3–17, 1987.
7. Corry RJ, West JC: Duct drainage through a long polyethylene catheter in Roux-en-Y limb. Transplant Proc 12 (Suppl 2): 93–94, 1980.
8. Groth CG, Lundgren G, Klintmalm G, Gunnarsson R, Collste H, Wilczek H, Ringdén O, Oestman J: Successful outcome of segmental human pancreatic transplantation with enteric exocrine diversion after modification in technique. Lancet 2: 522–524, 1982.
9. Tom WW, Munda R, First MR, Alexander JW: Physiologic consequences of pancreatic allograft exocrine drainage into the urinary tract. Transplant Proc 19: 2339–2342, 1987.
10. Dafoe DC, Campbell DA, Merion RM, Rosenberg L, Rocher LL, Vinik AI. Vine AK, Turcotte JG: Pancreatic transplantation – university of Michigan. Transplant Proc 19 (Suppl 4): 55–62, 1987.

130

11. Tom WW, Munda R, First MR, Alexander JW: Autodigestion of the glans penis and urethra by activated transplant pancreatic exocrine enzymes. Surgery 102: 99–101, 1987.

12. Sollinger HW, Belzer FO, Kalayoglu M: Transplantation of the intact pancreas organ: urinary drainage for pancreas transplantation. Transplant Immunol Lett 3: 1, 1986.

13. Corry RJ, Nghiem DD: Evolution of technique and results of pancreas transplantation at the university of Iova. Clin Transplantation 1: 52–56, 1987.

14. Illner WD, Gottwald Th, Abendroth D, Land W: Incidence of fistulas following human pancreas transplantation – positive influence of reabsorption of pancreatic secretions by the peritoneum. Transplant Proc 19: 2323–2324, 1987.

15. Kootstra G, van Hooff JP, Jörning PJG, Leunissen KML, van der Linden CJ, Beukers E, Buurman WA: A new variant for whole pancreas grafting. Transplant Proc 19: 2314–2318, 1987.

16. Calne RY, McMaster P, Rolles K, Duffy TJ: Technical observations in segmental pancreas allografting: observations on pancreatic blood flow. Transplant Proc 12 (Suppl 2): 51–57, 1980.

17. Brekke IB, Norstein J: Pancreatic transplant revascularization by dual arterial anastomoses. Transplant Proc 19: 3874–3875, 1987.

R. Schlumpf & F. Largiadèr
Universitätsspital
Departement Chirurgie
Rämistrasse 100
CH-8091 Zürich
Switzerland

6. Organ preservation

G. FLORACK

Introduction

Pancreatic transplantation as a procedure to achieve normalisation of the perturbed endocrine function in juvenile onset diabetics has increasingly drawn attention in recent years as demonstrated in reports given in this issue. Nevertheless, the frequency of pancreas transplants performed is still small when compared to that of other organs such as kidneys or livers. This discrepancy may be caused from the different intention for transplantation of various organs, since pancreas transplantation is not necessary for immediate life saving, but provides improvement in quality of life by halting the progression of impending secondary lesions associated with diabetes mellitus. In addition, technical problems with transplantation of the pancreas itself evolving from the characteristics of the gland with its complex two-fold endocrine and exocrine function has led to an initial reluctance of physicians to advice patients to undergo this procedure. In view of the recent data [1] reflecting the continuing improvement in the results of pancreas transplantation and the large reservoir of patients with type-1 diabetes as potential recipients, the demand on pancreatic organs for transplantation is likely to increase dramatically. In order to meet this request, it will be necessary to utilize all available cadaver organs through sharing and transportation between transplant centers.

To make a significant impact on widespread application of pancreas transplantation, reliable techniques of pancreatic graft preservation are needed. In case pancreas transplantation could be performed consistently successful after preservation periods of 12–36 hours, this time would be sufficient to complete the logistical maneuvers associated with organ transplantation.

J.M. Dubernard and D.E.R. Sutherland (eds.), International Handbook of Pancreas Transplantation, 131–154.
© *1989 by Kluwer Academic Publishers.*

Basic principles of organ preservation

Organ preservation is based on reduction of the metabolism at low temperatures. The consumption of oxygen, which is mandatory for energy supply, is significantly reduced during hypothermia. Levy [2] demonstrated that the oxygen consumption of canine kidneys during cooling at 10°C is only 5% compared to that at normal body temperatures. Both currently applied techniques of organ preservation utilize the effect of reduction in metabolism. The organ can either be flushed initially with cold preservation solution and is then stored in the same medium during the preservation period or a continuous or pulsatile machine perfusion of the graft is performed. The latter approach mimics, in vitro, a semi-physiologic situation combined simultaneously with hypothermic conditions. A criterion for organ preservation is the maintenance of the ion content in the extra- and intracellular space which therefore is of importance in the design of the preservation solutions. The extracellular space is rich in sodium (140 mEq/l), chloride (105 mEq/l) and bicarbonate (27 mEq/l), whereas intracellular potassium (90–150 mEq/l), magnesium (40 mEq/l) and phosphate (110 mEq/l) are dominant with a relatively low content of sodium and chloride. In order to maintain the ion distribution of the intra- and extracellular space, an electrochemical potential gradient exists over the cell membrane, mainly supported by energy-rich phosphates, the most important of which is adenosine-triphosphate (ATP). There is a continuous active potassium and sodium exchange between the cell interior and the external milieu (K^+/Na^+ ion pump) which requires energy. A disadvantageous effect of hypothermia is the reduction of the ATP level [3], resulting in an inactivity of the ion pump [4]. While the membrane potential disappears, a loss of intracellular potassium and magnesium occurs into the extracellular space in exchange with a higher intrusion of sodium and chloride into the cell, consequently followed by an uptake of water in order to equilibrate for the increased intracellular osmotic concentration. The final result is swelling of the cell [5, 6, 7, 8, 9].

The cell injury during hypothermia causes the 'no-reflow phenomenon' [10], which means the prevention of an immediate normal blood circulation through capillaries and small blood vessels of the transplanted graft.

The rationale in the composition of the flush solutions is to avoid both side effects of hypothermia, edema formation and potassium loss of the cells, by creating preservation solutions which are hypertonic and hyperkalemic [11, 12]. To achieve this goal various preservation solutions with different additives are recommended. Controversy exists concerning the amount of osmolality required for preservation solutions; the value in human plasma ranges around 290 mosm/l.

The theoretical considerations and experimental observations mentioned here were made initially with preservation of kidney grafts [13, 14, 15], but are useful also for other organs exposed to hypothermic conditions.

Experimental studies

Major problems encountered with pancreas preservation are related to the anatomical characteristics of the pancreas which is an organ with a complex double metabolic task, which develops rapidly intense edema even after minimal manipulation and which has, uncommon to the kidney, a low blood flow characteristic through its vasculature. Therefore most attempts to apply kidney preservation technology to the pancreas have produced less satisfactory results unless distinct modifications in technique were made.

The first systematic experimental investigations on preservation of the pancreas were undertaken by Idezuki et al. [16, 17] using a hyperbaric oxygen chamber for hypothermic storage of pancreaticoduodenal and segmental grafts. In their initial in vitro studies [16] they demonstrated a progressive decline in insulin response to glucose stimulation in grafts stored for 6 to 48 hours, which correlated with the outcome of pancreaticoduodenal canine allografts after transplantation. Graft viability was maintained up to 22 hours of preservation, whereas grafts preserved for longer periods became hemorrhagic shortly after restoration of blood flow [17]. The beneficial effect on graft survival after storage within a hyperbaric chamber (4 atmospheres) is probably related to the high pressure which helps to minimize edema and not to the oxygen supply. Since this technique was cumbersome and difficult to standardize it had no wide application for organ protection. Simple cold storage of segmental pancreas grafts was used by Serrou et al. [18]. They found that canine recipients of pancreas grafts stored in a protein gel for 8 hours survived longer than those receiving grafts stored in Collins solution (C4) or in polysaccharide gel for 8 hours. The average survival time was even longer after 24 hours graft preservation using the protein gel than with other solutions tested for shorter preservation periods. This example is typical of many experiments in which success or failure of a preservation technique was only monitored by the survival rate of the recipients of allografts, making differentiation between graft failure due to technical reasons from those of rejection extremely difficult. In few experimental designs reliability of hypothermic pancreas preservation was tested in an autotransplant model. Baumgartner [19] found a successful outcome with Collins solution for pancreas grafts preserved for 24 hours at 4° C, these results were confirmed by van Schilfgaarde et al. [20] using Euro-Collins. Slight deterioration of endocrine function after 4 weeks was attributed to the pancreatic duct management which caused graft fibrosis. Du Toit [21] showed similar good results when segmental pancreatic autografts were flushed with hypertonic citrate and stored on ice for 24 hours prior to transplantation. Although normoglycemia was achieved, a glucose intolerance was observed at 1 month which was thought to be an irreversible damage to the endocrine component of the graft due to hypothermia.

In our own experiments [22] we found that both Collins solution and a modified hyperosmolal silica gel filtered plasma (SGFP) solution – the composition of which is given later – were satisfactory in cold storage of pancreas grafts for up to 24 hours (67% and 75% long-term graft survival, respectively). When the preservation time was extended to 48 hours, SGFP was more reliable than Collins solution (Figure 1). If non-preservation complications were excluded, there were no preservation failures of grafts stored in SGFP for up to 48 hours, while 50% of the grafts stored in Collins solution were preservation failures (p = 0.015). Cold storage in SGFP for 24–48 hours resulted in a long-term function rate of 75% in all dogs, a success rate similar to that in recipients of unpreserved fresh transplants (80%). Pancreas preservation for 72 hours was possible in SGFP, but unpredictable graft losses occurred.

Recently there were reports on experimental studies in dogs that even after 72 hours of preservation consistently successful pancreas transplantation could be performed. Two of the newly introduced preservation solutions utilized the basic concept of high osmolal silica gel filtered plasma, but containing the additives KH_2PO_4 (1.05 g/l), K_2HPO_4 (3.7 g/l) and sucrose (40 g/l) [23] or, in contrast to the original solution, replacing glucose by mannitol [24]. These preservation solutions are modifications of SGFP currently already in clinical use at the University of Minnesota.

A third new preservation solution, experimentally applied in canine pancreases for 72 hours [25] contains potassium lactobionate, 110 mM; raffinose, 30 mM, KH_2PO_4 25 mM, $MgSO_4$, 5 mM; hydroxyethylstarch, 5 g%, adenosine, 5 mM; insulin and decadrone. This solution remains to be tested clinically.

Dafoe [26] used the recently advocated technique of pancreaticoduodenal allotransplantation in pancreatectomized pigs after cold storage of the grafts in Euro-Collins solution. In contrast to the promising results mentioned above he found that after 24 hours preservation the grafts failed uniformly and that already after 4 hours of cold storage a detrimental effect was noticed showing a higher incidence of technical complications, a marked plasma hyperamylasemia, a relative glucose intolerance with hypoinsulinemia, and an abnormal pattern of insulin secretion after i.v. GTT. Euro-Collins was accused for the high failure rate and regarded to be an improper solution for preservation of pancreaticoduodenal grafts.

Pulsatile or continuous organ perfusion is considered to be an alternative concept for pancreas preservation. However, a common feature of the perfu-

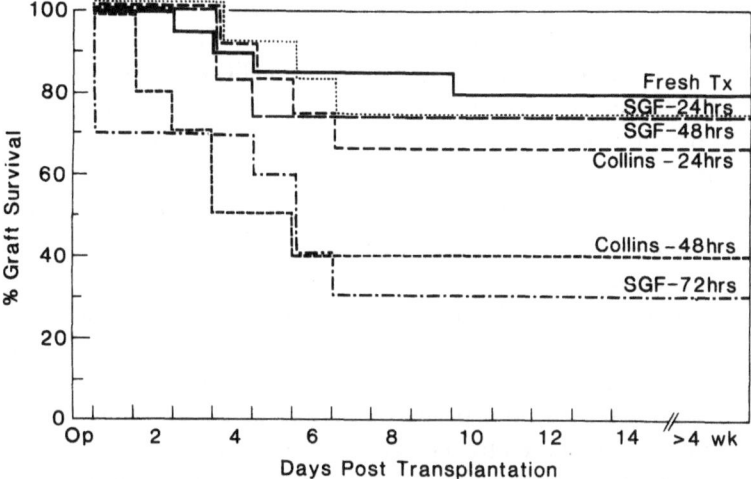

Figure 1. Functional survival of segmental pancreatic autografts preserved in either Collins solution or in hyperosmolal silica-gel-filtered plasma (SGF) prior to transplantation in totally pancreatectomized dogs.

sion machines currently in use is the provision of a high flow rate since these aggregates were originally designed for kidney preservation, an organ with a high blood flow characteristic. The pancreas, in contrast, has a low blood flow rate. Therefore when placing pancreas grafts on a perfusion machine distinct modifications in the technical set-up are required.

There are only few reports of experiments in which the investigators tried both cold storage and machine perfusion for pancreas preservation, and except from our own studies, all were done in allograft models. Brynger [27, 28] perfused canine segmental pancreas allografts with an albumin-containing extracellular electrolyte solution for 24 hours on a Gambro machine at a peak pressure of 50 mm/Hg and a high average flow rate of 95 ml/min. All grafts became edematous with weight gains of 135–275%, but 6 of 9 functioned after transplantation as did 4 of 8 grafts stored in a buffered invert sugar solution at 6–8° C for 24 hours.

De Gruyl et al. [29] and Westbroek et al. [30] transplanted whole pancreas duct-ligated canine allografts after 24 hours of either cold storage in Collins solution or perfusion with hyperosmolar cryoprecipitated dog plasma at a pressure of 60 mm Hg on a Belzer machine; all grafts functioned after transplantation.

Toledo-Pereyra et al. [31] cold stored or perfused whole pancreas duct ligated canine allografts with cryoprecipitated plasma (osmolarity: 310–330 mosm/l) on a Mox-100 machine at a pressure of 25–29 mm Hg for 24 hours.

4 of 6 grafts in each group functioned during the first week after transplantation. In later studies Toledo-Pereyra et al. [32] successfully used a colloid hyperosmolar solution (CHS) with an osmolality of 430–470 mosm/l for hypothermic storage of pancreas grafts for up to 48 hours. It was possible to extend the preservation time to 72 hours when a modified SGF solution was utilized [23].

In these studies it was not commented whether the high flow rates generated by the the organ perfusion machines caused any problems which may have led to subsequent organ loss.

When using a rat model Nolan [33] found cold storage to be consistently more successful than machine perfusion for pancreatic preservation. Despite adjusting the machine to a very low flow rate and using a hyperosmolar solution already after a 7 hour perfusion period the edema formation was a major problem, documented by the decreasing success rate.

In early experiments on pancreas preservation with the Mox-100 machine at Minnesota [34], segmental grafts were perfused with a silica gel plasma of normal osmolality (310 mosm/kg). Only after distinct adjustments of the perfusion machine which resulted in a low flow of 10–15 ml/min through the gland's vasculature, was a moderately successful 24 hour preservation rate achieved. However, all grafts failed when the preservation time was extended to 48 hours.

In follow-up experiments on pancreas preservation with pulsatile machine perfusion [35, 36] some of the techniques cited above were adapted, but further changes were made in the protocol, i.e., the graft was placed in a Petri dish and immersed in the perfusate solution, thus the graft received surface cooling at 7° C in addition to semiphysiologic pulsatile organ perfusion. The systemic machine flow was decreased but the peak perfusion pressure to the gland was kept at 30 mm Hg; and the osmolality of the perfusate was increased to 430 mosm/kg. After 24 hour organ preservation the results were fair, but the extension of the perfusion period to 48 hours led to an unacceptably high rate of immediate failure. Further modifications made to the perfusion solution such as increasing the osmolality to 470–500 mosm/kg, resulted in only a slight improvement in outcome after pancreas transplantation.

Pulsatile machine perfusion may inflict some damage to the pancreas that does not occur with cold storage alone. First, there is the rapid development of edema despite careful handling of the gland. Secondly, in the closed circuit system of a perfusion machine, pancreatic exocrine secretions pouring off the open ductal system are routed into the graft vasculature again which might be harmful. Thirdly, the profile of the pulse wave generated by the perfusion machine possibly also causes damage by disruption of tissue membranes.

In our study, flow rates in machine preserved grafts that functioned were lower (mean of 5 ml/min) than in those that failed (mean of 8.3 ml/min). Thus besides controlling the perfusion pressure it would be recommended to also continuously monitor and adjust the flow rate. In our experimental model the pure pancreas preservation failure rate with machine perfusion was between 30% and 40% at 24 to 48 hours. These results stand in contrast to the 0% preservation failure rate after 24 and 48 hours of cold storage in SGFP.

Of course a pancreas preservation technique by machine perfusion offers the advantages to perform physiologic and biochemical studies. It is certainly desirable to monitor viability parameters of the graft in vitro rather than placing the organ in cold storage and expecting it to work after transplantation. In search of an in vitro index of graft viability during pancreas preservation, Garvin et al. [37] recommended sequential perfusate amylase and blood gas determinations in order to predict future pancreatic transplant function. Also the historical studies by Idezuki [16] should be mentioned again where insulin production during organ perfusion was controlled.

On the other hand, most of the experimental work cited and the observations of our own studies show superior results after simple hypothermic storage compared to pulsatile machine perfusion for pancreas preservation. There is one convincing argument to favor one technique over the other for pancreas preservation, namely immediate and consistent graft function. Experimentally this can only be achieved with cold storage for at least 48 hours. Cold storage for pancreas preservation is also less complicated and less expensive than a continuous organ perfusion on an apparatus with its technical demands for maintenance and operation.

The colloid plasma solution, high osmolal SGFP, is recommended as persufate since it proved to be more reliable than the crystalloid solutions such as Collins' or Sacks'.

In addition to hypothermic preservation warm ischemia could affect the pancreatic graft. In experiments performed in dogs and rats [38, 39] it could be shown that at least the endocrine component of the pancreas has an amazingly long warm ischemia tolerance which is even greater than that of kidneys. However, the combination of warm ischemia (1 hour) plus cold storage (12–24 hours) was deleterious for the pancreas with some species-specific differences [40, 41]. There is evidence that the exocrine portion of the pancreas is more prone to the ischemic insult [42, 43]. Thus warm ischemia injury to the pancreatic graft must be avoided or reduced to a minimum especially when further cold ischemia periods are expected.

Clinical pancreatic organ preservation

Reports to the pancreas transplant registry

Preservation of human pancreatic allografts has shown to be disappointing when the period of cold ischemia is more than 6 hours. Therefore most transplant centers are reluctant to exceed this period of preservation for fear of irreversible ischemic damage to the pancreas graft [1, 44, 45, 46, 47, 48], however, in most instances the negative experiences have been made when pure electrolyte solutions for protection of the pancreatic organ were used. In early pancreas transplantation there are only anecdotal reports on pancreas preservation, mainly because there was the belief that any period of ischemia would harm the pancreatic allograft. At that time, still similar to the practice in many institutions today, or, in the situation of living related organ donation, the donor operation was carried out simultaneously with the recipient operation, allowing immediate transplantation of the pancreas after short cold flushing with heparinized Ringer's lactate. Between January, 1983 and August, 1986 information on pancreas transplant results according to duration of graft preservation are available through the transplant registry [44] on 617 pancreas grafts, most of which were preserved by cold storage in electrolyte solutions.

The functional survival rates for grafts stored <6 hours (45% at 1 year) were significantly higher than those stored from 6 to 12 hours (36% at 1 year), but there was no significant difference between those stored <6 hours and those stored >12 hours (40% at 1 year), nor between those stored 6 to 12 and those stored >12 hours (Figure 2). The technical failure rate was significantly higher for grafts stored 6 to 12 hours versus those stored < 6 hours (p = 0.004) but the difference between those stored for <6 hours vs >12 hours was not significant (p = 0.223). Thus, the lower functional survival rate for grafts stored 6 to 12 hours than those stored <6 hours or >12 hours may relate to a higher technical failure rate in the 6 to 12 hours group that was independent of preservation time; otherwise a higher technical failure rate could be expected in the >12 hour preservation group. On the other hand, the preservation solutions utilized may have had an impact on functional graft survival since most of the grafts preserved for <6 hours have been stored in simple electrolyte solutions while most of the grafts stored for >12 hours have been stored in hyperosmolar colloid solutions. At the intermediate time (6–12 hours), the pancreas grafts have been stored in both types of solution, and it may be that the detrimental effect of storage above 6 hours is seen only with the simple electrolyte solutions.

Patient survival rates did not differ according to pancreas graft preservation times (Figure 3).

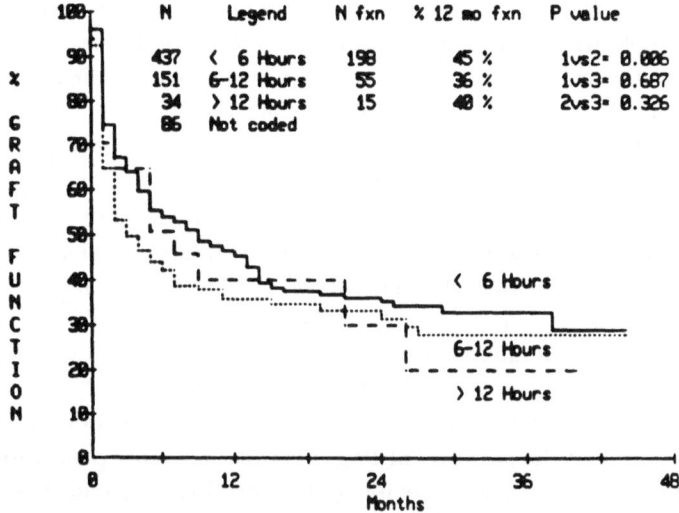

Figure 2. Graft function rates for cadaveric pancreas transplants (1. 1983 to 8. 1986) according to duration of graft preservation prior to transplantation. Pancreas Transplant Registry [44].

There are two different modalities of organ protection prior to transplantation, i.e., simple hypothermic storage or pulsatile respectively continuous machine perfusion at low temperatures. For kidney preservation there are controversial opinions as to which approach provides the best immediate and long term results [49, 50, 51], but general agreement exists for pancreas grafts,

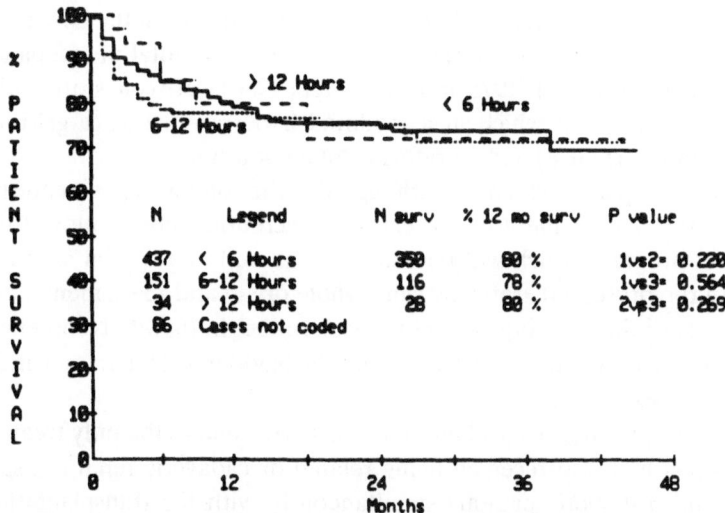

Figure 3. Patient survival rates for cadaveric pancreas transplants (1. 1983 to 8. 1986) according to duration of graft preservation prior to transplantation. Pancreas Transplant Registry [44].

that cold storage is the only appropriate technique. Similar to experimental findings, hypothermic perfusion of human pancreatic grafts has shown to be more expensive, technically demanding, and not effective for clinical pancreas preservation [42, 52]. It was therefore rarely used.

There are few individual reports on attempts to extend pancreas preservation for longer periods prior to transplantation, and so far, the experiences made have been disappointing. Since good initial graft function was a prerequisite for long-term success in pancreatic transplantation, Largiadèr et al. [53] emphasized that the warm ischemia time of pancreatic grafts should be short and the cold ischemia time should not exceed 10 hours. Tydén et al. [48] reported preservation failures due to pancreatitis in 3 of 13 grafts which had been preserved for longer than 6 hours. After changing their protocol, which also included performing of the pancreatic transplantation within 6 hours post harvesting, none of the subsequent 19 grafts were lost from pancreatitis.

In both institutions, the pancreatic grafts were hypothermically stored in intracellular-type electrolyte solutions (Euro-Collins and Perfadex solution).

At the University of Minnesota the preservation of pancreatic grafts is an integrated part of the pancreas transplant program, and attempts are made to continuously extend the safe preservation period. The results are given separately below.

Clinical experience with pancreas preservation at Minnesota

The most experience with transplantation of hypothermically preserved human pancreatic allografts to diabetic recipients is collected at the University of Minnesota [54, 55, 56]. 84 of 111 cadaveric grafts in a total of 165 pancreas transplants (between July 1978 until November 1986) were cold stored prior to transplantation, 82 of which in a modified hyperosmolal silica-gel-filtered plasma solution (SGFP) and 2 grafts in Collins solution.

Various transplant techniques with regard to the volume of pancreatic tissue used and the management of the exocrine secretion were employed in the transplant program which will be addressed as well in a special article (this issue). In the preserved grafts, 59 were whole organ and 25 segmental grafts. The pancreatic duct was injected with silicon rubber in 16, with Neoprene in 1, drained into a loop of the bowel in 36, into the bladder in 27, left open in 2 and ligated in 2 cases.

In 52 cases pancreas transplantation was performed as the only treatment. 27 recipients had also received living related or cadaveric renal transplants before, and 5 diabetic patients simultaneously with the transplantation of preserved pancreas grafts. The immunosuppressive regimen consisted of, in most cases, a triple drug therapy of cyclosporin, prednisone and azathioprine.

At the initiation of the pancreas transplant program at the University of Minnesota there was great reluctance to subject the pancreatic allograft to any period of ischemia. In this situation, the recipient and the donor were in adjacent operating rooms and the recipient was prepared for transplantation simultaneously with the donor pancreatectomy. The pancreas was transplanted immediately after cooling with heparinized Ringer's lactate solution. This procedure required careful synchronization of the donor and recipient operation, with the need to have two operative theaters and two transplant teams at the same time available. It also has limited the availability of cadaveric grafts for transplantation, since organ procurement in distant institutions with the unavoidable time delay was considered to be deleterious to the graft.

Based on the experimental work already cited with evidence that silica-gel-filtered plasma (SGFP) is appropriate for hypothermic pancreas preservation, this solution was adopted the first time in May 1981 for pancreas protection in humans. After initial occasional and cautious attempts with preservation, the cold ischemia period was later gradually extended. The confidence to rely on this preservation technique is emphasized by the fact that since September 1982 all cadaveric pancreas grafts were preserved prior to transplantation.

The silica-gel-filtered-plasma solution is similar to that tested in the animal model. The SGF-basic solution, which originally is iso-osmolal with 300 mosm/kg, was modified for hypothermic pancreas preservation.

Silica-Gel-Filtered Plasma (SGFP), modified hyperosmolal solution for cold storage pancreas preservation

SFG-plasma	400 ml
25% human albumin	100 ml
50% dextrose	10 ml
methyl prednisolone	250 mg
potassium chloride	20 mEq/l
magnesium sulfate	8 mEq/l
ampicillin	250 mg

The final osmolal concentration of the solution is 420 mosmol/kg and its electrolyte composition is:

Na, 135 mEq/l, K, 22.5 mEq/l, Cl, 85 mEq/l,

PO_4, 9 mEq/l, Mg, 8 mg/dl, Ca, 6 mg/dl,

glucose, 1180 mg/dl, albumin, 7.8 g/dl.

SGFP has been earlier applied successfully to kidney preservation and the advantages of the solution were already mentioned by the investigators [57, 58]. Almost all of the fibrinogen, cholesterol, lipoproteins and triglycerides can be precipitated. SGF has been shown to remove bacteria and herpes virus as well as any trace of red blood cell membranes, leukocytes and platelets. SGFP can be stored at room temperature. In the composition designed for cold storage pancreas preservation there are some characteristics which are considered to contribute to the success with modified SGFP.

- hyperosmolality, which is known to reduce cellular swelling and thus possibly improving the revascularization after transplantation by preventing the 'no-reflow phenomenon'.
- a moderately high potassium concentration as well as the presence of osmotic active ions ($MgSO_4$) within the extracellular space, which might reduce the migration of ions and other cellular constituents into the extracellular space, and thus, in turn preventing the intracellular uptake of sodium chloride and water.
- the high protein concentration with albumin which prevents vascular collapse during flushing and as an impermeant solute it prevents movement of fluid into the extravascular space, thus eliminating severe organ edema.
- methyl prednisolone stabilizes the cell membranes by inhibiting the release of lysosomal enzymes.
- glucose is a slow permeant compound and acts as a metabolic substrate. It increases the cellular ATP. Thus glucose could be a source of energy-supply if necessary at temperatures around 4°C.

All these factors may contribute to maintain cellular integrity during preservation. Most of the constituents of SGFP provide theoretical advantages, nevertheless, the design of the composition of the solution is still empirical. Although it was shown that SGFP is more reliable than other preservation solutions in experimental and clinical preservation of the pancreas there is no clear explanation why this is the case.

More recently, in a further modification of SGFP, glucose was replaced by mannitol, an agent which is not metabolized and acts by simple physical regulation of cell homeostasis. Whether this alteration results in an even better outcome of preserved pancreas grafts after transplantation must still be proven clinically.

The applied preservation technique is simple and similar to that used for hypothermic kidney preservation. Harvesting of the pancreas must be performed with minimal manipulation of the gland and with negligible warm ischemia exposition. The graft is then immersed in iced saline and is immediately flushed intra-arterially with cold SGFP solution. The fluid containing bottle is positioned about 3 feet above the organ in order not to create a too high perfusion pressure. 200 ml of SFGP solution are sufficient for cooling and getting the graft's venous effluent clear of blood. Flushing with more fluid could already cause edema. The graft is placed in a sterile plastic bag containing more SGFP, which for reasons of sterility and continuation of cooling is placed in two more ice-slush filled bags. This package can be stored and transported in an ice-filled styrofoam box or kept in the refrigerator until the time of transplantation.

With this simple technique, in many instances the pancreas was harvested from brain-dead donors in a distant hospital and flown to the transplant center for subsequent transplantation.

Of the 84 preserved pancreatic grafts in the Minnesota series, 82 were cold stored with the standard SGFP solution, whereas, 2 were stored with Collins solution. Of the latter, one graft was preserved for 6 hours. This case was done before the study on pancreas preservation was initiated. The other graft was recently offered from an other institution and was preserved in Collins solution for about 8.5 hours. Both grafts showed only poor or no endocrine function, respectively.

The cold storage time in SGFP ranged from 2–26 hours, mean 12 ± 5.4 hours ($\pm$ S.D.). Five of the pancreas transplants functioned but early losses occurred due to vascular complications or patient death; those cases are excluded from further analysis.

Two grafts showed poor endocrine function after transplantation presumably from ischemic injury with only slight increase in C-peptides, and the patients remained on insulin. In one case the preservation period was 26 hours, however, also vascular problems have occurred which made the reoperation with partial graft resection necessary. The other failed graft was subjected to longer than 1/2 hour warm ischemia, the only pancreas which was exposed to such an insult. In addition, the graft was hypothermically preserved for 11 hours before transplantation.

In two more cases the preservation technique was accused for the graft loss. These pancreases were cold stored for 10 and 12 hours, respectively, demonstrating normoglycemia after transplantation but both developed a severe and irreversible pancreatitis and had to be removed 25 and 14 days later despite sustained endocrine function. These examples might indicate that the exocrine portion of the pancreas is more vulnerable to ischemia than the endocrine portion.

All other preserved grafts functioned immediately after transplantation. Three pancreatic grafts transplanted recently after preservation times of 26 hours are functioning and the patients are insulin-independent.

Figures 4 and 5 illustrate the 24-hour metabolic profile, serum C-peptides, serum insulin and the oral glucose tolerance test before and at 1 month after transplantation in a patient who received a whole cadaver pancreas allograft which had been preserved for 11 hours.

In 1986 a study was carried out at Minnesota [56, 59] to investigate the effect of preservation on the early function and late outcome of human pancreas allografts which were transplanted after preservation in cold SGFP solution for various periods of 2–26 hours. 56 preserved cadaveric pancreas grafts

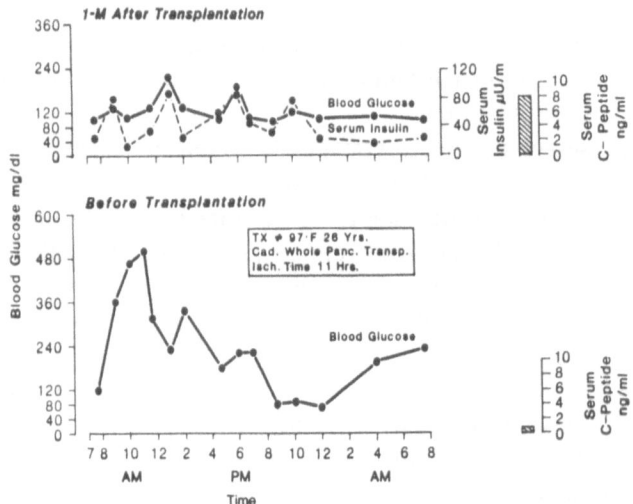

24-Hour Metabolic Profile

Figure 4. 24 hour metabolic profile, serum C-peptide, and serum insulin before and at 1 month following transplantation in a recipient of a pancreatic allograft preserved for 11 hours.

which were transplanted between August 1982 and June 1986 entered the analysis.

Pancreas transplants were subdivided into groups according to preservation periods of 2 to 6 hours (Group I), 6 to 12 hours (Group II), and 12 to 26 hours (Group III).

Early after transplantation the graft viability was assessed by incidence of primary non-function, insulin-independence within 2 weeks, function at 1 month and highest level of serum amylase. The results are depicted in Table 1. There was no statistical difference between any of the viability parameters measured with regard to the period of preservation.

Specific endocrine function tests, carried out 4–5 weeks after transplantation showed normal ranges in 85%, 72% and 78% of grafts for the 24 hour metabolic profile; in 43%, 83% and 68% for the glucose tolerance test, and in 100% for the serum C-peptides for groups I, II, and III.

The long-term outcome was influenced by factors other than length of preservation period, and major causes of graft loss were technical failure, rejection and patient death.

The results at Minnesota clearly show that preservation of pancreatic allografts can be successfully achieved for periods of at least 26 hours without serious damage to the organ. Providing the warm ischemia time is negligible, the graft viability and function are similar regardless of the period of preservation, at least during the first month after grafting, where the effect and the

Oral G.T.T.

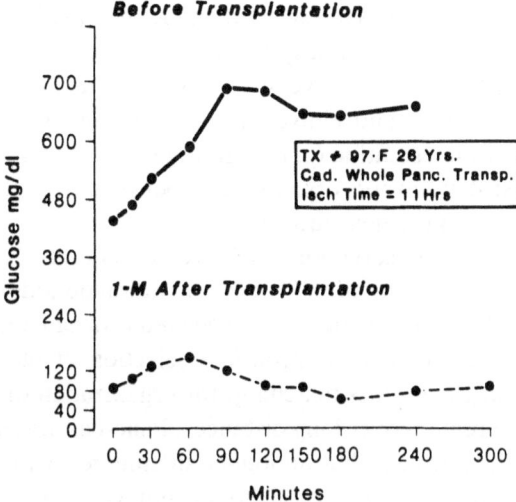

Figure 5. Oral GTT before and at 1 month following transplantation in the same patient as in Figure 4.

degree of preservation injury in pancreas transplantation is likely to become manifest. Although there was evidence in two cases that pancreatitis has occurred due to ischemic injury, this rate is low when compared to the data of other institutions [44, 48]. Graft pancreatitis is very common when intracellular-type electrolyte solutions are used for pancreas preservation for more than 6 hours.

Table 1. Viability of transplanted human pancreatic allografts after cold storage preservation in SGFP.

Group	Cold ischemia hours	No. of grafts	Primary non-function		Insulin independence within 2 weeks		Function at 1 month		Highest mean sr. amylase IU/L
			N	(%)	N	(%)	N	(%)	
I	2–6 (4.1 ± 1.3)	10	0	–	10	(100)	7	(70)	557 ± 661
II	6–12 (9.6 ± 1.5)	23	1	(4.3)	21	(91)	19	(82)	480 ± 690
III	12–26 (17.4 ± 4.1)	23	1	(4.3)	20	(87)	16	(70)	481 ± 425

146

In contrast to the data from the Transplant Registry [1, 44], recipients of pancreas grafts stored in SGFP for longer than 6 hours have remained insulin-independent and continue to have excellent endocrine function for up to three years post transplantation. Currently three transplant centers in the upper midwest region of the USA (University of Minnesota, Minneapolis, University of Iowa, Iowa City and University of Michigan, Ann Arbor) prefer SGFP as the preservation solution for cold storage of pancreas grafts [60]. This is probably the first step towards organ sharing between transplant centers (at least on a local basis) in the near future.

A reliable method for preservation of pancreatic allografts is of importance for clinical pancreas transplantation. The preservation periods achieved now, already simplify the logistical maneuvers associated with pancreas transplantation. This time is sufficient for appropriate selection of the recipient, for immunological typing and cross-matching, for organization of the operation and for organ procurement over long distances. Pancreas preservation makes transplantation still an urgent, but no longer an emergency procedure.

Pancreas preservation for up to 36 hours, not yet tested clinically, but reliably feasible experimentally, will facilitate organ sharing between transplant centers and thus make cadaveric pancreas grafts more widely available for transplantation.

References

1. Sutherland DER, Moudry KC: Clinical pancreas and islet transplantation. Transplant Proc 19: 113–120, 1987.
2. Levy MN: Oxygen consumption and blood flow in the hypothermic, perfused kidney. Am J Physiol 197: 1111–1114, 1959.
3. Martin DR, Scott DF, Downes GL, Belzer FO: Primary cause of unsuccessful liver and heart preservation: cold sensitivity of the ATPase system. Ann Surg 175: 111–117,1972.
4. Trump BF, Strumm JM, Bulger RE: Studies on the pathogenesis of ischemic cell injury. I. Relation between ion and water shifts and cell ultrastructure in rat kidney slices during swelling at 0–4°C. Virchow's Archiv (Cell Pathol) 16: 1–34, 1974.
5. Leaf A: On the mechanism of fluid exchange of tissues in vitro. Biochem J 62: 241–248, 1956.
6. Leaf A: Cell swelling. A factor in ischemic tissue injury. Circulation 48: 455–458, 1973.
7. Whittembury G, Proverbio F: Two modes of Na-extrusion in cells from guinea pig kidney cortex slices. Pfluegers Arch 316: 1–25, 1970.
8. Wilson TH: Ionic permeability and osmotic swelling of cells. Science 120: 104–105, 1954.
9. Grundmann R: Fundamentals of preservation methods. In: Toledo-Pereyra LH (ed) Basic concepts of organ procurement, perfusion and preservation; pp 93–120. Academic Press, 1982.
10. Flores J, DiBona DR, Beck CH, Leaf A: The role of cell swelling in ischemic renal damage and the protective effect of hypertonic solute. J Clin Invest 51: 118–126, 1972.
11. Collins GM, Bravo-Shugarman M, Terasaki PI: Kidney preservation for transportation. Initial perfusion and 30 hours' ice storage. Lancet 2: 1219–1222, 1969.

12. Keeler R, Swinney J, Taylor RMR, Uldall PR: The problem of renal preservation. Br J Urol 38: 653–656, 1966.
13. Collins GM, Halasz NA: Forty-eight hour ice storage of kidneys: Importance of cation content. Surgery 79: 432–435, 1976.
14. Collins GM, Green RD, Halasz NA: Importance of anion content and osmolarity in flush solutions for 48 to 72 hr hypothermic kidney storage. Cryobiology 16: 217–220, 1979.
15. Sacks SA, Petritsch PH, Kaufman JJ: Canine kidney preservation using a new perfusate. Lancet 1: 1024–1028, 1973.
16. Idezuki Y, Goetz FC, Kaufman SE, Lillehei RC: In vitro insulin productivity of preserved pancreas: a simple test to assess the viability of pancreatic allografts. Surgery 64: 940–947, 1968.
17. Idezuki Y, Goetz FC, Lillehei RC: Experimental allotransplantation of the preserved pancreas and duodenum. Surgery 65: 485–493, 1969.
18. Serrou B, Solassol C, Michel H, Gelis C, Pujol H, Romieu C: Eight- and twenty-four-hour canine pancreas preservation using a simple gel cooling technique. Transplantation 16: 398–402, 1973.
19. Baumgartner D, Sutherland, DER, Heil JE, Zweber B, Awad EA, Najarian JS: Cold storage of segmental canine pancreatic grafts for 24 hours. J Surg Res 29: 248–257, 1980.
20. van Schilfgaarde R, Gooszen HG, Bosman FT, Fröhlich M, Cramer-Knijnenburg GF, van der Burg MPM: Effects of 24-hour cold storage on the histology and long-term endocrine function of autografted canine left pancreatic segments. Transplant Proc 16: 809–810, 1984.
21. DuToit DF, Reese-Smith H: Citrate flushing and 24-hour cold storage of segmental canine pancreatic autografts. Transplantation 33: 202–204, 1982.
22. Florack G, Sutherland DER, Heil J, Zweber B, Najarian JS: Long-term preservation of segmental pancreas autografts. Surgery 92: 260–269, 1982.
23. Bock G, Toledo-Pereyra LH: Three-day pancreas preservation: Successful utilization of hyperosmolar colloid solution. Transplant Proc 18: 540–544, 1986.
24. Heise J, Sutherland DER: Successful hypothermic preservation of canine segmental pancreas grafts for 72 hours in SGFP. Personal communication, 1986.
25. Wahlberg JA, Love R, Landegaard L, Southard JH, Belzer FO: Seventy-hour preservation of the canine pancreas. Transplantation 43: 5–8, 1987.
26. Dafoe DC, Campbell Jr DA, Marks WH, Dorgstrom A, Merion RM, Berlin RE, Turcotte JG: Detrimental effects of four hours of cold storage on porcine pancreaticoduodenal transplantation. Surgery 99: 170–177, 1986.
27. Brynger H, Claes G: Behaviour of the duct-ligated canine pancreas during hypothermic albumin perfusion. Eur Surg Res 7: 287–296, 1975.
28. Brynger H: Twenty-four-hour preservation of the duct-ligated canine pancreatic allograft. Eur Surg Res 7: 341–354, 1975.
29. De Gruyl J, Westbroek DL, McDicken I, Ridderhof E, Verschoor L, van Strik, R: Cryoprecipitated plasma perfusion preservation and cold storage preservation of duct-ligated pancreatic allografts. Br J Surg 64: 490–493, 1977.
30. Westbroek DL, de Gruyl J, Dijkhuis CM, McDicken I, Drop A, Scholte A, Hulsman HAM: Twenty-four-hour hypothermic preservation perfusion and storage of the duct-ligated canine pancreas with transplantation. Transplant Proc 6: 319–322, 1974.
31. Toledo-Pereyra LH, Valjee KD, Chee M, Lillehei RC: Preservation of the pancreas for transplantation. Surg Gynec and Obstet 148: 57–61, 1979
32. Toledo-Pereyra LH, Chee M, Condie RM, Najarian JS, Lillehei RC: Forty-eight hour hypothermic storage of whole canine pancreas allografts. Improved preservation with a colloid hyperosmolar solution. Cryobiology 16: 221–228, 1979.
33. Nolan MS, Lindsey NJ, Ingram NP, Herold A, Slater DN, Fox M: Hypothermic preservation

of the rat pancreas with a view to maintaining endocrine function using either cold storage or pulsatile perfusion. Transplant Proc 16: 807–808, 1984.

34. Baumgartner D, Sutherland DER, Heil J, Zweber B, Awad EA, Najarian JS: Machine preservation of canine segmental pancreatic grafts. Surg Forum 31: 352–354, 1980.

35. Florack G, Sutherland DER, Squifflet JP, Morrow CE, Najarian JS: Preservation of segmental pancreatic autografts by pulsatile machine perfusion. Transplant Proc 15: 1314–1317, 1983.

36. Florack G, Sutherland DER, Heil J, Squifflet JP, Najarian JS: Preservation of canine segmental pancreatic autografts: Cold storage versus pulsatile machine perfusion. J Surg Res 34: 493–504, 1983.

37. Garvin PJ, Castaneda MA, Niehoff ML: In search of an in-vitro index of viability during pancreatic preservation. J Surg Res 40: 455–461, 1986.

38. Florack G, Sutherland DER, Ascherl R, Heil J, Erhardt W, Najarian JS: Definition of normothermic ischemia limits for kidney and pancreas grafts. J Surg Res 40: 550–563, 1986.

39. Schulak JA, Franklin WA, Stuart FP, Reckard CR: Effect of warm ischemia on segmental pancreas transplantation in the rat. Transplantation 35: 7–11, 1983.

40. Florack G, Sutherland DER, Dunning M, Zweber B, Najarian JS: Function of segmental pancreas grafts subjected to warm ischemia prior to hypothermic preservation. Transplant Proc 16: 111–114, 1984.

41. Schulak JA, Kisthard J: The effect of warm ischemia and cold storage preservation on rat pancreas transplantation. J Surg Res 36: 134–139, 1984.

42. Jones RT, Trump BF: Cellular and subcellular effects of ischemia on the pancreatic acinar cell. Virchows Arch B Cell Path 19: 325–336, 1975.

43. Slater DN, Bardsley D, Mangnall Y, Smythe A, Fox M: Pancreatic ischemia; sensitivity and reversibility of the changes. Br J exp Path 56: 530–536, 1975.

44. Sutherland DER, Moudry KC: Pancreas transplant registry report-1986. Clinical Transplantation 1: 3–17, 1987.

45. Sutherland DER: Current status of clinical pancreas and islet transplantation with comments on the need for an application of cryogenic and other preservation techniques. Cryobiology 20: 245–255, 1983.

46. Brekke IB, Dyrbekk D, Jakobsen A, Jervell J, Sodal G, Flatmark A: Improved pancreas graft survival in combined pancreatic and renal transplantation. Transplant Proc 18: 1125–1126, 1986.

47. Sollinger HW, Kalayoglu M, Hoffmann RM, Deierhoi MH, Belzer FO: Experience with pancreaticocystostomy in 24 consecutive pancreas transplants. Transplant Proc 17: 141–143, 1985.

48. Tydén G, Mellgren A, Brattström C, Öst L, Gunnarsson R, Östman J, Groth CG: Stockholm experience with 32 combined renal and segmental pancreatic transplants. Transplant Proc 18: 1114–1117, 1986.

49. Opelz G, Terasaki PI: Advantage of cold storage over machine perfusion for preservation of cadaver kidneys. Transplantation 33: 64–68, 1982.

50. Collins GM: The best method for renal preservation: cold storage. Transplant Proc 17: 1518–1520, 1985.

51. Belzer FO: Perfusion preservation versus cold storage. Transplant Proc 17: 1515–1517,1985.

52. Toledo-Pereyra LH: Pancreatic transplantation. Surg Gynecol and Obstet 157: 49–56, 1983.

53. Largiadèr F, Baumgartner D, Uhlschmid G: Ischemia tolerance of human pancreatic transplants. Transplant Proc 16: 1285–1286, 1984.

54. Sutherland DER, Goetz FC, Najarian JS: One hundred pancreas transplants at a single institution. Ann. Surg 200: 414–440, 1984.

55. Florack G, Sutherland DER, Chinn PL, Najarian JS: Clinical experience with transplantation

of hypothermically preserved pancreas grafts. Transplant Proc 16: 153–155, 1984.

56. Abouna GM, Sutherland DER, Florack G, Najarian JS, Moudry KC: Function of transplanted human pancreatic allografts after preservation in cold storage for 6–26 hours. Transplantation 43: 630–636, 1987.

57. Toledo-Pereyra LH, Condie RM, Malmberg R, Simmons RL, Najarian JS: A fibrinogen-free plasma perfusate for preservation of kidneys for one hundred and twenty hours. Surg Gynec and Obstet 138: 901–905, 1974.

58. Toledo-Pereyra LH, Condie RM, Moberg AW, Simmons RL, Najarian JS: Advantages of silica-gel-absorbed plasma perfusate for clinical renal preservation. Transplant Proc 7: 573–575, 1975.

59. Abouna GM, Sutherland DER, Florack G, Najarian JS, Moudry KC: Preservation of human pancreatic allografts in cold storage for 6–24 hours. Transplant Proc 19: 2307–2309, 1987.

60. Sutherland DER: Second international workshop on clinical pancreatic transplantation. Munich/Spitzingsee, 1986. Personal communication.

Commentary I

The safety and efficacy of pancreatic transplantation in select Type I diabetics has now been documented by several United States and European Centers with experience in this procedure. This success has gradually moved pancreatic transplantation from an experimental procedure to a therapeutic option in diabetic patients with significant secondary complications of the disease. Enthusiasm for pancreatic transplantation has been fueled by the increasing documentation that successful allografting can lead to a stabilization, or even reversal, of diabetic neuropathy, retinopathy, and nephropathy. Until recently, the major drawback to more widespread application of this procedure has been the inability to identify a method of short term preservation that would allow for predictable allograft function after cold ischemic times of greater than six hours. As a result, cadaveric donors were limited to situations where logistics were optimal, and sharing of pancreata among centers was virtually non-existent.

In addressing the shortcomings of pancreatic preservation, early experiments applied the principles utilized so successfully by Belzer and Collins in renal transplantation. The limitations of these techniques were soon realized. Cold storage preservation of the pancreas with Collins' solution, for even 24 hours, met with variable results by most investigators. Results with pulsatile perfusion of the pancreas were even less predictable. When the perfusion characteristics were modified to adapt to the low flow state of the ex vivo pancreas, and surface cooling and increased perfusate osmolarity were applied, results with perfusion preservation did improve. Despite these improvements, the overwhelming consensus is that, in the experimental setting, cold storage preservation is superior to pulsatile perfusion for pancreatic preservation. As a result, in clinical pancreatic transplantation, cold storage preservation has been utilized almost exclusively by most transplant centers. In addition, the major thrust of current laboratory investigations in pancreatic preservation has been directed towards improving the results of cold storage preservation. Towards this end, silica gel filtered plasma (SGFP) has been evaluated extensively as a flush solution for cold storage preservation. In the laboratory setting, immediate and consistent endocrine function, after hypothermic storage for 48 hours with modified hyperosmolar SGFP, has been demonstrated by Dr. Florack. Further modifications of this solution with the additives KH_2PO_4 and sucrose, or replacing glucose with mannitol, have resulted in successful 72 hour hypothermic preservation.

Although this experimental support for hypothermic preservation with modified SGFP is convincing, several unanswered questions remain to be addressed regarding pancreatic preservation. The disappointing results attained by most investigators following hypothermic storage with Collins' solution require further elucidation. It must be remembered that, in the experimental evaluation of pancreatic transplantation, several variables, other than the type of preservation solution can adversely affect graft function. In experiments involving pancreatic allografts, which many investigators have utilized, problems with rejection, as well as the effect of steroids and cyclosporin on glucose kinetics, can make an evaluation of preservation techniques difficult. Even in experiments involving autografts, the method of pancreatic duct management, and the variability in blood supply to the left lobe of the pancreas, especially in the canine model, can influence results. Only when these variables are controlled for, can true preservation failures be identified, and the optimal preservation solution be established. In addition, despite the inferior results, to date, with pulsatile perfusion preservation of the pancreas, this technique remains theoretically attractive in that it allows for continuous monitoring of various hemodynamic, physiologic, and metabolic parameters that may be predictive of post transplant graft function. If sensitive, and specific, indices of post transplant preservation failure, vascular thrombosis, and/or graft pancreatitis, can be identified, then modifications in the perfusate can be accomplished in an attempt to improve graft survival. Futhermore, the availability of such indices would prevent transplantation of grafts destined to fail. Therefore, despite the convincing evidence presented by Dr Florack that hypothermic preservation, with modified SGFP, is the optimal technique for both clinical and experimental pancreatic transplantation, further investigations are essential to allow for continued improvements.

Considerable evidence now exists that the islet cells are more tolerant to warm ischemic and preservation injury than the exocrine pancreas. In our laboratory, we also investigated the viability of islet cells after 24 hours of preservation by determining in vitro insulin release, in response to a standard glucose challenge, of pancreatic tissue slices removed sequentially from the left lobe of the canine pancreas [1]. These segments were taken pre harvest, after Collins' flush, after 24 hours of pulsatile perfusion and 15 minutes after autotransplantation. Autotransplants were classified as preservation successes or failures on the basis of post transplant intravenous glucose tolerance testing. When insulin release of the tissue slices obtained at these time intervals was compared for functioning versus non-functioning autografts, no significant differences in insulin kinetics were identified at any of these time intervals in the two groups. As a result, it seems most likely that the major limitation of pancreatic preservation is related to its effect on exocrine secretions. Following transplantation, this preservation 'injury' results in graft failure from progressive parenchymal damage secondary to pancreatitis.

With this background, we felt that the major thrust of our research efforts in pancreatic preservation should be directed towards identifying:
1. indices of viability during pancreatic preservation, to avoid transplantation of non functioning allografts, and,
2. effective methods of suppressing exocrine secretion to minimize preservation induced pancreatitis.

To address our first objective, 15 dogs underwent segmental pancreatic autografting after 24 hours of pulsatile perfusion and were divided into two groups on the basis of post transplant normoglycemia, or hyperglycemia. In our experience there were no differences in perfusion parameters between functioning and non functioning grafts. During preservation, functioning grafts demonstrated a significantly greater rate of amylase release. Although the reason for this remains to be determined, it is possible that a depletion of enzymes from the secretory granules may protect against the development of post transplant pancreatitis. In these experiments, we also found that non functioning grafts demonstrated increased oxygen extraction during preservation. This finding suggests that techniques to increase energy substrates (e.g., nucleotide enhancement techniques) may be beneficial in pancreatic preservation.

To address our second objective, the ability of various pharmacologic agents to suppress exocrine secretion is being evaluated both in vitro, utilizing pancreatic tissue slices, and in vivo, utilizing pancreatic autografts with functioning pancreaticocystostomies. To date, the effect of various concentrations of verapamil, somatostatin, dimethyl PGE_2 and terbutaline on octapeptide cholecystokinin (OP-CCK) stimulated exocrine secrection of canine pancreatic tissue slices has been evaluated. No significant inhibition of in vitro amylase release was demonstrated with any of these agents. The effect of various concentrations of verapamil and terbutaline on urinary amylase and bicarbonate levels in canine autografts wiht pancreaticocystostomies has also been evaluated. Preliminary findings demonstrate significant suppression of autograft amylase and bicarbonate release during terbutaline infusion. These studies are ongoing in anticipation of identifying agents that will improve the results of pancreatic preservation and transplantation.

In summary, it is obvious, from a review of this chapter, that significant progress has occurred in the field of pancreatic transplantation in general, and pancreatic preservation in particular. As we apply this expanding fund of knowledge to the clinical arena, we must not lose focus of the fact that much remains to be learned from continued investigations in pancreatic preservation.

Reference

1. Garvin PJ, Castaneda MA, Niehoff ML: In search of an in vitro index of viability during pancreatic preservation. Journal Surg Res 40: 455–461, 1986.

Paul J. Garvin
Transplant Service
Veterans Administration
Medical Center
St. Louis, Missouri 63106

Commentary II

Pancreas transplantation was started in 1982 at our institution. At present, about twenty transplants are performed annually with a one-year graft survival rate of approximately 65%. The operation is still done on an emergency basis and the pancreas is usually transplanted within six hours of harvest. Initially, pancreases were preserved in Collins' solution and, as discussed by Florack, this solution is reliable for only about six hours of storage. Recently, we developed a cold storage solution that is capable of preserving the pancreas in the laboratory for 72 hours [1]. We have begun to test this solution clinically, but have restricted preservation times to the same six hours so that we can determine if the new solution is equal to or better than Collins' solution for cold storage. Preliminary results indicate that the solution is at least comparable to Collins' solution for pancreas preservation and, in the near future, preservation times will be extended gradually on a case by case basis.

The need for extended quality pancreas preservation has been explained by Florack in this article. Florack, et al, have developed a solution for preservation of the pancreas for up to 48 hours. This solution is based upon silica-gel-filtered-plasma that is modified by the addition of human serum albumin,

65 mM glucose, 20 mM K and other additives that yield a hyperosmolar (420 mOsmoles/kg) solution. This solution is effective, but there are some theoretical and practical disadvantages to this solution. The solution is difficult to prepare and expensive to purchase because of the silica-gel-filtered-plasma. Also, because it is derived from natural plasma there may be considerable batch variations.

The success of this solution has been attributed to a number of factors discussed by Florack.

1. The solution is hyperosmolar and thus reduces cell swelling.

   Hyperosmolar preservation solutions have a disadvantage as compared to isoosmolar solutions. In hyperosmolar solutions, the extracellular and intracellular osmolality will reach equilibrium. Therefore, in a solution with an osmolality of 420 mOsm/kg the intracellular osmolality will equilibrate at 420 mOsm/kg by entry of the permeable osmotic agents into the cell and by shrinkage of cell volume. Thus, on reflow with blood (Osmolality = 290 mOsm/kg) there will be a tendency for the cells to rapidly swell to equilibrate intracellular osmolality with extracellular osmolality. This event may lead to reperfusion cell swelling and, if it occurs in the endothelium potentially lead to capillary compression and decreased blood flow. Thus, it is questionable if hyperosmolar conditions are required and beneficial for effective pancreas preservation.

2. The solution uses glucose as the primary impermeant to prevent cell swelling.

   Glucose is only semi-permeable in many organs such as the liver and pancreas. A saccharide, with a larger molecular weight, such as sucrose or raffinose would be a more effective impermeant. In addition, glucose can stimulate glycolysis and lead to an increase in tissue acidosis. The formation of lactic acid and an increase in hydrogen ions in the cell occurs even at hypothermia and acidosis is injurious to cell viability. A more favorable impermeant would be one that is nonmetabolizable. In a recent publication from the Minnesota Group [2], they have increased the pH of the flushout solution in an attempt to prevent intracellular acidosis.

3. The solution contains a high protein concentration for colloidal osmotic pressure.

   Although there is only suggestive evidence that colloids are necessary for effective cold storage of organs, there are theoretical advantages to including colloids in the flushout solution. The presence of colloids helps prevent expansion of the extracellular during flushout of the pancreas and may suppress compression of the capillaries. In addition, this may facilitate distribution of the flushout components throughout the organ resulting in a more effective preservation. For these reasons, we include a large molecular weight hydroxyethyl starch in our flushout solution.

154

The ideal flushout solution may also need to contain a number of other agents. These agents include an effective intracellular hydrogen ion buffer, a precursor for ATP resynthesis on reperfusion, and pharmacological agents to prevent oxygen free radial injury on reperfusion of damaged organs.

The work of Florack et al as well as our own is directed towards developing an ideal cold flushout solution for preservation of multiple organs. In the future, an ideal cold storage solution will be developed that is effective for preservation of all solid organs for at least thirty hours. The development of a universal cold flushout solution will require an understanding and application of the principles of anaerobic-hypothermic metabolism as applied to the various organs. The work presented here by Florack addresses some of these principles.

References

1. Wahlberg JA, Love R, Landegaard J, Southard JH, Belzer FO: 72-hour preservation of the canine pancreas. Transplantation 43: 1 5–8, 1987.
2. Abouna GM, Heil BS, Sutherland DER: Factors necessary for successful 48 hours preservation of pancreas grafts. Presented at the American society of transplant surgeons, May, 1987. Transplantation, in press.

F.O. Belzer and J.H. Southard
Department of Surgery
School of Medicine
University of Wisconsin, Madison, Wisconsin 53792

7. Pre-, per- and post-operative care of pancreas transplantation recipient

L.D. MONTI, P.M. PIATTI and D. LONG

Introduction

Diabetic patients undergoing surgery are a high risk group in term of both morbidity and mortality, even if the advent of insulin in 1921 radically changed the modalities of treatment. Different results are reported: Wheelock and Marble [1] reported a 3.7% mortality in a series of 2780 patients studied between 1965 and 1969, while Galloway and Shuman [2] found a 3.6% mortality and 17.2% morbidity in 667 cases. Mortality of diabetics undergoing renal transplantation reported to be two to four times the mortality of the non-diabetic patients undergoing renal transplantation [3].

Pancreas transplantation is mostly performed in uremic patients with a simultaneous kidney transplantation from the same donor. Uremic diabetic patients show a worse clinical status than diabetic patients submitted to pancreas transplantation alone, due to a higher degree of diabetic complications in the former group of patients. The majority of these patients are affected by proliferative retinopathy, peripheral vasculopathy, cardiomyopathy and neuropathy.

The major cause of mortality and morbidity was and still is myocardial disease. In our experience in 52 pancreas plus kidney transplantations performed at Lyon, 80% of patients shows cardiovascular complications before transplantation and the most important cause of death was cardiovascular disease.

The main aim of therapy must be to achieve rapid recovery from the surgical stress reducing intercurrent problems related directly to the metabolic disturbance, delayed wound healing or cardiovascular events. Diabetes mellitus may lead to complex biochemical disturbances, and the problems of diabetes and uremia are combined in patients submitted to kidney and pancreas transplantation. The metabolic problems related to pre-, per- and post-operative care during pancreas or pancreas plus kidney transplantation in insulin dependent diabetic patients will be discussed in this chapter.

155

J.M. Dubernard and D.E.R. Sutherland (eds.), International Handbook of Pancreas Transplantation, 155–165.
© *1989 by Kluwer Academic Publishers.*

Metabolic and hormonal changes in uremic diabetic patients

The kidney plays a part in the compensation for some metabolic and hormonal disturbances; for example, by increasing excretion of potassium when the plasma potassium rises and removing hydrogen ion and ketone bodies during ketoacidosis. Many complications of transplantation result from these disturbances; indeed hyperkalaemic cardiac arrest has been reported [4]. These facts prompted a decision to monitor the biochemical condition of a severe diabetic patient undergoing transplantation during and immediately after surgery.

Furthermore, kidney plays a central role in the clearance of low molecular weight peptides such as insulin, proinsulin, glucagon and c-peptide. These hormones are metabolized by the kidney in two pathways: the first one is glomerular filtration followed by uptake and degradation by the luminal border of the renal tubular cells, while, the second one involves uptake from the peritubular border and degradation in tubular cells, presumably by cytosolic enzyme systems [5].

In patients with advanced renal failure, basal plasma concentration of insulin, glucagon and c-peptide are elevated [6, 7], producing an alteration on glucose and metabolism, with reduced glucose response to administration of insulin [5]. On the other hand, most uremic patients have normal fasting glucose concentration, and it seems that the glucose intolerance of uremia is the result of impaired insulin action in target tissues. Westervelt [8] reported that uremia caused a blunted effect of insulin on glucose uptake in forearm perfusion studies, and De Fronzo et al. [9], used an euglycemic insulin clamp to demonstrate reduced glucose uptake in the peripheral tissues of uremic patients.

Insulin binding studies performed on adipocytes or hepatocytes of uremic rats show that insulin resistence associated with uremia may be primarily accounted for by altered postreceptor events that appear to result from a circulating factor [10, 11]. During uremia the relationship between c-peptide and insulin is abnormal [7]. The latter abnormality is due to greater renal clearance of c-peptide than of insulin, prevents use of plasma c-peptide concentrations as an index of insulin secretion in patients with renal failure.

The relatively abrupt decrease in insulin requirement often seen in type I diabetic patients as renal function deteriorates, probably results from a renal blood flow and insulin extraction, together with the eventual uremic depression of insulin degradation at extra-renal sites [12, 13]. Plasma immunoreactive glucagon is elevated in uremia, primarily due to decrease of catabolism rather than hypersecretion of this hormon [14]. Furthermore, cellular sensitivity to the hyperglycemic effect of physiological increments in glucagon is increased [14]. During pancreas and kidney transplantation the abnormal hormonal clearances discussed above are associated with a typical metabolic stress response which tends to override the normal homeostatic mechanisms. Catabolic response to surgery is characterized by increased metabolic rate, increased net protein breakdown and nitrogen loss, and glucose intolerance. The hormonal changes are well recognised [15]: there is an increase of catecholamine, ACTH and cortisol secretion. Glucagon [16] and growth hormone secretion may also be increased. These hormonal changes are associated with several interesting metabolic changes, while blood glucose concentrations increase during surgery. It was originally considered that extrahepatic glucose oxidation was decreased, but Long et al. [17] showed normal or increased peripheral glucose oxidation. The main defect appears to be inappropriately enhanced gluconeogenesis [18] which is non-suppressible by glucose [19]. The cause of this phenomenon and the relative insulin resistance have not been clearly documented.

There is a complex interplay between different catabolic hormones and the combined increase of circulating concentrations of the different hormones which probably account for the glucose changes. These are growth hormones and cortisol occurring principally in peripheral tissues and glucagon, catecholamines and cortisol occurring in the liver.

Anaesthetical management

Selection of anaesthetic agents does not appear to be a major factor in the safe outcome of a surgical procedure in diabetic patients. No agent is categorically contraindicated and none is specifically beneficial for diabetic patients. The choice of anaesthetic agents depends on the type of surgery, the medical status of patient, and the surgical risks.

Many anaesthetics are employed during surgery, such as alphaxalone, a steroid anaesthetic [20], neuromuscular relaxant drugs and anticholine esterases. The pharmacokinetics of several of newer muscular relaxants make them suitable for use in patients with chronic renal failure [21, 22]. Generally they do not appear to be dependent on the kidney or liver for their elimination, and these drugs may become the relaxant of choice in patients with impaired renal function.

The kinetics of benzodiazepines are altered in patients with acute or chronic renal failure. It is possible to have an increased volume of drug distribution together with an increased systemic clearance, probably due to an increase in the free, unbound drug function. All general anaesthetic agents are myocardial depressants, and may therefore reduce the cardiac output and blood flow to the transplanted kidney. Halothane, in low concentration is probably a safe supplement to nitrous oxide-oxygen anaesthesia, but it has no analgesic property and is liable to cause hypotension in patients receiving antihypertensive treatment or following recent hemodialysis.

Metabolic management

In patients submitted to pancreas transplantation the aim is to keep the blood glucose concentration between 6 and 8 mmol/l during pre-, per- and post-operative period. In the pre-, per- and early post-operative period, insulin therapy should be performed by intravenous route in order to avoid hypo- or hyperglycemic episodes with a careful control of infusion rate. A glucose controlled insulin infusion system (Biostator) has recently been developed. This instrument has a glucose electrode that continuously displays the blood glucose concentration. It is programmed to maintain normal blood glucose levels by infusing either 5 per cent glucose or regular insulin. The blood glucose level desired can be selected, and the computer automatically makes the appropriate adjustment. This instrument is a form of artificial pancreas and has been successfully used to control diabetes during surgery [23–25]. The duration of surgery in patients receiving simultaneous kidney and pancreas transplantation necessitates careful monitoring of the glucose and electrolytes, as well as attention to the maintainance of normothermia. Use of the artificial pancreas during operation makes all surgery considerably safer for the diabetic patients, and we believe that pancreatic transplantation in the labile diabetic constitutes an ideal indication. Since August 1983, Biostator has been routinely used during surgery at our Unit in Lyon. Prior to surgery, the artificial pancreas is brought into the operating theatre and calibrated, then patients are connected to the artificial pancreas which allows to control the hyperglycemic levels related to the surgical intervention. This is especially true after pancreatic-graft revascularization and the artificial pancreas reduces the possible hypoglycemic episodes occurring at the end of surgery.

Typical metabolic and hormonal patterns are shown in Figures 1 and 2. In the first patients, glycemic levels were high at the beginning of intervention, but were near normal at the end of surgery and persist in the normal range several hours after. The artificial pancreas gave a high rate of insulin in order to decrease glycemic levels. In spite of this, c-peptide rose from undetectable levels to very high levels at the revascularization stage, but decreased according to the pattern of the glycemic levels. The artificial pancreas gave glucose to maintain normoglycemia at the end of surgery.

Similar patterns are seen in Figure 2 in which glycemic levels were not so high as in the previous case, but in this case the patient was also normoglycemic at the end of surgery. C-peptide rose and remained high during the whole interval studied.

In Figure 3 is represented a case of one patient without steroid pulse before surgery. Glycemic levels were better with low insulin infusion rate from the artificial pancreas. This seems to demonstrate that pre-operative steroid treatment may contribute to the hyperglycemic answer during surgery. In fact,

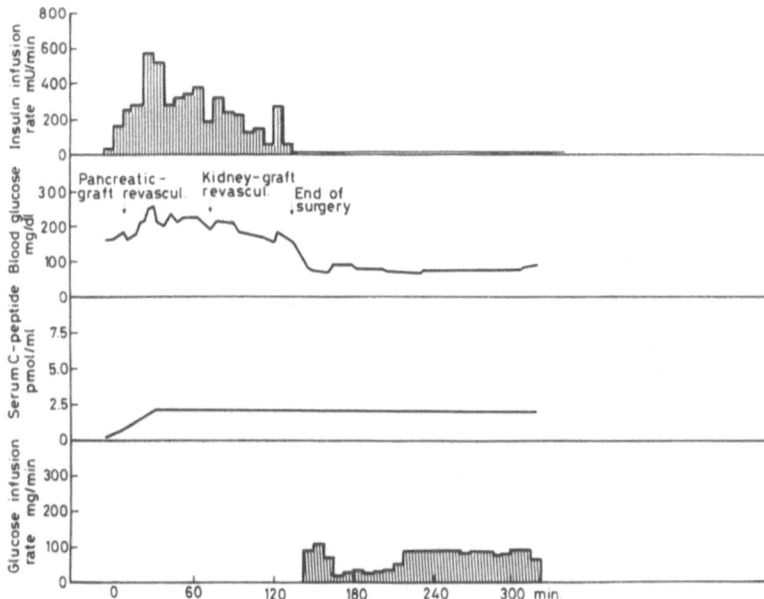

Figure 1. Use of the artificial pancreas to control plasma glucose in a patient submitted to pancreas plus kidney transplantation. A steroid pulse of 1 mg/kg of 6-methylprednisolone was performed before surgery.

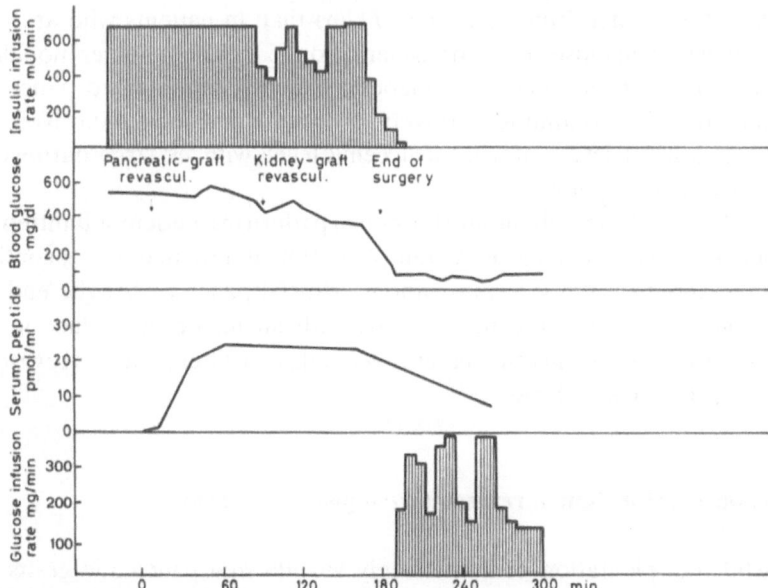

Figure 2. Use of the artificial pancreas to control plasma glucose in a patient submitted to pancreas plus kidney transplantation. A steroid pulse of 1 mg/kg of 6-methylprednisolone was performed before surgery.

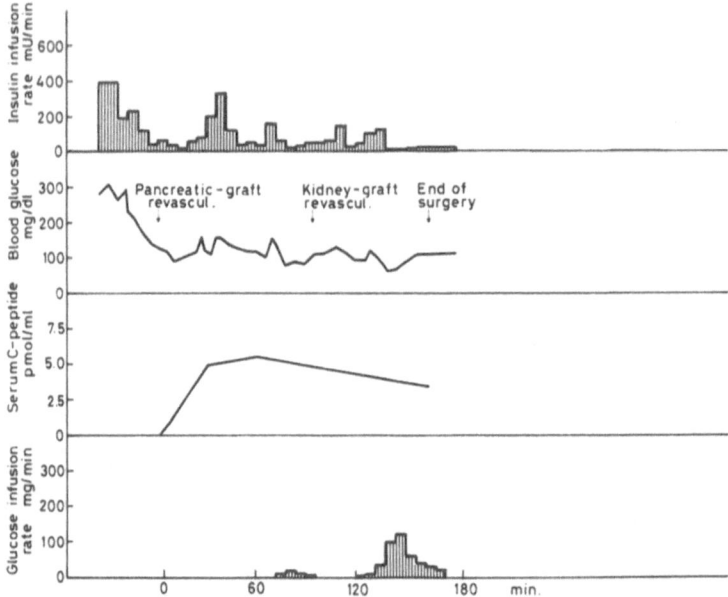

Figure 3. Use of the artificial pancreas to control plasma glucose in a patient submitted to plasma plus kidney transplantation. This patient was treated with cyclosporin alone starting at the beginning of surgery.

insulin infusion rate is higher in patients submitted to steroid pulse before transplantation (range from 15.3 to 38.7 U/h) than in patients who are not submitted to steroid pulse before transplantation (6.0 U/h). Another modality of treatment in insulin dependent diabetic patients submitted to pancreas transplantation, is a continuous intravenous insulin infusion with intravenous insulin pulses and strict monitoring of glycemic levels with test strips during the whole per-operative period.

Figure 4 shows the metabolic and hormonal pattern in a patient submitted to simultaneous pancreas and kidney transplantation and treated with a continuous intravenous insulin infusion without artificial pancreas. At the end of surgery, glycemic levels are near-normal with an important reduction of insulin-infusion rate. As in other cases, C-peptide rose after pancreas revascularization at a very high level.

Early endocrine function in revascularized pancreatic graft

Successful transplantation of immediately vascularized pancreatic grafts to animals made diabetic, uniformly restores plasma glucose to normal [26, 27], while several authors have noted a tendency for hyperinsulinemia and hypoglycemia to occur during the first few hours after transplantation [28–30]. In

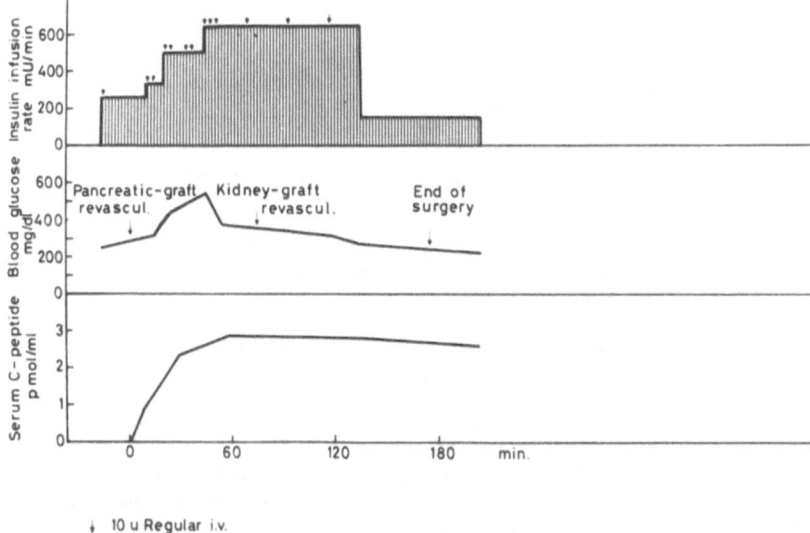

Figure 4. Use of continuous intravenous insulin infusion to control plasma glucose in a patient submitted to pancreas plus kidney transplantation. A steroid pulse of 500 mg of 6-methylprednisolone was performed before surgery.

order to define the role played by the transplanted pancreas in the hormonal changes seen in the per- and post-operative period after simultaneous kidney and pancreas transplantation, we have studied, at Lyon Unit, the hormonal and metabolic pattern in uremic non diabetic patients submitted to renal transplantation alone in comparison with uremic diabetic patients submitted to simultaneous pancreas and kidney transplantation.

We have demonstrated that c-peptide levels, almost undetectable in diabetic patients before pancreas-revascularization, rose at higher levels in comparison with controls, and remained at these levels during the whole intraoperative period. This happened in spite of the fact that the artificial pancreas, in diabetic patients, gave insulin in order to obtain normoglycemia and free insulin levels were higher in diabetic than in uremic patients during surgery. Plasma glucagon levels peaked immediately after pancreatic graft revascularization and were higher in diabetic patients than in uremic patients before renal graft anastomosis, but glucagon levels were comparable in both groups at the end of surgery (Figures 5 and 6).

In conclusion it seems that a prompt increase of endocrinepancreatic hormones occurs after successful pancreatic transplantation [31]. Nevertheless normoglycemia achieved later after surgery is probably due to the surgical stress and/or an inappropriate increase of glucagon levels.

The increase of glucagon levels does not seem the result of steroid [32] or anaesthetic drugs administration during surgery, since this increase does not

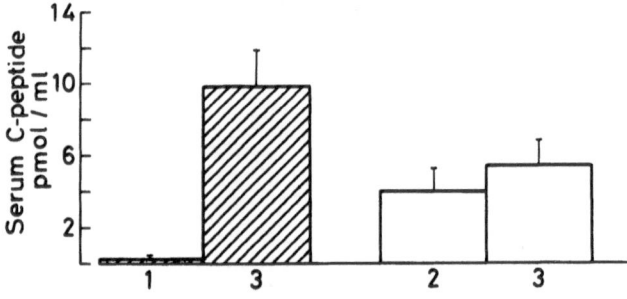

1 Before pancreatic - graft anastomosis
2 Before kidney-graft anastomosis
3 End of surgery

Figure 5. Serum c-peptide profile during surgery in 14 uremic diabetic patients submitted to pancreas plus kidney transplantation (shaded bars) and in 5 uremic non diabetic patients submitted to kidney transplantation alone (open bars).

occur in the uremic non diabetic patients (controls) submitted to the same drug treatment and to surgery for renal transplantation alone.

Conclusion

In diabetic patients submitted to pancreas transplantation, one of the most important anaesthetic problems is the acid-basis status and electrolytic imbalance as an elevation of potassium levels; that may cause problems in the

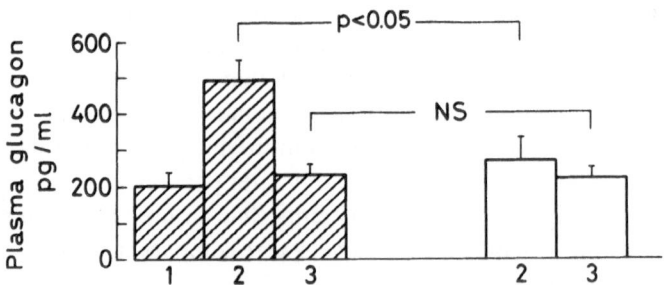

1 Before pancreatic-graft anastomosis
2 Before kidney-graft anastomosis
3 End of surgery

Figure 6. Plasma glucagon profile during surgery in 14 uremic diabetic patients submitted to pancreas plus kidney transplantation (shaded bars) and in 5 uremic non diabetic patients submitted to kidney transplantation alone (open bars).

adequacy of reversal of residual neuromuscular blockade at the end of anaesthesia. A reduction of this problem is obtained with routine dialysis of all patients before transplantation, of patients submitted to simultaneous kidney and pancreas transplantation, or with a good glycemic control before surgery of patients submitted to pancreas transplantation alone.

In our experience, the careful monitoring of acid-basic equilibrium, cardiovascular and glycemic parameters, during simultaneous pancreas and kidney transplantation seems not to increase the surgical risk in diabetic patients. The major problem seems to be correlated with the cardiovascular status of patients before transplantation. The majority of deaths is related to cardiovascular disease in the post-operative period.

Many approaches of insulin treatment are employed during surgery in order to obtain normoglycemia. These methods include avoiding glucose and insulin during surgery [33], or using intravenous glucose with low doses of subcutaneous retard insulin [34–36], or regular insulin given continuously during surgery [37–39], or glucose-insulin-potassium infusion [40]. These approaches were related to different degrees of mortality [35, 36]. In particular, the possibility of undetected hypoglycemia during general anaesthesia was underlined as a cause of death [41]. If the transplantation of pancreas and kidney are carried out together, the peroperative development of hypoglycemia may occur as a result of the production of endogenous insulin by the transplanted pancreatic tissue [28–30]. This may be further complicated by residual effects of any pre-operatively administered long-duration insulin preparation, as well as intraoperatively administered steroids given for immunosuppression. For this reason, other authors [23–25] have employed the artificial pancreas as an automatic feed-back control of plasma glucose during surgery.

In our experience, artificial pancreas is able to control glycemic levels during simultaneous pancreas and kidney transplantation, without hypoglycemic episodes at the end of surgery. In spite of high free insulin levels due to artificial pancreas, the pancreas graft is able to answer to hyperglycemia with a prompt release of insulin and c-peptide in the first minutes after revascularization. The concomitance of hyperglycemia and hyperinsulinemia strongly supports the presence of severe insulin resistance in the early post-operative period which probably is related to steroid treatment, uremic state, hyperglucagonemia and surgical stress.

References

1. Weelock FC jr, Marble A: Surgery and diabetes. In: Marble A, White P, Bradley RF, Krall LP (eds) Joslin's diabetes mellitus; p. 599. Lea and Febiger, Philadelphia, 1971.
2. Galloway JA, Shuman CR: Diabetes and surgery. A study of 667 cases. Am J Med 34: 177–181, 1963.

164

3. Kjellstrand CM, Simmons RL, Goetz FC, Clein MB, Buselmeier TJ, Najarian JS: Renal transplantation in patients with insulin-dependent diabetes. Lancet 2: 4–7, 1972.
4. Hirshman CA, Edelstein G: Intra-operative hyperkalemia and cardiac arrest during renal transplantation in an insulin-dependent diabetic patient. Anaesthesiology 51: 161–162, 1979.
5. Duckworth WC, Heinemann H, Goessling M: Enzymatic mechanisms for insulin and glucagon degradation by kidney. Clin Res 24: 359A, 1976.
6. Rubestein AH, Mako ME, Horowitz DL: Insulin and the kidney. Nephron 15: 306–326, 1976.
7. Jaspan JB, Mako ME, Kuzuya H, Blix PM, Horowitz DL, Rubestein AH: Abnormalities in circulating beta cell peptides in chronic renal failure: comparison of c-peptide, proinsulin and insulin. J Clin Endocrinol Metab 45: 441–446, 1977.
8. Westervelt FB: Abnormal carbohydrate metabolism in uremia. Am J Clin Nutr 21: 423–425, 1968.
9. Defronzo RA, Alvestrand A, Smith D, Hendler R, Hendler E, Warehn J: Insulin resistance in uremia. J Clin Invest 67: 563–568, 1981.
10. Maloff BL, McCaleb ML, Lockwood DH: Cellular basis of insulin resistance in chronic uremia. Am J Physiol 245: E178–E184, 1983.
11. Kauffman JM, Caro JF: Insulin resistance in uremia. J Clin Invest 71: 698–708, 1983.
12. Mondon CE, Dolkas CB, Reaven GM: Effect of acute uremia on insulin removal by the isolated perfused rat liver and muscle. Metabolism 27: 133–142, 1978.
13. Rabkin R, Unterhalter SA, Duckworth WC: Effect of prolonged uremia on insulin metabolism by isolated liver and muscle. Kidney Int 16: 433–439, 1979.
14. Sherwin RS, Basti C, Finkelstein FO, Fisher M, Black H, Hendler R, Felig P: Influence of uremia and hemodialysis on the turnover and metabolic effects of glucagon. J Clin Invest 57: 722–731, 1976.
15. Alberti KGMM, Gill GV, Elliott MJ: Insulin delivery during surgery in the diabetic patient. Diabetes Care 5: 65–77, 1982.
16. Russel RCG, Walker CJ, Bloom SR: Hyperglucagonemia in the surgical patient. Br Med J 1: 10–18, 1975.
17. Long CL, Spencer JL, Kinney JM, Geiger JW: Carbohydrate metabolism in man: effect of elective operations and major injury. J Appl Physiol 31: 110–114, 1971.
18. Giddings AEB: The control of plasma glucose in the surgical patient. Br J Surg 61: 787–792, 1974.
19. Gump FE, Long CL, Killian P, Kinney JM: Studies of glucose intolerance in septic injured patients. J Trauma 14: 378–383, 1974.
20. Strunin L, Strunin JM, Knights KM, Ward ME: Metabolism of 14C-labelled Alphaxalone in man. Brit J Anaesth 49: 609–614, 1977.
21. Duvaldestin P, Bertrand JC, Concina D, Herzel P, Lareng L, Desmonts JM: Pharmacokinetics of Fazadinium in patients with renal failure. Brit J Anaesth 51: 943–947, 1979.
22. Bevan DR, D'Souza J, Rouse JM, Caldwell J, Dring G, Smith RL: Clinical pharmacokinetics of Fazadinium Bromide in renal failure in man. Anaesth Analges 59: 529, 1980.
23. Massi Benedetti M, Puxeddu A, Calabrese G, Mercati U, Cortesini R, Santeusanio F, Alfani D, Trancanelli V, Antonella MA, Brunetti P: Use of the artificial endocrine pancreas during surgery. In: Brunetti P et al (eds) Artificial system for insulin delivery; pp 523–533. Raven Press, New York, 1983.
24. Marchal G, Mirouze J, Selam JL, Pham TC, Giordan J: Report of a clinical case of segmental pancreatic transplantation with the aid of the artificial pancreas. Transplant Proc 12: 95–97, 1980.
25. Schwartz SS, Horowitz DL, Zehfus B, Langer B, Moossa AR, Ribeiro G, Kaplan E, Rubestein AH: Use of a glucose controlled insulin infusion system (artificial beta cell) to control diabetes during surgery. Diabetologia 16: 157–164, 1979.

26. Kyriakides GK, Sutherland DER, Olson L, Miller J, Najarian JS: Segmental pancreatic transplantation in dogs. Transplant Proc 11: 530–532, 1979.
27. Papachristou DN, Fortner JG: Duct ligated versus duct obliterated canine pancreatic autografts: early postoperative results. Transplant Proc 11: 522–526, 1979.
28. Gunnarsson R, Arner P, Lundgren G, Ostman J, Groth CG: Assessment of pancreatic graft function. Transplant Proc 12: 107–111, 1980.
29. Lillehei RC, Simmons RL, Najarian JS, Weil R III, Uchida H, Ruiz JO, Kjellstrand CM, Goetz FC: Pancreatico-duodenal allotransplantation. Experimental and clinical experience. Ann Surg 172: 405–436, 1970.
30. Bewick M, Mundy AR, Eaton B, Watson F: The endocrine function of the heterotopic pancreatic allotransplant in dogs: II. The immediate post-transplant period. Transplantation 31: 19–22, 1981.
31. Piatti PM, Traeger J, Dubernard JM, Bosi E, Finaz J, Mongin-Long D, El-Yafi S, Secchi A, Pozet N, Monti LD, Pozza G: Hormonal evaluation of immediate pancreatic function in simultaneous kidney plus pancreas transplantation during artificial pancreas monitoring. Transplant Proc 17: 346–348, 1985.
32. Marco J, Calle C, Roman D, Diaz-Fierros M, Villanueva ML, Valverde I: Hyperglucagonism induced by glucocorticoid treatment in man. N Eng J Med 288: 128–131, 1973.
33. Flecter J, Langman MJS, Kellock TD: Effect of surgery on blood sugar levels in diabetes mellitus. Lancet 2: 52–54, 1965.
34. Moore FD: Metabolic care of the surgical patient. W.B. Saunders, Philadelphia, 1959.
35. Rossini AA, Hare JW: How to control the blood glucose level in the surgical diabetic patient. Arch Surg 111: 945–949, 1976.
36. Steinke J: Management of diabetes mellitus and surgery. N Engl J Med 282: 1472–1474, 1970.
37. Tailteman U, Reece EA, Bessman AN: Insulin in the management of the diabetic surgical patient; continuous intravenous infusion vs subcutaneous administration. JAMA 237: 658–660, 1977.
38. Thomas DJB, Platt HS, Smythe P: Assessment of continuous insulin infusion for the management of insulin dependent diabetics during and after surgery. Diabetologia 13: 436, 1977.
39. Woodruff RE, Lewis SB, McLeskey CH, Stefferson JL, Matsenbaugh SL: A reliable technique for strict intraoperative glucose control in insulin dependent diabetics. Diabetes 26: 423, 1977.
40. Husband DJ, Thai AC, Alberti KGMM: Management of diabetes during surgery with glucose-insulin-potassium infusion. Diabetic Medicine 3: 69–74, 1986.
41. Galloway JA, Shuman CR: Profile: Specific methods of management and response of diabetic patients to anaesthesia in surgery. Int Anaesthesiol Clin 5: 437–466, 1967.

8. Immunosuppression for pancreas transplant recipients

W. LAND

Introduction

When writing a chapter on immunosuppression for pancreas transplant recipients in 1986/87 one has to realize that the drug cyclosporin (CS) plays an important and major role in terms of a powerful immunosuppressive agent with regard to all protocols applied world-wide at the present time. At the moment, therefore, there appears to be no room for an exclusive use of conventional immunosuppressive therapy consisting of steroids and azathioprine in pancreatic transplantation. At the same time one has to state that an immunosuppressive protocol (including cyclosporin) in terms of a well-controlled large clinical trial with special emphasis on the particular situation of clinical pancreatic transplantation has not been worked out or even widely tested so far. Probably, the relatively small number of recipients transplanted at a few institutions are the major hint for the performance of such a clinical trial. Thus, the immunosuppressive protocols currently used in pancreatic transplantation necessarily have to be deduced from the large experience with the new drug cyclosporin in clinical renal transplantation. In fact, in the field of clinical renal transplantation, the use of cyclosporin has become meanwhile the method of choice in the vast majority of the international transplant centres. New methods of optimalization and modification regarding handling the drug and its reasonable application have lead to that development. Especially, the development of methods for reducing efficiently its main side-effect – nephrotoxicity – has made the use of cyclosporin easier and less hazardous for the patients. The recent observation of a 1-year graft survival rate of 90% under cyclosporin in cadaveric renal transplantation by several groups in the world implies a further landmark in the history of clinical renal transplantation.

Certainly, the accumulating experience with cyclosporin in renal transplantation has influenced the immunosuppressive protocols currently used in extra-renal transplantation. Therefore it is not surprising that nearly every

167

J.M. Dubernard and D.E.R. Sutherland (eds.), International Handbook of Pancreas Transplantation, 167–186.
© *1989 by Kluwer Academic Publishers.*

centre in the world involved in clinical pancreatic transplantation uses cyclosporin as major part of immunosuppressive protocols. However, it also has become evident that Azathioprine as the superior immunosuppressive drug in the past has maintained a firm place within all immunosuppressive protocols applied in pancreas transplantation.

According to that background information it appears to be wasting time and somewhat boaring to give a summary of historical data on immunosuppression in clinical pancreas transplantation during the past 10 years. In contrary, it seems of more importance to present ideas, assumptions and implements of optimal immunosuppression (including optimal use of CS) today with regard to clinical pancreatic transplantation. Since I recently collected data, points of consideration, immunosuppressive regimen, etc. concerning optimal use of cyclosporin in organ transplantation (published as a monograph in 1987 [1] I will not mention in detail all regimens and literature sources in the following chapter but rather would like to refer to this monography whenever possible in order to avoid repetitions.

Writing about immunosuppression in pancreatic transplantation another serious problem has to be mentioned at the very beginning. This problem lies in the fact that it is difficult or nearly impossible to work out valid data demonstrating the immunosuppressive potency of a given immunosuppressive regimen as revealed and reflected by the graft survival rates observed. (As known by everybody, in renal transplantation the immunosuppressive index of a given immunosuppressive regimen can be evaluated and assessed with regard to the graft survival rates observed). In pancreatic transplantation, however, the graft survival rates observed cannot be put in a clearcut relationship to the immunosuppressive index of the immunosuppressive regimen applied for the following reasons: There is still an uncertainty or even impossibility to detect a rejection episode of the pancreatic graft early enough; there is still a high percentage of (assumed) non-immunological graft losses; there is still a difficulty to discriminate between 'secondary' immunological loss or primary non-immunological graft loss (I come back to that problem later in this chapter); etc.

Thus, as a consequence of that dilemma, all immunosuppressive protocols currently used and thought to be optimal in the situation of pancreatic transplantation predominantly are based on theoretical considerations as well as on the experience with cyclosporin in the field of renal transplantation, rather than on a large experience with cyclosporin in clinical pancreatic transplantation.

Having mentioned these problems I would like to give some aspects of clinical immunosuppression in pancreas transplantation by discussing the following points:
- current concept of optimal use of cyclosporin in clinical organ transplantation;

- special aspects for an optimal use of cyclosporin in the situation of pancreatic transplantation;
- current immunosuppressive protocols and results in pancreatic transplantation with special reference to the Munich approach;
- trial of future perspectives of immunosuppression on pancreas transplantation.

Current concepts of optimal use of cyclosporin in clinical organ transplantation

Approaches to reduce cyclosporin-associated nephrotoxicity

From the very beginning, clinical (as well as experimental) studies showed very clearly the powerful immunosuppressive effect of cyclosporin. At the same time it become quite evident that this drug exerts a severe (almost always dose-dependent nephrotoxic effect (besides other side-effects not mentioned here).

The dilemma of early cyclosporin use in clinical organ transplantation consequently was characterized by the fact that a high (desired!) immunosuppressive index – only provided by a high dosage of cyclosporin, – was always associated with a high (undesired) nephrotoxic effect of the drug. This dilemma proved even more dramatic when it became obvious that pre-damaged kidneys (e.g.: co-existing renal injury as a consequence if ischemia of cadaveric renal transplants) are more susceptible to the toxic effect of cyclosporin.

Today in 1987, the solution of that dilemma has been achieved in a rather simple and logic way. Retrospectively it appears a little bit astonishing that it took several years to find this solution: namely to decrease the starting dose of cyclosporin to levels which are not nephrotoxic (e.g.: 4–6 mg/kg b.w. orally) – especially in cases with severe co-existing renal injury – and (because of the risk of underimmunosuppression) to add other non-nephrotoxic immunosuppressive agents in order to provide a sufficient immunosuppressive index to prevent rejection. These recent modifications of the early use of cyclosporin were of great importance and led to the development of socalled immunosuppressive combination therapy.

In contrast to that development, another approach was worked out and applied in the clinic with the same aim to optimize the use of cyclosporin in organ transplanted patients: the performance of pharmacokinetic and pharmacodynamic studies (besides routine therapeutic drug monitoring) in order to individualize cyclosporin treatment. It was especially the group of B. Kahan in Houston [2] who got involved in that kind of extremely interesting approach of optimal use of cyclosporin. Although of highly scientific value a general routine praxis of performing pharmacokinetic and pharmacodynamic studies in every patient appears to be not advisable because it is highly costly, time- and staff-consuming. Thus, only a few centres in the world have decided to do those studies routinely in their patients.

To my opinion, the most important approach to a reasonable immuno-suppression in pancreas transplanted patients today is the application of immunosuppressive combination therapy (= multiple drug treatment), which will be pointed out here a bit more in detail. For better understanding it seems reasonable to distinguish between: induction treatment, maintenance treatment and chronic renal dysfunction treatment:

Induction-/maintenance-/chronic renal dysfunction treatment

Induction treatment

Concerns the initial use of cyclosporin during the immediate post-transplant period for about 6 weeks. This period is characterized by an unstable graft function, almost always co-existing renal injury (= in all cases of combined cadaveric pancreatic and renal transplantation), increased alloreactivity, pro-longed period of intravenous application of cyclosporin and a decreased bowel motility (as a result of diabetic enteropathy plus the surgical intervention).

Maintenance treatment

Maintenance treatment concerns the use of cyclosporin following the phase of induction treatment. This period is characterized by an almost always stable graft function, normal or subnormal kidney function in case of simultaneous pancreatic and renal transplantation; increased bioavailability of cyclosporin (although diabetic enteropathy with reduced absorption of cyclosporin still exists in some patients). Alloreactivity is supposed to decrease steadily; acute rejection episodes become less.

Chronic renal dysfunction treatment

Chronic renal dysfunction treatment concerns the use of cyclosporin in cases of chronic progessive renal dysfunction. This may be either a consequence of a chronic nephrotoxic effect of cyclosporin (either to the renal transplant or to the native kidneys in case of pancreas transplantation alone) or a consequence of chronic rejection of the renal transplant (or even both events!).

Immunosuppressive combination therapy

Immunosuppressive combination therapy in terms of induction-treatment

Triple drug induction treatment. Triple drug therapy during induction period is based upon the conception (I) that acute nephrotoxic episodes as well as potentially – irreversible chronic – nephrotoxicity in cases of coexisting renal injury can only be minimized by administration of low-doses of cyclosporin at least during the period of coexisting renal injury until recovery, and (II) that two other immunosuppressive agents have to be added to low dose cyclosporin in order to avoid potential risk of underimmunosuppression.

Simultaneous kidney-function related therapy: Cyclosporin in low doses is given in combination with Azathioprine plus Prednisolon until a serum creatinine value below 3 mg% reflects recovery from co-existing renal injury. Then, by discontinuing Azathioprine cyclosporin dose is switched to appropriate doses according to target cyclosporin levels as desired. This regimen is – for instance – used in cadaveric renal transplantation by the Munich group. A quite similar protocol is used by the Basle group adding ATG instead of Azathioprine during that early period [3].

Simultaneous time-related = continued therapy: Cyclosporin in low doses is given initially in combination with Azathioprine and Prednisolone but then, continued in terms of triple drug maintenance treatment.

Quadruple drug induction treatment. Quadruple drug therapy during induction period can be divided into sequential kidney-function-related therapy and simultaneous time-related therapy.

Sequential kidney-function related therapy: The underlying conception of sequential quadruple therapy is based upon quite similar considerations as mentioned above with regard to simultaneous kidney-function related triple drug therapy with the exception that instead of low dose cyclosporin *no* cyclosporin is used during the immediate postoperative period until recovery from co-existing renal injury becomes evident. Thus, immunosuppressive treatment is started using ALG, Azathioprine and Prednisone, when renal function has recovered ALG is replaced by cyclosporin. This immunosuppressive protocol has been pioneered in pancreas transplantation by the Madison Group [4].

Simultaneous time-related therapy: Simultaneous time-related quadruple therapy is also being used in pancreatic transplantation, for instance by the Munich Group since 2 years, and recently by the Madison Group [5]. The Minneapolis protocol is similar except that ALG treatment is started one week posttransplant [6].

The conception again is that acute and potentially chronic nephrotoxicity can be only efficiently controlled by administration of low cyclosporin doses but that 3 more immunosuppressive agent should be added with regard to certain aspects in pancreatic transplantation as discussed in the next chapter. Such a protocol consists – for example – of low dose cyclosporin in combination with Prednisone, Azathioprine and either ALG/ATG or 04T3.

Immunosuppressive combination therapy in terms of maintenance treatment

Again various protocols of immunosuppressive combination therapy are widely being used in renal transplantation during the period of maintenance treatment. Besides combination regimens cyclosporin monotherapy is still being used in terms of single drug maintenance treatment and has been used by us 6 months posttransplant in every pancreas transplanted patient.

Single maintenance treatment. The conception of single drug maintenance treatment is based on the assumption that cyclosporin alone used in doses between 1,5 mg/kg and 6 mg/kg does prevent effectively chronic rejection as well as does not lead to major chronic nephrotoxicity.

Prerequisite for cyclosporin monotherapy is a careful therapeutic drug monitoring with the aim to keep the target trough CS levels in blood/serum within the therapeutic windows.

Double drug maintenance treatment. Double drug maintenance treatment consists of cyclosporin administration merely in conjunction with steroids. This approach represents the most common protocol of cyclosporin used at the present time specially in the U.S.A. It seems reasonable and desirable to perform routine therapeutic drug monitoring to adjust the daily oral dose (1,5 – 6 mg/kg) of cyclosporin to the target trough CS levels which should be within the proposed therapeutic windows.

Triple drug maintenance treatment. The conception of triple drug maintenance treatment (as for instance performed by the Minneapolis [6], Madison [5] is based upon the rationale (I) that side effects of each drug (particularly nephrotoxic effect of CS) administered in low doses is minimal, (II) that chronic rejection is better controlled by the synergistic – or better additive – effect of all three drugs.

Moreover, a strict adjustment of the daily cyclosporin dose to target trough CS levels seems not to be mandatory allowing to perform therapeutic drug monitoring in a more 'loose' way. Independent from this assumption it has to be stated, however, that the therapeutic windows for trough CS blood/serum concentrations under triple drug treatment have not been defined yet. Of course, they should be lower than the proposed windows for single or double drug therapy (see below).

Chronic renal dysfunction treatment

One of the main problems of cyclosporin therapy concerns chronic renal dysfunction either due to chronic rejection or chronic nephrotoxicity or even both. No hard data from single or multicentre control studies are available so far in order to give valid recommendations how to use cyclosporin during such chronic events. Thus, only some suggestions can be made at this point.

In case of predominantly chronic nephrotoxicity a modified triple drug therapy may be attempted consisting of low or even ultra-low CS doses in combination with Azathioprine and Prednisone. If unsuccessful, conversion to Azathioprine/Prednisone seems to be the last trial to overcome this problem. However, the potential risk of conversion-induced chronic rejection has to be kept in mind when performing such conversion procedure.

In case of predominantly chronic rejection again a modified triple drug protocol should be considered consisting of an increased CS dose adjusted to target levels up to 500 ng/ml in combination with Azathioprine and Prednisone which also should transiently administered with increased doses. It has to be stressed, however, that usually the prognosis of chronic rejecting organs is extremely poor regardless what efforts have been made for rescue.

Handling the drug (cyclosporin)

Since the immunosuppressive as well as the adverse effects of cyclosporin are supposed to be dose-dependent the daily cyclosporin dose administered is of great importance for an adeaquate use of the drug. Today, attemps have been undertaken to define more precisely high-, moderate-, low-, or even ultralow cyclosporin doses used during the daily praxis of immunosuppressive therapy (Table 1).

Obviously, recommendation about the cyclosporin dose can only be given in terms of a more or less arbitrary range. Nevertheless, the differentiation of

Table 1. Handling the drug: (Definition of doses; routes of application).

*	Daily dose:	
	High dose:	17–12 mg/kg orally = 6–5 mg/kg i.v.
	Moderate dose:	11– 7 mg/kg orally = 3–4 mg/kg i.v.
	Low dose:	6– 2 mg/kg orally = 1–2 mg/kg i.v.
	Ultra low dose:	– 1 mg/kg orally
*	Route:	
	I Intravenous:	short-term infusion/24 h-infusion
	II Oral:	daily dose divided into one, two or three doses
	III Double route:	intravenous/oral, at the same time

various dose ranges may be reasonable if either a high immunosuppressive index or – on the other hand – a minimal nephrotoxic effect is desired.

The problem of cyclosporin dosage with regard to the immunosuppressive index achieved becomes more difficult when multiple drug regimen are applied. In fact, it is impossible to define or measure the exact immunosuppressive effect of cyclosporin, whenever other immunosuppressive are added.

Concerning the route of administration cyclosporin is being used intravenously, orally or both ways. There is now accumulating clinical evidence that the intravenous route of cyclosporin is more toxic than oral administration. On the other hand, the use of a 24 h intravenous infusion combination with careful drug monitoring has reduced the possibility of severe nephrotoxic episodes drastically. Thus, according to the present experience, intravenous application of cyclosporin via a 24 h infusion seems to be the method of choice.

A particular problem of oral administration of cyclosporin in pancreatic transplant recipients is the fact, that due to the more or less advanced diabetic enteropathy absorption of cyclosporin may be disturbed thus requiring higher doses of the drug than in non-diabetic patients. Careful therapeutic drug monitoring is therefore mandatory in every pancreas transplanted patient to avoid underimmunosuppression due to decreased bioavailability.

Therapeutic drug monitoring

Therapeutic drug monitoring – in earlier times just an optional trial within the control trials has become more and more important and seems to be of extreme value especially in cyclosporin-treated recipients of pancreatic grafts. Meanwhile it is generally accepted that in the vast majority of cyclosporin-treated patients clearcut relationship between the blood/serum concentration of cyclosporin and both its toxic adverse effects and its immunosuppressive efficacy does exist (exception: multiple drug treatment). Therefore, it must be emphasized at the present time, that therapeutic drug monitoring has to be recommended as an aid to a rational, reasonable and efficient cyclosporin treatment in every organ-transplanted patient.

Using the Radioimmunoassay (RIA); high performance liquid chromatography (HPLC) and recently: a test using an monoclonal antibody) three methods are now available to monitor cyclosporin levels in whole blood or serum/plasma.

RIA's are widly used in clinical practice to monitor the drug plus several metabolites. A kit for this RIA is distributed by Sandoz Comp. Ltd.

There are some advantages for using RIA to measure the cyclosporin concentration in blood or serum: The possibility of rapidly processing large numbers of samples; simplicity; and ready standardization and computer-analysis of the data.

With HPLC only the parent compound is determined. Thus, it is the most specific technique to quantitate cyclosporin in blood or serum which reflects its major advantage. On the other hand, there are some disadvantages like its relatively lenghty per-sample, analysis time, complex instrumentation requiring special training of technicians, and others. Regardless those difficulties the application of HPLC rests seems to be mandatory in pancreatic transplant recipients with concomitant liver disease (liver dysfunction) in order to discriminate between the parent compound and the metabolites circulating in the blood.

Despite the difficulties, the use of HPLC (in combination with RIA) may be considered to be mandatory in cases of impaired liver function (= liver disorder) immediately after a liver or heart transplantation. Especially in such situations, the HPLC/RIA ratio provides important imformation about the parent drug and its metabolites. For instance, after a liver or heart transplantation, high RIA values can mimikry an adequate immunosuppressive index while HPLC simultaneously reveals the absence of the parent drug in the blood.

Recently, a monoclonal antibody that measures specifically native cyclosporin has been developed by Sandoz [7] (The new RIA kit is already available and, of course, has lead to a new 'therapeutic window': 100–300 ng/ml. Thus, for specific measurements (e.g. in liver or heart transplantation), the RIA kit based on this monoclonal antibody has advantageously replaced HPLC measurement. Parallel use of the non-specific measurements (cyclosporin + metabolites) will simplify the evaluation of metabolized drug.

Regardless the methods used for therapeutic drug monitoring the possibility to measure cyclosporin concentrations in blood/serum has allowed to elaborate on a therapeutic window of cyclosporin use. By trying to define more precisely an upper an lower limit of such a therapeutic window an apparent upper toxic threshold for nephrotoxicity could be worked out more firmly than the lower limit for a sufficient immunosuppressive index. In addition, there is accumulating evidence suggesting that cyclosporin target trough levels should be reduced with regard to time after transplantation according to the decreasing alloreactivity posttransplant (and perhaps with regard to saturation of peripheral compartments).

Thus, with the aim to minimize nephrotoxicity but provide an efficient immunosuppressive index several proposals of an optimal therapeutic window have been made during the past years which are shown in Figure 1.

I should be stressed, however, that the data shown in Figure 1 can only be used as guidelines for well-known reasons: (I) The therapeutic window seems to differ among patients (II) acute/chronic nephrotoxicity has been observed in patients with trough levels below the assumed upper toxic threshold; (III) acute/chronic rejection may occur in patients with apparently adequate drug

176

'Therapeutic windows' during CyA
(CyA/Pred.) therapy using the
'old' polyclonal RIA kit.

RIA: (whole-blood trough levels, oral administration)

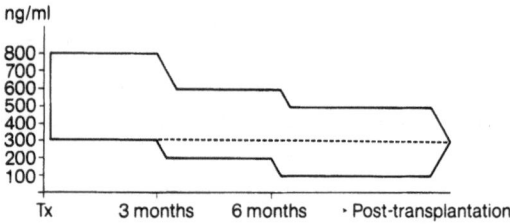

RIA: (serum trough levels, oral administration

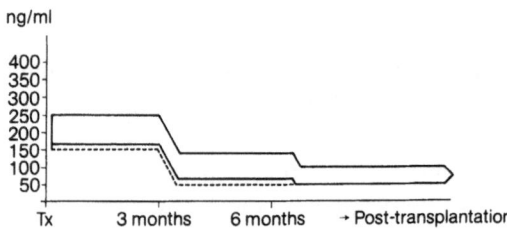

Figure 1. Proposals of 'therapeutic windows' during cyclosporin therapy alone or cyclosporin in conjunction with steroids.*

levels. For instance, acute late rejection episodes have been observed in patients with target whole blood levels below 300 ng/ml. Thus, to maintain and guarantee a safe immunosuppressive index one should try to exceed this value (dotted line in Figure 1).

Moreover, it should be stressed again that these therapeutic windows are of value only for cyclosporin monotherapy or cyclosporin therapy in conjunction with steroids.

Relevant features of pancreatic transplantation in relation to reasonable immunosuppression

There is general agreement that besides a basic concept of immunosuppression special aspects have to be taken into account depending on the underlying type of organ transplantation. In fact, in pancreatic transplantation, there are several pecularities which appear to be important with regard to a theoretical discussion of optimal immunosuppression. They will be mentioned briefly as follows:

* *N.B.*: Meanwhile another therapeutic window has been defined using Sandoz monoclonal RIA kits.

Pancreas transplantation in non-uremic/non-immunosuppressed recipients

As far as the timing of pancreas transplantation during the progressive course of the disease (= Type I Diabetes mellitus) is concerned first clinical manifestations of the late secondary syndrome (p.e. (pre)-proliferative diabetic retinopathy etc.) seems to be the ideal point for a reasonable indication for pancreas transplantation. Unfortunately, pancreas transplantation, according to this 'ideal' indication is still associated with poor results. Besides other problems not mentioned here acute severe rejection episodes are frequent and often irreversible indicating that immune alloreactivity against the pancreatic organ is high in those non-uremic, previously non-immunosuppressed patients. These preliminary – and still limited clinical observations have lead to the theoretical consideration that (I) whatever immunosuppressive protocol is being used it should provide an extremely high initial immunosuppressive index*, and (II) that subclinical diabetic damage of the native kidneys does not allow the application of high doses of cyclosporin. Taking those two points together the use of multiple drug induction treatment (= triple/quadruple drug induction treatment) appears to be the method of choice from the theoretical point of view. Since it becomes more and more obvious (from clinical observation in renal transplantation) that short-term initial administration of 3 or 4 immunosuppressive agents in low/moderate doses is safe (not leading to a higher incidence of infections diseases) it is justified to use that kind of induction treatment in type I diabetics undergoing single pancreas transplantation.

Simultaneous (combined) transplantation of the pancreas and the kidney in uremic (pre-uremic) diabetics

At the present time the simultaneous approach is the most common kind of pancreas transplantation in (pre)uremic diabetic patients. For still unknown reasons the incidence as well as the severity of rejection crises of the pancreatic transplant is surprisingly lower than those of the simultaneously transplanted kidney of the same donor. Some centres (Goteborg, Munich, and others) have observed a much higher immunological risk for the kidney than for the pancreas although in some cases both organs have been observed to be rejected at the same time.

Not only during the early phase post transplantation but also at a later stage (2–4 years post transplant) the kidney transplant seems to be more prone to an immunological attack than the simultaneously transplanted pancreas. There is accumulating clinical evidence suggesting that the incidence of chronic rejec-

* Perhaps the use of the new immunoclonal antibody BMA 031 (Land et al. [14] seems to be of interest in this situation.

tion of the kidney is higher than of the pancreatic organ and higher than that in kidney transplantation in non-diabetics.

This observation was at first made by the Munich group [8]* and meanwhile confirmed by the Stockholm group [9].

It is difficult at the present time to elucidate the reasons/factors leading to these events in cases of combined transplantation of the kidney and the pancreas in Type I-diabetics. Due to the still limited number of patients observed these observations may happen just by chance; on the other hand, some points of speculation can be made why it happens: the pancreatic graft is more protected by the cyclosporin-induced immunosuppression; there is an high degree of HLA-mismatches in the recipients (HLA matching is not performed in order to keep the cold ischemia time as short as possible!); triggering/potentiation of the immune response against the donor kidney by pharmacological mediator substances released from the donor pancreas; less DR-antigen expression of the pancreatic transplant (islet cells) compared to the renal transplant, etc.

One consequence of these preliminary clinical observations would be to start with an immunosuppressive protocol of high immunosuppressiv index: in this case to prevent early rejection of kidney and not the pancreas (as described in the previous sub-chapter). On the other hand, cyclosporin dose should be kept low with regard to the always more or less co-existing renal injury (ischemia!) making the renal graft more susceptibel to the toxic cyclosporin effect.

Thus, like in the situation of single pancreatic transplantation in non-uremic recipients also in combined transplantation of pancreas and kidney a multiple drug induction treatment appears to be the method of choice. Moreover, with regard to the clinical evidence of increased rate of chronic renal rejection a high immunosuppressive index in terms of immunosuppressive maintenance treatment has to be achieved (e.g. triple drug treatment).

Acute rejection episodes of the pancreatic transplant

Although based upon little experimental data one has to assume theoretically that acute rejection episode of a pancreatic organ is associated with some particular events not observed in rejection crisis of other organs. The theoretical background of this assumption is as follows:

The pancreatic transplant is known to be lost frequently due to venous thrombosis which represents a typical postoperative complication of that type of organ transplantation. Many factors are thought to contribute to that event of venous thrombosis, mainly: the low flow of the organ and the partially

* Meanwhile – using a triple/double (CS, 177a) drug maintenance treatment – the long-term results are far better (75% 3-year renal graft survival time).

intraparenchymal course of the splenic vein leading to mechanical venous compression during all events of swelling of parenchyma.

Acute rejection reaction represents one cause of inflammatory swelling of the pancreatic parenchyma which bears the risk of venous thrombosis due to mechanical compression of the vein. Thus, we are dealing with the following sequelae: primary acute rejection episode (which may be even mild and does not necessarily lead to immunological graft destruction)→ inflammatory swelling of the graft→ secondary venous thrombosis→ graft loss. In other words: a potentially 'harmless' acute rejection episode may lead to a graft loss via a secondary venous thrombosis.

If we take these theoretical thoughts into account with regard to basic immunosuppression as well as any kind of anti-rejection treatment in pancreatic transplant recipients the following therapeutical consequences should be discussed:

– The index of basic immunosuppression (particularly during the initial phase post transplant should be as high as possible with the aim to prevent even mild and moderate acute rejection episodes of the pancreatic organ.
– Anti-rejection treatment should be combined with a regimen of anticoagulation to prevent secondary venous thrombosis.

Those considerations imply at first that there is one more reason to use multiple drug induction treatment (with an high immunosuppressive index) in pancreatic transplantation and secondly that basic immunosuppression as well as anti-rejection treatment should routinely be associated with effective anticoagulation.

As mentioned already above earlier more clinical experience and experimental data are needed to confirm the suggestions made at that point; nevertheless, at the present time they might be of some aid to do a reasonable immunosuppression in the pancreas transplanted recipient.

Current immunosuppressive protocols and results in pancreatic transplantation with special reference to the munich approach

Introduction

The pancreas transplant graft survival rates worldwide have improved to over 40% at one year in the last few years regardless what surgical techniques have been used. Nevertheless, – as already mentioned – it is hardly possible to deduce those improved results only! To a better immunosuppression because too many other modifications have been carried out recently by almost all transplant groups. This conclusion is probably not in contradiction to the fact the Pancreas Transplant-Registry Report form 1986 [10] showed that pancreas allograft functional survival rates were significantly higher in the patients who received cyclosporin than in those who did not (42% versus 22% at one year). This report also showed a statistically significant higher graft survival rate in those patients receiving cyclosporin in combination with Azathioprine than in those receiving cyclosporin alone or with Prednisone. Looking at the immuno-suppressive protocols currently used by the different transplant groups it becomes evident that there is general agreement with the use of a multiple drug induction treatment. Thus, some groups [11, 12] start with a triple drug induction treatment, other groups [5, 6] with a simultaneous (time-related) quadruple drug induction treatment. As far as the daily doses of the different immunosuppressive agents are concerned the different protocols used differ only slightly. As one example of quadruple drug induction treatment the Munich protocol is mentioned here:

Cyclosporin is initially administered intravenously (= 24 h-infusion) at a dose of 1–2 mg/kg/day (desired target whole blood levels (RIA): 100–250 ng/ml); and is switched to oral administration around the 10th day post transplant (doses: 6–12 mg/kg/day adjusted to trough levels in the range of 300–500 ng/ml); Azathioprine is given at a dose of 2–1 mg/kg/day and has been discontin-ued 3 weeks posttransplant; methylprednisone is rapidly tapered from 250 mg/day to 30 mg/day; ATG (Fresenius®) or ALG (Behring-Company®) is admin-istered from postoperative day 1 to 10 at a dose of 4 mg/kg/day (Fresenius) and 20 mg/kg/day (Behring) respectively.*

In contrast to induction treatment there is no general agreement on the optimal immunosuppressive protocol used in terms of maintenance treatment. The most common use is double drug maintenance treatment consisting of cyclosporin and steroids (for instance = 11) but also triple drug maintenance treatment (cyclosporin: 2–10 mg/kg/day, Azathioprine: 1 mg/kg/day, predni-sone: 5–10 mg/day) is being applied Madison [5], Minneapolis [6].

The Munich group has used single drug (cyclosporin: 2–8 mg/kg) mainte-nance treatment from the 6th month posttransplant, but has very recently switched to either triple drug (cyclosporin, Azathioprine, Methylprednisone) or double drug (cyclosporin, Azathioprine) maintenance treatment in view of the poor long-term survival rate of the simultaneously transplanted kidneys.

One difficulty of multiple drug maintenance treatment is the uncertainty of optimal cyclosporin blood concentrations. Compared with the therapeutic window under cyclosporin treatment alone (or with Prednisone) (Figure 1) the blood/serum concentrations should be lower, (but how lower?). Most groups haven chosen a blood level (RIA) in the range of 100–300 ng/ml (using the monoclonal Sandoz RIA kits). Further experience is needed to define more precisely the lowest blood concentration of cyclosporin which gives a sufficient

* Recently we have used OKT3 instead of ALG or ATG over a period of 10 days.

long-term immunosuppressive index in combination with Azathioprine plus steroid therapy.

Anti-rejection treatment is almost always performed with poly- or (recently) monoclonal antibodies by all groups. With regard to the risk of early graft loss due to secondary venous thrombosis (as mentioned above) vigorous treatment should be started immediately which means that one should not waste time to start at first with steroid pulses only.

For the same purpose, any kind of anti-rejection treatment should be associated with anticoagulation for reasons mentioned earlier. (Heparin, Rheomacrodex, others). Although not proven efficiently from the scientific point of view the Munich protocol of anti-rejection treatment includes routinely the use of anticoagulants in cases of pancreatic transplant rejection.

Results

Graft survival rates

Apart from the data of the Pancreas Transplant Registry in 1986 it appears of utmost importance that in 1986 several groups (Stockholm, Madison, Iowa, Lyon, Munich, Innsbruck) have reported on a 1-year-graft-survival rate of more than 70% in recent subgroups of patients [13]. Interestingly enough, all patients out of these subgroups received cyclosporin in terms of multiple drug induction as well as maintenance treatment. Although the number of treated patients in each subgroup is still too small; altogether, these results seem to reflect that general improvement is at least in part influenced by the new immunosuppressive protocols used. In Figure 2 the current results of the Munich group are shown just as one example.

Acute nephrotoxicity

Using multiple drug induction treatment which implies application of low CS starting doeses the incidence of severe acute nephrotoxic episodes caused by SC can be prevented almost completely and is no problem of CS therapy any more according to our experience and the experience of other groups [5, 6, 13].

Moreover, the avoidance of severe toxic adverse effects or cyclosporin is even more exprissed during the phase of intravenous application of cyclosporin (which was characterized by a high frequency of acute nephrotoxic episodes in former times).

Incidence of severe (life-threatening) infections posttransplantation

It may be just by chance, that in a consecutive series of 122 non-diabetic kidney

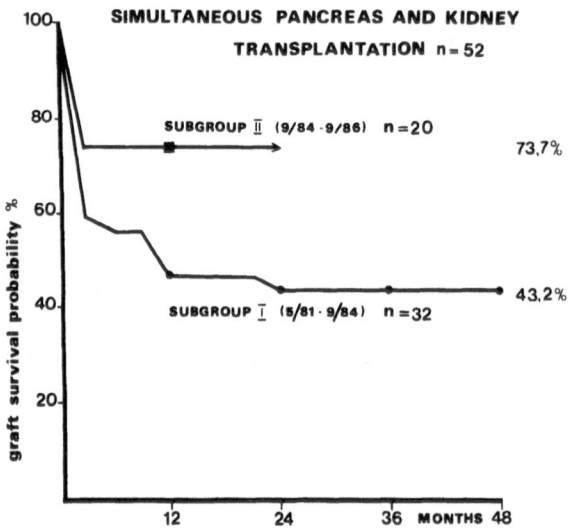

Figure 2. Results of the recent subgroup (= subgroup II) in pancreatic transplant recipients (compared to the results obtained before 1984) at the Centre of Munich (Dec. 1986). Only the pancreatic survival is depicted.

transplanted patients in 1986 no severe-life-threatening infection could be observed so far at our institution. Surpresingly, there was especially no case of severe CMV-infection. As also observed by other groups [6, 13] the incidence of severe infectious diseases posttransplant is reduced in pancreas-transplanted Type-I-diabetes using multiple immunosuppressive drug treatment. On the other hand, short-term initial heavy immunosuppression in a previously non-immunocompromized organism with a subsequent less incidence of severe acute rejection episodes (which otherwise would have been treated) may represent a particular kind of an immunosuppressive protocol which is safe with regard to the incidence of severe infectious diseases. The risk of manifestation of severe infections posttransplant seems to be more relevant in patients who are initially only moderately immunosuppressed over a certain period of time, who then develop severe acute rejection episodes (1–3 months posttransplant) requiring, then, heavy immunosuppression in term of efficient anti-rejection treatment (steroid pulses, poly- or monoclonal anti-lymphocyte antibodies). Certainly, one has to focus this observation more carefully in patients treated by multiple drug induction therapy in the new future.

Future perspectives

Future immunosuppressive therapy in pancreas transplanted recipients will probably stick to the current multiple drug combination protocols until a new

drug (2./3. generation of cyclosporin?) or methods for induction of transplantation tolerance will be available. In this respect, the new monoclonal
antibody BMA 031 [14] is of extremely high interest. With regard to the recent
results in cadaveric renal transplantation (even in immunological high risk
patients) the classical main problem of irreversible rejection seems to have
been overcome (only 5% irreversible graft losses in a consecutive series of
e.g.: ( ) 200 cadaveric renal transplantations at Munich in 1986).

Moreover, the previously severe side effect of cyclosporin – associated acute
nephrotoxicity has been meanwhile effectively controlled. There is still the
problem of late chronic progressive renal dysfunction which is thought to be
associated with a cyclosporin effect even if the blood levels are within the
normal range. Thus, better results of pancreatic transplantation in the near
future will be achieved rather by standardization of surgical techniques; optimal timing for a proper indication; a gaining expertise in the clinical management of pancreas-transplanted patients; etc., than by an improvement of the
immunosuppressive protocols currently used.

References

1. Land W: Optimal use of cyclosporin. An attempt at evaluation. In: Optimal use of Sand-
   immun in Organ Transplantation, ed. W. Land. Sandoz Ltd Basel and Springer Verlag Berlin,
   Heidelberg, 1987.
2. Kahan BB: Individualization of cyclosporin therapy using pharmacokinetic and pharmacodynamic parameters. Transplantation 40: 457, 1985.
3. Thiel G: Personal communication.
4. Sollinger HW, Deierhoi M, Kalayoglu M, Belzer EO: Sequential antilymphocyte globulin-
   cyclosporin therapy in cadaveric renal transplantation. Transpl Proc 18: 16, 1986.
5. Sollinger HW, Kalayoglu M, Hoffman M, Belzer FO: Quadruple immunosuppressive therapy in whole pancreas transplantation. Transpl Proc 19: 2297, 1987.
6. Sutherland DER, Goetz EC, Najarian JS: Improved pancreas graft survival by use of multiple
   drug combination immunotherapy. Transpl Proc 18: 1770, 1986.
7. Quesniaux V: The use of monoclonal antibodies to probe the surface of cyclosporines.
   Transpl Proc 18: (Suppl 5) 111, 1986.
8. Castro LA, Landgraf R, Hillebrand G, Land W: Causes of renal graft dysfunction in diabetics
   after simultaneous pancreas and kidney transplantation. Transpl Proc 18: 1733, 1986.
9. Groth CG: Personal communication.
10. Sutherland DER, Moudry K: Pancreas transplant registry. Transpl Proc 18: 1739, 1986.
11. Tyden G, Brattström C, Gunnarsson R, Lundgren G, Öst L, Östman J, Groth CG: Metabolic
    control 4 months to 4 years after pancreatic transplantation with special reference to the role
    of cyclosporin. Transpl Proc 19: 1987.
12. Dubernard JM, Faures JW, Gelet A, Martin X, Lefrancois N, Monti L, Similon B, Manzan
    K, Toraine JW, Traeger J: Simultaneous pancreas and kidney transplantation: long-term
    results and technical discussion. Transpl Proc 19: 1987.
13. II. Internat. workshop on clinical pancreatic transplantation: Munich, Spitzingsee, December
    1986. Discussion comments by: Corry R, Dubernard JM, Groth CG, Land W, Margreiter R,

Sollinger H, Sutherland DER. Papers published in Transpl Proc vol. 19, No 4 Suppl. 4 1987.

14. Land W, Hillebrand G, Illner WD, Abendroth D, Haucke E, Schleibner S, Hammer C, Racenberg J: First clinical experience with a new TCR/CD3 monoclonal antibody (BMA 031) in Kidney transplant patients. Transplant Int 1: 116, 1988.

Commentary

The author of the chapter on immunosuppression in pancreas transplant patients makes several points that deserve emphasis. Cyclosporine is best used in conjunction with other immunosuppressive drugs, since the synergism is greater for the therapeutic than for the toxic effects, as shown in experimental animal models by Squifflet et al. [1] years ago. At the University of Minnesota cyclosporin and azathioprine are used in combination for all organ transplant recipients [2–5] and this combination has been adapted by several other institutions [6].

Land emphasizes the nephrotoxic effect of high dose cyclosporin on transplanted kidneys but its effect on native kidneys should also be noted. At Munich, as at most transplant centers, the majority of pancreas transplants are performed in conjunction with a kidney transplant in uremic diabetic recipients. In this situation, the use of cyclosporin may augment renal graft injury manifested by a delay of function, and for that reason protocols have been devised in which the administration of cyclosporin is delayed until the kidney has recovered from the insult of transplantation. This strategy renders a pancreas vulnerable to early rejection, unless a potent alternative immunosuppression is used, such as antilymphocyte globulin (ALG).

At the University of Minnesota, the majority of recipients have been non-uremic, nonkidney transplant recipients of pancreas transplants alone [7], but almost all have had diabetic nephropathy of a moderately advanced degree, and cyclosporin may result in a further decrease in native kidney function [8]. Again, in such patients using maximal doses of azathioprine and prednisone allows cyclosporin to be used in doses that are non- or minimally nephrotoxic. With such a regimen, stable renal function can be maintained in the recipients [7, 8].

Land states that it is difficult to evaluate the effect of immunosuppressive strategies in preventing rejection of the pancreas grafts because there are so many failures for nonimmunological reasons. That statement is indeed true, but in the Registry, the analysis of graft survival rates have been done separately for technically failed grafts and technically successful grafts [9]. When grafts that fail because of local infection or early thrombosis are eliminated from the analysis, the advantage of using cyclosporin in combination with azathioprine over regimens that employ cyclosporin without azathioprine or azathioprine without cyclosporin is apparent. Land believes that thrombosis itself may be a manifestation of early, and even mild rejection, but there is no absolute proof that this is the case. Nevertheless, prevention of early rejection episodes appears to be important, and Land cites the multiple groups that are now using antilymphocyte globulin as part of a quadruple immunosuppressive strategy. At the University of Minnesota, we have given cyclosporin, azathioprine or prednisone from the time of transplant in recipients of pancreas transplants alone [3]. In recipients of simultaneous pancreas and kidney transplants, cyclosporin may be delayed until kidney graft function is established, but in that situation, we give ALG beginning the day after the transplant [10]. For recipients of pancreas transplants alone, renal function of the native kidneys is almost always sustained, and administration of ALG is delayed until the third day posttransplant, and its administration is contingent on the cultures of the graft duodenum (in the case of whole pancreas duodenal grafts), being negative. If the cultures are positive, ALG administration may be delayed until we are certain that there is no infection.

The diagnosis of rejection episodes in recipients of pancreas transplants alone is greatly facilitated by the use of a bladder drainage technique. At the University of Minnesota, the one year functional survival rate of bladder drained pancreas transplant in recipients on triple therapy has been 58% for all cases (n = 30) and 75% for technically successful cases (n = 24), primarily because of early treatment of rejection episodes [7, 11].

One contention of Land can be challenged, that the kidney is more susceptible to rejection than the pancreas. Although many groups have reported kidney rejection episodes occurring without any apparent rejection of a simultaneously transplanted pancreas from the same donor, it may mean only that the physiological manifestations occur earlier in the kidney than in the pancreas and that there is ongoing rejection in the pancreas which has been reversed by antirejection therapy initiated because of kidney transplant dysfunction. Careful monitoring will usually disclose dysfunction of the pancreas concomitant with that of the kidney [12]. Indeed, it may be that the pancreas is more susceptible to rejection than the kidney. In the Registry statistics, even when technically successful grafts only are analyzed, there are many more examples of long-term function of the kidney after loss of the pancreas than long-term function of the pancreas after loss of the kidney [9]. For technically successful cases where the pancreas has failed, one year after pancreas loss 30% of the kidneys transplants simultaneous with the pancreas are still functioning. In the analysis of technically successful pancreas transplant cases where the kidney failed, at the end of one year after kidney loss only 12% of the pancreas grafts were functioning. Thus, the pancreas may be more susceptible to rejection than the kidney even in doubly transplanted patients.

In recipients of pancreas transplants alone, rejection episodes have been

186

particularly frequent and severe [3]. In such patients high dose immuno-suppression must be given from the onset [7].

For widespread application of pancreas transplantation to be possible, antirejection treatment with less toxicity is needed. Eventually, regimens without the side effects of the agents currently employed will be devised. Meanwhile, the agents now available can be manipulated to give good graft survival rates in patients whose diabetic problems exceed those of chronic immunosuppression.

References

1. Squifflet JP, Sutherland DER, Rynasiewicz JJ, Field J, Heil J, Najarian JS: Combined immunosuppressive therapy with cyclosporin A and azathioprine. Transplantation 34: 315–318, 1982.
2. Simmons RL, Canafax DM, Strand M, Ascher NL, Payne WD, Sutherland DER, Najarian JS: Management and prevention of cyclosporin nephrotoxicity after renal transplantation: use of low doses of cyclosporin, azathioprine, and prednisone. Transpl Proc 17: 266–275, 1985.
3. Sutherland DER, Goetz FC, Najarian JS: Improved pancreas graft survival rates by use of multiple drug combination immunotherapy. Transpl Proc 18: 1770–1773, 1986.
4. Bolman RN et al. J Heart Transplantation 4: 315, 1985.
5. St. Cyr JA, Elick B, Freese D et al.: Use of triple therapy and percutaneous needle biopsy to minimize graft failure following liver transplantation. Transpl Proc 19: 2451, 1987.
6. Sollinger HW, Kalayoglu M, Hoffman RM: Quadruple immunosuppressive therapy in whole pancreas transplantation. Transpl Proc 19: 2297–2299, 1987.
7. Sutherland DER, Kendall DM, Moudry KC, Navarro X, Kennedy WR, Ramsay RC, Steffes MW, Mauer SM, Goetz FC, Dunn DL, Najarian JS: Pancreas transplantation in nonuremic, Type I diabetic recipients. Surgery 104: 453–464, 1988.
8. DeFrancisco AM, Mauer SM, Steffes MW, Goetz FC, Najarian JS, Sutherland DER: The effect of cyclosporin on native renal function in nonuremic diabetic recipients of pancreas transplants. J Diab Compl 1: 128–131, 1987.
9. Sutherland DER, Moudry KC: Report of the international pancreas transplant registry. In: Terasaki PI (ed) Clinical Transplants – 1987, pp. 63–101. UCLA Press, Los Angeles.
10. Sutherland DER, Goetz FC, Moudry KC, Najarian JS: Pancreatic transplantation – A single institution's experience. Diab Nutr and Metabolism1: 57–66, 1988.
11. Prieto M, Sutherland DER, Goetz FC, Rosenberg ME, Najarian JS: Pancreas transplant results according to the technique of duct management: bladder versus enteric drainage. Surgery 102: 680–691, 1987.
12. Margreiter R, Klima G, Bosmuller C: Rejection of kidney and pancreas after pancreatic-kidney transplantation. Diabetes (Suppl.) 37: 74–81, 1988.

D.E.R. Sutherland
Department of Surgery
School of Medicine
University of Minnesota
Minneapolis, Minnesota 55455

9. The diagnosis and treatment of pancreatic rejection

P. McMASTER

Introduction

The immunological response mounted by a recipient will, with very few exceptions, result in destruction of implanted cells or grafts. In man the process may be rapid even in patients receiving immunosuppressive agents, and for many years nearly half of all transplanted cadaveric kidneys were destroyed within 18 months. With improved immunosuppressive schedules and better patient monitoring and management, far fewer kidney grafts are now lost so that now over 75% of cadaveric grafts are expected to function well at 1 year. The diagnosis of kidney rejection is well defined by clinical, biochemical, cytological and histological parameters, and can usually be made with confidence and a treatment schedule introduced. In pancreatic transplantation this is not the situation. Clinical and biochemical parameters are uncertain and non-specific and there are many other causes of pancreatic dysfunction other than immunological assault and rejection. In the early reports in man [1] technical problems dominated the causes of graft loss and rejection was only clearly identified in a few cases. The techniques currently used for pancreatic implantation may well produce difficulties which can result in cessation of pancreatic graft function. The commonest of these problems are associated with the exocrine pancreatic secretion leading to infection or pancreatic abscess formation, or a progressive fibrosis and sclerosis of the graft after intraductal occlusion. Poor preservation techniques may lead to graft failure or subsequent development of pancreatitis and both venous and arterial trombosis which has occurred in 15% of segmental graft implants.

It is clear that pancreatic rejection is only one of several potential causes of graft dysfunction (table 1). In clinical practice the precise cause of graft dysfunction can only usually be identified by a careful process of evaluation and elimination and a clear diagnosis of rejection made. In the past if pancreatic grafting was undertaken simultaneously with kidney grafting it was often presumed that at the time of renal rejection the pancreas was also rejecting but

187

J.M. Dubernard and D.E.R. Sutherland (eds.), International Handbook of Pancreas Transplantation, 187–202.
© *1989 by Kluwer Academic Publishers.*

confirmation of this was often lacking. The first transplants of pancreatic grafts into non-uraemics however, clearly demonstrated [2] that immunological destruction of the pancreas does occur.

The diagnosis of pancreatic rejection

Experimental studies

Recent evidence in man shows that as with the kidney, pancreatic grafts between living related individuals have a better outcome than those from cadaver sources suggesting that MHC compatibility between donor and recipient may be a significant factor in the development of immunological responses. Klempnauer [3] confirmed the dominant role in MHC encoded histocompatibility antigen in eliciting rejection in both rat pancreas and heart models. In the vascularised pancreatic allografts, however, non MHC alloantigens also induced a strong immunological response and although as yet not really defined, may be an important factor in the rejection of pancreatic grafts. It remains possible that non MHC antigens situated in the exocrine part of the pancreas inevitably transfer at the time of pancreatic transplantation.

The histological features of rejection have also been studied in some detail in experimental rat models [4] but there may also be an increase in cellular infiltrate within pancreatic grafts following direct duct ligation independent of the presence of rejection. However, in the Lewis whole pancreatic allograft model the progressive ductal atrophy and sclerosis does not fundamentally alter the vascular and infiltrative picture of lymphocytes into the tissue in severe fulminant rejection.

Gotoh [5] noted that when pancreatic drainage went via the urinary system in mongrel dogs changes in serum and urinary amylase occurred at least 24 hours before abnormalities in blood sugar parameters were noted. These initial observations have been extended by Sollinger et al. [6] who have confirmed the significant early reduction in urinary amylase prior to serum biochemical changes also in canine models.

Sollinger et al. [7] also demonstrated that Indium-111 labelled platelets can

Table 1. Pancreatic graft 'failure'.

Rejection	Pancreatic Thrombosis
	Pancreatitis
Recurrent diabetes	Pancreatic Failure
	Sclerosis
	Infection

show a consistent and progressive infiltration into rejecting grafts, indicating rejection at an early stage prior to other clinical or biochemical parameters.

Attempts to develop an aspiration cytology diagnosis of graft rejection by Steiner et al. [8] have proved difficult and in contrast to the kidney where aspiration cytology is of benefit, it proved difficult to obtain adequate tissue in the pancreatic implants. Only 10% of aspiration biopsies were suitable for evaluation and complications and pancreatic fistulas were recorded following this. Attempts to define the prodromal biochemical symptoms of rejection more clearly were undertaken by Garvey et al. [9]. They compared fasting blood sugar and intravenous glucose tolerance tests. Fasting blood sugar levels of over 7.7 mmol/l correlated well with rejection and a K value (rate of disappearance of blood glucose) of less than 1.7 was associated with progressive graft failure in 6 of 7 treated animals.

The clinical diagnosis of rejection

Clinical features of pancreatic rejection have often been extremely difficult to differentiate from the development of local complications resulting in graft failure. While some groups have ascribed fever and swelling of the pancreatic graft associated with a high serum amylase [10] to rejection, others have seen a less clearly defined sequence of events. The rise in serum amylase has not always correlated well with the onset of pancreatic rejection, although the technique of ductal management may have significant influence on this. Where duct injection is used the serum amylase is normally elevated for 48 hours post-transplantation and minor fluctuations may also occur quite independently of pancreatic rejection. Where, however ductal drainage is established without complications hyperamylasaemia may be an early marker of rejection although not a consistent one.

In patients undergoing combined kidney and pancreatic transplantation, the development of renal rejection which is easily defined has often been taken as an index of active and concomitant pancreatic rejection. The fact that the results of combined kidney and pancreas grafting are better than the pancreas alone may suggest that the kidney does act as a true marker of pancreatic rejection, thus allowing simultaneous treatment of both grafts. However, the influence of uraemia and reduction of immune response may be more important than has perhaps previously been appreciated. It is also clear that while both grafts may reject simultaneously this is not inevitable and one or other graft may be lost from immunological destruction while the other continues to function without significant damage.

Biochemical parameters

By far the most consistent although not specific indication of pancreatic rejection is a rise in fasting blood glucose which can frequently be abrupt and unexpected. However, the elevation of fasting blood glucose is not specific and will also occur with other causes of pancreatic dysfunction. In order to try to overcome some of these difficulties Secchi et al. [11] measured 24 hour glycosuria related to creatinine clearance. When combined pancreatic and kidney grafting are undertaken the need to administer steroids to treat renal rejection will invariably lead to an associated rise in blood sugar making the interpretation of pancreatic function more difficult.

Of much more value would be a measurement of serum insulin as a direct measure of insulin output of beta cells within the pancreatic graft. However the presence of high levels of insulin antibodies often makes this impossible and plasma C-peptide levels may be the only indicator. Such measurements are rarely immediately available in the clinic because of the immunoassay techniques that are required, although they do suggest that a progressive fall in C-peptide production and a sharp fall at the time of rejection may occur [12]. Measurements of oral and intravenous glucose tolerance tests rarely give a consistent pattern even in the same patient and variation in glucose clearance makes their interpretation difficult. Nevertheless a progressive deterioration in the K value may be seen in a deteriorating pancreatic graft. However, again this is not specific and failure due to graft fibrosis may also produce similar results.

The use of the urinary tract as the mode of drainage either via the ureter or directly on to the bladder [6] allows urinary amylase to be used as a marker. Experimental studies in canine models and now in man confirm a significant fall in urinary amylase preceeding any overt clinical features of hyperglycaemia. Patients may be taught to monitor their urinary amylase using a home kit method, and to report in the moment levels start to fall precipitously. In the absence of other catastrophic events, this may yet prove one of the most simple and practical markers of early pancreatic dysfunction due to rejection.

Table 2. Diagnosis of rejection.

Kidney graft as 'marker'
Biopsy
Aspiration Cytology
Indium scanning
Biochemical changes
Arteriography

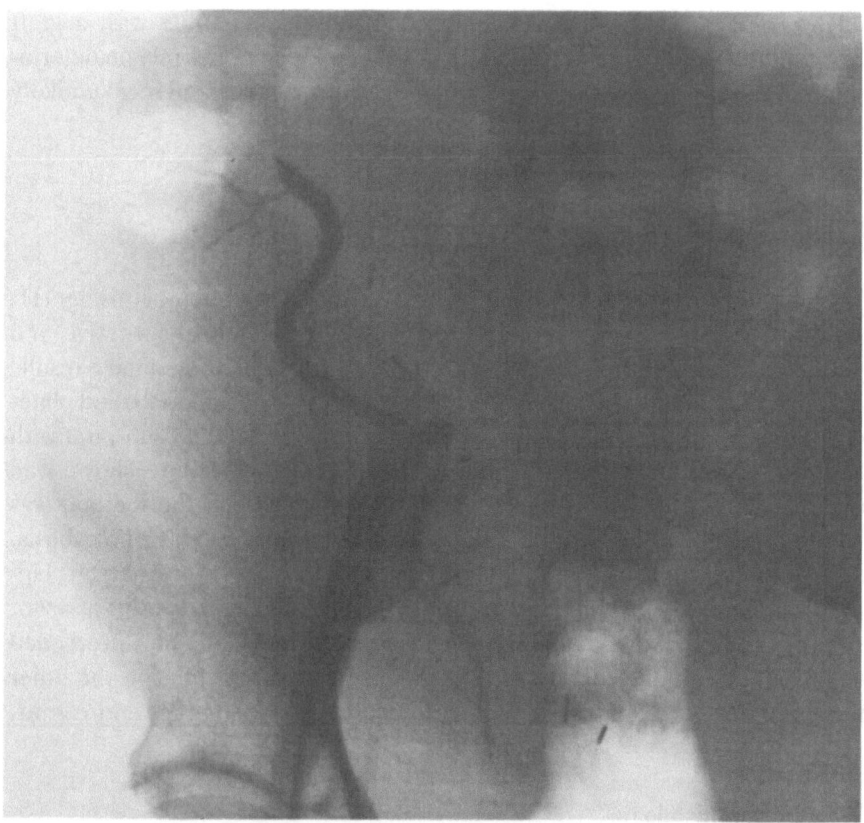

Figure 1. Arteriography showing pancreatic arterial thrombosis preceding acute graft failure and high serum glucose which was initially thought to be due to acute rejection.

Arteriography

Marked pancreatic dysfunction was often investigated in the early pancreatic grafts by arteriography. While failure was due to arterial thrombosis in many of these grafts, in some patients an angiographic picture suggestive of rejection was seen, and appeared similar to that found in renal grafts, [2]. With the introduction of digital subtraction angiography this mode of investigation may now warrant further study, but the need for an invasive approach to achieve high quality angiography has led to very little clinical utilisation.

Scintigraphy

Se 75I-Methionine has been used not only to confirm pancreatic viability but to demonstrate features of rejection [13]. Further modification of the technique by Jameson et al. [14] showed that in conjunction with 99m Tc DTPA it gave much clearer visualisation and indicated features compatible with a graft dysfunction due to rejection. However, both these techniques rely on deterioration of graft perfusion as a main marker of acute rejection and seem unlikely to detect early immunological events.

lll Indium platelets in monitoring pancreatic allografts in man

A promising technique has been studied in our department utilising 111-Indium labelled autologous platelets, which is based on quantitative and qualitative analysis of platelet uptake by the graft [15]. Preliminary results indicated that patients with insignificant accumulation of radio-labelled platelets in the pancreatic graft had an uneventful recovery and left hospital with satisfactory graft function. Patients who suffered graft failure showed an abnormal deposition of platelets within the pancreas and the method was helpful in detecting rejection as well as the early stages of graft thrombosis. Two distinctive patterns of pathological platelet accumulation emerged. Uptake of Indium-labelled platelets at the site of anastomosis presenting as a 'hot spot' on gamma camera images indicated early thrombosis and preceeded venous infarction due to venous obstruction. Acute rejection, on the other hand, manifested as a diffuse uniform accumulation involving the entire graft.

Cytology and histology

One of the major concerns in pancreatic grafting has been the fear that recurrent diabetes mellitus may occur due to immunological destruction of the beta cells from autoimmune antibodies. In 1982 Sutherland et al. [16] noted graft diabetes developing due to a beta cell insulitis in the absence of major features typical of both cellular and vascular rejection of the graft. The first recipient in whom this was noted was a living related identical sibling in whom it would not be anticipated that rejection would occur. A skin graft had confirmed HLA identity and the loss of beta cells with cellular islet cell damage clearly demonstrates that recurrent Type I diabetes due to 'auto islet antibodies' can occur [17].

Because of the risk of fistula formation, aspiration cytology for monitoring cellular changes has not been widely applied to the pancreas and its interpretation in the presence of cellular infiltrate associated with ductal management might make it in practice almost impossible. Percutaneous needle biopsy has also been somewhat infrequently undertaken although recent evidence suggests that the amount of leakage which can occur after biopsy may be less than had previously been feared. Open biopsy has most often been used to obtain histology.

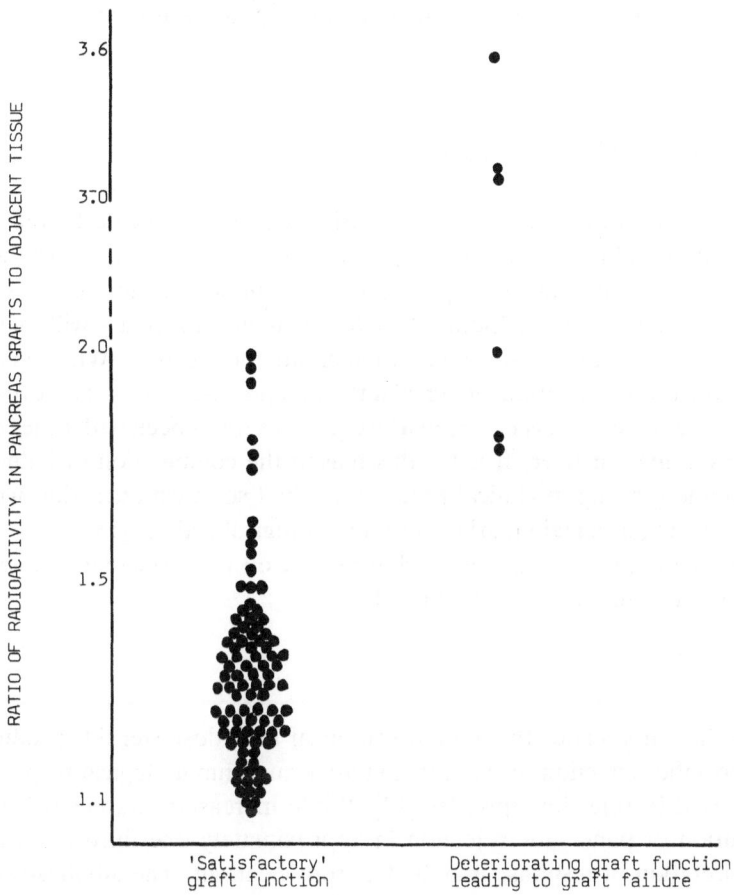

Figure 2. 111-Indium labelled platelets uptake in satisfactorily functioning and deteriorating pancreatic grafts.

Nuclear magnetic resonance and CAT scanning

Although both modalities offer considerable potential in evaluation of pancreatic grafts there is insufficient evidence at the moment to be able to adjudicate on their clinical value.

Conclusion

The diagnosis of pancreatic rejection remains a major clinical problem and often requires a combination of techniques to confirm the diagnosis (Table 3). Only by improving diagnostic techniques will the early introduction of effective treatment be possible and the patient spared the hazards of uneccessary and high immunosuppressive schedules when graft failure occurs from non-rejection causes.

Treatment of pancreatic rejection

It is now recognised that over 90% of islet cells need to be destroyed before frank abnormalities in plasma glucose will be recorded. Therefore the pancreas on its own – unless sophisticated techniques of monitoring such as cellular accumulation of Indium labelled platelets are used – will inevitably present at a relatively late stage in pancreatic destruction. With pancreatic rejection therefore often being a difficult and late diagnosis, reversal of pancreatic rejection has not been as frequent as it has been with other organs such as kidney or liver. It is for this reason the combination of kidney and pancreatic grafting in clinical practice has had so much attraction with the kidney acting as a main marker for immunological activity [18].

The main options available to clinicians faced with pancreatic destruction due to rejection are briefly outlined below.

Steroids

Since the early sixties the administration of high dose steroids producing a non-specific reduction in the inflammatory and immunological response has been used in rejection episodes [19]. While increasing steroids will lead to resolution of pancreatic rejection in approximately one third of cases, the interpretation of response may be far from clear cut. The administration of steroids in themselves can produce profound abnormalities in carbohydrate control and glucose tolerance which may persist for some days or weeks after treatment. Thus a clear cut and prompt response to steroids is not always encountered although ultimately between a quarter and one third of grafts demonstrating dysfunction purely attributable to rejection will respond. Where, however, pancreatic dysfunction is identified using cellular infiltration

Table 3. Clinical diagnosis of rejection.

	Non-specific	Specific
serum glucose	+++	−
urinary amylase	−	++
111–indium scan	−	++
biopsy	−	+++
kidney marker	+	−

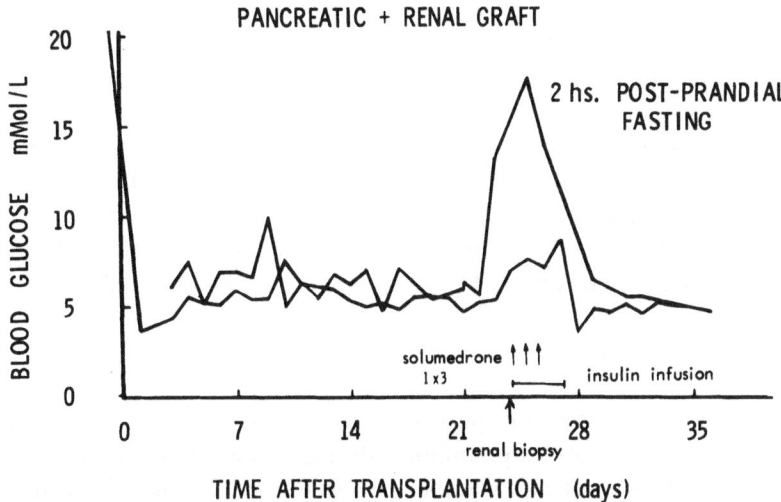

Figure 3. Serum glucose response to high steroids in the treatment of presumed pancreatic rejection.

monitoring or abnormalities in urinary amylase a higher response rate is normally anticipated with nearly half the grafts showing significant improvement with administration of steroids [16].

Cyclosporin

The absorption of cyclosporin in diabetics with autonomic gastro-intestinal dysfunction is potentially unreliable and erratic although Kahan et al. did not show any difference in bioavailability between diabetic and non-diabetic renal transplant patients [20]. In clinical practice if an intestinal loop has been used as part of the pancreatic reconstruction cyclosporin will normally be administered intravenously in the first week to ten days. It is also often accompanied by parenteral nutrition with its high lipid component causing further variability in cyclosporin utilisation.

Thus in the patient on cyclosporin as the prime mode of immunosuppressive treatment, when rejection occurs one of the immediate concerns must be to ensure that adequate concentrations of cyclosporin are being achieved. While it is now well recognised that the parent compound of cyclosporin probably contains the active component, many units have tended to rely on the RIA assay which is affected by cross-reacting metabolites. Levels between 700 and 1000 ngm/ml are usually required in the RIA metabolite estimation to ensure adequate parent compound levels and during acute rejection on cyclosporin unless these levels can be achieved and mentioned by oral administration on a twice daily basis then a continuous intravenous infusion of cyclosporin may well be required on an initial dose of 5 mg/kg/day. In more than half our patients experiencing early signs of rejection of the pancreas as monitored by cellular accumulation, adequate levels of CyA have not been achieved.

One alternative approach to immunosuppression in a patient on cyclosporin as the prime immunosuppressive mode would be the conversion from cyclosporin to Azathioprine. Little experience of this as a means of managing acute rejection has been accumulated but there does not appear to be much evidence to suggest that rejection taking place in patients on adequate levels of cyclosporin can then be aborted by conversion to Azathioprine [21].

ATG and OKT3

ATG has been used as part of post transplant immunosuppressive protocols and T cells have been carefully monitored during episodes of rejection [22, 23]. A clear cut pattern of efficacy has not been established and the administration of ATG in conjunction with cyclosporin is reported to be associated with a high incidence of lymphoproliferative disorders [25]. Nevertheless acute rejection can be aborted by a course of ATG in some patients although risks of over-immunosuppression and viral infections must always been borne in mind.

The introduction of monoclonal antibodies OKT3 (ORTHOCLONE) affords, in theory, a more specific approach to cellular manipulation in organ rejection. Again no prospective controlled trials in pancreatic grafting having been reported although anecdotal evidence suggests that monoclonal antibody appears less effective in resolving acute pancreatic rejection than in the kidney or liver.

Graft irradiation

Total lymphoid irradiation as part of a protocol of preparation has been undertaken in preparation for combined kidney and pancreatic grafting [26]. Although the incidence of acute rejection weas significantly less in this protocol, it was poorly tolerated by the diabetic and infective and overwhelming septic complications were frequently encountered.

There seems little evidence to suggest that local administration of radiotherapy has any significant role to play in the management of rejection episodes of pancreatic grafts but no controlled data are available.

Finally, with optimal treatment of pancreatic grafts now almost certainly comprising triple therapy with cyclosporin, Azathioprine and Prednisolone, the management of acute rejection episodes will now mostly by confined to the administration of increased steroids, and in a few selected centres the administration of OKT3 or ATG.

Conclusions

While the development of pancreatic grafting has been beset by major technical problems, ultimately success in grafting will be afforded when adequate immunological control can be achieved and graft destruction by rejection prevented. One of the major difficulties in pancreatic grafting has been the problem of identifying changes in a pancreatic graft due to immunological damage clearly and at an early stage. The use of the urinary drainage system allowing regular monitoring of the urinary amylase or alternatively the technique of cellular infiltrate monitoring with Indium labelled platelets both enable relatively early recognition of immunological assault on the pancreatic graft. With such techniques it is now becoming clear that acute rejection can be aborted by the administration of high dose steroids and adjustment of cyclosporin to more therapeutic ranges. The role of monoclonal antibodies in the treatment of rejection has yet to be defined.

References

1. Lillhei RC, Simmons RL, Najarian JS, Weil R, Uchida H, Ruiz JO, Kjellestrand CM, Goetz FC: Pancreatico-duodenal allotransplantation: experimental and animal experience. Ann Surg 172: 405–436, 1970.
2. Groth CG, Lundgren G, Arner P, Collste H, Hardesdt C, Lewander R, Ostman J: Rejection of isolated pancreatic allografts in patients with diabetes. Surg Gynae Obst 143: 933–940, 1976.
3. Klempnauer J, Hoins L, Steiniger B, Gunther E, Woinigeiit K, Pichlmayr R: Evidence for a differential importance of MHC and non-MHC alloantigens in pancreas and heart transplantation in the rat. Transplant Proc 16: 778–780, 1984.
4. Steiniger B, Klempnauer J, Brusch U, Wonigeit K: Histology of rejection in rat pancreas allografts with suppressed or preserved exocrine function. Transplant Proc 16: 783–784, 1984.
5. Gotoh M, Monden M, Motoki Y, Sakane O, Shima K, Okamura J: Early detection of rejection in the allografted pancreas. Transplant Proc 16: 781–782, 1984.
6. Sollinger HW, Kaylayoglu M, Hoffman RM, Belzer FD: Results of segmental and pancreatic cystostomy. Transplant Proc 17: 1149–50, 1985.
7. Sollinger HW, Lieberman LM, Kamps D, Warner T, Cook K: Diagnosis of early pancreatic rejection with Indium-111 oxine labeled platelets. Transplant Proc 16: 785–788, 1984.
8. Steiner E, Hammer C, Land W, Gruder P, Schneeburger H, Stangl M, Steiner W: Fine needle biopsy of canine pancreas graft: An attempt at cytologic diagnosis in graft rejection. Transplant. Proc 16: 789–90.
9. Garvey JFW, Deane SA, Grierson JM, Williamson P, McGill K, Eastman CJ, Duggin GG, Stewart GJ, Little JM: Effect of CyA on segmental pancreas allografts in the dog. Transplant Proc 16: 1043–45, 1984.
10. Largardier F, Ulschmid G, Binswanger U, Zaruba K: Pancreas rejection in combined pancreaticoduodenal and renal allotransplantation in man. Transplant Proc 19: 185–187, 1975.
11. Secchi A, Pontiroli AE, Traeger J, Dubernard JM, Touraine JL, Ruitton A, Blanc N, Pozza

G: A method for early detection of graft failure in pancreas transplantation. Transplantation 35: 344–348, 1983.

12. Ostman J, Arner P, Groth CG, Gunnarson R, Heading L, Lundgren G: Plasma C-peptide and serum insulin antibodies in diabetic patients receiving pancreatic transplants. Diabetologia 19: 25–30, 1980.

13. Svahn T, Lewander R, Hardstedt C, Lundgren G, Sundlein P, Groth CG: Angiography and scintigraphy of human pancreatic allografts. Acta Radiol Diagnos 19: 297–304, 1978.

14. Jamieson NV, McMaster P, Wraight EP, Evans DB, Calne RY: Radionuclide imaging in pancreas transplantation. Nuc Med Communication 1: 291–297, 1980.

15. Jurewicz WA, Buckels JAC, Dykes JGA, Chandler ST, Gunson BK, Hawker RJ, McCollum CN, McMaster P: 111-Indium labelled platelets in monitoring pancreatic allografts in man. Brit J Surg 72: 228–231, 1985.

16. Sutherland DER, Sibley R, Chinn P, Michael H, Srikanta S, Taub F, Najarian J, Goetz FC: Twin-to twin pancreas transplantation reversal and re-enactment of Type 1 diabetes. Clin Research 32: 561A, 1984.

17. Naji A, Silvers WK, Barker CF: Islet transplantation in spontaneously diabetic rats. Transplant Proc 13: 826–828, 1981.

18. McMaster P: What to expect from pancreas transplantation. Transplant Proc 16: 587–592, 1984.

19. Goodwin WE, Kaufman JJ, Mins MM, Turner RD, Glassock R, Goldman R, Maxwell J: Human renal transplantation J Urol 89: 13–19, 1963.

20. Kahan BD, Kramer WG, Wideman CA, Frazier OH, Lorber MI, Williams C, Flechner SM, Cooley DA, Van Buren CT: Analysis of pharmacokinetic profiles in 232 renal and 87 cardiac allograft patients treated with cyclosporin. Transplant Proc 18 (Suppl 5): 115–119, 1986.

21. Flechner SM, Van Buren CT, Jarowenko M, Kerman R, Kahan BD: The fate of patients converted from cyclosporin to Azathioprine to improve renal function. Transplant Proc 17: 1227–31, 1985.

22. Kelly GE, Sheil AGR: Treatment of Acute Rejection in recipients receiving CyA:ATG versus Prednisolone. Aust N Z Surg 56: 251–5, 1986.

23. Traeger J, Bosi E, Dubernard JM, Touraine JL, Piatti PM, Secchi A, Gelet A, Pozza G: Thirty months experience with CyA in human pancreatic transplantation. Diabetologia 27: 154–6, 1984.

24. Secchi A, Pontiroli AE, Bosi E, Piatti PM, Monti L, Traeger J, Dubernard JM, Gelet A, Pozza G: Effects of different immunsuppression treatment on the endocrine function of segmental neoprene injected pancreatic allografts. Transplant Proc 17 (Suppl 2): 136–40, 1985.

25. Ortho Multicenter Transplant Study Group: A randomized clinical trial of OKT3 monoclonal antibody for acute rejection of cadaveric renal transplant. New Eng J Med 313: 337–342, 1985.

Commentary

The most important point made by McMaster et al. in the chapter on treatment of pancreatic rejection are 1. the need for the good prophylactic immunosuppression so the need for treatment of rejection episodes is avoided; and 2. if rejection episodes do occur, the necessity of making the diagnosis early, since if one waits for hyperglycemia to occur more than 90% of the beta cell mass in the pancreas may have been destroyed and treatment will be futile.

In the early series at the University of Minnesota, graft biopsies were frequently performed [1]. From detailed immunohistopathologic examinations of biopsied and removed grafts, it is apparent that there are as many patterns of rejection in the pancreas as there are for the kidney [2]. Thus, there may be cases of rejection-induced dysfunction, in which beta cell mass is not destroyed, and treatment can restore normoglycemia. However, the most frequent form of rejection is vascular, and in such cases good graft function will be maintained until the islets die from ischemia.

Pancreas graft dysfunction, as opposed to actual destruction, appears to be manifested in the exocrine more than in the endocrine pancreas, and provisions to monitor graft exocrine function should be part of all modern pancreas transplant approaches. Two approaches are currently successful. One involves direct catheterization of the duct with external drainage for a temporary period, such as the first two months when the incidence of rejection episodes is the highest [3, 4]. This method can be used in conjunction with either enteric drainage [5] or delayed duct injection with a polymer [6]. The other method is urinary drainage [7]. The bladder drainage technique, as introduced by Sollinger [8] allows permanent monitoring of exocrine function by measurement of urinary amylase activity [9]. McMaster cites the first use of urinary amylase monitoring for diagnosis of rejection, and multiple authors has since confirmed its value [9–11]. Duct drainage with a catheter has been used by the group in Stockholm and Innsbruck not only for monitoring amylase in the pancreatic juice, but also for monitoring for appearance of mononuclear cells [5, 12]. The appearance of mononuclear cells in the pancreatic juice appears to be the earliest manifestation of rejection, and treatment at this point can generally reverse the process.

As McMaster points out, simultaneous kidney and pancreas transplants allow the kidney to be used for monitoring, with the manifestations of rejection in the kidney probably mirroring events in the pancreas in most cases [13]. However, there are exceptions and isolated rejection of either organ has occurred [12].

McMaster alludes to the fact that HLA matching may also reduce the incidence of rejection episodes, and the Registry data would seem to support this contention, with grafts in which there are few mismatches having higher functional survival rates than those in which there are several mismatches (See Registry Chapter).

I would disagree with McMaster that steroids compounds the difficulty in monitoring for rejection. In general, normoglycemia is achieved in the early posttransplant period even though high dose of steroids are administered. If during a rejection episode of a kidney, steroids are administered and hyperglycemia ensues, most likely the steroids are unmasking endocrine function dysfunction from ongoing rejection in the pancreas. Steroid induced diabetes most likely does occur in pancreas transplant recipients, as it does in kidney transplant patients [14], but the incidence is low (no more that 15% for kidney transplant recipients on triple therapy).

In regard to treatment of rejection, at the University of Minnesota the use of ALG or OKT3 has been highly effective, not only for the doubly transplanted patients, but also for recipients of pancreas transplants alone in which the bladder drainage technique has allowed early diagnosis of rejection [15]. The University of Wisconsin, has also reported a high rate of reversal of pancreas graft rejection episodes by administration of antiOKT3 [16].

The sophistication with which pancreas grafts can be monitored has increased. Biochemical monitoring of graft function is essential, and scanning techniques are only supplemental. With good prophylactic immunosuppression, rejection episodes will rarely occur during the initial hospitalization. Scanning techniques may be useful for confirming suspected rejection episodes when patients are admitted after deterioriation of biochemical parameters. Biochemical monitoring should be simple and able to be done at home or at any hospital. Measurement of urinary amylase fits this criteria. A home monitoring kit, alluded to by McMaster, now appears to be on the vurge of a reality [17]. The combination of aggressive prophylactic immunosuppressions, early diagnosis of rejection, and new antirejection agents have contributed to the improvements in graft survival rates that are reflected by reports from the individual institutions in this book, as well as from the Registry data.

The value of the early diagnosis of rejection is demonstrated by a report from the University of Minnesota cases comparing treatment initiated on the basis of hyperglycemia and enteric drained grafts versus a decline in urine amylase activity (with or without concurrent hyperglycemia) in urinary drained grafts [15]. Between November 1985 and February 1987, 14 recipients of enteric drained and 21 recipients of bladder-drained grafts were diagnosed to have rejection episodes. In four of the enteric drained cases, the occurrence of hyperglycemia was rapid and so severe that antirejection treatment was not initiated, while the other ten were treated. Hyperglycemia was reversed and an insulin-independent state re-established in only four cases (40%). In contrast, 17 patients in the bladder drained group had 1 and 4 had 2 multiple rejection episodes treated. All the patients treated more than once retained graft function and are insulin independent. Three primary rejection episodes were not reversed. In the other 14 patients treatment was followed by an increase in urinary amylase activity and a decrease in plasma glucose with maintenance or reversion to an insulin independent state.

These outcomes demonstrate the effectiveness of early treatment of rejection episodes based on a decline in exocrine function. The same objective may be achieved by external drainage of the pancreatic secretions via a catheter in the duct, but this advantage is maintained only for as long as the catheter remains in place, while with urinary drainage the exocrine function of the graft can be monitored indefinitely.

McMaster also mentions that graft dysfunction may occur because of recurrence of disease (autoimmune isletitits). Recurrence of disease has only been seen in recipients of isografts or allografts from HLA identical sibilings in which minimal immunosuppression is used [18]. Recurrence of disease has not been identified in grafts from cadaver donors [19], either because the process is MHC restricted, or because the degree of immunosuppression used for cadaver grafts also uniformly prevents the occurrence of disease [20]. For practical purposes, recurrence of disease is not an issue with current prophylactic immunosuppression.

References

1. Sutherland DER, Casanova D, Sibley RK: Role of pancreas graft biopsies in the diagnosis and treatment of rejection after pancreas transplantation. Transpl Proc 19: 2329–2331, 1987.
2. Sibley RK, Sutherland DER: Pancreas transplantation: an immunohistologic and histopathologic examination of 100 grafts. Am J Pathol 128: 151–170, 1987.
3. Tyden G, Brattstom G, Haggmark A: Studies on the exocrine secretion of human segmental pancreastic grafts. Surg Gynecol Obstet 164: 404–408, 1987.
4. Steiner E, Klima J, Niederwieser D et al.: Monitoring of the pancreatic allograft by analysis of exocrine secretion. Transpl Proc 19: 2336–2338, 1987.
5. Tyden G, Reinholt R, Brattstrom C, Lundgren G, Wilczek H, Bolinder J, Ostman J, Groth CG: Diagnosis of rejection in recipients of pancreatic grafts with enteric exocrine diversion by monitoring pancreatic juice cytology and amylase excretion. Transpl Proc 19: 3892–3894, 1987.
6. Baumgartner D, Bruhlmann W, Largarider F: Technique and timing of pancreatic duct occlusion with prolamine in recipients of simultaneous renal and intraoperative segmental pancreas allotransplants. Transpl Proc 16: 1134–1135, 1986.
7. Gliedman ML, Gold M, Whittaker J et al.: Clinical segmental pancreatic transplantation with ureter-pancreatic duct anastomosis for exocrine drainage. Surgery 74: 171–180, 1973.
8. Sollinger HW, Cook K, Kamps D et al.: Clinical and experimental experience with pancreaticocystostomy for exocrine pancreatic drainage in pancreas transplantation. Transpl Proc 16: 749, 1984.
9. Prieto M, Sutherland DER, Fernandez-Cruz L, Heil J, Najarian JS: Experimental and clinical experience with urine amylase monitoring for early diagnosis of rejection in pancreas transplantation. Transplantation 43: 71–79, 1987.
10. Fernandez-Cruz L, Esmatges E, Andreu J, Targarona EM, Prieto M, Gil-Vernet JM: Advantages and disadvantages of urinary tract diversion in clinical pancreas transplantation. Transpl Proc 19: 3895–3898, 1987.
11. van Hoof JP, Leunissen KML, Kingma PJ, Nieuwenhuyzen Kruseman AC, Degenaar CP, Menheere PPCA, Beukers EKM, Kootstra G: Urine amylase and insulin reserve capacity are valuable tools for diagnosing pancreas allograft rejection. Transpl Proc 19: 3899–3902, 1987.
12. Margrieter R, Klima G, Bosmuller C: Are kidney and pancreas rejected simultaneously after pancreatic-renal transplantation? Diabetes (Suppl) 37: in press, 1988.

13. Dubernard JM, Traeger J, Touraine L et al.: Patterns of renal and pancreatic rejection in double-grafted patients. Transpl Proc 13: 305, 1981.

14. Boudreaux JP, McHugh L, Canafax DM, Ascher M, Sutherland DER, Payne W, Simmons RL, Najarian JS, Fryd CS: The impact of cyclosporin and combination immunosuppression on the incidence of posttransplant diabetes in renal allograft recipients. Transplantation 4: 376–381, 1987.

15. Prieto M, Sutherland DER, Goetz FC, Najarian JS: Pancreas transplant results according to technique of duct management: Bladder versus enteric drainage. Surgery 102: 680–691, 1987.

16. Stratta RJ, Sollinger HW, D'Alessandro AM, Pirsch JD, Kalayoglu M, Belzer FO: OKT3 rescue therapy in pancreas allograft rejection. Diabetes 37 (Suppl): in press, 1988.

17. Prieto M, Collins W, Scott MH, Sells RA: Development of a method for home monitoring of urine amylase after pancreatic transplantation. Diabetes 37 (Suppl): in press, 1988.

18. Sibley RK, Sutherland DER, Goets F, Michael AF: Recurrent diabetes mellitus in the pancreas iso- and allograft. A light and electron microscopic and immunohistochemical analysis of four cases. Lab Invest 53: 132–144, 1985.

19. Sibley RK, Sutherland DER: Pancreas transplantation: An immunohistologic and histopathologic examination of 100 grafts. Am J Pathol 128: 151–170, 1987.

20. Sutherland DER, Goetz FC, Sibley RK: Recurrence of disease in pancreas transplants. Diabetes 38 (Suppl): in press, 1988.

D.E.R. Sutherland
Department of Surgery
School of Medicine
University of Minnesota
Minneapolis, Minnesota 55455

10. Pathology of pancreas grafts

R.K. SIBLEY

Introduction

During the past two decades, data on 1001 pancreas transplants have been entered into the International Pancreas Transplant Registry [1]. During these 20 years there has been continued improvement in graft survival, the most recent being 43% at one year. As reported to the Registry, technical factors (infection, thrombosis) are still major hazards to successful pancreas transplantation, accounting for the loss of 39% of grafts. Rejection and nondeterminate causes accounted for the loss of 45% of grafts, and 11% of grafts were lost because of death of the patient.

Between July, 1978 and July, 1987, 195 pancreas transplants were performed at the University of Minnesota Hospitals. Biopsy, transplantectomy and autopsy led to the histologic examination of 118 of these grafts. Only 13 of the 118 grafts remain functioning, in most cases following the institution of antirejection therapy following a diagnosis of biopsy-proven rejection. The cause of graft failure, or an hypothesis to explain the loss of the graft, was proposed in 99 of the grafts (Table 1), and these will be discussed in this report.

In the Minnesota series, infection, ascites, hemorrhage, and vascular thrombosis led to the loss of a significant proportion of the grafts [2, 3]. In the series of Dubernard et al. [4], the death of the patient was the major cause of loss of a functioning graft. If these factors can be overcome, the feasibility of pancreas transplantation as a highly successful and long-term therapy in the treatment of diabetes mellitus may come to fruition.

Pathology of the transplanted pancreas

Technical losses

Functioning graft losses. The demise of the patient, intractible ascites, and

203

J.M. Dubernard and D.E.R. Sutherland (eds.), International Handbook of Pancreas Transplantation, 203–223.
© *1989 by Kluwer Academic Publishers.*

infectious complications, such as intra-abdominal abscess, or peritonitis, led to the loss of 19 functioning grafts between 0 and 645 days (mean, 75 days) after transplantation in the Minnesota series. An acute or chronic peripancreatitis with fat necrosis was found in these cases and the endocrine and the exocrine pancreas were, for the most part, normal. Two of these grafts had infarction of the tail of the pancreas, which was secondarily infected leading to abscess formation. A third patient had graft removal at transplantation because of arterial bleeding; it demonstrated minor ischemic injury histologically. While an inflammatory infiltrate was quite difficult to find in the normal grafts, examination of several of these grafts with monoclonal antibodies against T and B lymphocytes and macrophages revealed a tenfold increase of cells as compared to biopsies from the donor pancreas at transplantation [3].

Table 1. Causes of pancreatic graft loss – 99 cases.

	Functioning grafts	Nonfunctioning grafts
Technical		
Abscess	10	
Ascites	3	
Hemorrhage	2	
'Abscess' – mucinous cystadenoma[a]	1	
'Pancreatitis' – infarction[b]	1	
Peritonitis	9	
Thrombosis-infarction		23
Vesico-cutaneous fistula	1	
Vascular anastomosis failure	1	
Viral		
Systemic CMV	1	
Gastrointest./bladder hemorrhage	4	
Infarction – IS[c] stopped		1
Type II diabetic[d]	1	
Death of patient	3	
Chronic pancreatitis/infarction		1
Recurrent disease		4
Recurrent disease/rejection		4
Rejection/thrombosis/infarction		6
Hyperacute rejection		1
Polymer duct obstruction		
Silicone		4
Silicone/infarction		1
Silicone/rejection		9
Silicone/rejection/infarction		6
Prolamine		1
Undetermined		1

[a] Mucinous cystademona found rather than abscess. [b] Clinically thought to have pancreatitis. [c] Immunosuppression. [d] high c-peptide, but patient insulin resistant.

A total of 65 needle or wedge biopsies of the transplanted pancreas, and five biopsies of the intestinal cuff of bladder drained transplants were performed at variable times in the posttransplant period. Six of these biopsies were performed on four patients with symptoms of hyperglycemia, but no histologic abnormality was apparent. Each of these patients currently has a functioning graft without any further therapy, excepting withdrawal of thiazides or beta blocking agents known to induce hyperglycemia, or the reduction in steroids the patient was receiving. One of these four patients (Case 65), currently $4^1/_2$ years posttransplantation, has mild impairment of glucose metabolism. He received a graft from an HLA-identical sibling. The second of three biopsies performed on this patient revealed a few T-lymphocytes in the islets, but no loss of beta cells. A repeat biopsy is being planned to determine whether this patient has developed histological evidence of recurrent disease [1, 3, 5].

Not surprisingly, these normal posttransplant tissues demonstrated a normal profile of histocompatibility antigens, although duct epithelium demonstrated an increase in Class II antigen expression [3]. In addition, frozen tissues available from the biopsies of one of the patients (Case 65) who had a minimal isletitis failed to demonstrate enhancement of either Class I or Class II major histocompatibility antigens on the islets or intraislet endothelium as seen in other patients who developed recurrent disease [5].

An additional 18 functioning grafts were lost primarily because of technical reasons – usually infectious – but these grafts were not normal histologically. Some showed histologic evidence of mild, subclinical, rejection. One resected graft, thought on the basis of radiographic studies to contain an intrapancreatic abscess, contained a $3^1/_2$ cm in diameter mucinous cystadenoma not recognized at the time of transplantation. Another patient with graft failure actually had a 'functioning' graft, based upon the finding of normal urinary C-peptide levels. This patient was discovered to be a Type II diabetic patient who was insulin-resistant. The graft was therefore removed and had evidence of mild acute rejection and entirely normal islets.

Infarction. One of the most serious problems which needs to be overcome if pancreas transplantation is to be as successful as other solid organ transplantations is primary arterial and venous thrombosis. Nearly 25% of the graft losses in our series were secondary to thrombosis with graft infarction; none of the implantation techniques, enteric, bladder, duct-injection, is immune to this serious complication.

The pathophysiology of the thrombotic episode is not exactly certain, but hemodynamic alterations, possibly secondary to vascular kinking, have been proposed. On the other hand, pancreatic enzyme damage to vascular endothelium might be a factor, perhaps secondary to ischemia or traumatic damage related to harvesting and implantation of the organ. It is of interest that acute necrotizing pancreatitis is associated with both arterial and venous thrombosis [6], presumably secondary to enzymatic digestion of vascular walls. Munda et al. [7] report that the complication of graft thrombosis could be resolved using a whole pancreas graft. However, the frequency of graft thrombosis is similar between whole and segmental grafts as reported to the Pancreas Transplant Registry [1].

Major thrombosis, usually arterial, may be superimposed upon acute or chronic vascular rejection; this occurred in at least 9 Minnesota grafts [3]. Several of these grafts had a known episode of previous rejection, but the thrombosis also occurred as a consequence of persistent subclinical rejection secondary to endothelialitis with chronic vascular rejection, eventually leading to serious blood flow alterations secondary to fibrointimal proliferative endarteritis.

As previously pointed out, arterial and venous thrombosis may occur in a setting of acute necrotizing pancreatitis. It is possible that transplanted patients with acute pancreatitis related to polymer duct injection or acute rejection could develop enzymatic damage to vessel walls as well, leading to focal thrombosis and segmental infarction, a not uncommon finding in biopsies and transplantectomies [3].

Distal venous and/or arterial thrombosis, with or without infarction of the distal pancreatic graft, is usually of little or no consequence. However, the infarcted segment may become secondarily infected, necessitating resection of a functioning graft.

Pancreatitis. Signs and/or symptoms of acute pancreatitis can be expected in the posttransplant period, since manipulation of the graft occurs during the harvesting, preservation and implantation procedures. Overt signs and symptoms of acute pancreatitis may be serious enough to result in the resection of a functioning graft because of sustained chemical peritonitis, intractable ascites or secondary infectious complications. In the Minnesota Series, histologic evidence of acute pancreatitis, characterized by a polymorphonuclear leukocyte rather than a mononuclear cell infiltrate, was found in 7 grafts: three biopsies, 3 pancreatectomies, and 1 autopsy [3]. One patient had severe intraabdominal hemorrhage secondary to the pancreatitis; one had a vesicocutaneous fistula associated with the acute pancreatitis; one, an abscess and acute pancreatitis. Biopsy of two silicone duct-injected grafts because of hyperglycemia in the early posttransplant period revealed acute pancreatitis related to the injected material. A third biopsy showed features of acute pancreatitis and acute rejection. One patient in the Minnesota Series, thought to have severe acute pancreatitis necessitating resection, was actually found instead to have venous thrombosis with early infarction. While symptoms of acute pancreatitis would seemingly be a feature of acute rejection because of the acinar damage secondary to the inflammatory infiltrate, in actual fact decreased urine amylase has been found to herald the onset of pancreatic rejection and appears to be a more reliable laboratory test than hyperglycemia in identifying early rejection, especially in the bladder implanted graft [8, 9]. Other authors, however, suggest that decreased urinary amylase is a late finding indicative of irreversible rejection [7].

The silicone and neoprene duct-injected grafts examined in the first week posttransplant show histologic evidence of acute pancreatitis as well as a prominent acute peripancreatitis. In an experimental setting, Gebhardt and Stolte [10] found that prolamine duct injection was not associated with the provocation of acute pancreatitis, and Land et al. [11] have reported a lack of acute complications related to polymer duct injection in human pancreas transplants. However, a chronic destructive pancreatitis is the long-term result of polymer duct injection, which occurs in experimental models [12–14] and human auto- and allograft transplantation [12].

Chronic rejection may be difficult to separate from chronic pancreatitis. Both are characterized by exocrine pancreatic loss with fibrosis, lymphocytic and plasma cell infiltrates, and coalescence of the islets. In several of our enteric drained grafts, a loose, edematous fibroproliferative onionskin-like change occurred around large ducts – changes reminiscent of those seen in the liver in patients with biliary duct obstruction. The most helpful finding in separating chronic pancreatitis from chronic rejection is that of fibroproliferative endarteritis, a feature of chronic organ transplant rejection.

Infectious complications. Bacterial peritonitis and abdominal abscesses are a serious hazard in the pancreas transplant. These complications are usually treated with antibiotics, surgical drainage, and, if necessary, transplantectomy.

Serious viral associated gastrointestinal or bladder hemorrhage occurred in 5 patients in the Minnesota series. In one of these cases, a duodenal cuff biopsy of a bladder implanted graft revealed cytomegalovirus duodenitis and, because of persistent hemorrhage, the graft was removed 13 days later and demonstrated CMV pancreatitis as well. Four functioning enteric-drained grafts were also resected, and CMV inclusions within the mucosal epithelium and endothelial cells were associated with severe inflammation and ulceration (Figure 1) [3]. This phenomenon – cytomegalovirus-associated gastrointestinal hemorrhage – is a well-known hazard in the immunosuppressed transplanted patient [15]. Overall, cytomegalovirus inclusions were found in the grafts of 13 patients. The islets were involved in 2 patients, the exocrine pancreas in 12 patients. A mononuclear cell infiltrate of variable intensity, histologically similar to that seen in acute rejection occurred in most of the grafts, and several had improvement in function following the institution of anti-rejection therapy.

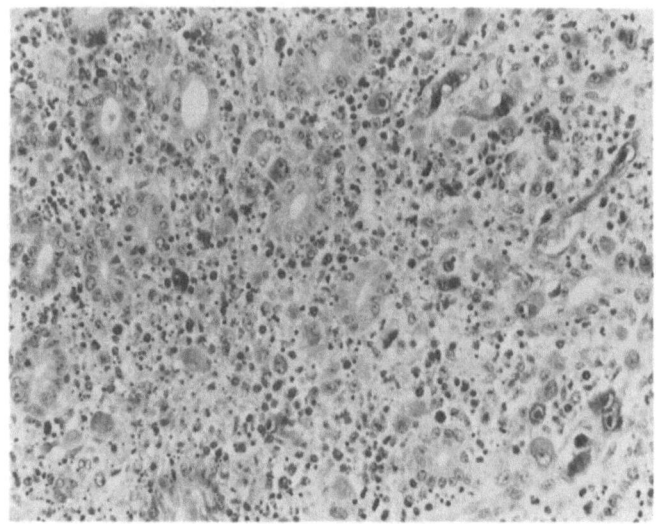

Figure 1. Cytomegalovirus associated gastrointestinal hemorrhage or urinary tract hemorrhage occurred in five patients. The mucosa at the anastomotic site was infested with CMV which resulted in ulceration (immunoperoxidase, anti-CMV × 150).

Rejection

Hyperacute. The diagnosis of hyperacute rejection is especially difficult in the pancreas transplant because of the frequency of graft failure in the early post-transplant period secondary to vascular thrombosis. One patient in the Minnesota series had laboratory and pathologic features compatible with hyperacute rejection. Clinically there was initial graft function, but within hours, there was evidence of a failing graft, and a transplantectomy was performed at 3 days. The original negative cross-match demonstrated 80% positivity at this time, a feature which does not occur in grafts with venous or arterial thrombosis. Histologically, there was margination of polymorphonuclear leukocytes in small vessels, with extensive fibrin thrombosis of small and medium-sized veins and arteries.

Acute and chronic rejection. Acute rejection in the pancreatic graft, as in other transplanted organs, is characterized clinically by variable degrees of graft malfunction. The earliest sign of graft malfunction in pancreas transplantation has been either that of hyperglycemia or decreased urine amylase production. As in other transplanted organs, there are other causes of graft malfunction: altered glucose metabolism related to the steroids the patient is receiving, or thiazides and beta blocking agents known to be associated with hyperglycemia [9]; vascular insufficiency; perhaps an allogeneic inflammatory infiltrate associated with paracrine effects of Interleukin-1 [16, 17] caused by obstructive pancreatitis or CMV pancreatitis. That some factor other than loss of beta cell mass appears to be the cause of hyperglycemia in acute rejection can be demonstrated by biopsy, where immunohistochemical staining typically demonstrates normal islets. In chronic rejection, however, a majority of islets may be destroyed, explaining the graft failure.

A histologic diagnosis of acute and/or chronic rejection was made in 37 grafts in 36 patients in the Minnesota series [3]. Acute rejection is characterized by a pleomorphic infiltrate of transformed small lymphocytes with angulated hyperchromatic nuclei and smaller number of lymphoblasts with round vesicular nuclei and nucleoli (Figure 2). Macrophages, polymorphonuclear leukocytes, eosinophils and plasma cells also infiltrate the exocrine pancreas. A few lymphocytes may also be found in the islets [3]. Similar infiltrates occur in transplanted pancreatic nerves. Most helpful in the recognition of acute rejection is the finding of an endovasculitis consisting of subendothelial infiltrates of lymphocytes and macrophages (Figure 3). Fibrinoid necrosis and a necrotizing arteritis may also occur (Figure 4).

The diagnosis of acute rejection may be difficult, especially in duct injected grafts, even when a transplantectomy has been performed. In the duct-injected graft, acute rejection may be suspected if there is an especially intense infiltrate of transformed lymphocytes, or endovasculitis, or nerve infiltration by lymphocytes is evident.

The inflammatory cell infiltrates in acute rejection are primarily composed of CD2+ T-lymphocytes with CD8+ cells predominating. CD38+ reactive cells and macrophages were also evident. There were 50 times as many inflammatory cells in these tissues as compared to the normal donor biopsies. MHC antigens were either induced or there was marked increase in their expression by the exocrine pancreas in acute rejection (Figure 5), but similar features were seen in duct-obstructed grafts which did not show definite histologic features of rejection [3].

The histologic separation of chronic rejection from chronic pancreatitis can be extremely difficult. Certainly a patient could have both, as commonly occurs in the duct injected graft. The most reliable histologic feature in the diagnosis of chronic rejections is fibrointimal endarteritis, characterized by variable concentric fibrous narrowing of arterial lumens (Figure 6).

Biopsy of the cystoscopically visualized intestinal cuff of grafts with bladder drainage may be of use in the diagnosis of graft rejection. We examined 11 biopsies of the duodenum (7 donor, 4 posttransplant) but could not differentiate between donor and posttransplant biopsies because the donor biopsies demonstrated variable ischemic damage and mononuclear cell infiltrates, while posttransplant biopsies revealed the following: no abnormality in a patient with hyperglycemia and reduced urinary amylase; crypt abscesses,

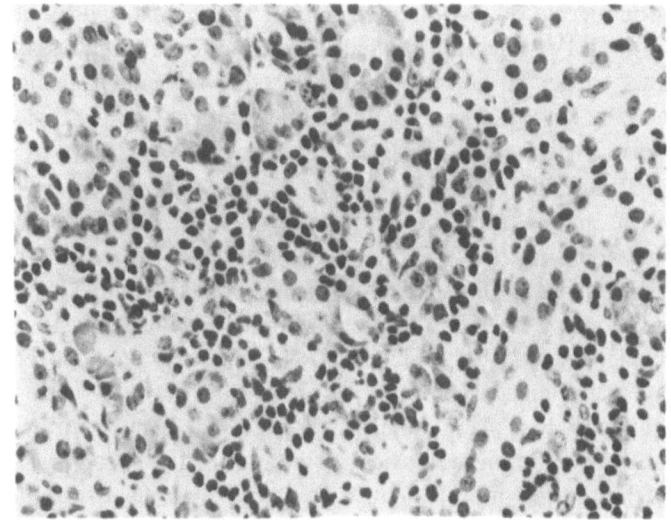

Figure 2. The major feature of acute rejection is a mononuclear inflammatory infiltrate consisting predominantly of transformed lymphocytes which infiltrates the exocrine pancreas. (H&E × 300).

ischemic damage, and mild mononuclear cell infiltrates in a patient with a normal graft undergoing surgical revision from bladder to enteric drainage because of intractable cystitis; changes identical to severe graft-vs.-host disease in a patient with hyperglycemia who eventually lost graft function; and

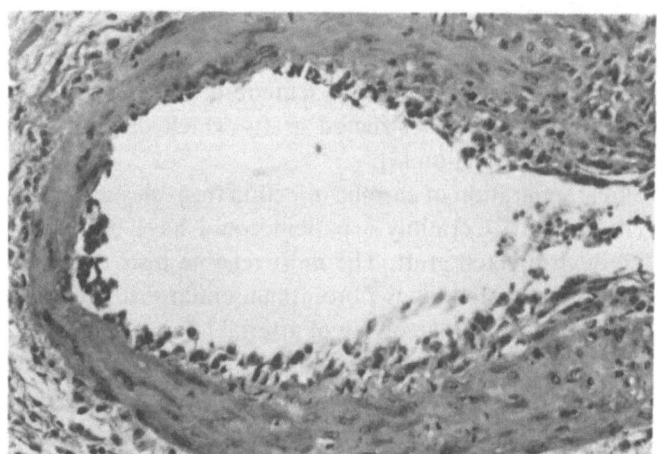

Figure 3. The finding of endovasculitis is helpful in the identification of acute rejection in pancreases where the differential diagnosis includes chronic pancreatitis, CMV associated pancreatitis, and polymer duct-obstructed pancreatitis. (H&E × 300).

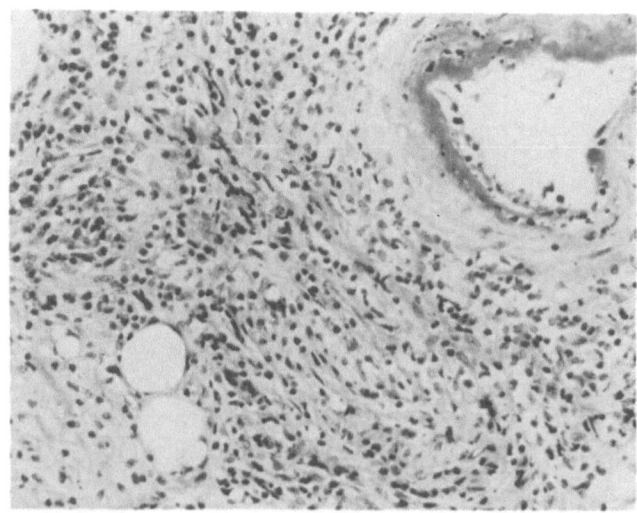

Figure 4. Necrotizing vasculitis with fibrinoid necrosis occurred in this silicone duct injected graft with acute rejection. (H&E × 150) (From: Sibley RK: In: Groth CG (ed) Pancreatic transplantation. Grune & Stratton Ltd, London, 1988.

severe graft-vs-host disease-like changes with cytomegalovirus inclusions in a patient with bladder hemorrhage but normal graft function.

Examination of small bowel mucosa and muscularis in pancreatectomy specimens is generally of little help in differentiating the cause of graft loss, but some cases have demonstrated a marked polymorphonuclear and mononucle-

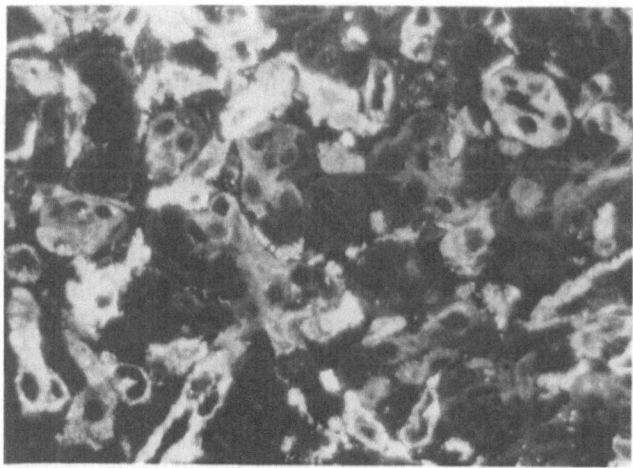

Figure 5. Induction and/or marked increase in Class II antigen expression is seen in the exocrine pancreas in patients with acute rejection (Immunofluorescence, HLA-DR, × 185) (From Sibley RK, Sutherland DER, Am J Pathol 128, 151, 1987.

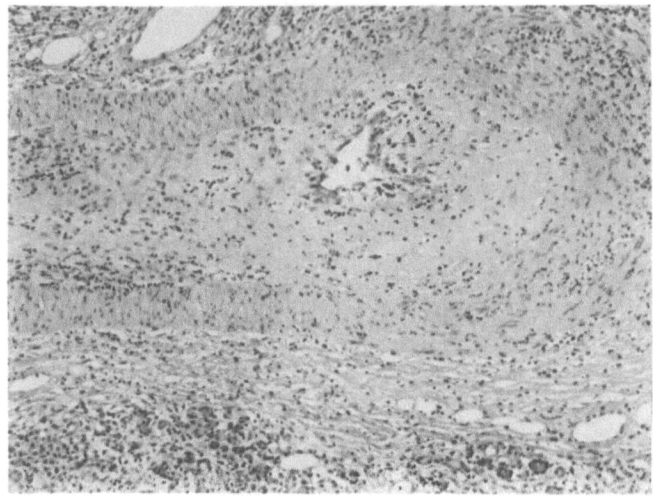

Figure 6. Fibroproliferative endarteritis allows the recognition of chronic rejection. (H&E ×
120).

ar cell infiltrate in the mucosa and muscularis propria in cases with histologic
evidence of rejection in the pancreatic tissues. We are therefore not presently
convinced that small bowel mucosal biopsy is useful in the management of
pancreatic transplant patients.

Recurrent diabetes mellitus

Nine patients developed clinical and pathologic evidence of recurrent disease
in the Minnesota series. Clinical features include progressive hyperglycemia
requiring insulin treatment, the return of C-peptide levels to pretransplant
baseline levels, or the intermittent use of insulin and C-peptide levels reduced
from initial posttransplant levels. The major histologic features are an isletitis
characterized by an infiltrate of T-lymphocytes and macrophages, hyperex-
pression of Class I major histocompatibility antigen by islet cells, and the
selective destruction and loss of beta cells [3, 5, 18]. The clinical course and
pathologic features of these cases have been presented in detail [3, 5, 18].

Each patient was a Type I diabetic of long duration who received a segmental graft from an HLA-identical twin (cases 16, 67, 69 and 79), or HLA-
identical sibling (cases 30, 34, 48, 51, and 71). All but one case were enteric
drained, the exception being a prolamine duct-injected isograft (case 16) [3, 5].
Three of the HLA-identical twin recipients received no immunosuppressive
therapy; one HLA-identical twin received low-dose azathioprine; the HLA-
identical siblings all received low-dose cyclosporin and prednisone in addition

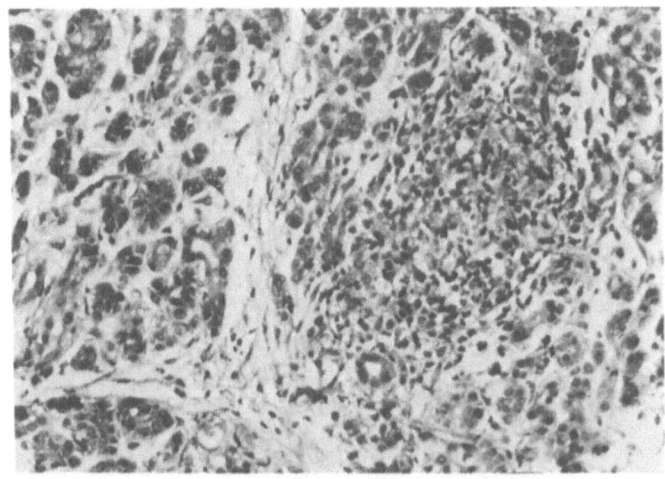

Figure 7. A prominent mononuclear cell infiltrate occurred in the islets of biopsies from patients with evidence of recurrent diabetes (H&E × 130) (From: Sibley RK et al, Lab Invest 53, 132, 1985).

in three cases. Each patient was insulin-independent for 1 to 32 months posttransplant, when clinical evidence of graft malfunction became apparent. Three of the isografts (cases 16, 67, 69) and one of the allograft recipients (case 34) developed clinical signs of graft insufficiency 1 to 2 months posttransplant and biopsies in 3 of these cases (cases 16, 67, 69) were performed at that time. An intense mononuclear cell infiltrate centered upon the islets was found which was associated with variable architectural disarray, and beta cell degranulation or destruction (Figures 7, 8) [3, 5]. Immunohistochemical studies revealed intense Class I antigen expression by the islet cells (Figure 9) and an increased Class II antigen expression by intra-islet endothelial cells. There were numerous Ia-positive mononuclear cells in the islets. These were mostly CD2+ T-lymphocytes, which when further examined consisted of a few CD4+ and CD38+ T cells and large numbers of CD8+ T-lymphocytes [3, 5]. Similar, but not identical, features have been reported in the islets of Type I diabetic patients of recent onset in tissue examined at autopsy [19, 20].

The biopsy in case 16 performed 51 days posttransplant contained fewer inflammatory cells in the islets than evident in cases 67 and 69 and, in addition, many islets were already devoid of beta cells. There was resolution of the isletitis and decreased expression of Class I antigen in the islets lacking beta cells.

The histologic features in biopsies obtained 6 to 12 months posttransplant when there was either a partially functioning (case 69) or nonfunctioning graft (cases 34, 67) revealed not only a lack of isletitis but also the lack or near lack of beta cells in the islets, features identical to those seen in the end-stage Type I

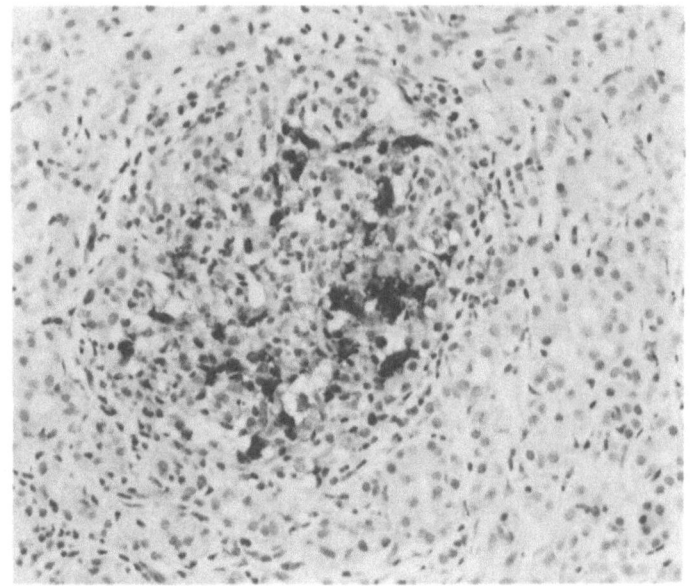

Figure 8. Immunohistochemical staining for insulin and glucagon revealed marked disarray of islet architecture and, even in biopsies with early evidence of recurrent disease, decreased number of beta cells. (Immunoperoxidase, insulin × 190) (From: Sibley RK et al, Lab Invest 53, 132, 1985).

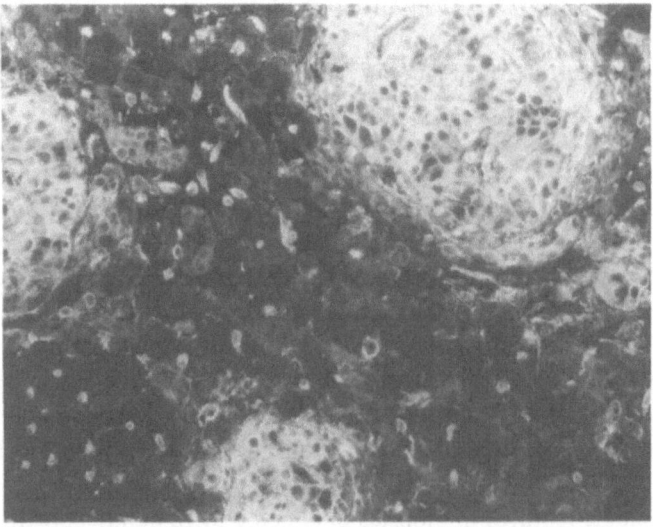

Figure 9. A marked increase in Class I antigen involving all islet cells was found in patients with isletitis and recurrent diabetes. (Immunofluorescence, HLA-A, B, C × 64) (From: Sibley RK, Sutherland DER, Am J Pathol 128, 151, 1987).

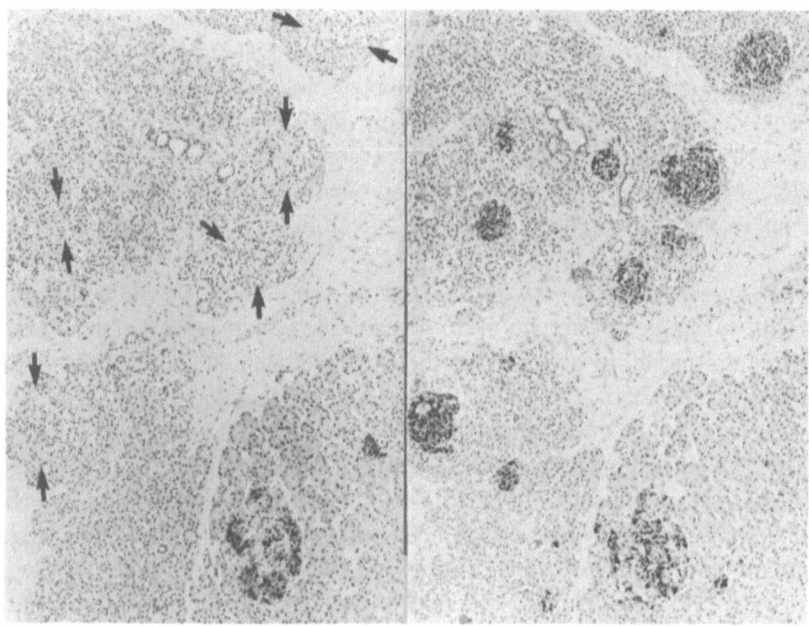

Figure 10a, b. In failed grafts with recurrent disease, the islets were devoid of insulin (arrows) and showed replacement of the islets by glucagon. (A: Immunoperoxidase, insulin, × 53) (B: Immunoperoxidase, glucagon, × 76) (From: Sibley RK et al, Lab Invest 53, 132, 1985).

diabetic patient (Figure 10a, b) [21–23] and the BB rat [24, 25]. In addition, the increased major histocompatibility antigen expression found in the earlier biopsies had disappeared.

Case 79 has had a clinical course different from the previous described four cases. She underwent a prospective biopsy approximately two months posttransplant because of the development of recurrent disease in the previous three isografts. She had been placed on azathioprine and at the time of the biopsy had entirely normal function. The biopsy, however, revealed a mild isletitis and marked Class I antigen expression in the islets was evident. The beta cells appeared normal. No modification of the immunosuppressive regimen was made and the patient remained well until mild hyperglycemia was noted 38 months posttransplantation. Repeat biopsy demonstrated the lack of beta cells in nearly 90% of the islets; the remainder contained beta cells, no inflammatory cells, and there was normal major histocompatibility antigen expression by endocrine and endothelial cells. Cyclosporin was added to her immunosuppressive regimen and she now requires insulin intermittently, 51 months posttransplantation.

The remaining 4 patients (cases 30, 48, 51 and 71) with morphologic evidence of recurrent disease, unlike the preceding cases, had morphologic evidence of rejection as well. These patients developed clinical evidence of graft malfunction 7, 9, 23 and 21 months posttransplantation, and became insulin dependent 58, 15, 29 and 21 months posttransplant respectively. Loss of function was likely the result of recurrent disease in cases 30 and 51, for biopsies revealed an isletitis and prominent loss of beta cells, while cases 48 and 71 most likely lost function on the basis of chronic rejection, for only mild beta cell loss was apparent in the transplantectomy specimens [3].

Polymer duct injection associated pancreatitis. Obliteration of the pancreatic duct with subsequent destruction of the exocrine pancreas was shown in the experimental model to be a safe method for management of the pancreatic exocrine secretions [10, 26]. Several different substances have been utilized in different centers, the most common being neoprene, prolamine, and silicone.

At the University of Minnesota 36 silicone, 4 prolamine, and 1 neoprene duct-injected transplants were performed between March, 1980 and March, 1986. Only 4 of these grafts are still functioning from $4^{1}/_{2}$ to 7 years after transplantation. Thirty of the 41 cases were examined in the pathology laboratory via 25 biopsies from 21 cases, 14 transplantectomies, and 3 autopsies.

Silicone rubber injection. Tissue samples obtained soon after transplantation in silicone injected grafts demonstrate an acute pancreatitis with extravasated foreign material in the interstitial tissues. Perilobular edema and a mild chronic inflammatory infiltrate is also apparent. In later biopsies or pancreatectomies, there is chronic pancreatitis of variable severity. In the milder cases there is irregular atrophy of lobular exocrine units with perilobular fibrosis and edema and a mild pleomorphic inflammatory infiltrate of lymphocytes, plasma cells, eosinophils, polymorphonuclear leukocytes, macrophages, and a foreign body giant cell reaction to the silicone (Figure 11). Even though a biopsy usually was obtained because of hyperglycemia, the islets were almost always remarkably normal. More severe damage is characterized by extensive to total destruction of the exocrine pancreas, which is replaced by fibrous tissue of varying densities (Figure 12). In some cases there is a mononuclear cell infiltrate of lymphocytes, plasma cells and macrophages, while in others there is dense fibrosis with few inflammatory cells excepting the foreign body giant cells. In other cases the variably atrophic gland is further damaged because of vascular thrombosis with secondary infarction [3].

In 13 patients, 16 biopsies were performed to determine the cause of hyperglycemia. There was variable chronic pancreatitis in each of these grafts and in 8 a diagnosis of superimposed acute rejection was made based upon a more pronounced lymphocytic infiltrate, and in most cases, endovasculitis. The presence of a vasculitis is most helpful in establishing the presence of acute rejection in a duct-injected graft. Fibrinoid necrosis of vessels, however, is not

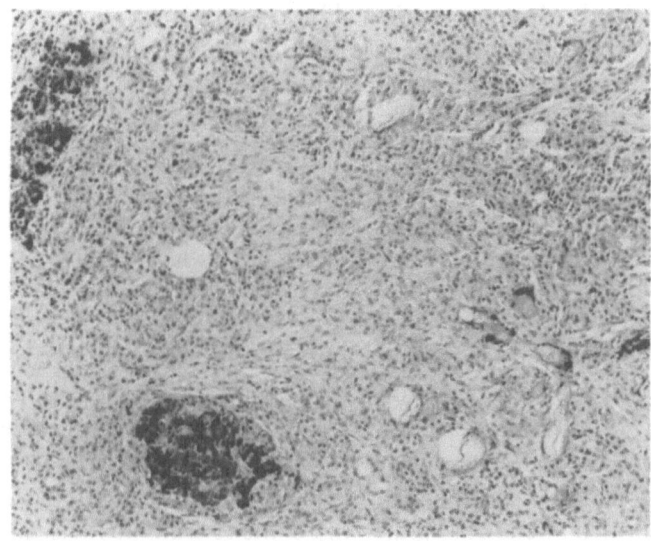

Figure 11. Silicone duct-injected grafts demonstrated aggregates of the foreign substance with a mixed inflammatory infiltrate including foreign body giant cells. Identification of acute rejection in these cases is difficult. (Immunoperoxidase, insulin, × 75.)

specific for rejection, for similar changes can be found in cases of acute necrotizing pancreatitis [6]. Antirejection treatment was associated with long-lasting graft function in only one of these patients [1, 9]. The beta cells were normal in all of these patients with hyperglycemia except one, where the

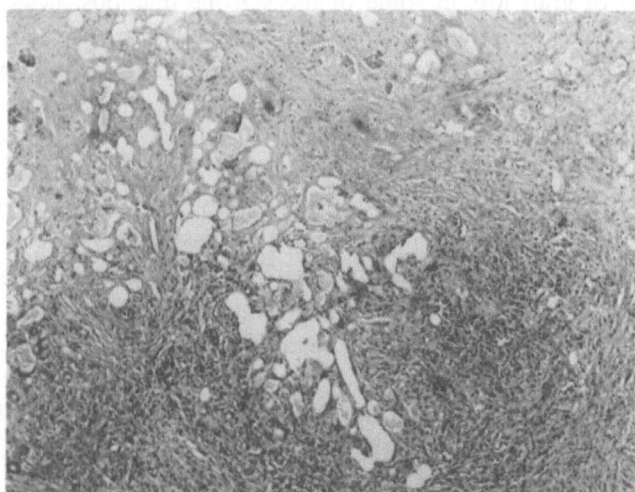

Figure 12. Delayed effect of silicone duct injection is marked exocrine atrophy, a pleomorphic inflammatory infiltrate secondary to the extravasated silicone, and, as in this case, destruction of the islets as well. A portion of the graft was also infarcted. (H&E × 48.)

biopsy contained only infarcted tissue [3].

In 4 patients the grafts were no longer functioning when the biopsy was obtained. Each graft showed moderate to severe pancreatitis and, in addition, one showed zones of infarction and another, superimposed acute rejection. Neither of the latter 2 grafts contained any islets, while the islets in the other 2 cases contained normal beta cells.

In 2 further grafts the biopsy was incidentally obtained when there was incision and drainage of an intraabdominal abscess and a pseudo-cyst in one patient each. The islets of both cases were found to be normal. One of these grafts is still functioning nearly 5 years after transplantation, but the other was removed because of unsuccessful treatment of the abdominal abscess.

Thirteen of 14 patients undergoing transplantectomy no longer had a functioning graft when it was removed. In addition to moderate to severe chronic pancreatitis, acute and/or chronic rejection and variable infarction occurred in 8 grafts, chronic pancreatitis and infarction in 2 grafts, and arterial or venous thrombosis with infarction in 2 grafts. In 9 of the 13 grafts no islets, and thus no beta cells, were found; in 4 grafts, some islets contained nearly normal numbers of beta cells (Figure 13), while other islets had reduced numbers of beta cells [3]. Similar alterations in islet morphology have been reported in patients with long-term chronic pancreatitis [27].

Two of 3 patients dying in the Minnesota series had nonfunctioning grafts at their demise. One patient had normal appearing islets, the second, reduced numbers of beta cells in the islets which were set in a dense cicatrix in addition to the presence of acute and chronic rejection and zones of infarction.

The cause of graft loss in some of the silicone duct-obstructed grafts is obvious – destruction of the islets, and thus beta cells, in the setting of severe chronic pancreatitis, and acute and/or chronic rejection and infarction. The cause of hyperglycemia in grafts with normal numbers of beta cells, and the complete 'loss of function' in grafts with normal islets are hard to understand. Perhaps the release of Interleukin-1 by the inflammatory infiltrate related to chronic pancreatitis and/or acute rejection is responsible for the hyperglycemia; perhaps alterations of the microcirculation of islets plays a role in the loss of function in the nonfunctioning grafts with severe chronic pancreatitis.

Immunohistochemical studies of 6 silicone injected grafts revealed no significant difference in the major histocompatibility antigen expression by the exocrine pancreas between the duct-injected grafts and those with acute rejection. The number of CD4+ and CD8+ cells was also similar, but more activated T cells were present in the duct injected grafts [3].

Prolamine injection. The 2 prolamine injected grafts demonstrated severe exocrine atrophy and a moderate lymphocytic, plasma cell and macrophage infiltrate. The islets were often surrounded by large numbers of what appeared

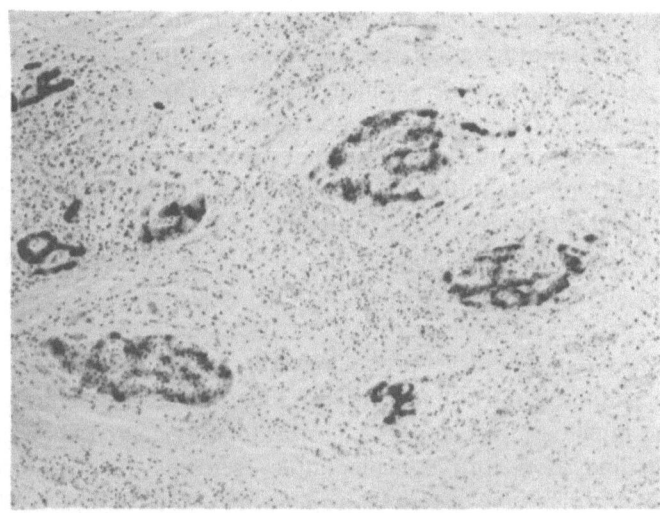

Figure 13. This failed silicone duct-injected graft demonstrates severe exocrine atrophy, a scattered mild inflammatory infiltrate, and numerous islets containing abundant numbers of beta cells. (Immunoperoxidase, insulin × 48.)

to be proliferating ductules and/or simplified acini (Figure 14). Similar findings were reported by Land, et al. [28]. During the first months posttransplant there is ductal epithelial destruction with concomitant destruction of acini and interstitial fibrosis. After 4 months the graft usually consists of islets surrounded by loose connective tissue and there is disappearance of the foreign materi-

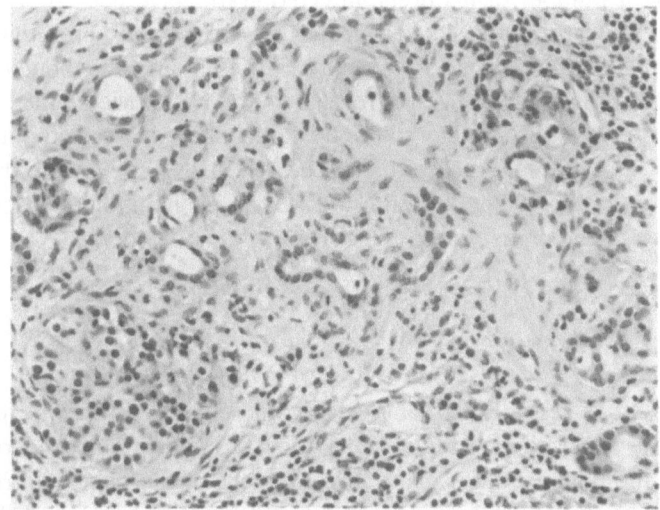

Figure 14. Prolamine duct-injected grafts contain simplified acini or ductules, and islets surrounded by an edematous and fibrotic stroma containing chronic inflammatory cells. (H&E × 150.)

al. A variable but usually mild inflammatory infiltrate is evident [28].

Both of the Minnesota cases were no longer functioning when examined. One had entirely normal islets which were encompassed by loose fibrous connective tissue, and the second demonstrated evidence of recurrent diabetes (see case 16, recurrent diabetes). Whether prolamine-injected grafts will be more successful long-term than other techniques is still uncertain. However, the one-year graft survival of 74% reported by Land et al. [28] in cases transplanted since late 1984, is higher than the 42% reported to the Transplant Registry for all techniques combined for 1985–86 [1].

Neoprene injection. The 8 neoprene-injected grafts, received as a courtesy from Dr N. Blanc-Brunat of Lyon, France, showed changes similar to those in the silicone-injected grafts: focal acute necrotizing pancreatitis was seen in tissues obtained soon after transplantation, whereas the long-term grafts demonstrated progressive exocrine atrophy with extensive fibrosis, large aggregates of neoprene with a focal foreign-body giant cell reaction and scattered plasma cells and lymphocytes. In most instances, there were variably sized islets amongst the cicatrix and foreign material (Figure 15). These features have been described in the dog model [12, 13] and in human transplants [12, 29, 30]. Immunoperoxidase for insulin revealed that most islets contained abundant beta cells as well as scattered islets containing only a few alpha and beta cells (Figure 16). Some grafts, in addition, demonstrated superimposed vascular thrombosis and resultant infarction or features of acute rejection, perhaps related to reduced immunosuppression in the days prior to transplantectomy.

The largest number of neoprene-injected grafts have been performed by Dubernard and Traeger and colleagues, who have reported an actuarial one-year survival of 25% in 52 grafts [4]. None of these grafts was thought to have failed on the basis of graft fibrosis related to neoprene. Metabolic investigations of long-term functioning grafts, however, show increasing numbers of patients with abnormal glucose tolerance tests [31]. It is possible that these features are secondary to alterations of islet microcirculation caused by the cicatrization of the pancreatic graft.

Summary

Criteria have been established for the diagnosis of acute and chronic rejection, foreign body induced pancreatitis, infectious complications, and recurrent disease in the pancreas transplant. Management of the pancreas transplant patient can be enhanced by biopsy and histologic examination of the graft. Unfortunately biopsy of the pancreas graft is not as simple as in the renal, hepatic and cardiac transplant, in which biopsy is a standard component of post-transplant care.

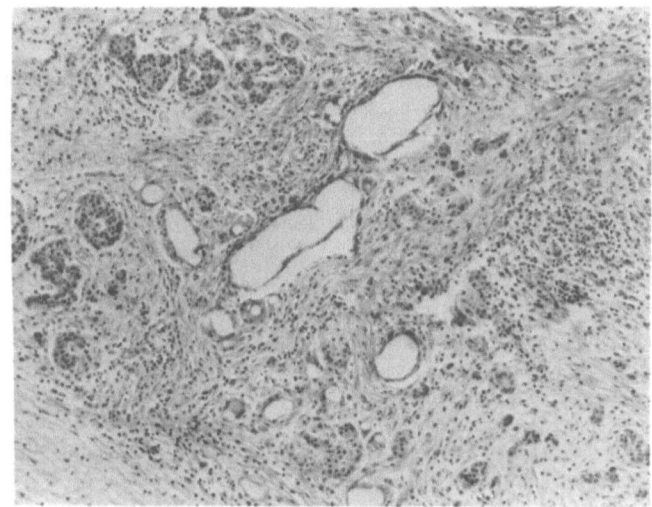

Figure 15. The neoprene duct-injected grafts showed features similar to those in the silicone duct-injected grafts. There is marked exocrine atrophy, and a mixed inflammatory infiltrate with marked fibrosis and clustering of islets. (H&E × 75.)

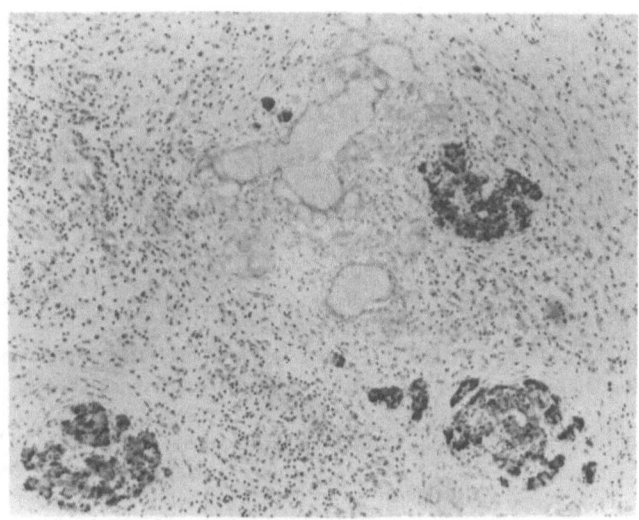

Figure 16. This neoprene duct-injected graft demonstrates total destruction of the exocrine pancreas, numerous beta cell rich islets, and extravasated polymer. (Immunoperoxidase, insulin × 75).

222

References

1. Sutherland DER, Moudry KC: Pancreas transplant registry: history and analysis of cases 1966 to October 1986. Pancreas 2: 473–488, 1987.
2. Sutherland DER, Goetz C, Najarian JS: Pancreas transplantation at the University of Minnesota: donor and recipient selection, operative hand postoperative management, and outcome. Transplant Proc 19: 63–74, 1987.
3. Sibley RK, Sutherland DER: Pancreas transplantation. Am J Pathol 128: 151–170, 1987.
4. Dubernard JM, Traeger J, Piatti PM, Gelet A, El Yafi S, Martin X, Devonec M, Henriet M, Kamel G, Canton F, Codas H, Touraine JL: Report of 54 human segmental pancreatic allografts prepared by duct obstruction with neoprene. Transplant Proc 17: 312–314, 1985.
5. Sibley RK, Sutherland DER, Goetz F, Michael AF: Recurrent diabetes mellitus in the pancreas iso- and allograft. Lab Invest 53: 132–144, 1985.
6. Phat VN, Guerrieri MT, Alexandre JM, Camilleri JP: Early histological changes in acute necrotizing hemorrhagic pancreatitis. Path Res Pract 178: 273–279, 1984.
7. Munda R, First MR, Weiss MA, Alexander JW: Pancreas transplantation – University of Cincinnati. Transplant Proc 19 (Suppl 4): 17–23, 1987.
8. Prieto M, Sutherland DER, Fernandez-Cruz L, Heil J, Najarian JS: Experimental and clinical experience with urine amylase monitoring for early diagnosis of rejection in pancreas transplantation. Transplantation 43: 73–79, 1987.
9. Sutherland DER, Casanova D, Sibley RK: Role of pancreas graft biopsies in the diagnosis and treatment of rejection after pancreas transplantation. Trans Proc 19: 2329–2332, 1987.
10. Gebhardt C, Stolte M: Pankreasgang-okklusion durch injektion einer schnellhartenden aminosaurenlosung. Langenbecks Arch Chir 346: 149–166, 1978.
11. Land W, Landgraf R, Illner WD, Wirsching R, Jensen U, Gokel M, Castro LA, Fornara P, Burg D, Kampik A: Improved results in combined segmental pancreatic and renal transplantation in diabetic patients under cyclosporin therapy. Transplant Proc 17: 317–324, 1985.
12. Blanc-Brunat N, Dubernard JM, Touraine JL, Neyra P, Dubois P, Paulin C, Traeger J: Pathology of the pancreas after intraductal neoprene injection in dogs and diabetic patients treated by pancreatic transplantation. Diabetologia 25: 97–107, 1983.
13. Gooszen HG, Bosman FT, van Schilfgaarde R: An analysis of long-term histologic changes leading to decreased endocrine function after duct obliteration of the canine pancreas. Transplant Proc 16: 776–777, 1984.
14. Land W, Gebhardt C, Gall FP, Weitz H, Gokel MJ, Stolte M: Pancreatic duct obstruction with prolamine solution. Transplant Proc 12 (Suppl 2): 72–75, 1980.
15. Foucar E, Mukai K, Foucar K, DER 1, Van Buren CT: Colon ulceration in lethal cytomegalovirus infection. Am J Clin Pathol 76: 789–801, 1981.
16. Mandrup-Poulsen T, Egeberg J, Nerup J, Bendtzen K, Nielsen JH, Dinarello CA: Ultrastructural studies of time-course and cellular specificity of Interleukin-1 mediated islet cytotoxicity. Acta path microbiol immunol scand 95: 55–63, 1987.
17. Comens PG, Wolf BA, Unanue ER, Lacy PE, McDaniel ML: Interleukin-1 is potent modulator of insulin secretion from isolated rat islets of Langerhans. Diabetes 36: 963–970, 1987.
18. Sutherland DER, Sibley RK, Za, XZ, Michael A, Srikanta S, Taub F, Najarian J, Goetz FC: Twin to twin pancreas transplantation: reversal and reenactment of the pathogenesis of type I diabetes. Trans Assoc Amer Phys 97: 80–87, 1984.
19. Bottazzo GF, Dean BM, McNally JM, McKay EH, Swift PGF, Gamble DR: In situ characterization of autoimmune phenomena and expression of HLA molecules in the pancreas in diabetic insulitis. NEJM 313: 353–360, 1985.
20. Foulis AK, Farquharson MA, Hardman R: Aberrant expression of class II major histocom-

patibility complex molecules by insulin containing islets in type I (insulin-dependent) diabetes mellitus. Diabetologia 30: 333–343, 1987.

21. Gepts W: Pathologic anatomy of the pancreas in juvenile diabetes mellitus. Diabetes 1: 619–633, 1965.

22. Gepts W, Lecompte PM: The pancreatic islets in diabetes. Am J Med 70: 105–115, 1981.

23. Foulis AK, Liddle CN, Farquharson MA, Richmond JA, Weir RS: The histopathology of the pancreas in Type 1 (insulin-dependent) diabetes mellitus, 1986: a 25-year review of deaths in patients under 20 years of age in the United Kingdom. Diabetologia 29: 267–274, 1986.

24. Nakhooda AF, Like AA, Chappel CI, Murray FT, Marliss EB: The spontaneously diabetic Wistar rat: metabolic and morphologic studies. Diabetes 26: 100–112, 1977.

25. Marliss EB, Nakhooda AF, Poussier P, Sima AAF: The diabetes syndrome of the 'BB' Wistar rat: possible relevance to type I (insulin-dependent) diabetes in man. Diabetologia 22: 225–232, 1982.

26. Dubernard JM, Traeger J, Neyra P, Tourceine JL, Tranchant D, Blanc-Brunat N: A new method of preparation of segmental pancreatic grafts for transplantation: trials in dogs and in man. Surgery 84: 633–639, 1978.

27. Klöppel G, Bommer G, Commandeur G, Heitz P: The endocrine pancreas in chronic pancreatitis. Anat Histol 377: 157–174, 1978.

28. Land W, Landgraf R, Illner W-D, Abendroth D, Kampik A, Jensen U, Lenhart FP, Burg D, Hillebrand G, Castro LA, Landgraf-Leurs MMC, Frey L, Gokel M, Schleibner St., Nusser J, Ulbig M: Clinical pancreatic transplantation using the prolamine duct occlusion technique – the Munich experience. Trans Proc 19 (Suppl 4): 75–83, 1987.

29. Dubernard JM, Traeger J, Bosi E, Gelet A, El Yafi S, Devonec M, Piatti PM, Chiesa R, Martin X, Mongin-Long D, Touraine JL, Pozza G: Transplantation for the treatment of insulin-dependent diabetes: clinical experience with polymer-obstructed pancreatic grafts using neoprene. World J Surg 8: 262–266, 1984.

30. Munda R, Alexander JW, First MR, Knowles HC, Weiss MA: Synchronous transplantation of a kidney and duct-obliterated segmental pancreas: report of a case. Trans proc 12: 98–102, 1980.

31. Cantarovich D, Traeger J, LaRocca E, Monti LD, Lefrancois N, Cantarovich F, Betuel H, Blanc-Brunat N, Faure JL, Gelet A, Dubernard JM, Pozza G, Touraine JL: Evolution of metabolic and endocrine function in ten neoprene-injected segmental pancreas allografts at three to 54 months after transplantation, versus preliminary results in nine whole pancreas allografts with enteric diversion. Trans Proc 19: 2310–2313, 1987.

11. Endocrine function of the pancreatic graft

G. POZZA and A. SECCHI

Introduction

The aim of pancreatic allotransplantation is to provide a source of insulin which is able to respond to the physiological insulinogenic stimuli in order to restore normal glycemic homeostasis [1].

From a theoretical point of view this approach seems to be promising, substituting traditional treatments, such as multi injection regimen or continous insulin infusion, which very often are unable to bring metabolic control back to normality [2]. The achievement of a good metabolic control shows a major relevance in insulin-dependent diabetic patients since there is growing evidence that degenerative complications of diabetes are the long term consequence of metabolic derangement [3].

Transplanted pancreas contains a certain amount of well vascularized islets of Langerhans, which seem to keep their endocrine activity. The exocrine secretory function can either be inactivated (duct injection with polymers or duct ligation) or diverted (enteric, urinary or peritoneal). So far, the transplanted pancreas is able to release not only insulin, but also glucagon and, presumably, somatostatin and pancreatic polypeptide [6].

There is evidence that the transplanted pancreas is able to release insulin through a self regulated system, and to normalize glucose metabolism [7].

Short term endocrine function

The revascularization of the pancreatic graft, usually anastomized to the iliac vessels, leads to an immediate release of pancreatic hormones, mainly insulin and glucagon [8].

This had been demonstrated in animals, submitted to pancreatic autografts: a prompt insulin release was observed in dogs with very low levels of insulin before surgery [9].

225

J.M. Dubernard and D.E.R. Sutherland (eds.), International Handbook of Pancreas Transplantation, 225–238.
© *1989 by Kluwer Academic Publishers.*

In man the same studies were performed with the determination of C peptide levels. The C peptide levels, nearly undetectable at the beginning of surgery, rise immediately after graft revascularization reaching the value of 10 pmol/ml at 60 minutes, as shown in Figure 1 [8]. In these patients free insulin levels are constantly elevated throughout surgery as a consequence of exogenous insulin administration (Figure 1). A reduction of exogenous insulin requirement is observed after graft revascularization, when these patients are connected during surgery to an artificial pancreas (Biostator, Miles), in order to achieve a good metabolic control during the whole surgery period [8]. The time of cold or warm ischemia does not seem to influence C peptide levels during surgery: C peptide levels remain sustained during the whole intraoperative period, and blood glucose levels tend to be lower at the end of surgery (Figure 1). An immediate increase in glucagon levels is observed after graft revascularization; in fact, glucagon rises from 150 pg/ml before transplantation to 43 pg/ml at 5 minutes.

Half-term endocrine function

Segmental pancreatic transplantation, when the surgery has been technically successful, restores within a few weeks a satisfactory metabolic control. Nevertheless during the first days after surgery, high blood glucose levels are often present in concomitance with high C peptide levels, ranging from 5 to 20 pmol/ml [10]. Several factors can be taken into consideration in order to explain these findings. Among them, high doses of steroids, administered for immunosuppression [11] are probably the main cause of such condition. A second reason could be the total parenteral nutrition, which is administered during the first two weeks after surgery, in order to prevent stimulation of the exocrine pancreatic function from gastrointestinal hormones, commonly released when nutrients are ingested. All regimens of total parenteral nutrition contain high quantities of glucose and tryglycerides, which respectively increase blood glucose and insulin resistance.

The frequent finding of hyperglycemia during the immediate postsurgical period, have pointed out some interpretative problems, since hyperglycemia can be the consequence of the previously exposed reasons but it can also represent a reduction of the endocrine function in the transplanted pancreas, both due to a rejection, or to a vascular complication, such as thrombosis. In these conditions, the best way to assess the endocrine function of the transplanted beta cell is the assay of plasmatic and urinary C peptide levels: in the presence of high C peptide levels these episodes can be related to extrapancreatic factors, as previously reported [12]. Unfortunately C peptide assay remains currently a long time requiring procedure, not always useful for the

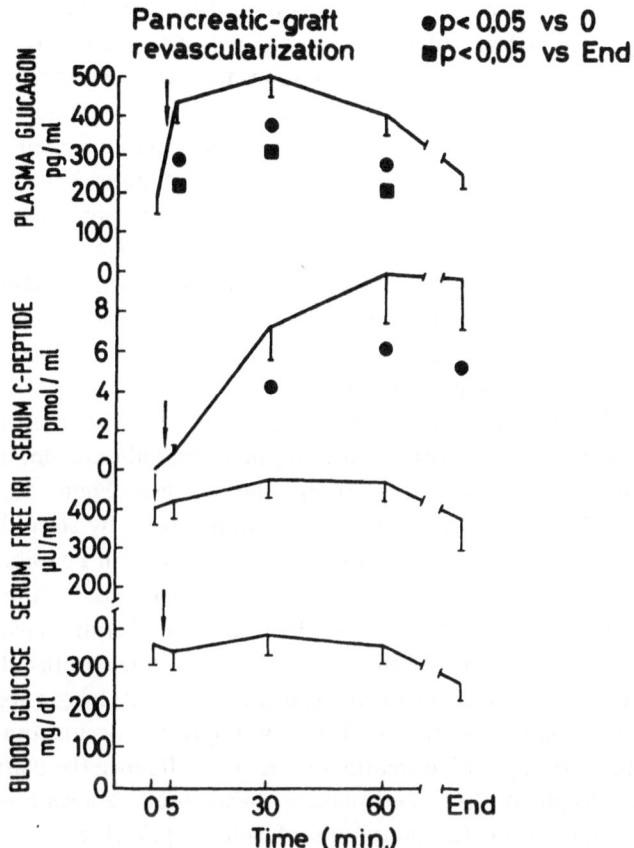

Figure 1. Intra-operative profiles of Plasma Glucagon (pg/ml), Serum C Peptide (pmol/ml), Serum Free Insulin (μU/ml), Blood Glucose (mg/dl) in 9 IDD patients during pancreatico-renal transplantation.

immediate assessment of the pancreatic endocrine function.

An other simple method to detect daily the graft function, particularly during the period of parenteral nutrition, consists in the withdrawal both of the parenteral nutritions, and of the i.v. insulin infusion, during a two-hour period early in the morning, several hours after the last steroid administration. The observation of the blood glucose behaviour, detected at the beginning and at the end of this interval can be helpful: during this period an increase in the blood glucose values can be interpreted as a deterioration of the endocrine function and it requires further investigations (ultrasonography, scintiscan, C peptide assay and eventually arteriography), while decreased or unmodified blood glucose levels can be explained as an indication of good graft function.

In the following weeks there is a restoration of the blood glucose levels, both fasting and postprandial, and during this period the beta cell shows a satisfactory response, in term of insulin and C peptide release, to several insulinogenic stimuli. The oral glucose tolerance test shows a good, but delayed insulin release, while blood glucose levels, in the normal range at baseline, return to normal values only at 180 minutes, showing an impaired glucose tolerance, according to the WHO criteria [6, 13, 14] (Figures 2 and 3). In these patients, the withdrawal of steroids from the immunosuppressive treatment does not seem to ameliorate the glycemic or insulinemic response to oral glucose [13]. A good insulin release is observed when glucose is abministered i.v., with a prompt increase immediately after glucose infusion (Figure 4), only slightly lower than in non diabetic controls, and Conard's K of glucose disposal shows normal or borderline values [6, 13].

The transplanted pancreas also shows a good insulin response to insulinogenic stimuli other than glucose, such as arginine and tolbutamide. In fact, the arginine-induced insulin release is prompt and byphasic (Figure 5), as in non diabetic controls, and it does not seem to be impaired by steroid administration [13]. The same response can also be observed when 1 g tolbutamide is administered i.v. [6, 13]: insulin levels reach 75 μU/ml at the 5th minute.

It is difficult to assess the function of the transplanted alpha cells, since the original pancreas maintain its function. However, a few months after transplantation, basal plasma glucagon and its response to oral glucose appear to be in the normal range (Figure 6), that is to say suppressed or not stimulated [6, 13]). The immunosuppressive treatment does not influence the plasma glucagon response to glucose p.o. and plasma glucagon also shows a normal response when aminoacids (arginine) are infused i.v. [13] (Figure 7). The normality of glucagon basal levels shows that the transplanted alpha cells respond correctly to the physiologic inhibition, although the mass of the alpha cells is almost doubled, including both the original and the transplanted pancreas.

The transplanted alpha and beta cells show to respond correctly to the inhibitory action of somatostatin, when exogenously administered, as demonstrated by the infusion of somatostatin during an arginine test [6].

The insulin response to the previously described insulinogenic tests shows that the transplanted pancreas keeps the possibility to secrete insulin, although not always according to the normal pattern, as shown after oral glucose, where a delayed insulin release is observed, perhaps due to the paraphysiologic condition of the transplanted pancreas. In fact, the transplanted pancreas does not respect the functional and morphological situation of the original pancreas. Firstly the amount of transplanted beta cells is reduced, due to several reasons, such as the 'segmental' technique, the possible presence of undetected rejections and of warm ischemia, leading to some necrosis and damage of the endocrine tissue. Furthermore it is known that the suppression of the exocrine function in animals reduces the insulin secretion and impairs

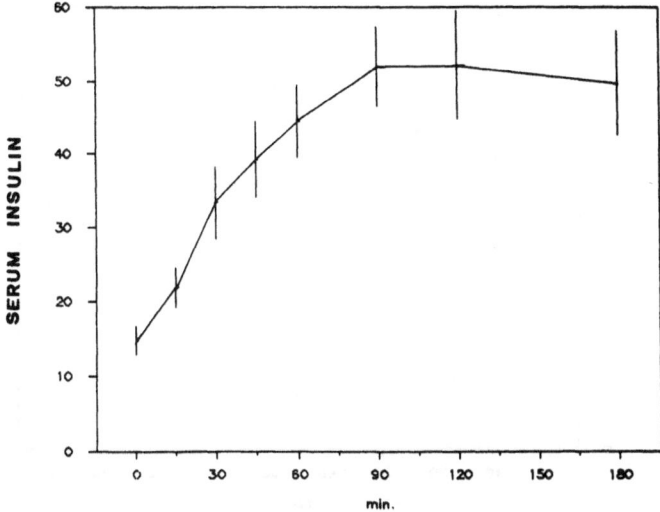

Figure 2. Serum Insulin levels (μU/ml) after Oral Glucose Tolerance Test (75 g p.o.) in 14 IDD uremic patients submitted to kidney and pancreas transplantation. See text.

glucose tolerance [15]. The transplanted pancreas is also denervated and the role played by the vagus nerve [16] and by acetylcholine [17] on insulin response to glucose is well described in animals, although it is not completely clarified in man [18]. Furthermore, the pancreas is transplanted eterotopically and it secretes insulin in the peripheral circulation, rather than in the portal

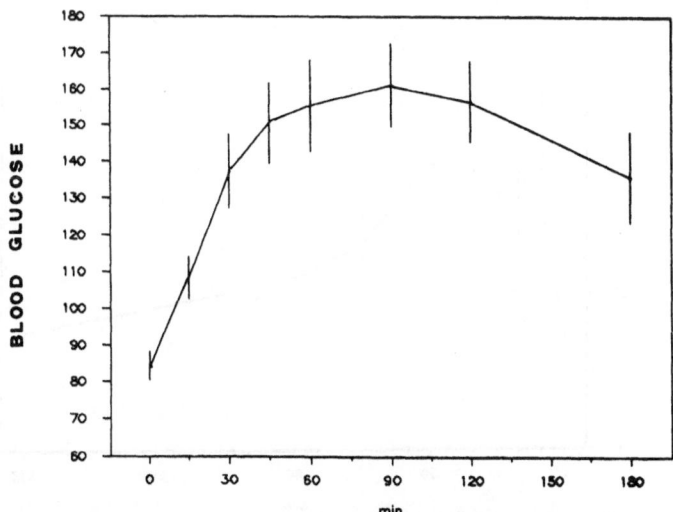

Figure 3. Blood Glucose levels (mg/dl) after Oral Glucose Tolerance Test (75 g p.o.) in 14 IDD uremic patients submitted to kidney and pancreas transplantation. See text.

230

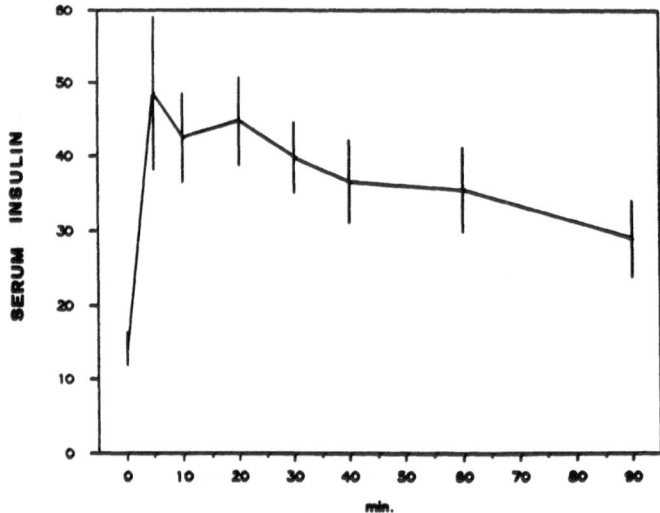

Figure 4. Serum Insulin levels (μU/ml) after Intra Venous Glucose Tolerance Test (0.5 g/kg i.v.) in 15 IDD uremic patients submitted to kidney and pancreas transplantation. See text.

circulation: therefore, insulin reaches the liver, main target organ of its action, only after a total body circulation, having developed its action at the level of the muscular and adipose tissues. The transplanted pancreas is also far from its physiological location and the gastrointestinal hormones are known to stim-

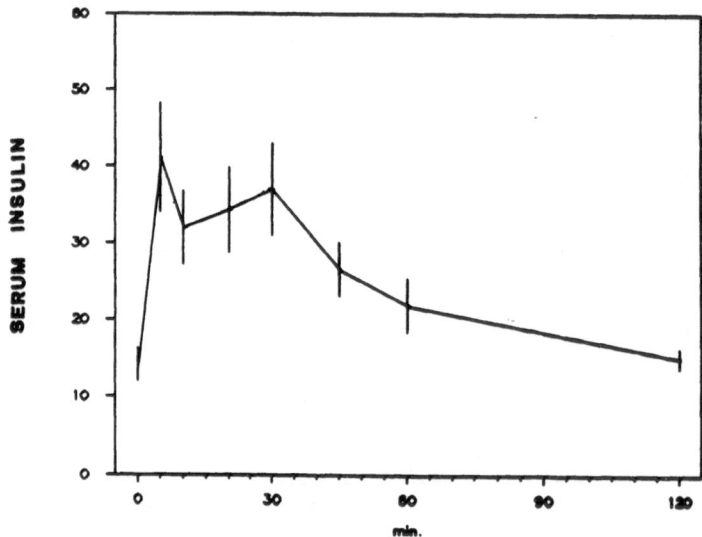

Figure 5. Serum Insulin levels (μU/ml) after arginine test (30 g i.v. over 30 min) in 8 IDD uremic patients submitted to kidney and pancreas transplantation. See text.

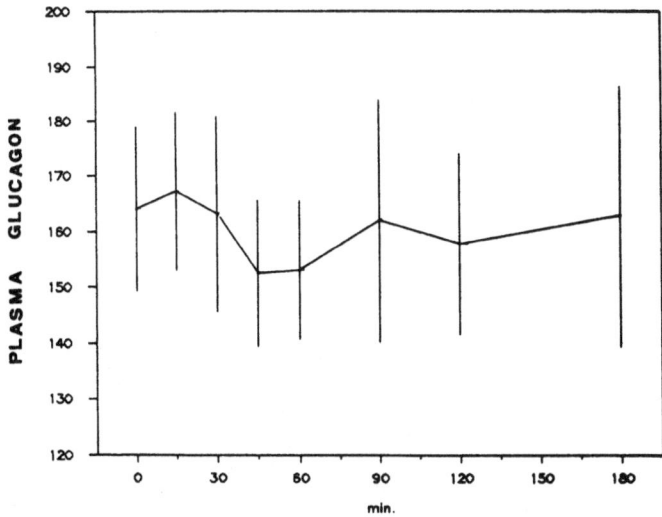

Figure 6. Plasma Glucagon levels (pg/ml) after oral glucose tolerance test (75 g p.o.) in 14 uremic IDD patients submitted to kidney and pancreas transplantation. See text.

ulate insulin and glucagon release in experimental animals [19, 20].

During insulin infusion the alpha and beta cells response to insulin-induced hypoglycemia shows an inhibition of C peptide secretion, which continues during the post-infusional period (Figure 8). In some instances a glucagon increase is not always observed, suggesting an impairment of alpha cell function [21].

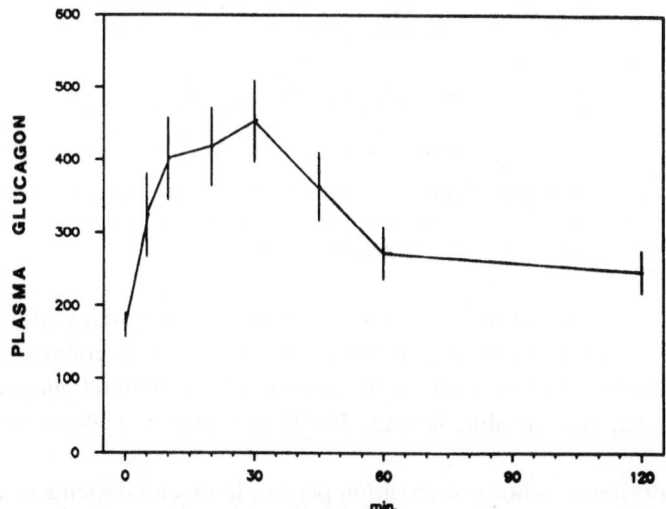

Figure 7. Plasma Glucagon levels (pg/ml) after arginine test (30 g i.v. over 30 min) in 8 uremic IDD patients submitted to kidney and pancreas transplantation. See text.

232

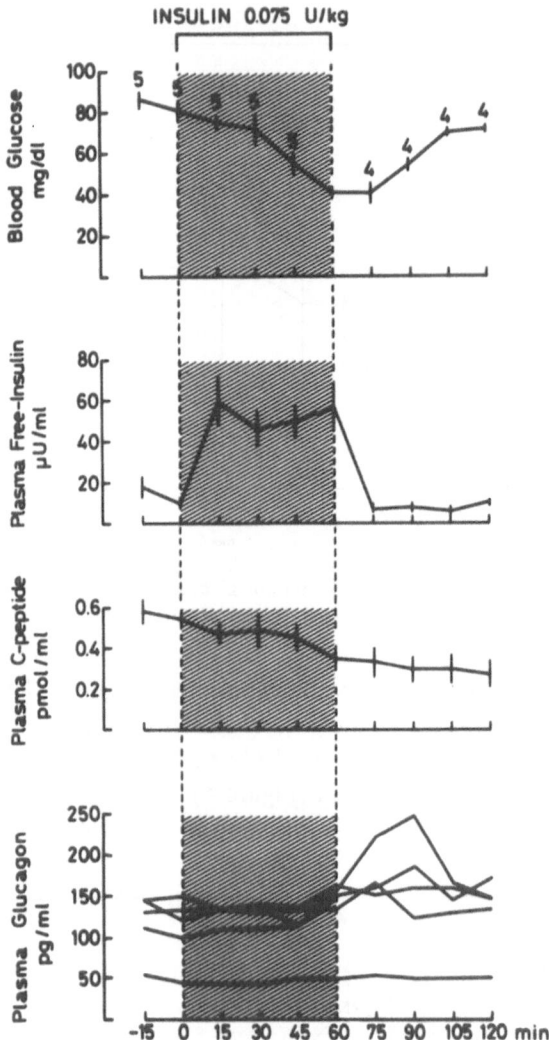

Figure 8. Blood Glucose (mg/dl), Plasma Free Insulin (μU/ml), Plasma C Peptide (pmol/ml) and Plasma Glucagon (pg/ml) during insulin test (0.075 U/kg over 60 min) in 4 uremic IDD patients submitted to kidney and pancreas transplantation. See text.

Pancreas transplantation, when successful, leads some weeks after surgery to complete insulin-independence, while endocrine and metabolic patterns remain in the normal range. This is shown by the 24 hour metabolic profile for blood glucose, free insulin, lactate, B-OH butyrate and glucagon [7, 22] (Figure 9).

In fact, during a 24-hour observation period, in insulin-dependent diabetic patients following as closely as possible their usual daily routines, blood glucose levels show minimal variations in the fasting and in the postprandial

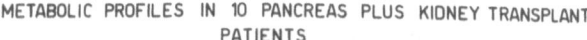

METABOLIC PROFILES IN 10 PANCREAS PLUS KIDNEY TRANSPLANT
PATIENTS

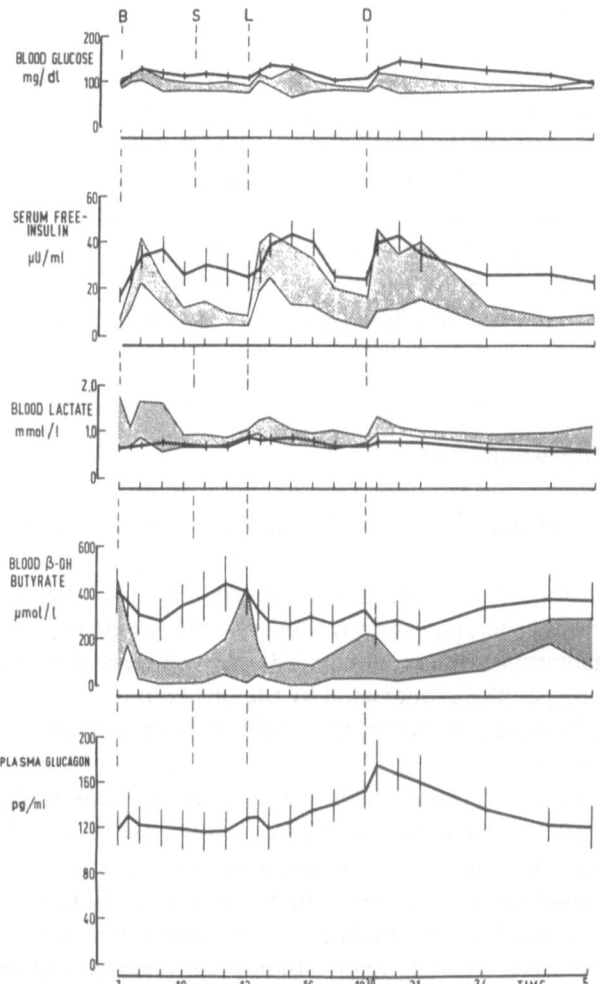

Figure 9. 24 hours metabolic profiles for Blood Glucose (mg/dl), Serum Free Insulin (μU/ml),
Blood Lactate (mmol/l), Blood B-OH Butyrate (μmol/ml) and Plasma Glucagon (pg/ml) in 10
uremic patients submitted to kidney and pancreas transplantation. See text.

state, ranging between 4 and 10 mmol/l. During the same observation period
insulin levels show a physiological increase, although delayed, in the postprandial period, reaching 40 μU/ml, while a mild hyperinsulinemia is present
in the fasting period (night). This could be due both to steroid administration,
and to the peripheral rather than portal delivery of insulin from the transplanted pancreas. Blood lactate concentrations are always in the normal
range, during the 24-hour observation, while B-OH butyrate is higher than in
controls, although an inverse relation with the pattern of insulin secretion is

present. This mild hyperketonemia could be due to a low concentration of insulin at the hepatic level, unable to completely control ketone body production.

24-hour glucagon patterns remain in the normal range, although the alpha cell mass is almost doubled after pancreas transplantation, showing that alpha cells correctly respond to the physiologic feed-back system [7].

In summary, at the half term period, pancreas transplantation leads to insulin independence and to the disappearence of the symptoms and signs of diabetes bringing blood glucose and intermediary metabolites back to normality. The minor differences from normality in hormonal and metabolic patterns could be due to the peculiar physiology of the pancreas graft, as previously discussed.

Long term endocrine function

The insulin-dependent diabetic patient undergoing pancreas transplantation is generally a patient with a long history of diabetes, presenting late complications of the disease, such as retinopathy, neuropathy, macroangiopathy and nephropathy, and in fact, pancreas transplantation is frequently associated to kidney transplantation in these patients [23]. Nevertheless, these patients are frequently young people, as indicated by the selection criteria used in many centres. So far, in these patients the transplanted pancreas has to demonstrate a long term function.

Several technical and immunological factors in pancreas transplantation could be responsible for late failures, as frequently observed.

Among these factors, as reported by many authors, the chronic rejection of the pancreatic tissue and the suppression of the exocrine function, mainly by polymers, were considered the main causes of long term insufficiency of the transplanted beta cell. So far, many studies were carried out in order to evaluate the long term function of pancreatic grafts [14, 22, 24, 25].

When a classical insulinogenic stimulus, such as oral glucose, is studied one year after transplantation, glucose tolerance remains normal and insulin secretion seems to be more physiological, with an higher peak at 30 minutes [25] (Figure 10). The same amelioration is observed during a 24-hour observation period, investigated two years after transplantation: blood glucose levels tend to be lower than in the immediate postoperative period, insulin release seems to be more physiological, and intermediary metabolites remain normal (Figure 11). In particular B-OH butyrate returns to the normal range, showing that the transplanted pancreas restores its capacity to control ketone bodies production, probably with an higher concentration of insulin at the hepatic level [25].

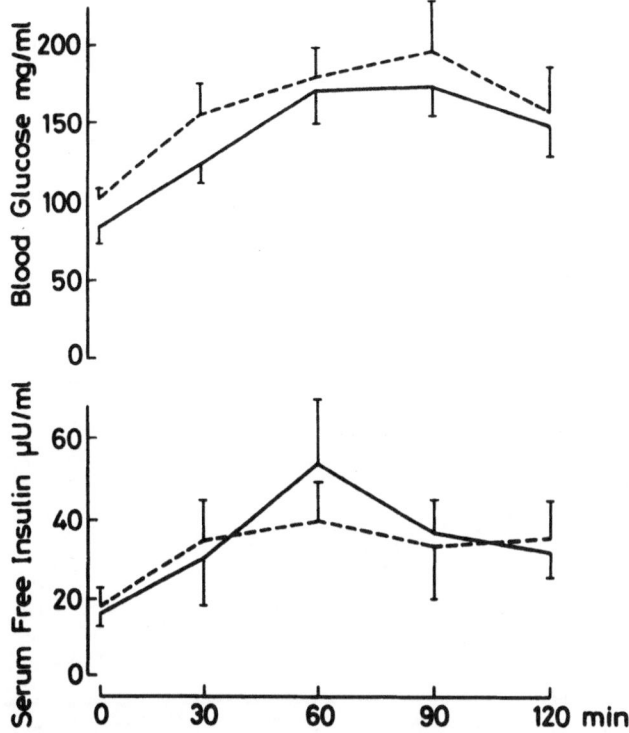

Figure 10. Blood Glucose (mg/dl) and Serum Free Insulin (μU/ml) after Oral Glucose Tolerance Test (75 g p.o.) in 6 IDD patients 3 months (---) and 1 year (——) after pancreas allotransplant.

The amelioration of the glucose metabolism in the long term follow-up is confirmed by the analysis of glucosilated hemoglobin, with a reduction from the pretransplant values of 10.1% to 5.9% at 3 years [25].

As to the effects of different immunosuppressive treatments on the endocrine function of the transplanted pancreas, the availability of cyclosporin, a potent immunosuppressive agent, led to the reduction or suppression of steroid doses, which could be helpful particularly in the long term period, in order to reduce a potential diabetogenic stress on the transplanted pancreas. In fact in some instances steroids has to be reduced to very low doses (5 mg every other day) in order to achieve a satisfactory metabolic control, unachievable in the same patient with 10 mg/day of prednisone (G. Pozza, unpublished).

On the other hand there are some data in the literature referring a 'diabetogenic' effect of cyclosporin, particularly when associated with steroids, both in man [26] as in animals [27], although there is no general agreement at this regard. In our experience the administration of cyclosporin alone is accompanied by a 24 hr metabolic profile for blood glucose closer to physiological values than in patients treated with steroids [28, 29].

236

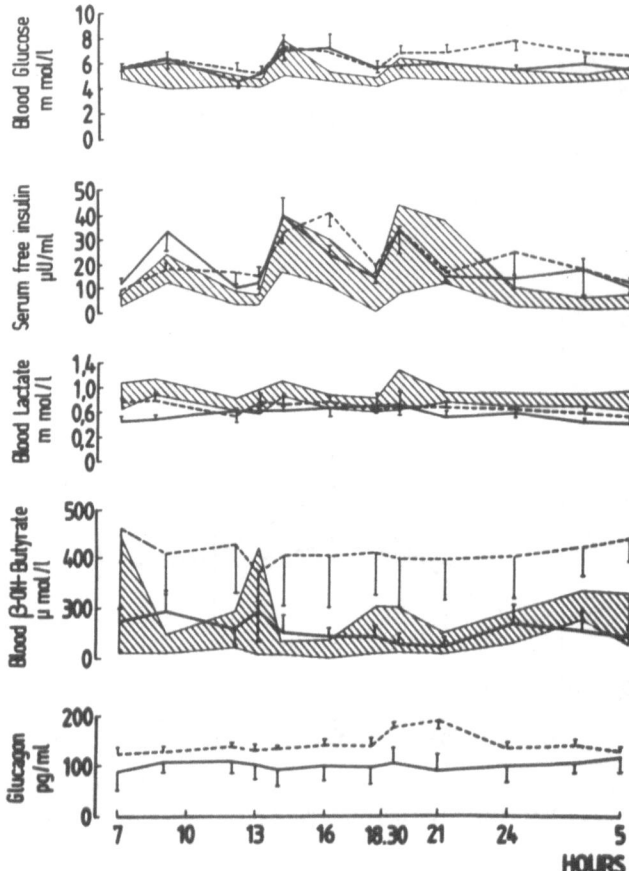

Figure 11. 24 hours metabolic profiles for Blood Glucose (mg/dl), Serum Free Insulin (μU/ml), Blood Lactate (mmol/l) and Blood B-OH Butyrate (μmol/l) and plasma Glucagon (pg/ml) in 3 IDD patients 6 months (---) and 2 years (——) after pancreatic allotransplant.

Conclusions

Pancreas transplantation leads to restoration of glucose homeostasis in patients affected by insulin-dependent diabetes mellitus, particularly in their every-day life. Furthermore it is also able to develop a near-normal response when maximal stimuli are applied, such as glucose or arginine.

These near-normal responses are achieved although the pancreas is transplanted eterotopically, far from its physiologic environment, it is denervated and its exocrine function is suppressed, when the segmental-duct obstruction technique is employed.

So far pancreas transplantation comes up to our expectations, leading diabetic patients to insulin-independence, although further development of the surgical technique, with a more respectful preservation of the physiology of the transplanted pancreas, could amaliorate these results.

References

1. Sutherland DER, Moudry K: Pancreas transplant registry report. Transplant Proc (in press) 1986.
2. Tattersall R: Brittle diabetes. Clinical endocrinology and metabolism 6: 403–19, 1977.
3. Pirart J: Diabetes Care 168: 252, 1978.
4. Dubernard JM, Traeger J, Neyra P, Touraine JL, Tranchant D, Blanc Brunat N: New method of preparation of a segmental pancreatic graft for transplantation. Trials in dogs and in man. Surgery 84: 633–639, 1978.
5. Sutherland DER: Pancreas and islet transplantation. Diabetologia 20: 435–450, 1981.
6. Pozza G, Traeger J, Dubernard JM, Secchi A, Pontiroli AE, Bosi E, Malik MC, Ruitton A, Blanc N: Endocrine responses of type 1 diabetic patients following successful pancreas transplantation. Diabetologia 24: 244–48, 1983.
7. Pozza G, Bosi E, Secchi A, Piatti PM, Touraine JM, Gelet A, Pontiroli AE, Dubernard JM, Traeger J: Metabolic control of type 1 diabetes after pancreas transplantation. Br Med J 291: 510–13, 1985.
8. Piatti PM, Traeger J, Dubernard JM, Bosi E, Finaz J, Mongin-Long S, El Yafi S, Secchi A, Pozet N, Monti L, Pozza G: Hormonal evaluation of immediate pancreatic function in simultaneous kidney plus pancreas transplantation during artificial pancreas monitoring. Transplant Proc 17: 346–48, 1985.
9. Papachristou DN, Agnati N, Fortner GJ: Duct ligation versus duct obliteration of canine pancreatic autografts: early post-operative results. Transplant Proc 11: 522–526, 1979.
10. Traeger J, Dubernard JM, Piatti PM, Bosi E, El Yafi S, Lenfrancois N, Cantarovich D, Secchi A, Gelet A, Kamel G, Monti LD, Touraine JL, Pozza G: Cyclosporin in double simultaneous pancreas plus kidney transplantation. Transplant Proc 17: 336–39, 1985.
11. Traeger J, Bosi E, Dubernard JM, Touraine JL, Piatti PM, Secchi A, Gelet A, Pozza G: Thirty months' experience with cyclosporin in human pancreatic transplantation. Diabetologia 27: 154–56, 1984.
12. Secchi A, Pontiroli AE, Traeger J, Dubernard JM, Touraine JL, Ruitton A, Blanc N, Pozza G: A method for early detection of graft failure in pancreas transplantation. Transplantation 35: 344–348, 1983.
13. Secchi A, Pontiroli AE, Bosi E, Piatti PM, Monti L, Traeger J, Dubernard JM, Gelet A, Pozza G: Effect of different immunosuppressive treatments on the endocrine function of segmental neoprene-injected pancreatic allografts. Transplant Proc 17: 136–40, 1985.
14. Landgraf R, Landgraf-Leurs NNC, Burg D, Kampik A, Land W: Follow up of simultaneous kidney and pancreas transplantation in type 1 diabetes. Transplant Proc 15: 687–91, 1984.
15. Heptner W, Neubauer HP, Schleyerbach R: Glucose tolerance and insulin secretion in rabbits and dogs after ligation of the pancreatic duct. Diabetologia 10: 193–96, 1974.
16. Bloom SR, Vaughan NJA, Russel RCG: Vagal control of glucagon release in man. Lancet 2: 546–49, 1974.
17. Katinuma H, Kaneto A, Kuzuya T, Nakao K: Effects of methacoline on insulin secretion in man. J Clin Endoc Metab 28: 1384–88, 1968.
18. Lund B, Aagaard P, Deckert T: Effect of vagotomy on insulin release after oral and intravenous glucose administration. Scand J Gastroent 10: 777–80, 1975.
19. Creutzfeld W: The incretin concept today. Diabetologia 16: 75–85, 1979.
20. Unger RH, Eisentraut AM: Entero-insular axis. Arch Int Med 123: 261–66, 1969.
21. Bosi E, Secchi A, Piatti PM, Pontiroli AE, Gelet A, Touraine JL, Dubernard JM, Traeger J, Pozza G: Insulin induced hypoglycaemia test in pancreatic transplant patients: effect on C-peptide and glucagon secretions. E J Clin Invest 14: 22, 1984.
22. Sutherland DER, Najarian JS, Greenberg BZ, Senske BJ, Anderson GE, Francis RS, Goetz

238

FC: Hormonal and metabolic effects of a pancreatic endocrine graft. Annals Int Med 95: 537–41, 1981.

23. Traeger J, Dubernard JM, Bosi E, Piatti PM, Gelet A, El Yafi S, Beutel H, Secchi A, Touraine JL, Pozza G: Patient selection and risk factors in organ transplantation in diabetics: experience with kidney and pancreas. Transplant Proc 16: 577–82, 1984.

24. Blanc-Brunat N, Dubernard JM, Touraine JL, Neyra P, Dubois P, Paulin C, Traeger J: Pathology of the pancreas after intraductal neoprene injection in dogs and diabetic patients treated by pancreatic transplantation. Diabetologia 25: 97–107, 1983.

25. Traeger J, Dubernard JM, Monti LD, La Rocca E, Piatti PM, Cantarovich D, Lefrancois N, Bosi E, Secchi A, Pontiroli AE, Touraine JL, Pozza G: Clinical experience with long term studies on degenerative complications in pancreatic graft in man. Transplant Proc (in press) 1986.

26. Gunnarsson R, Klintmalm G, Lundgren G, Wilczeck H, Ostman J, Groth CG: Deterioration of glucose metabolism in pancreatic transplant recipients given cyclosporin. Lancet 2: 571–572, 1983.

27. Hahn HJ, Laube F, Lucke S, Kloting I, Kohnert KD, Warzock R: Toxic effects of cyclosporin on the endocrine pancreas of Wistar rats. Transplantation 41: 44–47, 1986.

28. Pozza G, Traeger J, Dubernard JM, Secchi A, Bosi E, Pontiroli AE: Cyclosporin and glucose tolerance in pancreas allotransplantation. Lancet 2: 1080, 1983.

29. Pozza G, Secchi A, Pontiroli AE, Bosi E, Traeger J, Dubernard JM, Gelet A: Immuno-suppressive treatment after pancreas transplantation. Immunology in Diabetes. Ed Andreani, Di Mario, Federlin, Heding. London. 203–208, 1984.

12. Exocrine function of the pancreas graft

G. TYDÉN and C.G. GROTH

Introduction

For many years the majority of graft losses following pancreas transplantation were attributable to complications related to the exocrine pancreas such as graft pancreatitis and leakage of pancreatic digestive enzymes with ensuing pancreatic fistulas and infections. Because of this different techniques regarding the handling of the exocrine pancreas were evaluated the most drastic being obstruction of the pancreatic duct with a synthetic polymer leading to atrophy and cessation of function of the exocrine portion of the graft. Indeed, this simple technique was for many years the one most commonly used. However, in recent years there has been a renewed interest in the exocrine pancreas since it has become clear that the transplantation of a pancreas graft with intact exocrine function has several advantages in spite of its potential hazards. The atrophy of the exocrine part that follows duct obliteration may eventually lead to impairment of the endocrine part of the graft. Such an impairment of the endocrine function with time has not been found in grafts with intact exocrine function [1]. Perhaps even more important is the fact that in pancreatic graft rejections the exocrine portion seems to be involved at an earlier stage and to a much greater extent than the endocrine part [2]. Consequently monitoring of the pancreatic exocrine function would make it possible to identify and treat rejection episodes before the endocrine part is impaired. This is of course only possible in grafts with intact exocrine function. Furthermore, pancreas transplants with preserved exocrine function have been found to constitute an interesting experimental model making possible unique studies on the physiology of the exocrine pancreas.

In this chapter the current knowledge regarding the exocrine function of pancreas grafts is reviewed. Furthermore some studies regarding the effects of gastrointestinal hormones on the output and the enzyme content of the pancreatic juice are referred to as well as studies regarding the penetration of drugs to the pancreatic juice.

239

J.M. Dubernard and D.E.R. Sutherland (eds.), International Handbook of Pancreas Transplantation, 239–255.
© *1989 by Kluwer Academic Publishers.*

The exocrine pancreas graft in the immediate postoperative period

Hyperamylasemia post transplantation

Immediately after transplantation there is almost invariably an elevation in the serum amylase. The level usually rises to reach a peak after 24–48 hours. The degree of postoperative hyperamylasemia will depend on several factors but of these the degree of ischemic injury afflicted on the graft is probably the most important one. Thus, a correlation between the magnitude of the postoperative hyperamylasemia and the cold ischemia time was found by Lundgren et al. [3] (Figure 1). Likewise in a recent Stockholm series [4] a sixfold increase in the serum amylase level was found when mean cold ischemia time was 7.4 hours while the increase in serum amylase was only threefold when the mean cold ischemia time was brought down to 4.6 hours.

Another factor influencing postoperative amylase levels is the technique used for exocrine handling. When exocrine diversion has been provided for the peak value is usually 3–5 fold the normal value, the level then falls exponentially to reach normal range after 4–7 days. With duct occluded grafts the peak value is usually somewhat higher, 5–10 times normal and normalization often takes longer. Some patients may maintain a moderately elevated level for several months.

Another possible factor inducing hyperamylasemia immediately after transplantation is the manipulation of the gland during the transplant procedure be it in conjunction with the retrievel in the donor during the backtable work or during the recipient operation. Obviously such operative trauma should be kept to a minimum and some investigators have advocated a non-touch technique. In our experience, however, the pancreas may be handled and touched albeit with nimble fingers.

Postoperative pancreatic sweat

For many years the placement of pancreatic grafts was almost exclusively extraperitoneally in the right or left inguinal fossa. However, with pancreatitis or any pancreatic injury a fluid high in amylase and other enzymes sips out from the pancreatic graft and accumulates around the gland, a phenomenon often referred to as pancreatic sweating. With extraperitoneal placement of the graft this fluid was not reabsorbed but eventually gave rise to fistulas, which often became contaminated with bacteria necessitating removal of the graft. Several different techniques were proposed to solve this problem, such as fenestrating the peritoneum adjacent to the pancreas, placing the pancreas with the vascular anastomosis extraperitoneally and the tail intraperitoneally through a hole in the peritoneum and wrapping up the pancreas with the

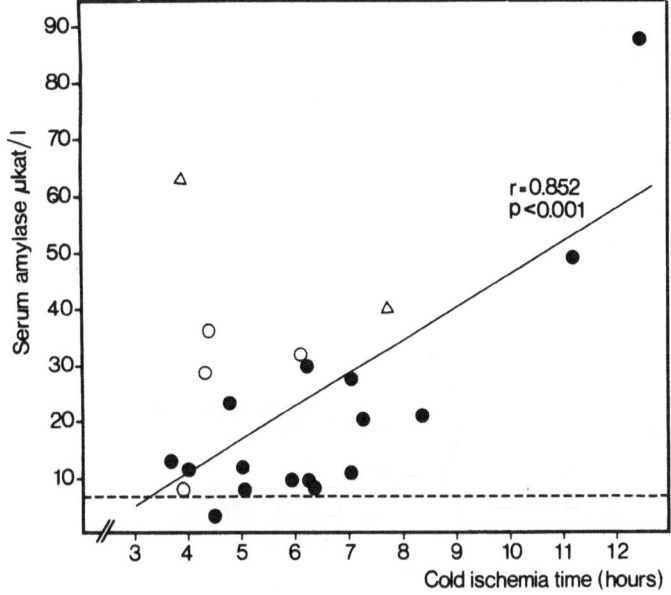

Figure 1. Effect of cold ischemia time on postoperative serum amylase levels. ● grafts perfused with Perfadex and with enteric diversion. △ grafts perfused with Sach's solution and with enteric diversion. ○ duct ligated grafts perfused with Perfadex. The regression line concerns the 16 grafts perfused with Perfadex and with enteric diversion.

omentum. Nowadays it has become more common to place the whole graft intraperitoneally since the peritoneum has the capability of absorbing the peripancreatic transudate. Recently the peripancreatic fluid was studied by following the discharge from an abdominal drain tube that had been placed at the graft [5] (Figure 2). It was found that during the first days the amount of fluid drained was almost half a litre, the output thereafter gradually declined to 100 ml after 5 days at which time the tube was usually removed. The amylase activity in this fluid was initially 17 times higher than that concomitantly found in the serum. During the following days the amylase activity in the fluid rapidly decreased to reach the same level as that in serum after one week. Thus it seems clear that during the first postoperative days the pancreatic graft sweats a fluid rich in pancreatic digestive enzymes, this probably being a consequence of ischemic injury to the graft. This finding emphasizes the importance of applying drainage at the graft site. Also it speaks in favour of intraperitoneal placement of pancreas grafts since the peritoneum is capable of absorbing such fluid collections.

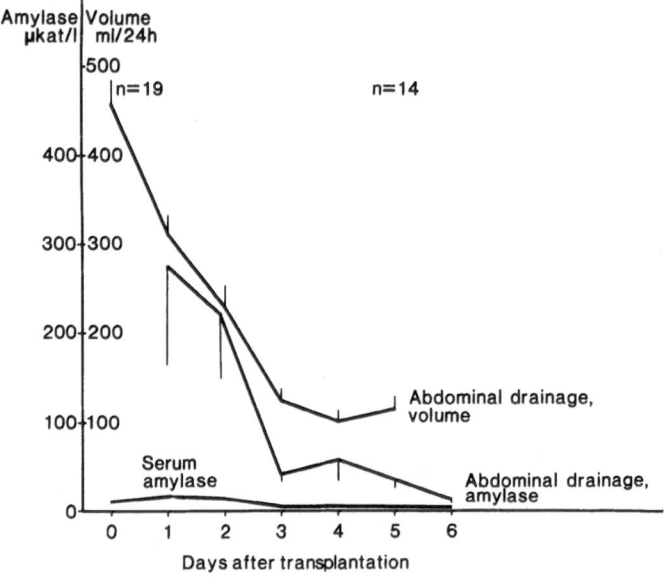

Figure 2. Flow rate of the fluid drained via an abdominal drain tube placed with its tip at the pancreatic graft and amylase activity in the fluid. Also shown is the serum amylase activity. Normal value for serum amylase is 1.5–6.0 μkat/l. Vertical lines indicate standard error of the mean. By permission of Surgery, Gynecology & Obstetrics.

Volume and composition of the pancreatic juice

With the technique used in Stockholm in pancreatic transplantation the segmental graft is anastomosed to a jejunal Roux-en-Y-loop and a pancreatic duct catheter is used to temporarily (3–4 weeks) divert the pancreatic juice to the exterior, thus promoting healing of the pancreatico-enteric anastomosis [6]. This technique makes it possible to monitor the enzyme content and the secretion rate of the pure pancreatic juice and thus determine the functional status of the grafts. Thus it has been shown that the volume of pancreatic juice is low in the first postoperative days but then rises to reach a plateau level of 500–600 ml/24 h after 4 days [5] (Figure 3). During this time the patients were given parenteral nutrition only. When allowed to eat after 1 week the volume of pancreatic juice again increased to reach a new plateau of 700–800 ml/24 h (range 250 ml–850 ml/24 h). The amylase activity and the lipase concentration were very high during the first postoperative days but then gradually decreased to reach a steady level after 4–7 days (Figure 3). The finding of a low volume of a highly concentrated juice in the immediate postoperative period is probably attributable to ischemic graft injury. It also points out the value of diverting the exocrine juice to the exterior for the first postoperative days to protect the

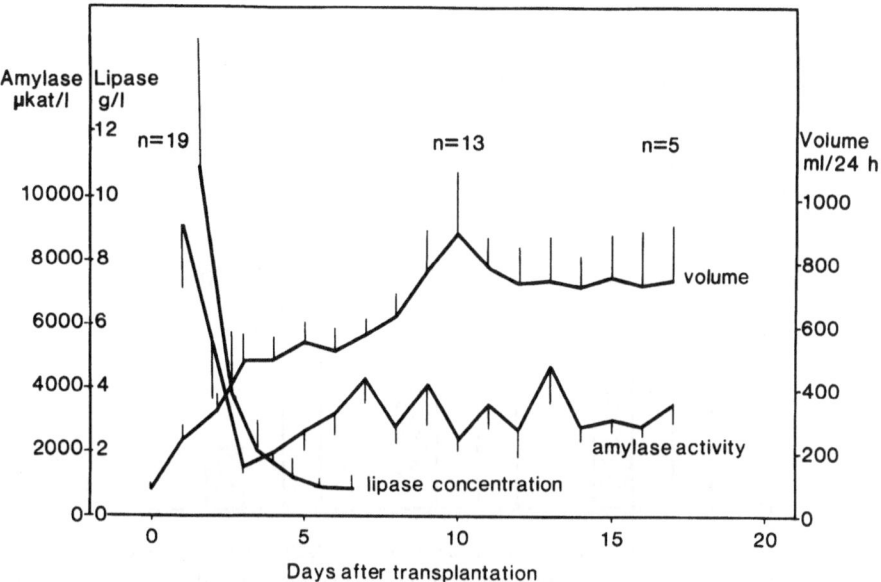

Figure 3. Rate of secretion of pancreatic juice in the pancreatic duct catheter and the amylase activity and lipase concentration in the juice after segmental pancreatic transplantation. Vertical lines indicate standard error of the mean. By permission of Surgery, Gynecology & Obstetrics.

pancreatico-enteric anastomosis. As the ischemic graft injury healed the volume of pancreatic juice increased to reach a new plateau of 500 ml/day. This seems to be a normal output taking into account that the graft consists of approximately half the pancreas. As might be expected when oral feeding was commenced on the 8th postoperative day the daily output of pancreatic juice again increased to reach a new plateau. Since the graft has no nerve supply this increase in pancreatic juice output must be hormonally mediated. Indeed in the same study, the intravenous administration of a bolus dose of secretin showed that the grafts were capable of a sixfold increase of the pancreatic juice output. Also it was found that the administration of intravenous somatostatin was able to reduce not only the basal pancreatic juice volume output but also the output of amylase and lipase (Figure 4). This finding gives support to the concept that somatostatin may be of value in pancreatic transplantation. Indeed in a patient with a duct ligated intraperitoneally placed graft a favourable effect of somatostatin on exocrine secretion has previously been reported [7] and some groups use somatostatin routinely during the first postoperative week [8, 9]. However, it must be borne in mind that somatostatin has other effects that are less desirable in this context such as reducing pancreatic blood flow [10] and inhibiting insulin and glucagon release [11].

244

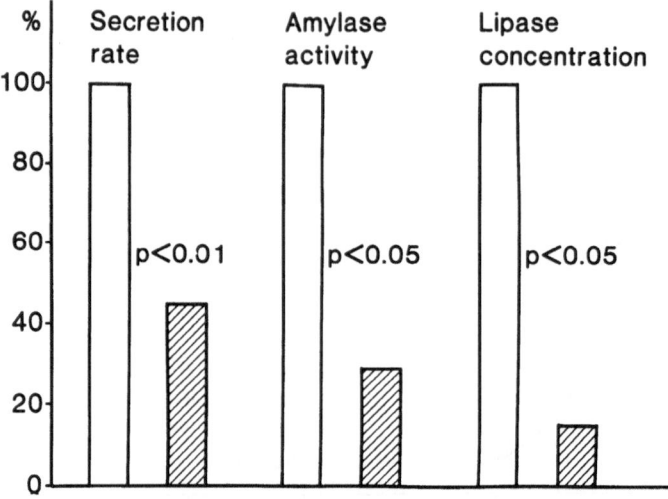

Figure 4. The effect of an intravenous infusion of somatostatin (250 µg/hour) on the secretion rate of the pancreatic juice and the amylase activity and lipase concentration in the juice measured in recipients of segmental pancreatic grafts. By permission of Surgery, Gynecology & Obstetrics.

Late episodes of hyperamylasemia

Episodes of hyperamylasemia may occur months to years following the transplantation. In some cases such episodes have been found to precede chronic graft rejection but in others the ethiology remains obscure. Thus, a transient elevation in the serum amylase may appear with no concomitant sign of endocrine impairment as judged from blood glucose levels and serum C-peptide levels. However, in one patient that presented with a mild hyperamylasemia but clear cut symptoms of pancreatitis 3 months after transplantation and who underwent laparotomy and graft biopsy the biopsy showed marked acute rejection. In a few patients episodes of graft pancreatitis have been diagnosed several years following the transplantation with increased serum amylase levels and severe pain at the graft site. These have all resolved on conventional treatment and the endocrine function of the grafts have remained intact. An explantation for these attacks may be temporary obstruction of the pancreatic duct due perhaps to mucosal overgrowth from the jejunal Roux-loop. However, in one patient with repeated episodes of graft pancreatitis there was a clear cut correlation with emotional stress and in another to viral infection. Also trauma to the pancreatic graft might cause late hyperamylasemia. One remarkable such case has been seen in Stockholm where a patient developed severe pancreatitis following pelvic examination [12]. The examiner was not aware of the fact that the pancreas could be felt in the pelvic fossa and palpated the mysterious mass for some time. The next day serum amylase was $200\,\mu kat/l$ (ref value below $5.2\,\mu kat/l$). Hyperamylasemia persisted for 2 weeks. Graft function then deteriorated and insulin had to be reinstituted.

Serum amylase/isoamylase pattern following pancreas transplantation

It may seem surprising that the serum amylase level eventually falls to the pretransplant level since, after heterotopic segmental pancreatic transplantation, the recipient carries two functioning exocrine pancreatic glands, the native pancreas and the pancreatic graft. Assuming that the amylase appearing in the blood is simply an effect of acinar cell leakage, the serum amylase level would be expected to increase after the addition of a pancreas transplant. Furthermore, when a functioning pancreatic graft is removed because of a local complication or when a graft ceases to function abruptly because of arterial thrombosis, the serum amylase level immediately falls below normal. After this drop the amylase level again gradually rises to normal after 3–5 days [13]. An explantation of this phenomenon has been given by studies on the isoamylase pattern in these patients [14]. Prior to transplantation, amylase in serum consist of two major components, salivary and pancreatic, in approximately the same proportions. Following transplantation it was found that although the serum amylase level was unchanged the isoenzyme pattern had changed. Thus, there was a drastic increase in pancreatic amylase with a concomitant fall in salivary amylase (Figure 5). It seems therefore that when the pancreatic amylase is increased by the addition of a pancreatic graft there is a depression in the release of salivary amylase. It was found that when a pancreatic graft function was abruptly lost, the drop in the serum amylase level was due to a decrease in the pancreatic amylase. During the following days when the serum amylase level gradually again increased to reach the normal value the increase was due to a reappearance of salivary amylase (Figure 6). Thus, it seems that the amylase found in the blood is not simply an effect of leakage from the pancreas and the salivary glands but is due to a carefully controlled release into the blood stream. If the release of pancreatic amylase is increased there is a concomitant decrease in the release of salivary amylase. Likewise, if pancreatic amylase is decreased there is an increase in salivary amylase. Based on these findings it seems worthwhile to not only follow the serum amylase levels but also to study the isoamylase pattern when the function of the exocrine portion of the pancreas is assessed. Thus, a finding of a very high proportion of pancreatic amylase as compared to the salivary amylase would indicate intact function of the exocrine part of the pancreatic graft. On the other hand, if a normal value of salivary amylase is found there would be a suspicion of poor pancreatic graft exocrine function.

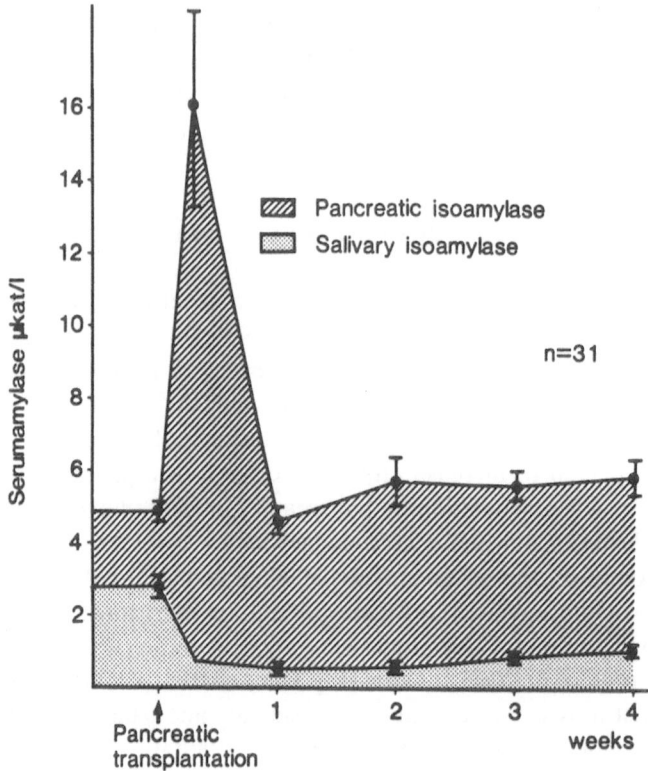

Figure 5. Serum amylase and isoamylase pattern during the first month following pancreatic transplantation. Note that pancreatic isoamylase has, to a large extent, replaced the salivary isoamylase after transplantation. The peak during the first week after transplantation is due to graft ischemic injury.

The exocrine pancreas during rejection episodes

Severyn et al. [15] have reported on biopsy findings in dogs subjected to combined renal and free draining pancreatic transplantation. At the onset of kidney rejection but before functional impairment of the pancreas was noted (hyperglycemia), renal graft biopsies revealed generalized mononuclear infiltration while biopsies of the pancreas showed diffuse interstitial infiltration but the islet of Langerhans appeared to be spared. Likewise, Schulak et al. [2] examined in the rat daily speciments from the time of pancreas transplantation to determine the earliest histological sign of rejection. Histological evidence of rejection was present by day 3 as a perivascular lymphoid infiltration while the islets remained normal. Extensive cellular rejection of the exocrine tissue occurred by day 6 when most recipients where still normoglycemic. Antirejection treatment instituted at this stage was successful in some cases, but was never effective when hyperglycemia was present. Thus, it seems that

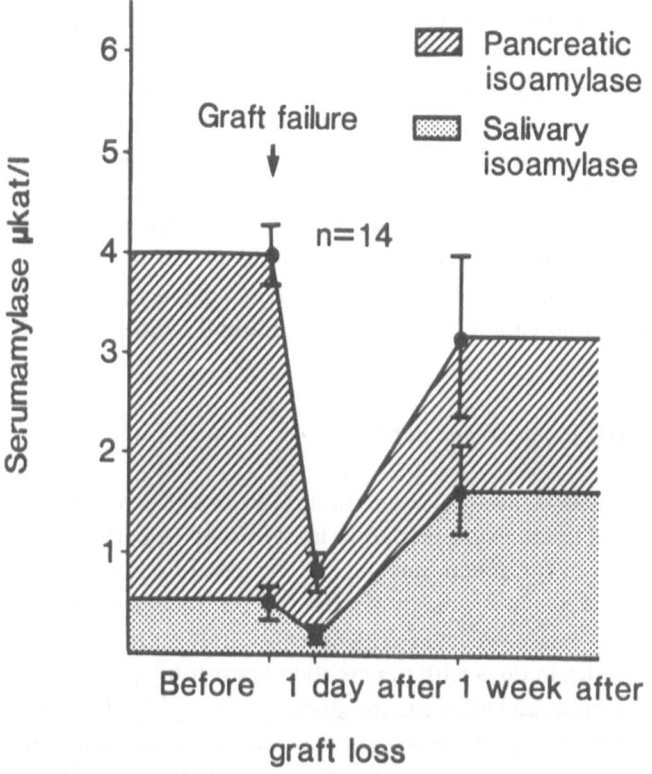

Figure 6. Serum amylase and isoamylase pattern in conjunction with sudden loss of a functioning graft. The graft loss is accompanied by a sudden decrease in serum amylase. Recovery is accomplished by pancreatic as well as salivary isoamylase returning to normal levels.

during pancreatic graft rejection the exocrine part of the gland is mainly involved, the endocrine part being afflicted only at a later and more irreversible stage of the rejection. Monitoring of the exocrine part of the pancreas graft therefore seems to be essential in the diagnosis of rejection.

Serum amylase

Serum amylase could be expected to serve as an indicator of injury to the exocrine pancreas. This is true of course only for pancreatic grafts with preserved exocrine function i.e. with exocrine drainage as opposed to duct obliterated grafts. Indeed the Zürich group has reported a transient elevation of serum amylase preceding rejection episodes in recipients of combined renal and pancreatic grafts [16, 17]. Similar findings have been reported from Stockholm [18, 19]. In some but not all of the patients a slight transient elevation in serum amylase preceded pancreatic rejection episodes by 1–2 days. In the Minnesota series, however, serum amylase levels have not proven to be helpful in diagnosis of rejection [20]. This discrepancy may be explained by the fact that the serum amylase consists of pancreatic amylase from the native pancreas as well as the pancreatic graft and of salivary amylase from the salivary glands. Thus, the serum amylase level is a reflection not only of the state of the pancreatic graft but also of the native pancreas and the salivary glands. Furthermore, the serum amylase level is also affected by renal function and probably also by steroids. A more consistent finding noted by Tydén et al. [13] is that when the pancreatic graft is suddenly lost due to thrombosis or irreversible rejection there is usually a sharp decline in serum amylase levels, often to subnormal values, followed by a gradual increase to normal levels over 3–5 days.

Amylase activity in pancreatic juice

As has been discussed above it seems that rejections afflicting the pancreas are mainly confined to the exocrine part at least during the early reversible stage. Determinations of the functional state of the exocrine portion should therefore be of great value in the diagnosis of rejection. Indeed clear cut reductions in the amylase excretion from a pancreatic graft were first noted during rejection episodes in dogs with pancreatico-cystostomy [21].

When the technique with exocrine drainage to the bladder was introduced clinically, it was also speculated that the urinary amylase would be an important tool for diagnosing acute rejection episodes [22]. Shortly thereafter Gil-Vernet [23, 24] did indeed observe that a marked drop in urine amylase did occur in conjunction with renal graft rejection in recipients of combined renal and pancreatic grafts. Subsequently this finding has been confirmed by others [25] and today many centers use urinary amylase as the prime marker for pancreatic graft rejection, especially in recipients of single pancreatic grafts. Since variations in the amylase content of the urine are reflected in variations in pH, the simple measurement of the urinary pH has proven to be a parameter which can be monitored by the patient himself even at home. Still, some difficulties might exist with the interpretation of the amylase data, for instance when there are great variations in urinary output [26].

The possibility of diagnosing acute rejection episodes by urinary monitoring has prompted many groups to adopt the bladder for exocrine diversion. It is clear, however, that similar, or perhaps even better information, can be obtained by measuring amylase in the pancreatic juice itself if the juice is diverted to the exterior after transplantation [27, 28]. Such a diversion has been accomplished with grafts with pancreatico-enteric anastomosis, but also as a preliminary step for grafts subsequently to undergo duct occlusion [28].

When the exteriorized pancreatic juice was monitored in Stockholm, it was found that a marked reduction in the amylase activity in pancreatic juice did indeed occur during pancreatic graft rejection episodes, while the fasting blood glucose, the serum C-peptide and the serum amylase were essentially unaffected (Figure 7). Following antirejection treatment with methylpred-nisolone the amylase activity recovered. A characteristic drop in the amylase content of the juice, which was reversible on steroid medication, has now been recorded in several Stockholm patients (Figure 8) [29].

A problem with this technique for diagnosing rejection is of course the fact that the pancreatic juice is available for monitoring only for a limited time usually until discharge at which time the catheter will have to be removed. However, the majority of all acute rejection episodes will occur during this time period.

Pancreatic juice cytology

When the pure pancreatic juice is diverted to the exterior, daily determinations of the pancreatic juice cytology can be performed. This has been shown to be of great value in the diagnosis of rejection and may be more sensitive than the variations in pancreatic juice amylase. The pancreatic juice contain large amounts of granulocytes for the first postoperative days probably as a reflection of the ischemic graft pancreatitis. However, subsequently the pancreatic juice becomes completely devoid of cells until a rejection episode occurs. Then monocytes appear in the juice followed by the occurrence of lymphocytes and lymphoblasts. This phenomenon has been found to precede the decline in serum amylase by 1 or 2 days. Following antirejection treatment the lympho-blasts disappeared and the pancreatic juice again was totally devoid of cells (Figure 7) [29]. Thus, pancreatic juice cytology may prove to be the most sensitive measure of pancreatic graft rejection hitherto described.

The penetrations of drugs into the pancreatic juice

The purpose of diverting the pancreatic juice to the exterior as is done with the technique employed in Stockholm was originally to promote healing of the pancreatico-enteric anastomosis and thus avoid the hazards of pancreatic fistulas. However, this technique also makes it possible to perform studies on the penetration of drugs to the pancreas. Of special interest in the field of pancreatic transplantations is the penetration of immunosuppressive drugs such as cyclosporin to the graft. Normally the dosage of cyclosporin is based on the whole blood or plasma trough levels. However, the blood levels do not necessarily reflect the concentration in the organs [30]. Brattström et al. [27] performed simultaneous measurements of cyclosporin in plasma and pancreatic juice in patients subjected to pancreatic transplantation with the pan-

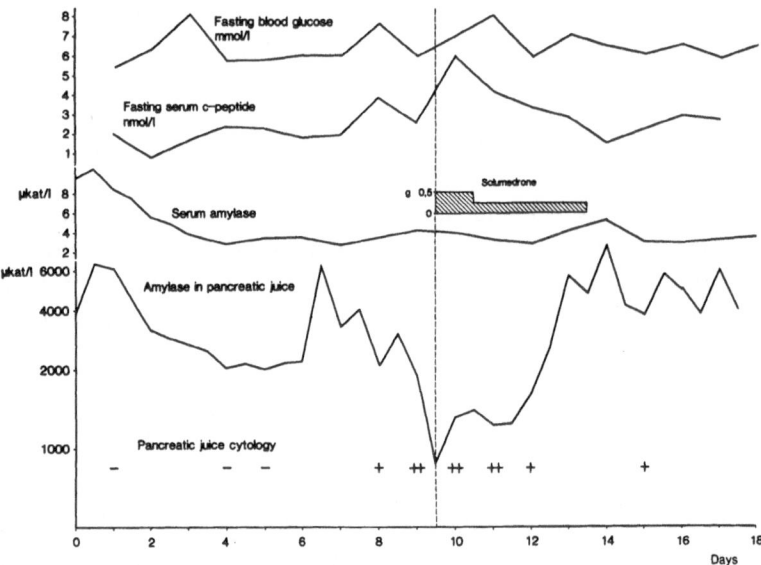

Figure 7. Fasting blood glucose level, fasting serum C-peptide, serum amylase, amylase content in the pancreatic juice and the findings from pancreatic juice cytology during a suspected rejection episode in a patient with a single pancreatic graft. The pancreatic juice cytology was defined as negative when there were no cells or only granulocytes and positive when monocytes and/or lymphoblasts appeared. Noted the marked drop in the amylase content of the juice occurring simultaneously with the occurrence of inflammatory cells. Following administration of Solu-Medrone these abnormalities disappeared. Serum amylase was unaffected.

creatic juice temporarily diverted to the exterior. They found the concentration of cyclosporin in pancreatic juice to be about 30% of that in plasma as determined by radio immuno assay. This relationship was similar on HPLC analysis (Figure 9). Since the protein content of pancreatic juice is only 10% of that in plasma and cyclosporin is highly bound to protein the concentration of cyclosporin in pancreatic juice was unexpectedly high. The high concentration probably reflects a high tissue concentration of cyclosporin in the pancreas [30] and may explain the diabetogenic effect of cyclosporin which has been reported [31].

Another group of drugs where penetration to the pancreatic graft is of special interest is the antibiotics. If any therapeutic effect is to be expected following antibiotic treatment of pancreatic infections the chosen antibiotic should have good penetration into the pancreas and also be effective against the bacteria commonly isolated in pancreatic infections. In a study performed by the Stockholm group the concentration of clindamycin, piperacillin and cefoxitin in the pancreatic juice was studied following pancreatic transplantation [32]. Clindamycin is especially effective against anaerobic bacteria, pipe-

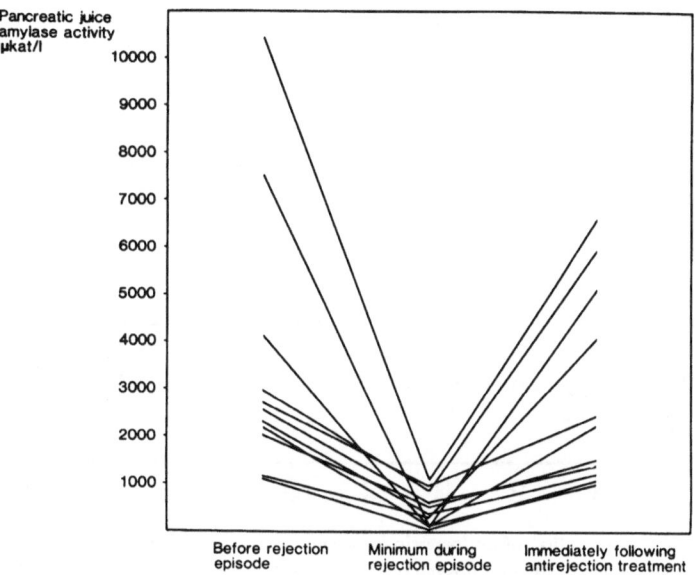

Pancreatic juice
amylase activity
µkat/l

Figure 8. Amylase activity in the pancreatic juice before, during and immediately after 11 suspected pancreatic graft rejection episodes.

racillin against enterococcus and gram-negative bacteria and cefoxitin against anerobic bacteria and most enterobacteria found in pancreatic infections. In this study clindamycin was found to reach therapeutic levels in the pancreatic juice well above the minimum inhibitory concentration for all anerobic bacteria and most streptococci (Figure 10). Clindamycin therefore seems to be a suitable antibiotic for the treatment of pancreatic infections. However, since both enterococcus and the enterobacteria which are commonly found in pancreatic infections are resistent to clindamycin some antibiotic active against these bacteria should be used in combination with clindamycin. However, it was found that the penetration of cefoxitin and piperacillin, which would be suitable drugs to be used in combination with clindamycin, did not penetrate into the pancreatic juice in therapeutic concentrations although adequate concentrations were achieved in the serum. These two drugs therefore seem to be less suitable in this respect. In another study the penetration of two quinolones to the pancreatic juice was studied following oral administration [33]. The concentration of ciprofloxacin in pancreatic juice was 30% of that in serum and the corresponding figure for ofloxacin was around 100%. Thus the level of ofloxacin in pancreatic juice exceeded the minimum inhibitory concentration for most gram-negative enteric pathogens during several hours after administration of a single oral dose. It seems therefore that ofloxacin also would be a good alternative in the treatment of severe infections

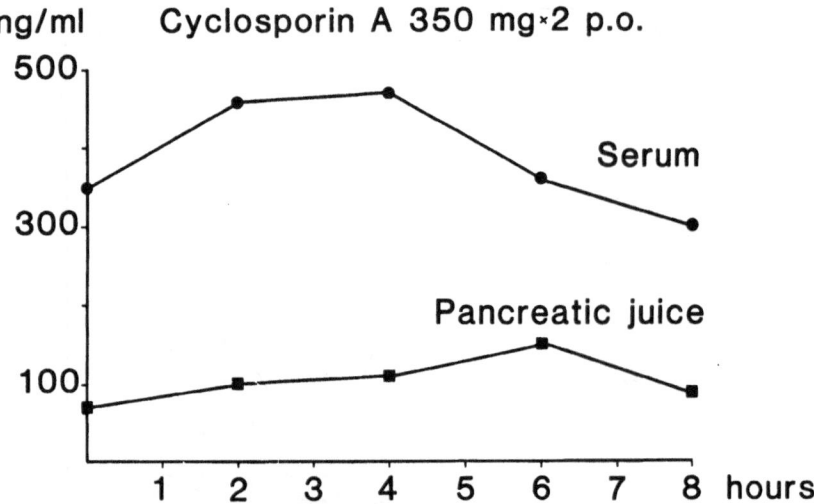

Figure 9. The concentration of cyclosporin in plasma and pancreatic juice determined by RIA. Cyclosporin was given orally at a dosage of 350 mg b.i.d.

in pancreatic grafts. Concerning ciprofloxacin only the peak concentration succeeded in reaching the minimum inhibitory concentration values for the enteric pathogens.

Conclusions

Following pancreatic transplantation, a fluid rich in amylase escapes from the graft during the first several days. This finding emphasizes the importance of draining the graft site, also it speaks in favour of intraperitoneal placement of the graft since the peritoneum appears to be able to absorb some of the fluid.

Serum amylase is a good marker of ischemic injury and also of posttransplantation pancreatitis, both conditions being reflected by hyperamylasemia. Low serum amylase levels occur immediately after a sudden loss of a functioning pancreatic graft, for instance because of thrombosis. An interesting relationship exists between the pancreatic and salivary isoamylase with some mechanism working to keep the sum of the two at a constant level, this level constituting the serum amylase.

The temporary use of a pancreatic duct catheter leading to the exterior has proven to be of great value. Not only is the pancreatic anastomosis protected from the digestive forces of the juice, but monitoring of the exocrine function of the graft is possible on a minute to minute basis. Also, it is now established that acute pancreatic graft rejection is accompanied by a marked fall in the

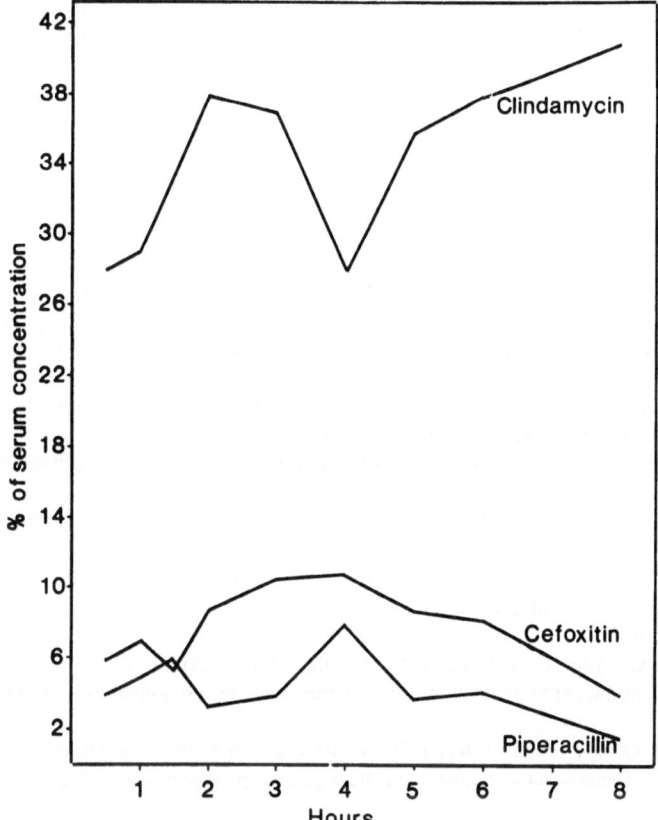

Figure 10. The penetration of clindamycin, piperacillin and cefoxitin into pancreatic juice. The concentrations in pancreatic juice are expressed as percentages of those in serum.

amylase content of the juice. The pancreatic duct catheter has also made possible studies on the effects of gastrointestinal hormones on pancreatic excretion as well as on the penetration of various drugs to the pancreatic gland.

References

1. Tydén G, Brattström C, Gunnarsson R, Lundgren G, Öst L, Östman J, Groth CG: Metabolic control 2 months to 4.5 years after pancreatic transplantation with special reference to the role of cyclosporin. Transplant Proc 19: 2294–2296, 1987b.
2. Schulak JA, Drevyanko TF: Experimental pancreas allograft rejection: correlation between histologic and functional rejection and the efficacy of antirejection therapy. Surgery 98: 330–336, 1985.
3. Lundgren G, Wilczek H, Klintmalm G, Tydén G, Groth CG: Procurement and preservation of human pancreatic grafts. Transplant Proc 16: 681–683, 1984.

254

4. Tydén G, Mellgren A, Brattström C, Öst L, Gunnarsson R, Östman J, Groth CG: Stockholm experience with 32 combined renal and segmental pancreatic transplantations. Transplant Proc 18: 1114–1117, 1986.

5. Tydén G, Brattström C, Häggmark A, Groth CG: Studies on the exocrine secretion of human segmental pancreatic grafts. Surg Gynecol & Obstet 164: 404–406, 1987.

6. Groth CG, Lundgren G, Klintmalm G, Gunnarsson R, Collste H, Wilczek H, Ringdén O, Östman J: Successful outcome of segmental human pancreatic transplantation with enteric exocrine diversion after modifications in technique. Lancet 4: 522–524, 1982.

7. Groth CG, Collste H, Lundgren G, Ringdén O, Thulin L, Wilczek H, Gunnarsson R, Östman J: Surgical techniques for pancreatic transplantation. A critical appraisal of methods used and a suggested new modification. Horm Metab Res 13: 37–41, 1983.

8. Lenhart FP, Unertl K, Jensen U, Landgraf R, Land W: Postoperative management after simultaneous segmental pancreas and kidney transplantation. Transplant Proc 16: 713–714, 1984.

9. Cortesini R, Alfani D: Clinical experience with kidney and pancreas transplantation in diabetic patients. Diab Nephropathy 4: 127–130, 1985.

10. Samnegård H, Tydén G, Thulin L: Effect of somatostatain on regional splanchnic blood flows in man. Angiographic studies. Acta Chir Scand, 500: 71–73, 1980.

11. Eféndic S, Lins PE, Uvnäs-Wallensten K: Extrahypophyseal effects of somatostatin. Ann Clin Res 10: 151–156, 1978.

12. Tydén G, Groth CG: Pancreatic graft failure due to pelvic examination. Lancet 1: 812, 1987.

13. Tydén G, Groth CG: Interaction between pancreas transplant and native pancreas. Lancet 1: 1514–1515, 1985.

14. Brattström C, Tydén G, Tollemar J, Bergström K, Groth CG: Serum amylase/isoamylase ratio as a determinant of pancreatic graft exocrine function. Transplant Proc 19: 3876–3879, 1987.

15. Severyn W, Olson L, Miller J, Kyriakides G, Rabinovitch A, Flaa C & Mintz D: Studies on the survival of simultaneous canine renal and segmental pancreatic allografts. Transplant 33: 606–612, 1982.

16. Largiadér F, Uhlschmid G, Binswanger U, Záruba K: Pancreas rejection in combined pancreaticoduodenal and renal allotransplantation in man. Transplant 19: 185–187, 1975.

17. Baumgartner D, Largiadér F, Uhlschmid G, Binswanger U: Rejection episodes in recipients of simultaneous pancreas and kidney transplants. Transplant Proc 15: 1130–1331, 1983.

18. Groth CG, Lundgren G, Arner P, Collste H, Hårdstedt C, Lewander R, Östman J: Rejection of isolated pancreatic allografts in patients with diabetes. Surg Gynecol & Obstet 143: 933–940, 1976.

19. Tydén G, Lundgren G, Gunnarsson R, Östman J, Groth CG: Laboratory findings during rejection of segmental pancreatic allografts. Transplant Proc 16: 715–717, 1984.

20. Sutherland DER, Goetz FC, Najarian JS: One hundred pancreas transplants at a single institution. Ann Surg 200: 414–440, 1984.

21. Gotoh M, Monden M, Motoki Y, Sakane O, Shima K, Okamura J: Early detection of rejection in the allografted pancreas. Transplant Proc 16: 781–782, 1984.

22. Sollinger HW, Cook K, Kamps D, Glass NR, Belzer FO: Clinical and experimental experience with pancreaticocystostomy for exocrine pancreatic drainage in pancreas transplantation. Transplant Proc 16: 749–751, 1984.

23. Gil-Vernet JM, Fernández-Cruz L, Andreu J, Figuerola D, Caralps A: Clinical experience with pancreatico-pyelostomy for exocrine pancreatic drainage and portal venous drainage in pancreas transplantation. Transplant Proc 17: 342–345, 1985.

24. Gil-Vernet JM, Fernández-Cruz L, Caralps A, Andreu J, Figuerola D: Whole organ and pancreaticoureterostomy in clinical pancreas transplantation. Transplant Proc 17: 2019–2020, 1985.

25. Prieto M, Sutherland DER, Goetz FC, Najarian JS: Pancreas transplant results according to technique of duct management: Bladder versus enteric drainage. Surgery (in press) 1987.

26. Munda R, First MR, Josse SN, Alexander JW: Experience with pancreatic allografts in renal transplant recipients. Transplant Proc 17: 353–354, 1985.

27. Brattström C, Tydén G, Lundgren G, Öst L, Groth CG: Studies of the exocrine secretion of segmental pancreatic grafts with special reference to the diagnosis of rejection and to the penetration of drugs into the pancreatic juice. Transplant Proc 19: 2294–2296, 1987.

28. Steiner E, Klima G, Niederwieser D, Köningsrainer A, Herold M, Margreiter R: Monitoring of the pancreatic allograft by analysis of exocrine secretion. Transplant Proc 19: 2336–2338, 1987.

29. Tydén G, Reinholt F, Brattström C, Lundgren G, Wilczek H, Bolinder J, Östman J, Groth CG: Diagnosis of rejection in recipients of pancreatic grafts with enteric exocrine diversion by monitoring pancreatic juice cytology and amylase secretion. Transplant Proc 19: 3892–3894, 1987.

30. Ried M, Gibbons S, Kwok D, Van Buren CT, Fleckner S, Kahan BD: Cyclosporin levels in human tissues of patients treated for one week to one year. Transplant Proc 15: 218–221, 1983.

31. Gunnarsson R, Klintmalm G, Lundgren G, Tydén G, Wilczek H, Östman J, Groth CG: Deterioration in glucose metabolism in pancreatic transplant recipients after conversion from azathioprine to cyclosporin. Transplant Proc 16: 709–710, 1984.

32. Brattström C, Malmborg A-S, Tydén G: Penetration of clindamycin, cefotixin and piperacillin into pancreatic juice in man. Surgery 103: 563–567, 1988.

33. Brattström C, Malmborg A-S, Tydén G: Penetration of ciprofloxacin and ofloxacin into human pancreatic juice. J Antimicro Chemother 22: 213–219, 1988.

13. Effect of pancreas transplantation on secondary complications of diabetes

D.E.R. SUTHERLAND

Introduction and statement of the problems

The major reason to perform pancreas transplantation is to ameliorate the secondary complications of diabetes affecting the eye, nerve, renal and other systems. The purpose is to prevent the appearance, halt the progression or induce regression of the lesions that lead to renal failure, impaired vision, and loss of limb function or viability.

Pancreas transplantation performed solely to obviate the need for insulin injection is usually not justified, because generalized immunosuppression is needed to prevent rejection and antirejection therapy has complications of its own. If pancreas transplantation does not influence the course of secondary complications, it should not be applied, at least in nonuremic, nonkidney transplant patients, until fully effective, nontoxic immunosuppression is available. In patients with end stage diabetic nephropathy, immunosuppression is obligatory, and a pancreas transplantation is justified to avoid the need for insulin, and the improvement in life style that ensues, even if other secondary complications are advanced. However, even in these patients, secondary complications may be favorably influenced, and the evidence that this is so is summarized in this chapter.

Almost all patients with end stage diabetic nephropathy also have lesions of retinopathy and neuropathy [1]. Correction of both diabetes and uremia may have a greater influence than the correction of uremia alone on the symptoms from and progression of the lesions. In addition, recurrence of diabetic nephropathy may be prevented in the newly transplanted kidney [2].

Nonuremic, nonkidney transplant recipients of a pancreas transplant should have secondary complications that are, or are progressing to a stage, more serious than the potential side effects of the antirejection therapy. Because of the uncertainty as to which patients are in this category, very few have been transplanted [3]. According to the Pancreas Transplant Registry, through May of 1987, 883 of 1,077 recipients of primary pancreas grafts had also received

257

J.M. Dubernard and D.E.R. Sutherland (eds.), International Handbook of Pancreas Transplantation, 257–289.
© *1989 by Kluwer Academic Publishers.*

primary kidney transplants (82%), 685 simultaneous (64%) and 183 before the pancreas transplant (17%). Only 194 recipients of primary pancreas transplants did not have end stage diabetic nephropathy (18%).

Thus, information on the effect of correction of the diabetic state alone on pre-existing secondary complications is limited, and there is need for more information in this group as well as the uremic recipients of both a pancreas and a kidney transplant. So much effort has been focused on establishing pancreas transplantation as a successful technique, it is only recently that information on secondary complications has begun to emerge. Studies on such patients, however, are extremely important. It is still an hypothesis that the complications of diabetes are secondary to disordered metabolism, and pancreas transplantation is the only technique that can establish a constant, euglycemic state in diabetic patients. All studies in nontransplant diabetic patients have had to rely on imperfect methods of exogenous insulin administration, and episodes of hyperglycemia (and of hypoglycemia) were inescapable [4].

There is considerable evidence from clinical and animal studies to support the hypothesis that retinopathy, neuropathy, nephropathy and the lesions in other systems are secondary to disordered metabolism [5, 6], justifying the application of pancreas transplantation at this time to selected nonuremic, nonkidney transplant patients with emerging or established secondary lesions of diabetes [7]. Retrospective and prospective observations in diabetic patients have tended to show that both the frequency and severity of the lesions affecting the eyes, nerves and kidneys are increased in in patients who tended to have 'poor' as opposed to 'good' control of diabetes [5, 8, 9]. There are, however, always exceptions, and some patients with what is considered 'good' control develop secondary complications, while some with 'poor' control do not [10]. It is apparent that factors others than the degree of hyperglycemia influence whether or not a patient will develop lesions, including genetic susceptibility and environmental influences. Even the patients with good control do not have perfect control, and in some animal models lesions of nephropathy and neuropathy have developed even when there has been a very mild diabetic state [11].

Animal studies fully support the concept that nephropathy, retinopathy and neuropathy are secondary to disordered metabolism, with lesions developing after induction of diabetes that resemble those in human diabetics [12]. Furthermore, the development of the lesions can be prevented by pancreas or islet transplants, and established or early lesions can be reversed [13–17]. These observations provide further impetus to the clinical application of pancreas transplantation for treatment of diabetes.

Studies of the effect of pancreas transplantation, or indeed of intensified insulin treatment [9], must be divided in those in which the goal is primary prevention or secondary intervention. In regard to pancreas transplantation, studies on primary prevention have not been tenable because of the risks of immunosuppression and the fact that not all diabetic patients develop secondary complications [1]. Thus, pancreas transplantation performed soon after the diagnosis of diabetes, or before there is any evidence of secondary lesion, would subject some patients not destined to develop secondary complications of diabetes to the risks of immunosuppression. For this reason, pancreas transplantation is almost always performed in patients who already have lesions. In this case, pancreas transplantation is a secondary intervention.

If reliable markers existed to predict which patients were at high risk to develop the lesions before their appearance, primary intervention could be performed, but at this time there are no such markers. Once the lesions appear, there are certain features which predict progression. For example, albuminuria predicts that diabetic nephropathy will progress to uremia, only the rate being uncertain [18].

Thus, in almost all cases pancreas transplantation is a secondary intervention. It is a primary intervention only in a special sense for combined pancreas and kidney transplant in uremic diabetics. A transplanted kidney is at risk to develop recurrence of diabetic nephropathy, and this process is prevented by a successful pancreas transplant [2]. Indeed, if pancreas transplantation did not prevent recurrence of disease in a transplanted kidney, all theories as to pathogenesis of diabetic nephropathy would be upset.

The major problem with the studies on the effect of pancreas transplantation on established complications is that secondary intervention may be too late. Thus, even if an effect is not seen, the hypothesis that the lesions are secondary to disordered metabolism may still be correct. The intervention may have been too late, at a time when the lesions are self-perpetuating independent of metabolic control. Ideally, recipients of pancreas transplant should be stratified into those with early or late lesions in order to discern a point where the lesions may pass from a stage of being reversable, or able to be stabilized, to a stage where they are irreversible or self-perpetuating independent of metabolic control.

Pancreas transplantation is, of course, not the only way to study new problems, and in recent years several trials of secondary intervention with intensified insulin treatment regimens have been conducted [9, 19–22]. Currently, an NIH sponsored Diabetes Control and Complications Trial of primary prevention, assessing both retinopathy and nephropathy, is ongoing [22, 23].

The secondary intervention trials with intensified insulin treatment regimens in patients with established retinopathy or proteinuria tend to support the conclusion that such intervention can retard the progression of retinopathy [9]. Urinary albumin excretion may also decline, but progression has also been noted in many patients, and even accerelated retinopathy has occurred during the first several months after intensified insulin treatment [9, 23]. The problem with the clinical studies is the inability to achieve perfect control, and it may take near perfect control for clear cut differences between groups of patients to be seen. For example, streptozotocin induced diabetic rats, in whom perfect metabolic control is restored by pancreas transplantation do not develop neuropathy, while rats giving islet transplantation by a technique that gives lese than perfect control develop lesions [17], and similar observations have been made on the development or reversal of nephropathy in the rat model [16].

Thus, pancreas transplantation is unique in its ability to induce a constant euglycemic insulin independent state, with no effort on the part of the patient, except to take immunosuppression! Theoretically, studies in pancreas transplant recipients should be superior to other studies to address the question of the effect of diabetic control on secondary complications.

However, the fact that the pancreas transplant recipients must take immunosuppression introduces another variable, the effect of immunosuppression itself on either abetting or ameliorating the lesions independent of the metabolic effect of the pancreas transplant. Thus, cyclosporin might exacerbate the renal dysfunction of diabetic nephropathy, either by directly accerelating diabetic lesions, or by introducing a separate effect on the kidney [24]. On the other hand, successful pancreas transplantation might induce an amelioration of the diabetic renal lesion, without an improvement in function because the beneficial effect of the transplant was masked by the detrimental effect of cyclosporin on the kidney [25]. Any study on function of native kidneys must take into account the effects of cyclosporin, not only on function but on morphology, and functional studies can be extremely difficult to interpret without morphology. Not only might creatinine clearance be decreased, even as the diabetic lesons are ameliorated, but albuminuria might be decreased by the effect of cyclosporin itself on the kidney rather than because the diabetes was corrected.

Illustrations can be given for the other immunosuppressants as well as for other lesions. For example, prednisone might affect muscle strength, compounding the evaluation of neuropathy. Prednisone and cyclosporin, both induce hypertension, and hypertension is also a known accelerator of diabetic lesions [25]. Thus a pancreas transplant simultaneous with correction of hypertension, either by a kidney transplant or by medication, followed by improvement of specific lesions, would leave uncertain which of the interventions were responsible, unless comparison is made to a control group undergoing only one of the interventions. On the other hand, if hypertension did not exist before a pancreas transplant, but was induced after the pancreas transplant because of the antirejection medications (cyclosporin, prednisone), and it was not treated, one might see a worsening of lesions that were otherwise destined to improve because of the correction of diabetes.

Even the technique of pancreas transplantation could influence the evaluation of secondary complications. For example, the use of urinary drainage technique for management of graft exocrine secretions will make a comparison of proteinuria before and after the transplant difficult to interpret. Most of the protein in the urine will be that excreted directly from the pancreas, unless one separates the proteins into the various components. Measurement of urinary albumin excretion may be valid, but total urine protein could not be used as an index of renal function.

Studies on secondary complications are also compounded as to whether they are conducted in the recipients of pancreas transplants alone or recipients of pancreas and kidney transplants, for several reasons. First, uremia itself influences the secondary complications, exacerbating both neuropathy and retinopathy [27, 28]. In recipients of simultaneous pancreas and kidney transplant, uremia and diabetes are corrected simultaneously, making it difficult to distinguish the contribution of one over another if amelioration of the secondary lesions of diabetes occurs. From the patient's standpoint, and from a practical standpoint, the differentiation may not be important, but from a study standpoint, when attempting to understand the pathogenesis of the lesions, it is extremely important. For purposes of a study, uremic diabetic patients ideally should be randomized to receive a kidney plus a pancreas transplant versus a kidney transplant alone, with the course of pre-existing complications involving the eyes and nerves compared in both groups of patients.

For uremic diabetic patients who receive a kidney transplant first followed later by a pancreas, lesions involving the eyes and nerves and other systems could be quantitated both pre- and post-kidney transplant, providing a new baseline after uremia has been corrected. The effect of correction of uremia can be discerned, followed by discernment of the effect of correction of diabetes. In addition, for the study of some lesions, the group of patients receiving sequential kidney and pancreas transplants can be pooled with the nonuremic, nonkidney transplant recipients of pancreas transplants alone, studying the course of lesions from a nonuremic baseline. The nonuremic, nonkidney transplant recipient of a pancreas transplant alone are more likely to have lesions in a relatively early stage, an advantage from a study standpoint, but to date the smallest proportion of pancreas transplant recipients have been in this group.

Study of the effect of pancreas transplants on the secondary complications of diabetes is further compounded by the problem of failed grafts. If patients were randomized to receive a pancreas transplant versus no transplant, the transplant patients would include those with failed grafts. On the other hand, in nonrandomized studies, the failed transplant patients can become the control group. If a pancreas transplant fails early, either from rejection or from technical problems, such patients could be followed long-term and the eye, kidney and nerve lesions in these patients compared to those who have had continuous graft function. This approach has been used in some studies, particularly in the Minnesota series [7, 29].

Review of the studies of the effect of pancreas transplantation on secondary complications is difficult and complex. There have been no randomized studies to date. There have been only a few studies in which patients with failed grafts have been used as controls. The range of severity of complications within a given organ system has also been extreme. Retinopathy and neuropathy are rarely mild in uremic recipients of kidney transplants, and in many the lesions may be too advanced to be helped. In the nonuremic, nonkidney transplant patients, the severity of the lesions ranges the entire spectrum, both within and between systems. For example, some patients have normal renal function with no proteinuria, while others have heavy proteinuria with creatinine clearance in the preuremic phase [30]. Some patients are referred for pancreas transplantation because of progressive retinopathy, which may itself by too advanced to help, but have renal lesions or neuropathic lesions ranging from absent to mild to moderately advanced, and the study of these lesions may be of greater value than the study of original lesions which prompted the patient or the patient's physician to seek pancreas transplantation.

In most studies, the mix with which lesions have occurred in individual patients has not been disclosed. How many patients were blind from retinopathy with normal kidneys, while how many patients with uremia (almost all have retinopathy) had nearly normal vision should be stated. In general, the studies have focused on one lesion, independent of the others.

In this chapter, the data that has been published on the course of nephropathy, retinopathy, neuropathy and macrovascular disease in pancreas transplant patients will be reviewed. Almost no patients have had a pancreas transplant as primary preventive therapy for the development of lesions in all systems, but in some patients intervention that was secondary for lesions of one system fortuitously allowed observations on the effect of pancreas transplantation as primary prevention of lesions in another system. An attempt will be made to discern difference in the effect on primary prevention and on secondary intervention. An attempt will also be made to sort out the effect of correction of diabetes alone versus correction of both uremia and diabetes, and an attempt will be made to discern the effect of immunosuppression on the course of the lesions.

There are no perfect studies, but the information that is available is useful in devising strategies for future studies in pancreas transplant patients. Since a constant euglycemic state is restored by pancreas transplantation [31, 32], the information from imperfect studies in these patients can complement the information from the intensified insulin treatment trials on the question of whether control of diabetes does influence the progression of secondary lesions [9]. The observations in the pancreas transplant patients will not fully answer the question of whether attempts at intensified insulin treatment are equally worthwhile, because even if a favorable effect is shown, the price of intensified insulin treatment (hypoglycemic episodes), could be too high, particularly if near perfect control is required to influence the lesions. Likewise, in the nonuremic, nonkidney transplant patients, the side effects of anti-rejection therapy must be balanced against the effect, if any, on secondary complications, to discern whether the benefits of pancreas transplantation sufficiently outweigh the risks of chronic immunosuppression given the current state-of-the-art. In the following sections, the information available on the course of secondary complications after pancreas transplantation are considered separately for each of the organs and tissues affected by diabetes.

Effect of pancreas transplantation on diabetic nephropathy

Diabetic nephropathy is the one secondary complication where information on primary prevention is available, all be it in a transplanted kidney, as opposed to secondary intervention for lesions in native kidneys. The effect of cyclosporin on renal function and morphology must be distinguished from the effect of diabetes (or lack thereof) in either situation. The effect of pancreas transplantation on recurrence of diabetic nephropathy in transplanted kidneys is considered first.

Recurrence of diabetic nephropathy on transplanted kidneys

The recurrence of diabetic nephropathy in normal kidneys transplanted to diabetic recipients has been amply documented. Mauer et al. described the appearance of light microscopic lesions with afferent and efferent arteriolar hyaliumosis [33], linear immunofluorescent staining for IgG and albumin on glomerular and tubular basement membranes [34], and, in electron microscopic quantitative studies, an increase in glomerular mesangial volume [35], the latter the one lesion correlating with renal function [36]. Glomerular basement membrane thickening also occurs after transplantation of the kidney into a diabetic recipient [35], but this lesion does not seem to relate to function [36]. Microscopic lesions are rarely seen before two years post-kidney transplant, and the frequency, rapidity, and severity by which the lesions recur is high variable [12], perhaps influenced by the same factors that are operative in their occurrence in native kidneys, depending on the degree of glycemic control posttransplant, hypertension, and the genetics of susceptibility of the donor of the transplanted kidney to damage from hyperglycemia, some being more susceptible than others [37].

Recurrence of diabetic nephropathy in transplanted kidney has largely been a morphological finding only. Very few diabetic recipients followed long-term have had kidneys fail for recurrence of disease. Microscopic lesions are readily apparent, but most graft failures have been from chronic rejection or death with functioning grafts [38]. However, a few patients followed greater than 10 years posttransplant have developed lesions to the extent that the grafts failed [39]. Recurrence of disease is a definite problem, and with the very large number of diabetic recipients of kidney transplants in recent years, it can be anticipated that graft failures from this process will increase in frequency [40].

No prospective studies have compared recurrence of disease in patients randomized to have or not have pancreas transplants. However, two groups (Stockholm and Minnesota) have examined kidney transplant biopsies obtained from diabetic renal allograft recipients at various times after pancreas transplantation, and have compared the results to posttransplant biopsies of kidney in diabetic patients who did receive pancreas transplants as well as to nondiabetic recipients of kidney transplants alone, with quantitative electron microscopic measurements of glomerular mesangial volume and basement membrane [41, 42]. It should also be noted that one of the very first pancreas transplant recipients to have long term function, a patient of Gliedman et al. [43], had a kidney transplant a few months after a pancreas transplant, and at death four and one-half years later there was no evidence of recurrence of diabetic nephropathy in the transplanted kidney. It is also relevant to note the case report of Abouna et al. [44] on the regression of light microscopic lesions of diabetic nephropathy in a kidney transplanted from a diabetic cadaver donor to a nondiabetic recipient, with reappearance of the lesions following subsequent development of de novo diabetes in the recipient [45]. The rapidity with which the lesions disappeared and reappeared is surprising, and unfortunately electron microscopic studies were not carried out in the case study of Abouna et al. [44, 45].

In another anecdote, light microscopic lesions of diabetic nephropathy present in a kidney several years after transplantation to a diabetic recipient have also been noted to regress after a subsequent successful pancreas transplant (Minnesota series, S.M. Mauer, et al., personal communication). Indeed, the patient with the longest functioning pancreas transplant is in this series [46]. This patient received a kidney transplant from her mother in 1973, at which time a biopsy of the transplanted kidney was normal. A repeat biopsy in 1978, at the time of a cadaveric pancreas transplant, showed an increase in the glomerular mesangium. A biopsy two years after successful pancreas transplantation showed a reduction in mesangium, and serial biopsies in this patient, now nearly 10 years postpancreas transplant, have continued to show a normal kidney.

Recent studies have used quantitative electron microscopic morphometric techniques [47] to assess diabetic nephropathy in transplanted kidneys. Those of Bohman et al. [41], from the Stockholm series, were in diabetic recipients of simultaneous pancreas and kidney transplants from the same donor. Those of Bilous et al. [42], from the University of Minnesota, were in recipients of pancreas transplants after a previous kidney transplant from a different donor.

In the study of Bohman et al. [41] 9 renal allograft biopsies were obtained from 5 patients between 13 and 50 months after combined kidney and segmental pancreas transplantation. The results were compared to 29 biopsies in 29 diabetic recipients of kidney transplants alone, and 2 biopsies in 4 nondiabetic kidney transplant recipients. Biopsies performed before 18 months after transplantation showed no detectable changes of diabetic nephropathy on light microscopic examination and in any recipients. In diabetic recipients of kidney transplants alone examined at more than two years posttransplant a wide range of lesions was observed, from slight hyaline arteriosclerosis to rather pronounced diabetic glomerular intravascular lesions. Some recipients were immunosuppressed with cyclosporin and some with azathioprine. When those with cyclosporin were excluded, a very weak correlation was found between the light microscopic diabetic nephropathy score and the patient's serum creatinine level at the time of the biopsy ($r = 0.68$) and there was also a weak correlation between the nephropathy score and blood pressure control ($r = 0.4$) but not with metabolic control, proteinuria or duration of diabetes at the time of transplantation.

Linear immunofluorescent staining for IgG along glomerular and tubular basement membranes was carried out in only three of the biopsies examined by Bohman et al. [41]; and all were positive (the earliest was 26 months posttransplant). In the report no distinction was made between the diabetic renal allograft recipients with or without pancreas transplants in regard to the immunofluorescent or light microscopic findings of the transplanted kidneys. Distinction between the pancreas and non-pancreas transplant recipients was made only on the electron microscopic studies of the renal transplant biopsies (Figure 1). In diabetic recipients of kidney transplants alone, basement membrane thickness was normal in biopsies obtained between 13 and 27 months after transplantation, and was above normal in all but one of the 12 biopsies obtained more than 27 months after transplantation. In contrast, biopsies in nondiabetic recipients and in diabetic recipients of combined kidney and pancreas transplants showed basement membrane thickness to be within the normal range in all cases. Serial biopsies taken at yearly intervals in two patients showed no changes in basement membrane thickness with time (Figure 1).

Bohman et al. [41] also measured the relative volume of the glomerular mesangium, and it ranged between 20% and 31% in 14 biopsies in patients

266

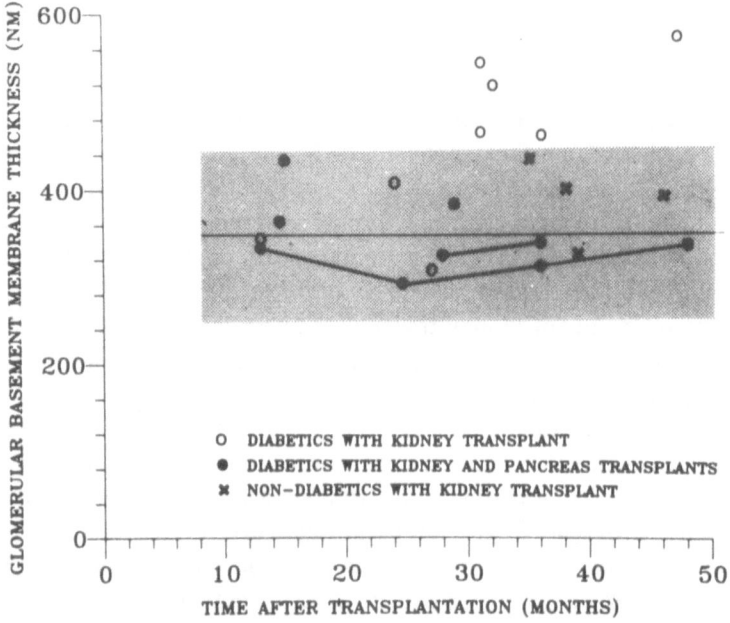

Figure 1. Glomerular basement membrane thickness determined by electron microscopic morphology in renal allograft biopsies from: diabetic recipients of renal grafts only (open circles); diabetic recipients with combined kidneys pancreas transplantation (closed circles); and non-diabetic recipients of renal allografts (x). Points connected by lines indicate serial biopsies in the same graft. Shaded area indicates mean ± 2 SD normal basement membrane thickness as reported by Steffes et al. [39]. From Huddinge Hospital, Stockholm, Bohman et al., Transpl Proc 19: 2290–2292, 1987 [41].

without a pancreas transplant, while it ranged between 7% and 26% in five biopsies in patients who had a pancreas transplant, close to the normal range according to measurements reported by Steffes et al. [47]. The studies by Bohman et al. [41] are fragmentary and not complete, but are consistent with the expectation that diabetic nephropathy should not recur in the kidneys transplanted to recipients of simultaneous pancreas transplants as long as the pancreas continues to function. Unfortunately, the studies are hampered by not having pretransplant biopsies and by not having their own normal controls, having to rely on comparison to other studies [47].

The results of the study of Bilous et al. [42] in the Minnesota recipients of a pancreas transplant after a previous kidney transplant are also consistent with the hypothesis that recurrence of diabetic nephropathy in a transplanted kidney should be prevented by a successful pancreas transplant. In the Minnesota studies, renal allograft biopsies were obtained at the time of the pancreas transplant and two years after a successful pancreas transplant in 9 insulin dependent Type I diabetic patients. Baseline biopsies showed mesangial volumes within normal limits and only minimal glomerular basement membrane thickening. At followup, no significant changes were detectable in mean glomerular volume (1.28 ± 0.20 whole versus $1.36 \pm 0.30 \times 10^6\,\mu m^3$); mesangial volume per glomerulus (0.20 ± 0.8 versus $0.25 \pm 0.10 \times 10^6\,\mu m^3$); filtration surface per glomerulus (0.15 ± 0.4 versus $0.16 \pm 0.04 \times 10^6\,\mu m^3$; or glomerular basement membrane (GBM) width (440 ± 58 versus 493 ± 123 nm). The rate of change of GBM thickening decreased in three or four patients in whom biopsies were performed at the time of and serially after the renal transplant and at the time of and serially after the pancreas transplant. The pancreas transplant recipients had significantly less mesangial expansion (0.24 ± 0.10 versus $0.55 \pm 0.21 \times 10^6$ mM; $p<.01$) than a group of 11 diabetic patients who were matched for age of onset of diabetes, duration of diabetes prior to kidney transplant, and survival of the renal allograft. Thus, in the Minnesota studies, recipients of pancreas transplants that functioned for >2 years had significantly less severe glomerularopathy in renal allografts than in those transplanted to diabetic recipients who did not receive a pancreas transplant.

The studies of Bohman et al. [41] and Bilous et al. [42] support the hypothesis that glycemic correction can prevent the development of nephropathy in renal allografts in man. Any other outcomes of course, would have been astounding and would have upset all theories as to the pathogenesis of diabetic nephropathy.

Effect of pancreas transplantation and of cyclosporin on diabetic nephropathy in native kidneys or nonuremic, nonkidney transplant recipients

The only information available in this category of recipients is from ongoing studies in the Minnesota series, and only a preliminary analysis has been reported [25]. The results are consistent with the hypothesis that restoration of the euglycemic state has a saluatory effect on the diabetic lesions, but at the expense of decreased renal function in patients on cyclosporin.

Bilous et al. [25], in an abstract, reported the results of quantitative morphometric measurements of glomerular volume, mesangial volume and basement membrane induced in biopsies in 7 patients before and greater than 2 years after successful pancreas transplantation (Table 1). In all patients, glycosylated hemaglobin was normal posttransplant ($7.6 \pm 0.9\%$ at the time of the biopsy versus $10.2 \pm 1.1\%$ pretransplant, $p<.01$). Comparing pre and post transplant biopsies, there was a significant reduction in mean glomerular volume (from 2.01 ± 0.80 to $1.5 \pm 0.83 \times 10^6\,\mu m^2$, $p<.01$) and in mesangial volume per glomerulus (0.65 ± 0.36 to $0.42 \pm 0.38 \times 10^6\,\mu m^2$, $p<.05$) mean glomerular basement thickness was not changed, compared to a control group of insulin treated diabetic patients with serial native kidney biopsies, the rate of basement thickness decreased significantly after transplantation. Five of the 7 pancreas transplant recipients also had a decrease in fractional urinary albumin excretion. However, there also was a decrease in creatinine clearance, from a mean of $90.2 \pm 21.3 \pm 23$ ml/minute to 60.0 ± 14.1 ml per minute (p<.01). The morphological changes are unlikely due to cyclosporin, but the functional changes most likely are. It is extremely unlikely that cyclosporin is responsible for the disappearance of diabetic lesions in the native kidneys, because cyclosporin cannot prevent their appearance in kidneys transplanted to diabetic recipients [35].

The question of the effect of cyclosporin on function in nonuremic, nonkidney transplant recipients has also been examined in some detail in the Minnesota series [7, 24]. De Francisco et al. [24], in a study of 33 cyclosporin treated recipients with functioning pancreas grafts followed for varying periods of time showed that there was an increase in serum creatinine and a decrease in creatinine clearance within a few weeks of the transplant, but the patients followed long-term remained stable (Table 2).

In a recent report on the total Minnesota experience with pancreas transplants alone in 111 nonuremic, nonkidney transplant recipients [7], the spectrum of diabetic lesions pretransplant was catalogued and effect of cyclosporin on function was re-examined. Pretransplant, the mean serum creatinine level was 1.02 ± 0.3 mg/dl, and were <1.0 in 46%, 1.1–1.5 in 43%, and 1.6–2.0 mg/dl in 10% of the recipients. The mean creatinine clearance pretransplant was 90.8 ± 27.7 ml/min and were 26–50 in 7%, 51–75 in 27%, 76–100 in 36% and >100 ml/min in 30%. Microscopic lesions of diabetic nephropathy pretransplant, as assessed by the proportion of glomerular volume that was mesangium (47), were classified as mild (<.2), moderate (.2 to .3) and severe (>.3) in 8%, 33% and 58% of the recipients, respectively (mean of $.28 \pm .12$).

In this series, 35 patients have had a pancreas transplant alone function for >1 year, and at the time of analysis 10 additional patients had grafts that were functioning for <1 year (7). All but 3 of the patients with grafts functioning for

Table 1. Glomerular structure and function in native kidneys after successful pancreas transplantation in seven nonuremic recipients followed more than two years in the clinical research center at the university of Minnesota[a].

Mean ± SD	Pretransplant	Posttransplant	p
Glomerular volume ($\times 10^6 \mu m^3$)	2.01 ± 0.80	1.51 ± 0.83	<0.01
Mesangial vol/glomerulus ($\times 10^6 \mu m^3$)	0.65 ± 0.36	0.42 ± 0.38	<0.05
GBM thickness (nm)	594 ± 106	605 ± 129	NS
Creatinine clearance (ml/min/1.73 m^2)	90 ± 21	60 ± 14	<0.05
HbA1 (%)	10.2 ± 1.1	7.6 ± 0.9	<0.01

[a] From Bilous et al., Diabetes 36: 43A, 1987 [25].

Table 2. Paired analysis of mean (± SD) serum creatinine and creatinine clearance before and at various timepoints after transplantation in 33 cyclosporin-treated nonkidney transplant diabetic recipients with functioning pancreas grafts studied in the clinical research center at the university of Minnesota[a].

	(n = 28) PreTx	2 Wks PostTx	Mean change%	(n = 13) PreTx	6 mos PostTx	Mean change%	(n = 11) PreTx	1–2 Yrs PostTx	Mean change%	(n = 4) PreTx	>2 Yr PostTx	Mean change%
Serum creatinine (mg/dl)	1.0 ± 0.3	1.5 ± 0.6	27 ± 19	1.0 ± 0.3	1.4 ± 0.4	27 ± 16	0.9 ± 0.3	1.4 ± 0.5	33 ± 18	0.9 ± 0.3	1.5 ± 0.2	36 ± 17
Creatinine clearance (ml/min)	90 ± 34	55 ± 23	− 39 ± 18	93 ± 21	62 ± 22	− 33 ± 25	94 ± 20	58 ± 13	− 37 ± 13	108 ± 17	63 ± 16	− 41 ± 13

P values for difference between levels before transplantation and those at all time points after transplantation: serum creatinine <0.05; creatinine clearance <0.02.

P values for difference between levels at 2 weeks versus those at six months, one-two years or more than two years after transplantation for both serum creatinine and creatinine clearance were > .2.

[a] From De Francisco et al., J Diab Compl 1: 128–131, 1987 [24].

>1 year were on cyclosporin. In these 3 patients, renal function remains stable in 2 (both with pretransplant creatinine clearance of >100), but had declined from 47 to <30 ml/minute over a 6 year period in the other. In patients on CsA, blood level targets were 200 ng/ml for the first six months, 159 ng/ml for second six months and 100 ng/ml thereafter. In 25 patients with long-term graft function, the mean serum creatinine pre and one year posttransplant were 1.10 ± 0.37 and 1.76 ± 0.5 mg/dl, and the corresponding creatinine clearance values were 94 ± 30 versus 52 ± 19 ml/min (p<.001). In 10 patients with measurements at baseline and values 1 and 2 years posttransplant, mean serum creatinine levels were 1.10 ± 0.44, 1.46 ± 0.28 and 1.38 ± 0.32 mg/dl. For most patients, after the initial increase in serum creatinine and decline of creatinine clearance values tended to remain stable, and the values in patients with multiple serial determinations during the first two years posttransplant are shown in Figure 2. However, two CsA treated patients with pretransplant creatinine clearances of 55 and 70 ml/min had exceptional courses, with declining creatinine clearance during the first year posttransplant to less than 25 ml/min; both underwent successful kidney transplants at that time [7].

Pancreas transplants in nonuremic, nonkidney transplant recipients treated with cyclosporin are performed under the assumption that cyclosporin nephrotoxicity will not be progressive, and that end stage renal disease will be prevented by cessation of progression of diabetic nephropathy. If the diabetic nephropathy is self-perpetuating, independent of metabolic control, or if cyclosporin nephrotoxicity becomes progressive, and the patients develop end stage renal disease in spite of a functioning pancreas graft, presumably they are no worse off than if they had not had a pancreas transplant without the pancreas transplant, progression of diabetic nephropathy to end stage renal disease was inevitable anyway. Both of the patients in the Minnesota series who required kidney transplants after a pancreas transplant [7], were in the category of having markers predicting progression of nephropathy [18].

Full assessment of the effect of pancreas transplantation on diabetic nephropathy awaits the development of an effective immunosuppressive therapy that does into include cyclosporin or other nephrotoxic agents. Meanwhile, most patients with early, but otherwise predictably progressive diabetic nephropathy, appear to have stable renal function after an initial decline, tolerate the cyclosporine necessary to prevent pancreas rejection, and have an improvement in microscopic lesions of their native kidneys [25].

Effect of pancreas transplantation on diabetic retinopathy

Assessment of the effect of pancreas transplantation on diabetic retinopathy is compounded by the fact that the treatment of retinal lesions is usually not

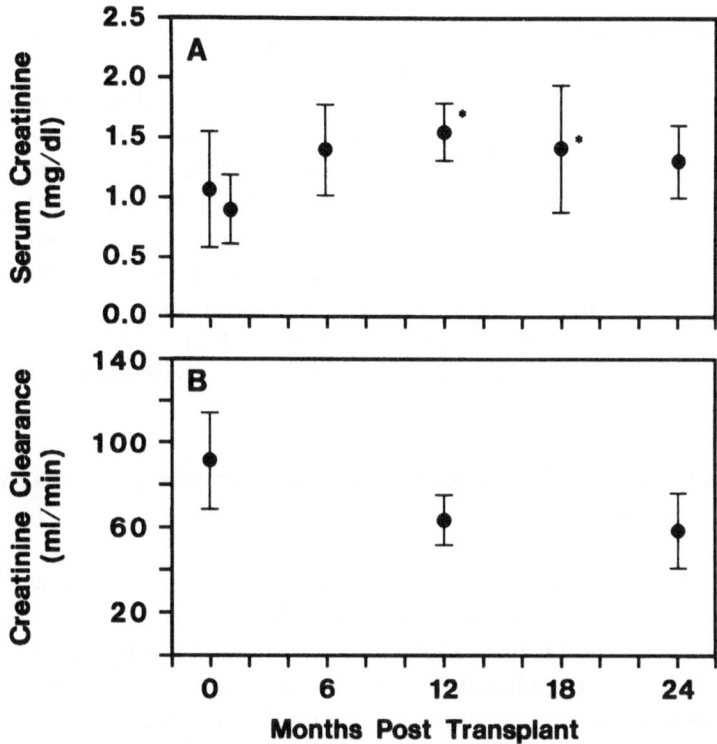

Figure 2. Mean (±) S.D. serum creatinine (A) and creatinine clearance (B) in 9 cyclosporin treated nonuremic, nonkidney recipients of pancreas transplants with functioning grafts in whom measurements were made at each of the indicated time points. There is approximately a 40% increase in serum creatinine and a 40% decrease in creatinine clearance after transplantation, but long-term the levels remain stable in most patients. From the University of Minnesota, Sutherland et al., Surgery 104: 453–464, 1988 [7].

withheld after a pancreas transplantation, when laser or other interventions are indicated. Assessment of visual acuity is also hampered because pre-existing aneurysms may bleed, even if no new ones are formed, and temporarily, if not permanently, impair vision even if retinopathy per se stabilizes. Vitrectomy and other interventions may also be performed.

In patients with end-stage diabetic nephropathy, the analyses are further compounded by the effect uremia may have on exacerbating the course of retinopathy [27]. Correction of uremia by kidney transplant alone has been reported to slow the progression of diabetic retinopathy in some recipients [48]. Thus, progression, or lack of progression of retinopathy in recipients of simultaneous pancreas and kidney transplants is difficult to interpret in the absence of a control group of recipients of kidney transplants alone. Unfortunately the studies to date in the recipients of simultaneous pancreas and kidney transplants have not included such controls [49]. Any apparent alter-

alterations on a course of retinopathy may be due to the correction of uremia as well as diabetes.

In recipients of pancreas transplants alone, however, either in nonuremic, nonkidney transplant recipients or in recipients of a previous kidney transplant, unexpected deviation from the baseline obtained at the time of the pancreas transplant will be due to correction of the diabetes itself [41].

The information available from studies of eyes in pancreas transplant recipients are reviewed in the following subsections, in the case of simultaneous transplants from the Munich experience [49], and in the case of pancreas transplants alone from the Minnesota experience [29]. In both studies, the analyses were compounded by the wide range of severity of retinopathy at the time of transplantation.

The influence of combined pancreatic and renal transplantation on advanced diabetic retinopathy

The University of Munich group has followed 34 patients with successful combined pancreas and kidney transplants, all with advanced diabetic retinopathy, but with useful vision in at least one eye [49]. Thirty patients had laser treatments before transplantation, with 35 eyes receiving pan retinal photocoagulation, and 19 incomplete or focal coagulation; only 13 eyes were not treated. Two of the patients were blind in one eye before transplantation. Two patients had also had a vitrectomy of an eye before transplantation. Fifty-six eyes had proliferative diabetic retinopathy, and 10 eyes had preproliferative changes. Features studied in these patients included objective and subjective visual acuity, frequency of vitreous hemorrhages, frequency of laser treatments, grading of retinopathy by fundus photographs, and fluorescene angiography.

Eight patients were followed for a mean of 21 months, but information on the range of followup is not given. Objectively, 20 patients (59%) had no alteration in visual function during the posttransplant observation, 13 (38%) had an improvement, and 1 (3%) had deterioration. Objectively, visual acuity after combined pancreatic and renal transplantation was improved by at least one line in at least one eye in 19 of 34 patients (56%), remained stable in 11 patients (32%) and deteriorated in 4 patients (12%). Deterioration occurred in one because of a cataract, in 2 because of vitreous hemorrhage, and in 1 because of a proliferative process with vitreous hemorrhage. The authors compare the changes in visual acuity to those reported by Khaluli et al. [50] in 45 diabetic recipients of renal transplants alone, in which 37 were stable (84%), 2 improved (4%), and 3 worsened (11%). Again the duration of followup is not given, and may not be comparable. In the Munich experience, the patients with graft function for more than 12 months had no further deterioration of visual acuity, but the number in this category is not given.

Pretransplant vitreous hemorrhage occurred in 46 of the 67 eyes at risk (69%). During the early posttransplant period, 16 of 67 eyes (24%) had vitreous hemorrhage, and of 43 eyes followed for more than 10 months, 5 had hemorrhage (12%). A life-table type analysis was not performed. In addition, there were no controls [49]. Thus, it is impossible to know whether the course after pancreas/kidney transplantation in the Munich cases [49] differed from what would be expected after kidney transplantation alone [48, 50]. The antecdoctal data presented by these authors is interpreted as showing an additional favorable effect of the pancreas transplant over and above that seen with kidney transplantation alone, but the conclusions are tentative and the investigators themselves remain cautious [49].

Course of diabetic retinopathy after pancreas transplant alone

The only studies reporting the course of diabetic retinopathy after pancreas transplant alone are from the University of Minnesota [7, 29]. In the studies comparisons were made between patients who had a successful pancreas transplant with grafts functioning for >1 year to a group of control patients in which the graft failed early. In patients followed through the Clinical Research Center at the University of Minnesota, detailed comparisons were made of visual acuity and retinopathy grade, using actuarial, life-table analytic techniques [29].

In the Clinical Research Center study [29], progression of diabetic retinopathy over at least the first year was similar between patients with failed and with functioning grafts, but after three years the group with functioning pancreas transplants had less deterioration than the control group. There were 22 patients with functioning pancreas transplants who were serially followed, with a mean hemaglobin A1C of 7.0% at the time of the followup analysis, and 16 in whom a transplant was unsuccessful (failed at less than 3 months), and in whom the mean glycosolyated hemaglobin at the time of followup exam was 12.0%. The patients included both nonuremic, nonkidney transplant recipients of pancreas grafts as well as those who had a pancreas transplant one year or more after a kidney transplant. Thus, all were nonuremic at baseline. Diabetic retinopathy and visual acuity was graded according to the criteria of the national diabetic retinopathy study group [51]. The time of progression to retinopathy or loss of visual acuity was assessed by life table analysis, thus compensating for differences in length of followup. Progression of retinopathy was defined as an increase in two or more grades in retinopathy in score, and a decrease in visual acuity was defined as a change of 2 or more lines on standard reading charts.

The results of pre and posttransplant metabolic profiles on oral glucose tolerance tests are shown for the patients with functioning grafts, all insulin-independent after the transplant, in Figure 3, and for the control group (those whose grafts failed early) in Figure 4. Recipients with functioning grafts were euglycemic and their mean glucose tolerance test results were within the normal range, while those with failed grafts were hyperglycemic with extreme glycemic excursions both pre and posttransplant.

At the baseline eye exam pretransplant, 10 of the 22 study group patients had irreversible blindness in one eye due to diabetic retinopathy. Therefore 34 eyes could be evaluated. During followup of patients with functioning grafts, visual acuity remained unchanged from baseline in 16 eyes (47%), improved by one or more lines of acuity in 6 eyes (18%) and decreased by one or more lines in 12 eyes (35%). In the patients with failed grafts (controls), visual acuity remained unchanged in 10 eyes (36%), improved in 3 (11%) and deteriorated in 15 (53%). A life table analysis in which time the loss of two or more lines of visual acuity was used as the end point did not show any significant differences between the two groups in the rate of deterioration in visual acuity [41].

In regard to retinopathy, at the pretransplant evaluation of the 34 eyes in the study group (functioning grafts), the severity of disease ranged from minimal nonproliferative (grade P0) to end stage proliferative retinopathy (Grade P13); the mean grade of retinopathy was P6.09. During followup, the condition of 19 of the 34 eyes (56%) remained unchanged, while 15 eyes (44%) progressed to a more advanced grade of retinopathy (Figure 5).

In the 28 control group eyes, the grade of retinopathy had similar distribution at the baseline examination (Grade 6.7). During followup, 13 eyes (46%) remained unchanged (46%), 14 (50%) progressed and 1 (4%) improved (Figure 6). Of the one improvement in the retinopathy score in the control group, there is an explanation. The eye had opaque media (grade P14) at baseline. The vitreous hemorrhage cleared spontaneously during followup, and the repeat exam showed quiescent retinopathy (grade P13).

A comparison of the groups for the end point of an increase by 2 or more grades in retinopathy score showed no significant differences during the first three years of followup (Figure 7). Thereafter the patients with nonfunctioning continue to deteriorate, while those with functioning grafts remained stable (Figure 7).

The relatively stable condition of the eyes with advanced retinopathy, observed in both the study and control groups, was presumably due in part to photocoagulation therapy. Before pancreas transplantation, all 15 eyes with advanced retinopathy in the study group received pan retinal photocoagulation and 14 of the 18 eyes with advanced disease in the control group had been treated. Among patients with mild retinopathy at baseline, 5 of 19 in the study group were treated while none of 10 eyes in the control group were so treated.

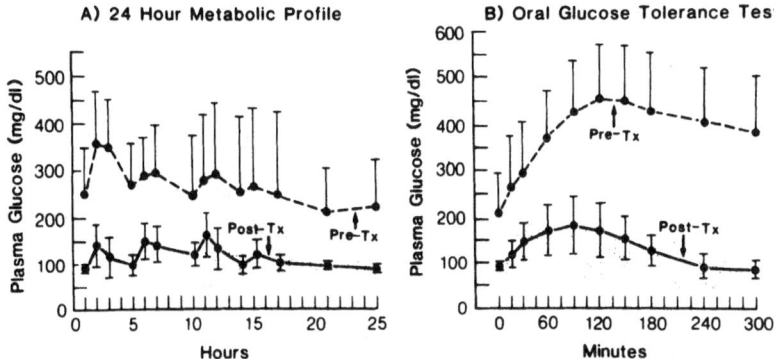

Figure 3. Mean plasma glucose concentrations (± S.D.) before and ≥1 year posttransplant during 24 hour metabolic profiles (A) and oral glucose tolerance tests (B) in 22 patients with functioning grafts assess for visual acuity and retinopathy grade at both time points (see Figure 5). None of the patients were taking insulin post-transplant, and mean glucose values were with the normal range (shaded area). From the University of Minnesota, Ramsay et al., New Engl J Med 318: 208, 1988 [29].

Although at first glance these results may seem disappointing, with no difference in progression of retinopathy between patients with functioning grafts versus those whose grafts failed, the observations are similar to those made intensified insulin treatment trials, where the natural history of the disease continues to occur during the first year after the intervention, while

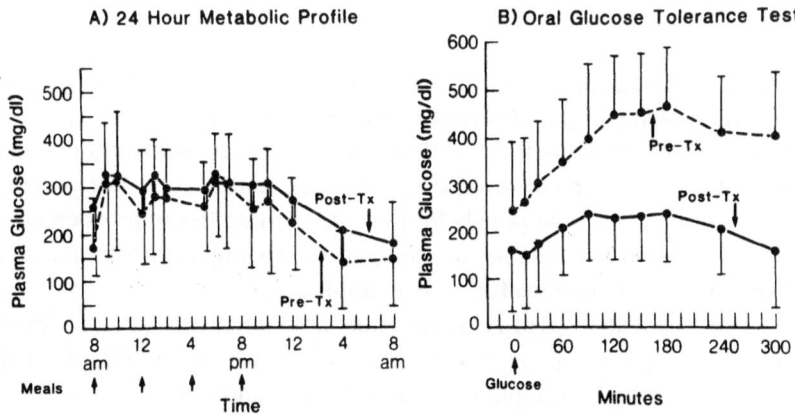

Figure 4. Mean plasma glucose concentrations (± S.D.) during 24 hour metabolic profiles (A) and oral glucose tolerance tests (B) before and at ≥1 year after transplantation in 16 patients whose grafts underwent early failure (≤3 months). At the time of the posttransplant study the patients were all on insulin and were hyperglycemic. These patients also had evaluation of visual acuity and retinopathy grade before and ≥1 year posttransplant (see Figure 6) and were compared to the patients in Figures 3 and 5. From Ramsay et al., New Engl J Med 318: 208, 1988 [29].

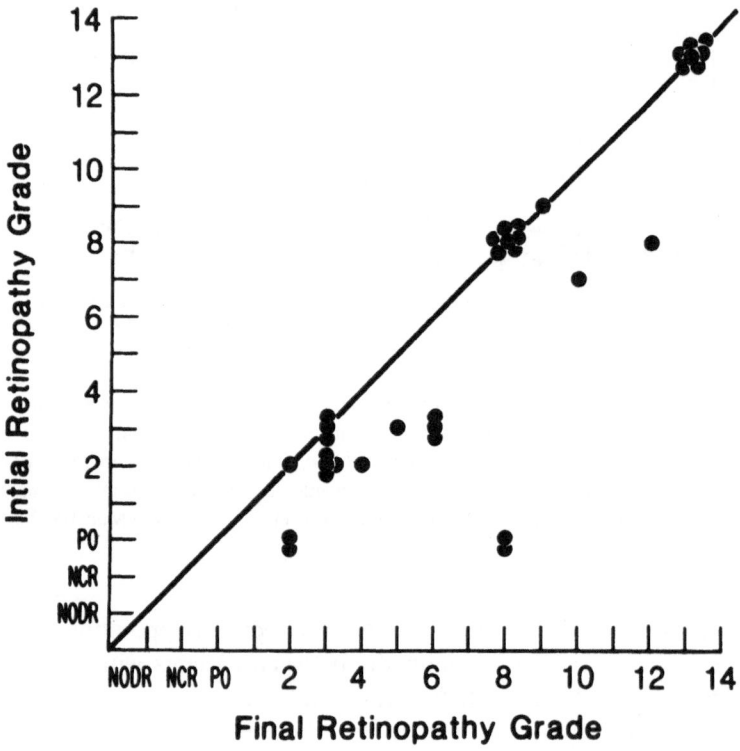

Figure 5. Retinopathy grades pretransplant versus one year posttransplant in 34 eyes of recipients with functioning pancreas transplants in the Minnesota series [29]. Compare to Figure 6.

late followup shows stability in the well controlled patients [9]. In addition, most of the patients in the Minnesota series had advanced retinopathy [29], and it may very well be that intervention with pancreas transplants must occur earlier in the course of the disease to influence retinopathy. For pancreas transplantation to be applied solely for this reason, immunosuppression needs to be improved, but the stability in retinopathy seen long-term after pancreas transplantation is an impetus for such an application.

In a more recent analysis of 111 nonuremic, nonkidney transplant recipients of pancreas transplants alone at the University of Minnesota [7], all of the recipients studied had retinopathy to some degree, and was relatively mild in only 36% of they eyes, (microaneurysms present, or nonproliferative retinopathy). Proliferative retinopathy or neovascularization was present in 36% (p 3–11), and involutional retinopathy (P12–13) in 28%. Following transplantation, 42 eyes in patients with functioning grafts were re-examined at one year. Retinopathy did not regress in any eyes, the grade remained the same in 23 (59%) and advanced by greater than one grade in 16 (41%). However, of 18

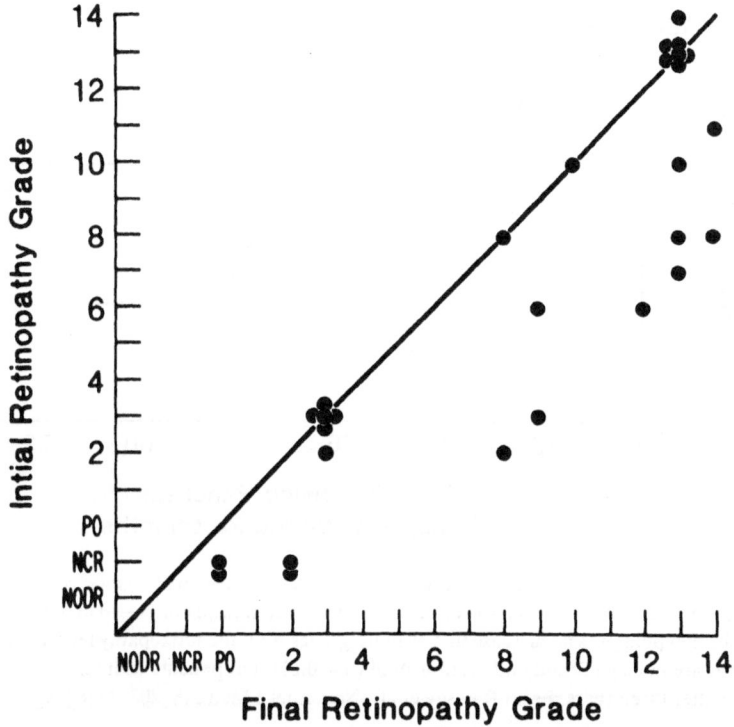

Figure 6. Retinopathy grades pretransplant, one year posttransplant in 28 eyes of Minnesota pancreas transplants recipients whose grafts failed early [29]. Compare to Figure 5.

eyes studied at two years, visual acuity was unchanged in 15 (83%) and retinopathy remained stable in 10 (55%).

These findings indicate that pancreas transplantation, as treatment of diabetic retinopathy should be applied early in the course of the disease. For such an approach to become routine, immunosuppression needs to be improved. If retinopathy is advanced, the natural history is not altered in the immediate post-transplant period, although long-term, retinopathy remains stable in pancreas transplant recipients.

Effect of pancreas transplantation on course of diabetic neuropathy

Assessment of the effect of pancreas transplantation on diabetic neuropathy is in some ways easier and in other ways more difficult than the assessment of the effect of nephropathy and retinopathy. Cyclosporin can have neuropathic effects. On the other hand, there are no interventions for neuropathy that treats the process as effectively as laser and other surgery treat diabetic

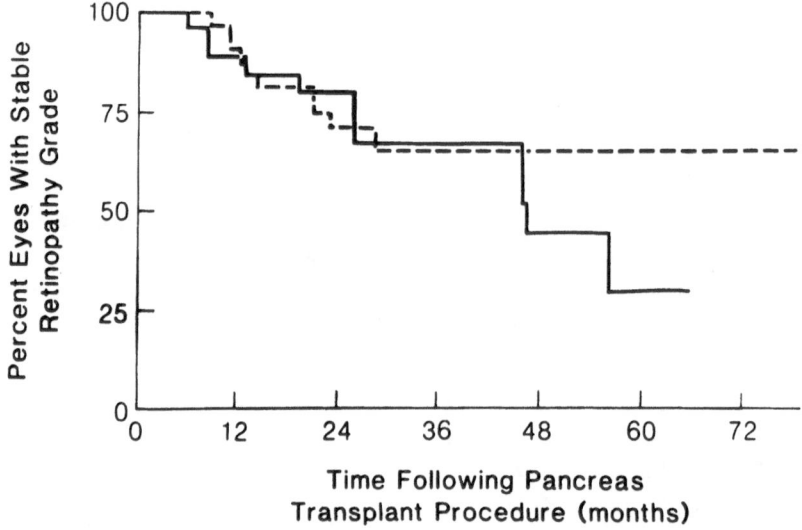

Figure 7. Percent of pancreas transplant recipients with stable retinopathy grade versus time for those with successful transplants (---) versus those with failed transplants (——) in the Minnesota series. The end point was an increase in 2 or more grades from the retinopathy level at baseline. The curves are not significantly different overall (p = 0.67), but patients with functioning grafts stabilized after three years. From Ramsay et al., New Engl J Med 318: 208, 1988 [29].

retinopathy. Hence, the natural history can be followed without the compounding effect of treatment.

As with retinopathy, uremia exacerbates diabetic neuropathy, and correction of uremia by kidney transplantation alone has been reported to favorably influence the course of neuropathy [27, 28]. Thus, reports of alterations in the course of neuropathy after combined kidney pancreas transplantation to not allow the investigator to distinguish between the effect of correction of uremia versus the correction of diabetes, unless a control group with kidney transplant alone is included.

Another problem with evaluation of neuropathy is need for multiple of tests to assess both autonomic and somatic motor and sensory function, some tests being objective and others subjective. In the following subsections, the results of objective studies are summarized, and are divided into those performed in uremic recipients of simultaneous kidney and pancreas transplants and those performed in nonuremic recipients of a pancreas transplant alone, either after or without a previous kidney transplant.

Course of neuropathy in uremic recipients of simultaneous kidney pancreas transplants

Solders et al. [52] compared the results of electroneurographic and autonomic function studies in diabetic recipients of combined kidney and pancreas versus recipients of kidney transplants alone in the Stockholm series. Thirteen patients with combined kidney and pancreas transplants that functioned for longer than 12 months were compared to 16 diabetic recipients of kidney transplants alone or of combined transplants in which the pancreas failed. Fifteen nondiabetic recipients of kidney transplants alone were included as another control group. The groups were comparable in regard to renal function, but the recipients of successful pancreas transplants had normal glycosolyated hemoglobin values (less than 8.5%). In the diabetic patients with functioning renal grafts only, glycosolyated hemoglobins were elevated (greater than 11.4%). Motor nerve conduction velocity (MCV) and distal latency (DL) in the median and peroneal nerves, and sensory nerve conduction velocity (SCV) and the amplitude of sensory nerve action potentials (SMAP) in the distal and proximal parts of the median and sural nerves were measured. The degree of polyneuropathy was expressed as an index, ENeG-IX, calculated by taking the deviation of each of the 10 variables from the normal age matched laboratory control and dividing the sum of these deviations by 10.

Autonomic neuropathy was assessed by measuring the beat to beat variation of the electrocardiogram (R-R variation) plotting against time. The R-R variation relative to the mean R-R interval was calculated during the one minute of deep breathing at six breaths per minute.

Before transplantation, all three groups had evidence of polyneuropathy, but it was much more advanced in the two diabetic groups (Figure 8). After transplantation nerve conduction improved slightly in all three groups, but did not return to normal in either of the diabetic patients, whether with a kidney transplant alone functioning or with both the kidney and the pancreas transplant functioning, the improvement was similar in both of these groups.

Similarly, the R-R variation during deep breathing was significantly lower in all diabetic patients on age match controls, while in the nondiabetic control group the mean value was within the normal limits. None of the three groups showed improvement in RR variation by two years after transplantation (Figure 9). Thus, at least in this study [52], an improvement in somatic neuropathy was noted following kidney transplant alone or a combined kidney and pancreas transplantation, similar to what has been described by other groups for diabetic recipients of kidney transplants alone [28].

In the other studies of kidney transplants alone, nerve conduction velocities have remained unchanged after successful kidney transplantation (usually low to start with), but evoked muscle action potential amplitudes have generally

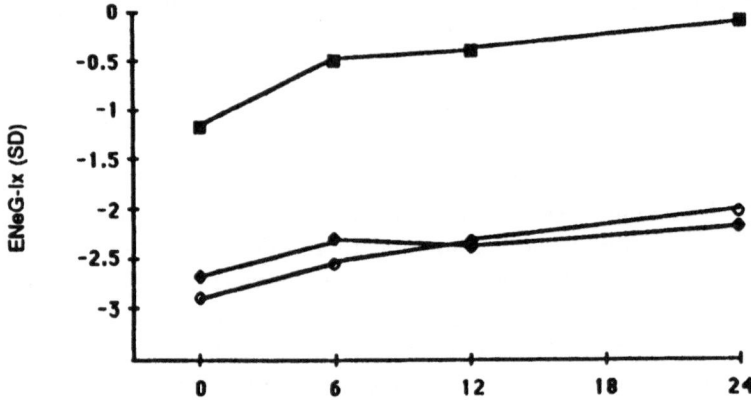

Figure 8. Electroneurographic polyneuropathy index (EneG-Ix) as a mean of the standard deviation from normal controls before and serially after transplantation in diabetic recipients of simultaneous pancreas and kidney transplants (solid diamonds) versus diabetic recipients kidney transplants alone (open diamonds), with comparison to nondiabetic recipients of kidney transplants (solid squares). A slight improvement occurs in all groups, but the diabetic recipients do not normalize during the two years of followup. From Huddinge Hospital, Stockholm, Solders et al., Lancet 2: 1232, 1987 [52].

continued to progressively decrease, even after uremia is corrected [28]. In the study by the Stockholm group, data on this specific parameter was not reported [52]. In a study by the Minnesota group, pancreas transplantation was found to halt the otherwise progressive decrease in muscle action potentials even though no improvement occurred in nerve conduction velocities [53].

The Munich group has reported the results of studies of diabetic autonomic neuropathy in 5 recipients of simultaneous pancreas and kidney transplants [54]. Unfortunately, no tests were conducted pre-transplantation, so a change from baseline could not be detected. Recipients of combined pancreas and renal transplants, as well as recipients of kidney transplants alone, had R-R intervals that were closer to normal than those of uremic nontransplanted patients, but there was no difference between the two transplant groups [54], an observation similar to that made in the Stockholm study [53].

Course of neuropathy in nonuremic recipients of pancreas transplants alone

The only reported studies on the course of diabetic polyneuropathy after pancreas transplant in non-uremic recipients are from the University of Minnesota [7, 53]. The first study was on a group of 34 patients examined at one year and 11 patients at two years after successful pancreas transplantation [53]. Of the 34 patients, 12 had received a functioning renal allograft more than one year previously, while the others were nonuremic, nonkidney transplant pa-

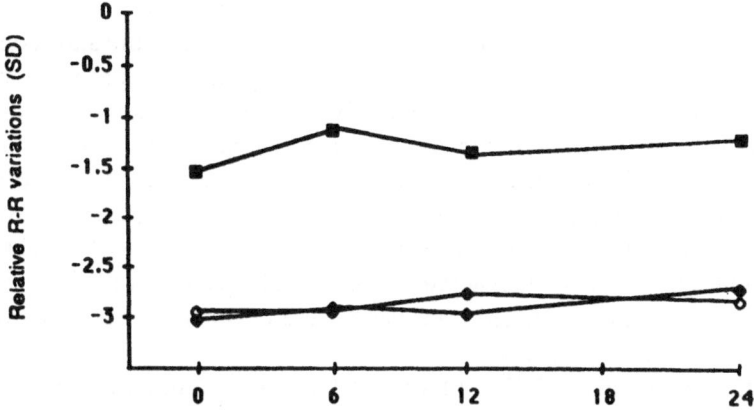

Figure 9. Mean relative R-R variation during deep breathing (in standard deviations) as an index of autonomic neuropathy before, and serially after transplantation in diabetic recipients of combined pancreas and kidney transplants (closed diamonds), versus diabetic recipients of a kidney transplant alone (open diamonds), with comparison to nondiabetic recipients of kidney transplants (solid squares). There are no changes after transplantation in any of the groups. From Huddinge Hospital, Stockholm, Solders et al., Lancet 2: 1232–1234, 1987 [52].

tients. The patients were pooled for the analysis. Before pancreas transplantation, clinical evidence of polyneuropathy was present in all patients. The motor nerve conduction velocities (NCV) were below normal and the mean amplitude of the evoked muscle action potentials (MAP) were in the low normal range. Following pancreas transplantation, abnormalities of muscle strength and tendon reflexes did not progress (Table 3). Motor nerve conduction velocities improved slightly, and MAP amplitudes were essentially unchanged (Table 4). The fact that MAP amplitudes do not decline is thought to be significant, since other studies of the natural history of diabetic neuropathy has shown inexorbably progression deterioration in this parameter [27, 28].

In another Minnesota study [7], only those who were nonuremic and did not receive a kidney transplant were included, and two groups were compared,

Table 3. Tendon reflexes in diabetic patients studied in the clinical research center at the university of minnesota before, and 1 and 2 years after successful pancreas transplantation[a].

Reflexes[b]	Pre-transplant	Year 1	Year 2
Biceps	-1.4 ± 0.3 (65%)	-1.0 ± 0.3 (43%)	-1.7 ± 0.5 (86%)
Quadriceps	-1.6 ± 0.3 (69%)	-1.3 ± 0.3 (65%)	-2.3 ± 0.6 (86%)
Achilles	-2.9 ± 0.3 (88%)	-2.5 ± 0.3 (86%)	-2.9 ± 0.6 (86%)

[a] From van der Vliet et al., Transplantation 45: 368, 1988.
[b] The values are mean scores ± standard errors. The percentages of patients with decreased reflexes are shown in parenthesis.

those who had continuous graft function for more than one year, and those who had early failure of pancreas grafts. All were studied before and at one or two years posttransplant. Comparisons pre- and post-transplant were made for motor nerve conduction velocities (NCV) in both upper and lower extremity curves; evoked compound muscle action potential (MAP) with the values in the upper and lower extremities averaged to facilitate comparisons; sensory nerve action potential (NAP) amplitudes and distal latency (LAT) measured orthodromically in the median and sural nerves; and sensory (NCV) evaluated antidromically in the median nerve. At one year 24 patients with functioning transplants and 14 with failed transplants were examined, and at two years there were 11 in each group.

Pretransplant, mean NCV, MAP and NAP amplitudes were below the lower limits of normal, and mean distal latencies were prolonged (Table 5). In patients with functioning grafts, motor and median sensory nerve conduction parameters showed a mild improvement and serial NAP amplitudes were only slightly decreased. In the patients with failed transplants, the mean NCV did not change, the MAP amplitudes decreased significantly, and sensory MAP amplitudes tended to decrease with time. The changes from pretransplant were significant within each group, and the differences at one and two years between successfully and unsuccessfully transplanted patients were also significant. There was a tendency for a higher percentage of patients with function-

Table 4. Motor nerve conduction parameters in pancreas transplant recipients with functioning grafts studied in the clinical research center at the university of Minnesota[a].

Nerve		Pretransplant (n = 34)	Year 1	Pretransplant (n = 11)	Year 2
Ulnar	NCV m/s	47.1 ± 0.8	48.8 ± 0.9[b]	46.4 ± 1.7	48.1 ± 1.4
	DL ms	2.8 ± 0.1	2.8 ± 0.1	2.9 ± 0.3	2.8 ± 0.2
	MAP mV	8.8 ± 0.6	9.0 ± 0.6	9.4 ± 1.2	9.7 ± 1.2
Median	NCV m/s	48.4 ± 0.6	49.8 ± 0.7[c]	48.7 ± 1.3	37.6 ± 1.4
	DL ms	3.9 ± 0.1	3.8 ± 0.1	3.7 ± 0.2	4.1 ± 0.2
	MAP mV	7.4 ± 0.6	7.5 ± 0.6	7.8 ± 0.9	2.7 ± 0.6
Peroneal	NCV m/s	37.2 ± 1.1	38.3 ± 1.1[c]	37.3 ± 1.4	37.6 ± 1.4
	DL ms	4.8 ± 0.2	4.4 ± 0.2	5.0 ± 0.4	4.1 ± 0.2
	MAP mV	2.6 ± 0.4	2.6 ± 0.4	2.9 ± 0.9	2.7 ± 0.6
Tibial	NCV m/s	36.6 ± 0.9	38.2 ± 1.0[d]	36.1 ± 1.1	38.6 ± 1.8
	DL ms	6.0 ± 0.2	5.7 ± 0.2	6.1 ± 0.3	5.7 ± 0.3
	MAP mV	3.3 ± 0.4	3.6 ± 0.4	4.0 ± 0.8	3.5 ± 0.8

[a] From van der Vliet et al., Transplantation 45: 368, 1988.
[b] p<0.005.
[c] p<0.01.
[d] p<0.05.

Table 5. Comparison of motor and sensory nerve conduction pre and posttransplant in nonuremic diabetic patients with functioning and nonfunctioning pancreas grafts studied in the clinical research center at the university of Minnesota[a].

Mean ± S.D.	Parameter	One year followup				Two year followup			
		Functioning pancreas [24]		Failed transplants [14]		Functioning pancreas [11]		Failed transplants [11]	
		Pre	Post	Pre	Post	Pre	Post	Pre	Post
Motor									
U.E.	NCV m/s	48.4 ± 4.8[a]	50.7 ± 5.3[a]	48.0 ± 4.4	48.9 ± 4.9	50.4 ± 3.6	51.6 ± 2.3[d]	48.1 ± 4.0	47.5 ± 3.6[d]
	MAP mV	8.3 ± 2.3	8.7 ± 2.2[b]	8.9 ± 2.6[c]	7.1 ± 2.3[b, c]	9.1 ± 2.1	9.6 ± 1.9[e]	8.6 ± 1.6	7.4 ± 1.4[e]
L.E.	NCV m/s	38.0 ± 5.1	39.5 ± 5.6	37.1 ± 5.0	36.6 ± 4.5	37.7 ± 5.3	38.6 ± 5.9	37.3 ± 5.3	36.5 ± 5.2
	MAP mV	3.0 ± 2.1	3.2 ± 2.3	3.2 ± 2.3	1.9 ± 1.8	2.6 ± 1.9	3.1 ± 2.1	2.5 ± 1.9[f]	1.8 ± 1.9[f]
Sensory									
Median	NCV m/s	51.2 ± 3.6[g]	53.5 ± 3.3[g]	50.1 ± 4.4	51.5 ± 2.0	51.1 ± 3.3	53.8 ± 2.7[j]	50.1 ± 5.2	49.7 ± 3.1[j]
	LAT ms	3.7 ± 0.7[h]	3.4 ± 0.5[h]	3.5 ± 0.5	3.4 ± 0.4	3.6 ± 0.7[k]	3.3 ± 0.4[k]	3.6 ± 0.5	3.6 ± 0.7
	NAP uV	7.9 ± 5.2[i]	10.2 ± 5.2[i]	10.4 ± 9.3	7.4 ± 5.6	8.8 ± 5.6[l]	12.3 ± 5.1[l]	9.0 ± 6.2	8.7 ± 6.7
Sural	LAT ms	3.5 ± 0.2	3.5 ± 0.3	3.2 ± 0.3	3.5 ± 0.3	3.5 ± 0.6	3.5 ± 0.7	3.3 ± 0.8	3.5 ± 0.7
	NAP uV	3.3 ± 3.8	3.0 ± 3.9	1.8 ± 3.4	1.5 ± 2.7	2.9 ± 3.7	1.2 ± 2.7	1.5 ± 1.9	1.2 ± 3.0

[a] From Sutherland et al., Surgery 104: 453, 1988 [7].

[b, g, i, j, k, l] p<0.05.

[a, c, d, e, f, h] p<0.0005.

U.E. = Upper extremity nerves; L.E. = Lower extremity nerves; NCV = Nerve Conduction Velocity; MAP = Muscle Action Potential; NAP = Nerve Action Potential; LAT = Nerve Distal Latency.

ing grafts to have an increase and a lower percentage to have a decrease in motor NCV in the amplitudes of the evoked MAPs at one and two years posttransplant when compared to patients with failed transplants (Table 6). The differences between the two groups was significant for MAP in the upper extremities at one year and the lower extremities at two years. Again, the fact that the evoked muscle action potentials stabilized in the successfully transplanted patients is significant, when compared to the inevitable progression in nontransplant patients.

Detailed studies of autonomic neuropathy in non-uremic recipients of pancreas transplants alone have yet to be reported. It appears, however, that pancreas transplantation has a beneficial effect on at least somatic neuropathy.

Course of diabetic microangiopathy after simultaneous pancreas and kidney transplantation

There are no reported studies on the course of macroangiopathy after pancreas transplantation, but the Munich group has applied some innovative techniques to the study of microangiopathy in recipients of simultaneous pancreas and kidney transplants [55]. Again, the studies suffer from the fact that the patients have both uremia and diabetes corrected simultaneously, a

Table 6. Percent of nonuremic recipients of pancreas transplants studied in the clinical research center at the university of Minnesota with changes[a] in motor nerve conduction velocities (NCV) and amplitude of evoked muscle action potentials (MAP) from baseline in the upper (U) and lower (L) extremities (E) for those with[b] versus those without[c] functioning (FXN) grafts[d].

	MAP-UE		MAP-LE		NCV-UE		NCV-LE	
	Fxn	No Fxn	Fxn	No Fxn	Fxn	No Fxn	Fxn	No Fxn
One year F/U								
Increase	39	7	52	29	74	50	70	50
No change	26	14	9	14	13	21	4	21
Decrease	35	79	39	57	13	29	26	29
P value	0.03		0.37		0.32		0.23	
Two Year F/U								
Increase	55	18	55	0	45	36	45	30
No change	27	18	9	9	27	9	18	30
Decrease	18	64	36	91	27	54	36	40
P value	0.08		0.01		0.35		0.72	

[a] By 1 mV for MAP and 1 m/sec for NCV.
[b] Functioning at 1 year (n = 24) and at 2 years (n = 11).
[c] Nonfunctioning at 1 year (n = 14) and at 2 years (n = 11).
[d] From Sutherland et al., Surgery 104: 453, 1988 [7].

group with failed grafts is not included and neither is a group of patients kidney transplants alone included. In addition, the followup time was extremely variable, and the analyses were done in a static fashion rather than by life table. Nevertheless, the results indicate that diabetic microangiopathy is improved after transplantation. In 18 patients, measurements were made pre and 12 months after transplantation, transcutaneous oxygen tension was measured, telethermography of the lower extremity was performed, and blood flow in the skin was measured using the laser speckle method. Thermoregulatory behavior improved. In 5 patients, studied by the laser speckle method, blood flow to the skin was normalized. The tcpO$_2$ values rose from 44 ± 2 to 64 ± 4 mm mercury (p<.01), and reoxygenization time decreased from 205 ± 8 to 113 ± 3 seconds, the latter within the normal range (Figure 10).

The relative contribution of correction of diabetes versus correction of uremia remains to be discerned, and the tests need to be applied in uremic diabetic recipients of kidney transplants alone as well as the nonuremic recipients of pancreas transplants alone. Nevertheless, the results suggest that diabetic microangiopathy is favorably influenced by the pancreas and kidney transplant.

Summary and conclusions

Normalization of plasma glucose levels by pancreas transplantation generally has a favorable effect on the course of pre-existing secondary complications in diabetic recipients. In recipients of simultaneous kidney transplants, it is not always possible to distinguish between the contribution made by correcting uremia, versus that of correcting diabetes.

Successful pancreas transplantation prevents recurrence of diabetic nephropathy in a transplanted kidney, as expected [2, 41, 42]. Pancreas transplantation alone, in nonuremic, nonkidney transplant recipients, can induce regression of microscopic lesions of diabetic nephropathy [25], but in cyclosporin treated recipients renal function may deteriorate because of cyclosporin [24]. In most cyclosporin treated recipients of pancreas transplants alone, after in initial decline renal function remains stable [7]. The evidence to date would suggest that in most patients with early nephropathy, progression to renal failure will be avoided by a successful pancreas transplant. However, there is a critical level of function, below which cyclosporin cannot be tolerated, and advanced nephropathy may be self perpetuating independent of metabolic control. Patients in whom pancreas transplantation would appropriately be applied to prevent progression of diabetic nephropathy would be those with albuminuria, a creatinine clearance of >70 ml/min, and mild to moderately advanced lesions on renal biopsy.

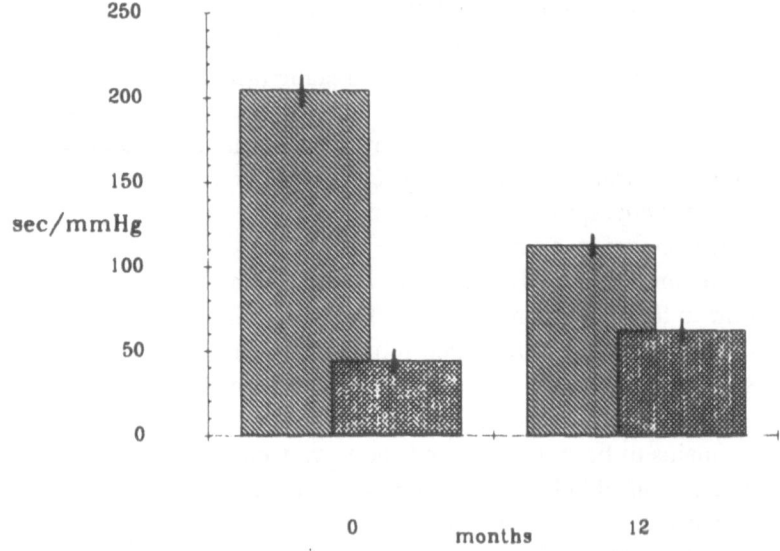

250

200

150

sec/mmHg

100

50

0

0   months   12

Figure 10. Characteristics of reoxygenation time and tcp0₂ values before and at 12 months after kidney and pancreas transplantation in uremic diabetic recipients. There was a significant (p<.01) decrease in reoxygenation times (hatched bars to the left at each of the time points), and tcp0₂ values increased (stippled bars to the right of each of the time points). From the University of Munich, Abendroth et al., Transpl Proc 20: 874, 1988 [55].

In regard to retinopathy, almost all recipients with pancreas transplants who have been studied had advanced retinopathy [29, 49]. In recipients of pancreas transplants alone, the course of retinopathy at least during the first year post-transplant is similar for those with and without graft function [29]. Long-term, the patients with functioning grafts appear to be more stable than those without.

In regard to neuropathy, the somatic motor and sensory systems appears to be favorably influenced by a functioning pancreas transplant, with stabilization of evoked muscle amplitude potentials, and improvement in some other parameters [7, 52, 53]. The autonomic system remains stable [52, 54].

Ideally, pancreas transplantation should be applied early in order to favorably influence the course of secondary complications. Because current immunosuppressive regimens have side effects, most recipients selected for pancreas transplantation have had advanced lesions and most have been uremic recipients of combined kidney and pancreas transplants. The non-uremic recipients of pancreas transplants alone have also usually had complications that were rapidly progressing. Nevertheless, the data from the few patients in whom pancreas transplantation has been applied at an early stage shows that a beneficial effect on diabetic lesions is achieved, but application before there is any evidence of secondary complications awaits the development of more effective and less toxic immunosuppressive regimens. When such a regimen is available, prospective studies can be designed that can address the questions currently so difficult to study in trials employing intensified exogenous insulin treatment regimens [9, 23]. Meanwhile, pancreas transplantation can be performed in patients with secondary complications of diabetes that are, or are progressing to a stage, more serious than the side effects of current immunosuppressive treatment. Patients will benefit and investigators can expand and extend the studies described in this chapter.

References

1. Harris MI, Entmacher P: Mortality from diseases. In: Harris MI, Hamman RF (eds) Diabetes in America; Ch 29, pp 1–48. U.S. Dept Health and Human Services, NIH pub No 85–1468, 1985.
2. Bohman SO, Tyden G, Wilczek H et al.: Prevention of kidney grafts diabetic nephropathy by pancreas transplantation in man. Diabetes 34: 306–307, 1985.
3. Sutherland DER, Moudry KC: Pancreas transplant registry. Pancreas 2: 473–488, 1987.
4. Ungar RH: Meticulous control of diabetes: benefits, risks and precautions. Diabetes 31: 479, 1982.
5. Tchoubroutsky G: Relation of diabetic control to development of microvascular applications. Diabetologia 15: 143–152, 1978.
6. Sutherland DER: Pancreas and islet transplantation: I. Experimental studies. Diabetologia 20: 161, 1981.
7. Sutherland DER, Kendall DM, Moudry KC et al.: Pancreas transplantation in nonuremic, Type I diabetic recipients. Surgery 104: 453–464, 1988.
8. Pirart J: Diabetes mellitus and a degenerative complications: a prospective study of 4400 patients observed between 1947 and 1973. Diabetes Care 1: 168–263, 1978.
9. Hanssen AF, Dohl-Jorgenson K, Lauritzen T et al.: Diabetic control of microvascular applications: the near normal glycemic experience. Diabetologia 29: 677–84, 1986.
10. Raskin P, Rosenstock J: Blood glucose control and diabetic complications. Ann Intern Med 105: 254–63, 1986.
11. Orloff MJ, Mitsito N et al.: Prevention, stabilization and reversal of the metabolic disorders and secondary complications of diabetes by pancreas transplantation. Transpl Proc 20: 868–873, 1988.
12. Mauer SM, Steffes MW, Brown DM: Studies of diabetic nephropathy in animals and man. Diabetes 25: 850–857, 1976.
13. Mauer SM, Steffes MW, Sutherland DER, Najarian JS, Michael AF, Brown DM: Studies of the rate of regression of the glomerular lesions in diabetic rats treated with pancreatic islet transplantation. Diabetes 24: 280–285, 1975.
14. Steffes MW, Brown DM, Basgen JM, Mauer SM: Amelioration of mesangial volume and surface alterations following islet transplantation in diabetic rats. Diabetes 29: 509–515, 1980.
15. Orloff MJ, Yamanaki N, Greenleaf G et al: Reversal of mesangial enlargements in rats with long standing diabetes by whole pancreas transplantation. Diabetes 35: 347–355, 1986.
16. Orloff MJ, Mitsito C, Mitsito O et al.: Comparison of controlling nephropathy and metabolic disorders of diabetes whole pancreas and pancreatic islet transplantation in rats. Ann Surg 206: 324–334, 1987.
17. Orloff MJ et al.: Effect of pancreas transplantation on diabetic somatic neuropathy in rats. Surgery 104: 437–444, 1988.

288

18. Viberti GC, Hill RD, Jarre HRJ et al: Microalbuminuria as a predictor of clinical diabetic nephropathy. Lancet 1: 1430–1432, 1982.
19. Kroc colaborative study group. Blood glucose control and the evolution of diabetic retinopathy and albuminuria: a preliminary report of a multicenter trial. New Engl J Med 311: 365–72, 1984.
20. Lauritzen T, Frost-Larsen K, Larsen HW, Deckert T, Steno study group: Two year experience with continuous subcutaneous insulin infusion in relationship to retinopathy and neuropathy. Diabetes 34 (Suppl 4): 74–79, 1985.
21. Feldt-Rasmussen B, Mathiesen ER, Deckert T: Effect of two year strict metabolic control on progression of incipient nephropathy in insulin dependent diabetes. Lancet 2: 1300–1304, 1986.
22. Diabetes control and complications trial research group. Design of methodologic considerations for the feasibility phase. Diabetes 35: 530–45, 1986.
23. DCCT research group. Are continuing studies in metabolic control of microvascular complications in insulin dependent diabetes mellitus justified? New Engl J Med 318: 246–250, 1988.
24. De Franciso AM, Mauer SM, Steffes MW, Goetz FC, Najarian JS, Sutherland DER: The effect of cyclosporin on native renal function in non-uremic diabetic recipients of pancreas transplants. J Diab Compl 1: 128–131, 1988.
25. Bilous RW, Mauer SM, Sutherland DER et al.: Glomerular structural function following treatment of pancreas transplantation for insulin dependent diabetes mellitus. Diabetes 36: 43A, 1987.
26. Christensen CK, Mogensen CE: Antihypertensive treatment: Long-term reversal of progression of albuminuria in incipient diabetic nephropathy. A longitudinal study of renal function. J Diab Compl 1: 45–52, 1987.
27. Friedman EA, L'Esperance FA (eds) Diabetic renal retinal syndrome 3. Grune and Stratton Inc, Orlando, 1986.
28. van der Vliet JA, Navarro X, Kennedy WR et al.: Diabetic polyneuropathy and renal transplantation. Transpl Proc 19: 3597–3599, 1987.
29. Ramsay RC, Goetz FC, Sutherland DER: Progression of diabetic retinopathy after pancreas transplantation for insulin dependent diabetes mellitus. New Engl J Med 318: 208–214, 1988.
30. Steffes MW, Mauer SM, Sutherland DER, Goetz FC: Renal function and pancreas transplantation. Transpl Proc 18: 1778–1779, 1986.
31. Sutherland DER, Najarian JS, Greenberg BZ, Senske BJ, Anderson GE, Francis RS, Goetz FC: Vascularized segmental transplantation on the pancreas in insulin-dependent patients: hormonal and metabolic effects of an endocrine graft. Ann Int Med 95: 537–541, 1981.
32. Pozza G, Traeger J, Dubernard JM, Serdri A, Pontiroli AE, Boss E, Malik MC, Ruitton A, Blanc N: Endocrine responses of type I (insulin-dependent) diabetic patients following successful pancreas transplantation. Diabetologia 24: 244, 1983.
33. Mauer SM, Barbosa J, Vernier RL: Development of vascular diabetic lesions in kidneys transplanted in the diabetic patients with diabetes mellitus. New Engl J Med 295: 916–920, 1976.
34. Mauer SM, Miller K, Goetz FC: Contact of renal extracellular membranes in kidney transplantation in patients with diabetes mellitus. Diabetes 25: 709–712, 1976.
35. Mauer SM, Steffes MW, Conet J et al.: Development of lesions in the glomerular basement membrane and mesangium after transplantation of the normal kidneys to diabetic patients. Diabetes 32: 948–952, 1983.
36. Mauer SM, Steffes MW, Ellis EN et al.: Structural functional relations in diabetic nephropathy. J Clin Invest 74: 1143–1155, 1984.
37. Mauer SM, Goetz FC, McHugh LE, Sutherland DER, Barbosa J, Najarian JS, Steffes MW: Long-term study of normal kidneys transplanted into patients with type I diabetes. Diabetes 38: 516–523, 1989.

38. Sutherland DER, Bentley FR, Mauer SM, Menth L, Nylander W, Goetz FC, Barbosa J, Ascher NL, Simmons RL, Najarian JS: A report of 26 diabetic renal allograft recipients alive with functioning grafts at 10 or more years after primary transplantation. Diabetic nephropathy 3: 39–43, 1984.
39. Bentley FR, Sutherland DER, Mauer SM, Nylander W, Ascher N, Menth L, Simmons RL, Najarian JS: The status of diabetic renal allograft recipients who survive for 10 or more years after transplantation. Transpl Proc 17: 1573–1576, 1985.
40. Sutherland DER, Fryd DS, Payne WD, Ascher N, Simmons RL, Najarian JS: Kidney transplantation in diabetic patients. Transpl Proc 19: 90–94, 1987.
41. Bohman SO, Wilczek H, Tyden G et al: Recurrent diabetic nephropathy in renal transplants placed in diabetic patients in the protective effect of simultaneous pancreatic transplantation. Transpl Proc 19: 2290–2292, 1987.
42. Bilous RW, Mauer SM, Sutherland DER et al: Effects of pancreas transplantation on kidney allograft glomerular structure in Type I diabetes. Diabetes 38 (Suppl. 1): 262, 1989.
43. Gliedman ML, Tellis VA, Soberman R et al.: Long-term effects on pancreatic transplant function in patients with advanced juvenile onset diabetes. Diabetes Care 1: 1–9, 1978.
44. Abouna GM, Al-Adnani MSA, Kremer GM et al.: Reversal of diabetic nephropathy in human category kidneys after transplantation of nondiabetic recipients. Lancet 2: 1274–1276, 1983.
45. Abouna GM, Al-Adnani MSA, Kremer MSA et al: Fate of transplanted kidneys with diabetic nephropathy. Lancet 1: 622–623, 1986.
46. Sutherland, DER, Goetz FC, Najarian JS: One hundred pancreas transplants at a single institution. Ann Surg 200: 414–440, 1984.
47. Steffes MW, Barbosa J, Basgen JM et al.: Quantitative glomerular morphology of the human kidney. Lab Invest 49: 82–86, 1983.
48. Ramsay RC, Cantrill HC, Knobloch WH, Goetz FC, Sutherland DER, Najarian JS: Visual parameters in diabetic patients following renal transplantation. Diabetic nephropathy 2(1): 26–29, 1983.
49. Ulbig N, Kampick A, Landgraf R et al.: The influence of combined pancreatic and renal transplantation on advanced diabetic retinopathy. Transpl Proc 19: 3554–3556, 1987.
50. Khauli RB, Novick AC, Steinmuller DR, Buszta C, Nakamoto S, Vidt DG, Magnusson M, Schreiber M: Comparison of renal transplantation and dialysis in rehabilitation of diabetic end-stage renal disease patients. Urology 27: 521–525, 1986.
51. Diabetic nephropathy study group. Manual of operations, Baltimore diabetic retinopathy coordinating center, 1972.
52. Solders G, Wilczek H, Gunnarson R et al.: Effects of combined pancreatic and renal transplantation on diabetic neuropathy: A two year followup study. Lancet 2: 1232–1235, 1987.
53. van der Vliet JA, Navarro X, Kennedy WR et al.: The effect of pancreas transplantation on diabetic polyneuropathy. Transplantation 45: 368–379, 1988.
54. Schafferhans E, Heidbreder E, Land W et al.: Diabetic autonomic neuropathy after simultaneous pancreas and kidney transplantation. Transpl Proc 18: 1136–1138, 1986.
55. Abendroth P, Landgarf R, Milner WD et al.: Course of diabetic microangiopathy after simultaneous pancreas and kidney transplantation. Transpl Proc 20: 874–875, 1988.

14. Pancreas transplant registry

D.E.R. SUTHERLAND and K.C. MOUDRY

Introduction

The International Pancreas Transplant Registry was founded at a meeting held in Lyon, France in 1980 [1]. The American College of Surgeons/National Institutes of Health (ACS/NIH) Organ Transplant Registry forwarded information on 57 on pancreas transplants performed between 1966 and June 30, 1977 to the new Registry [2]. Information on all other cases known to have been performed up to that time, including 3 from 1976 (one primary and two secondary) that had not been reported to the ACS/NIH Registry, were also incorporated into the new Registry [1]. Since 1980, all institutions performing pancreas transplants have submitted data to the Registry on age of the recipient, duration of diabetes, HLA typing, technique of transplantation, duration of preservation, type of immunosuppressive regimen, duration of graft function, and causes of graft failure.

Several previous reports of the Registry have been made [3–9]. The results of analyses performed on May 11, 1987 are summarized in this chapter.

Number of pancreas transplant and method of analysis

Between December 17, 1966, to April 24, 1987, 1157 pancreas transplants in 1077 diabetic patients were reported by 93 institutions to the registry, 570 in 44 North American, 572 in 40 European, and 15 in 9 other located institutions. The number has increased nearly every year, and 892 (76%) of the cases have been performed since 1982 (Figure 1).

Cadavers donated 1093 (1017 primary, 65 secondary and 10 tertiary and 1 quaternary) and living relatives 64 pancreas grafts (60 primary, 4 secondary). Primary kidney transplants were performed simultaneous with the pancreas in 685, before the pancreas in 183, and after the pancreas in 14, while 194 (28%) patients were recipients of primary pancreas transplants alone.

291

J.M. Dubernard and D.E.R. Sutherland (eds.), International Handbook of Pancreas Transplantation, 291–322.
© *1989 by Kluwer Academic Publishers.*

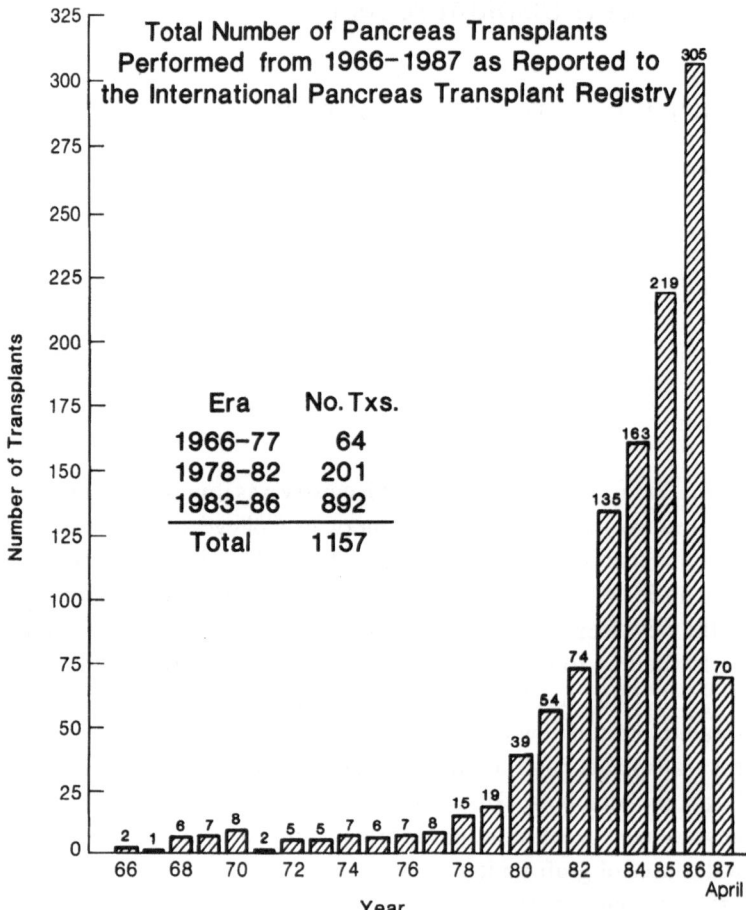

Figure 1. Number of pancreas transplants as reported to the Registry by year between December 17, 1966 and April 24, 1987.

Graft and patient survival rates were calculated by the actuarial technique, and the significance of differences between groups were determined by the Gehan test [11]. The significance of differences in incidences of events were determined by the Chi-square test. Pancreas grafts were counted as functioning only if the recipients were reported to be insulin independent.

Because the results of pancreas transplantation significantly improved with time, separate analyses of outcome according to multiple variables were performed for the 892 cases (438 in 36 North America and 445 in 35 European institutions) reported to the Registry since January 1, 1983 (855 cadaver, 37 related donor transplants; 829 primary, 53 secondary, 9 tertiary grafts and 1 quaternary).

Overall results for all 1966–87 cases

The fate and functional classifications of all pancreas transplant cases according to length of followup at the time of the analysis are given in Table 1. Of 271 grafts known to have functioned for ≥1 year, 196 are currently listed as functioning (the longest for >8 years). Of 341 technically successful grafts listed as having failed because of rejection or undetermined causes, 58 (17%) did so at >1 year posttransplant. Of 300 grafts counted as technical failures, all but 4 were lost at >1 year. Of 121 recipients of technically successful transplants who died with functioning grafts, 14 (12%) did so at >1 year posttransplant. Of the 762 total grafts that failed, 75 (10%) did so at >1 year posttransplant. The 395 grafts currently listed as functioning were all transplanted after 1977. Of the 857 technically successful cases, the 1 year actuarial insulin-independent rate in the recipients was 51%.

The patient and graft functional survival rates at one year for all 1966–87 cases in the Registry were 76% and 37%. Overall patient and graft survival rates were similar (p>0.15) for North America and European recipients (Table 2).

The analysis, of 1966–87 cases also showed that recipient and graft survival rates after retransplantation (n = 80) were not significantly different (p>0.15) than those after primary transplantation (n = 1077), 33% versus 38% for graft function and 84% versus 75% for patient survival at one year.

The overall graft and recipient survival rates have significantly improved with time (Figure 2). Graft survival rates for 1985–87 cases (n = 594) were

Table 1. Classification of all 1966–87 pancreas transplant cases in the registry.

Classification	Years post-transplant			Totals (%)
	<1	1–4	4–8	
No failed	687	69	6	762 (66%)
Tech failures[a]	296	4	–	300 (26%)
Lost function (TS)[b]	282	53	6	341 (29%)
DWFG[c]	108	13	–	121 (11%)
No functioning[d]	199	176	20	395 (34%)[e]
Total	886	245	26	1157 (100%)

[a] Technical failures are grafts that failed within 3 days of the transplant or at anytime from local infection primary thrombosis, bleeding or other such problems leading to graft removal.
[b] Technically successful (TS) grafts that were ultimately rejected or failed for unknown reasons.
[c] DWFG = Recipient died with functioning graft.
[d] Insulin-independent.
[e] By technique, [No. functioning]/[No. cases] is 125/418 duct injected, 116/360 enteric drained, 151/328 urinary drained 1/21 open duct intraperitoneal, and 0/20 ligated.

47% at one year, significantly higher (p<0.04) than the 38% one year function rate for 1983–84 cases (n = 248). The recipient survival rates were significantly higher for 1985–87 than for 1983–84 cases (p<0.03).

Kidney graft functional survival rates in pancreas transplant recipients also significantly improved with time (Figure 3A). In the overall analysis of 1966–87 cases, kidney graft survival rates were significantly higher in recipients of a subsequent pancreas transplant than in those receiving a pancreas simultaneous with a kidney (Figure 3B). This difference is expected, since the former group consists of selected patients who survived after a kidney to receive a pancreas transplant.

Results of 1983–87 cases

The classification of 1983–87 pancreas transplant cases according to multiple variables are summarized in Table 3. Of 892 pancreas transplants in this era,

Table 2. Pancreas transplant registry data for North America and Europe.

Category	North America		Europe	
	No Txs	1 Yr survival Graft (patient)	No Txs	1 Yr survival Graft (patient)
All cases 1966–87	570	35% (78%)	572	40% (76%)
1983–87 Cases	438	41% (81%)	445	47% (81%)
Technique				
Duct injected	29	19%[a]	248	50%[a]
Enteric drainage	140	42%	137	47%
Urinary drainage	261	45%	53	34%
Type				
Whole	316	42%	44	39%
Segmental	122	39%	401	48%
Preservation				
<6 hours	238	42%[b]	316	52%[b, c, d]
6–12 hours	76	33%	94	46%[c, e]
>12 hours	62	41%[f]	6	0%[d, e, f]
Immunosuppression				
Aza + CsA ± Pred	310	44%[g]	241	58%[g, h, i]
CsA ± Pred	99	37%	166	39%[h]
Aza + Pred	27	30%	31	29%[i]
Assoc. with kidney				
Px + kidney	192	46%	371	51%[j]
Px after kidney	139	38%	24	36%
Px alone	101	38%[k]	50	21%[j, k]

Comparisons with p values <0.05 indicated by lettered superscripts.

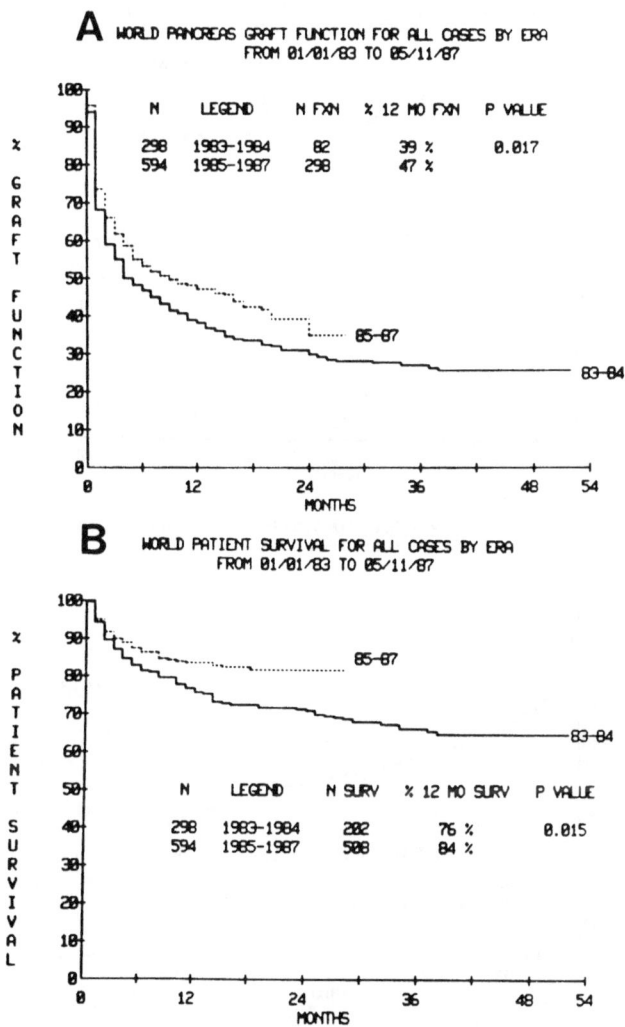

Figure 2. (A) Graft and (B) patient survival rates for all pancreas transplant cases reported to the Registry by era of transplantation through April 24, 1987.

380 were listed as functioning (181 at >1 year) and 512 as failed (47 at >1 year). Of the failed grafts, 285 were technically successful: of these, 218 lost function because of rejection of undetermined causes (37 at >1 year posttransplant), while 67 maintained an insulin-independent state until the recipients died with functioning grafts (7 at >1 year posttransplant).

The 1 year graft and patient survival rates for all 892 cases reported to the Registry for the 1983–87 era were 43% and 81% respectively (Figure 4). The

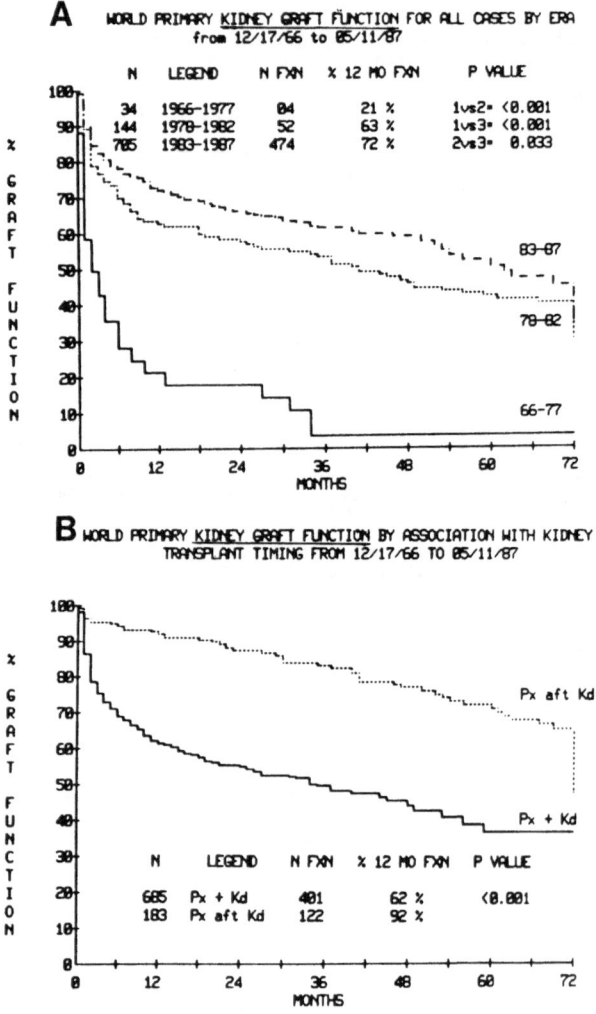

Figure 3. Renal graft functional survival rates in pancreas transplant recipients with end-stage diabetic nephropathy according to (A) era of transplantation and (B) according to timing of kidney transplant relative to the pancreas for all cases since 1966.

graft and patient survival rates in this era were not significantly different for North American and European cases (Table 2).

Primary transplantation versus retransplantation

The pancreas graft survival rate after retransplantation was not significantly different than after primary transplantation for 1983–87 cases (Figure 4A). The recipient survival rate after retransplantation however, was significantly higher that after retransplantation than after primary transplantations (Figure 4B).

Table 3. Transplant results in various categories for 1983–87 cases.

Variable	No cases	No tech failures (%)	No failed (all causes)[a] Time posttransplant		No ins-independent Time posttransplant		1 Yr[b] Fxn rate
			<1 year	>1 year	<1 year	>1 year	
Technique							
Duct-injection	281	57 (20%)	142	72	53	64	46%
Enteric drainage	281	87 (31%)	152	18	37	74	43%
Intestine	253	74 (29%)	134	15	36	68	44%
Stomach	28	13 (46%)	18	3	1	6	35%
Urinary drainage	315	74 (23%)	158	7	108	42	42%
Bladder	297	70 (24%)	143	6	108	40	44%
Ureter	18	4 (22%)	15	1	0	2	17%
Method							
Whole	364	92 (25%)	195	12	97	60	41%
Segmental	528	135 (26%)	270	35	102	121	45%
Spleen included							
Yes	27	7 (26%)	17	1	5	4	32%
No	865	220 (25%)	448	46	194	177	44%
Preservation time							
<6 hours	557	125 (22%)	272	33	126	126	47%
6–12 hours	173	57 (33%)	102	9	28	34	39%
>12 hours	69	21 (30%)	40	3	18	8	35%
Immunosuppression							
CSA ± Pred	268	79 (29%)	164	7	15	66	38%
CSA + AZA ± Pred	555	132 (24%)	253	18	182	102	49%
AZA + Pred	69	15 (25%)	41	5	–	13	31%
HLA mismatches (A, B, DR)							
≤3	163	50 (31%)	92	7	39	56	49%
≥4	361	105 (29%)	210	22	72	61	39%
No data	317	69 (22%)	159	18	78	64	47%
Association c Kid Tx							
Px + Kid	565	133 (24%)	265	30	142	128	49%
Px after Kid	165	50 (30%)	98	8	30	29	37%
Px alone	156	44 (28%)	100	9	24	23	32%
Px before Kid	5	– –	1	–	3	1	50%
Retransplants							
Yes	63	17 (27%)	36	3	13	11	40%
No	829	210 (25%)	424	44	186	170	49%
Total	892	227 (25%)[c]	465 + = 512	47	199 + = 380	181	43%

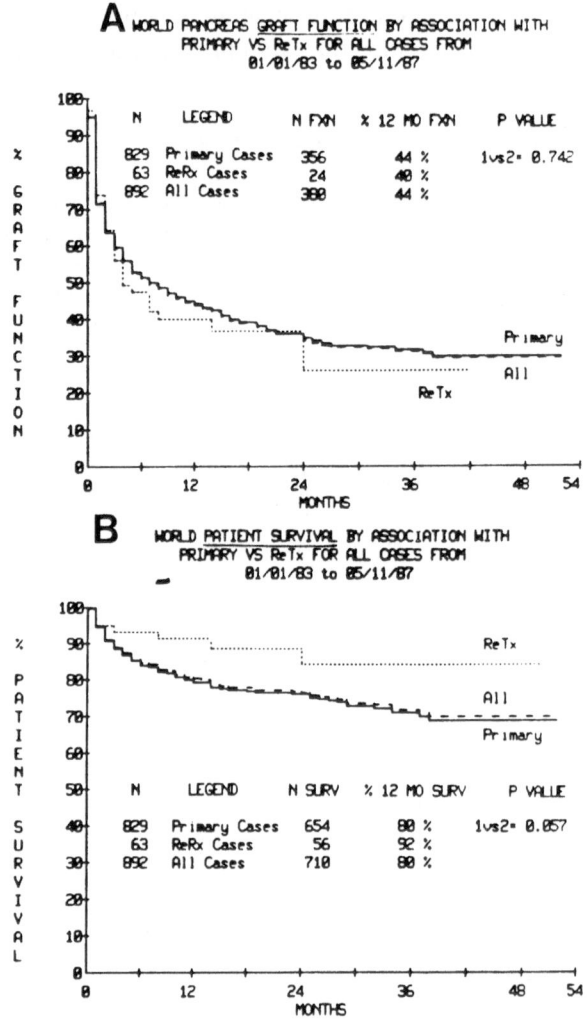

Figure 4. (A) Graft and (B) recipient survival rates for primary transplant, retransplant and all pancreas transplant cases reported to the Registry from January 1, 1983 to April 24, 1987.

Results according to duct management technique

The number of transplants and the graft survival rates at one year in each of the most common duct management categories are given in Table 2. The graft survival rates were almost identical for duct injection, bladder drainage and intestinal drainage, and in each of these categories were significantly higher compared to ureter drainage. The results with stomach drainage were not significantly different than in the other categories.

The incidence of technical failures according to method of pancreas duct management, are given in Table 3. The technical failure rates were significantly different ($p<0.05$) for duct injection versus intestine and stomach and for bladder versus stomach drainage.

The 227 technical failures included 112 thromboses (12.5% incidence) and, 56 infection (6.2% incidence). The number (and incidence) of failures from thrombosis, infection and other technical causes in the various categories were 33 (12%), 15 (5%) and 9 (3%) for duct injection; 33 (13%), 21 (8%) and 20 (8%) for intestinal drainage; 8 (28%), 4 (14%) and 1 (4%) for stomach drainage; 35 (12%), 13 (4%) and 22 (7%) for bladder drainage; and 0 (0%), 1 (6%) and 3 (23%) for ureter drainage.

Figure 5A depicts the graft survival rate curves for recipients in the three most common duct management categories, polymer injection, enteric drainage (intestine and stomach combined) and urinary drainage (bladder and ureter combined). The results according to method of duct management are shown separately for North American and European cases in Table 2. Urinary drainage was the most common method of duct management in North America (71% of cases), while polymer injection was most common in Europe (56% of cases). Enteric drainage was the second most common method on both continents. Within each continent, the graft survival rates were highest for the duct management method used most frequently and lowest for that used least frequently, but the differences were not significant ($p>0.25$). Between continents, the graft survival rate was significantly ($p = 0.047$) higher for duct injection in Europe than in North America; just the opposite was the case for urinary drainage, but the difference was not significant ($p = 0.674$).

Polymer injection, enteric drainage, and urinary drainage heve their own variations, and the graft survival curves for each variation are shown in Figure 6. In the duct injection category, the functional survival rates are significantly higher for neoprene and prolamine than for polyisoprene injected grafts (Figure 6A). Grafts survival rates were not significantly different for recipients of grafts injected immediately versus those in which duct injection was delayed until after a period of external drainage of the exocrine secretions via a catheter (Figure 6B). In the enteric drainage category, the functional survival rate was insignificantly higher for grafts anastomosed to the small intestine than to the stomach (Figure 6C). For urinary drainage, however, the functional survival rate was significantly higher for grafts anastomosed to the bladder than to the ureter (Figure 6D).

Patient survival rates were nearly identical for recipients in the three most common duct management categories (Figure 5B). In the urinary drainage category, however, the one year patient survival rate was significantly lower ($p\leq0.004$) for the recipients of grafts managed by ureter than by bladder

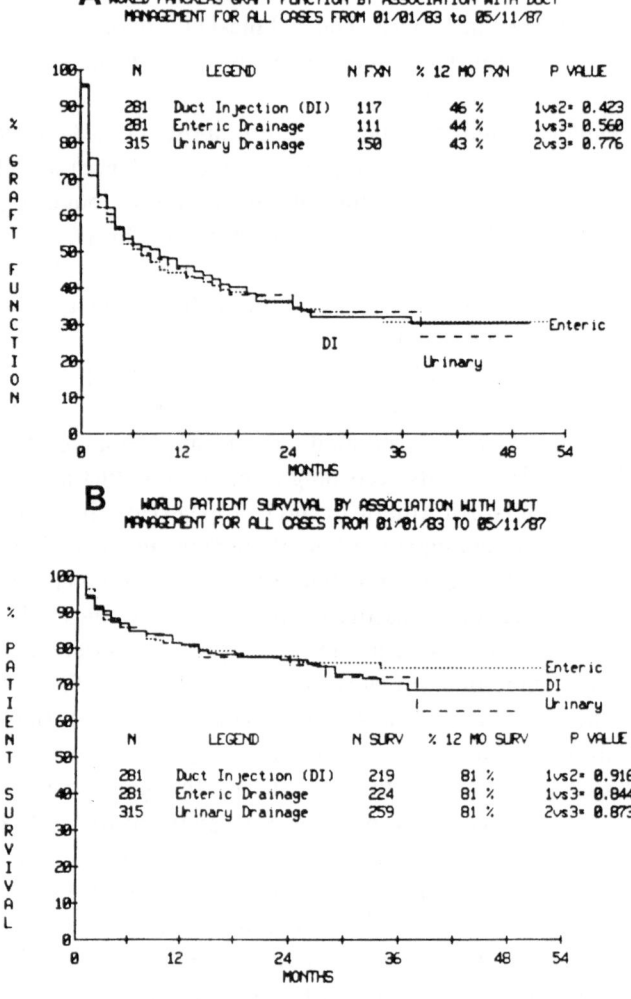

Figure 5. (A) Graft and (B) patient survival rates for 1983–87 recipients of pancreas transplants according to three different duct management techniques.

anastomosis (50% vs 84%). Within the enteric drainage category, however, the patient survival rates were not significantly for recipients of grafts managed by stomach than by intestimal anastomosis (76% vs 82%).

Segmental versus whole pancreas transplant results

Of the 892 transplants for the 1983–87 era, 528 (29%) were segmental and 364

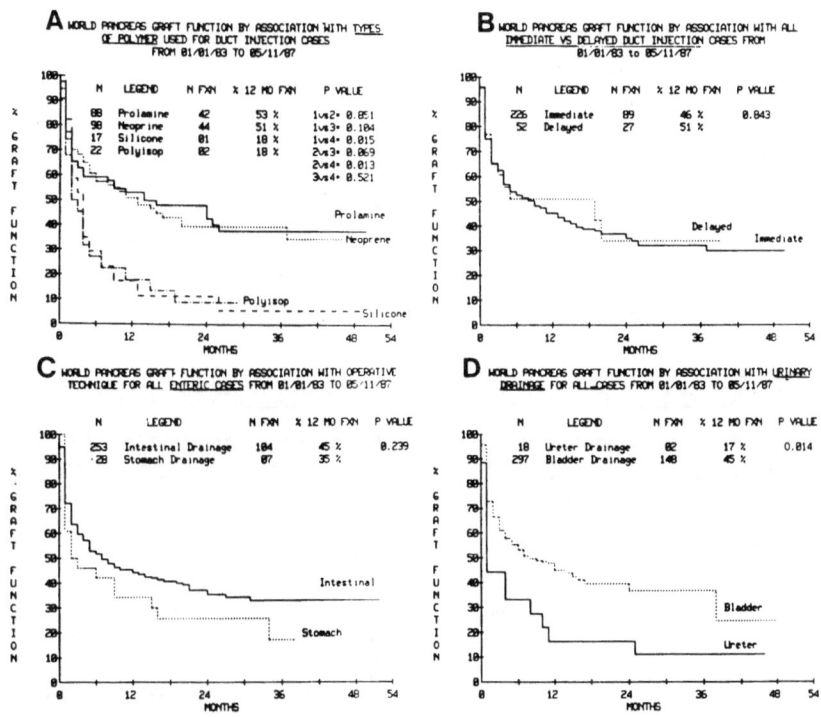

Figure 6. Functional survival rates for 1983–87 pancreas transplant recipients of (A) duct-injected grafts according to type of polymer used; (B) duct-injected grafts according to whether the polymer (all types) was injected immediately or delayed (all prolamine) until days or weeks after the transplant; (C) enteric-drained cases according to whether drainage was into the small intestine or the stomach; and (D) urinary-drained cases according to whether drainage was into the ureter or bladder.

(59%) were whole pancreas grafts. The overall technical failure rate was similar (p = 0.921) for both types of grafts (Table 2), and there were no significant differences (p>0.15) in the incidences of thromboses (12.5% vs 12.6%) or infections (6.8% vs 5.4%).

Functional survival rates were also similar for recipients of segmental and whole grafts, whether analyzed for all cases (Figure 7A), or technically successful cases only (61% at 1 year for 393 segmental and 56% for 272 whole organ grafts, p = 0.627). There also were no significant differences in functional survival rates between recipients of segmental and whole grafts in the various duct management categories (Figure 7B–D). In the enteric drainage category, the functional survival rates at one year were 44% for recipients of segmental (n = 187) and 43% for recipients of whole (n = 94) grafts. Since, all stomach drained grafts) were segmental, a comparison of segmental and whole

302

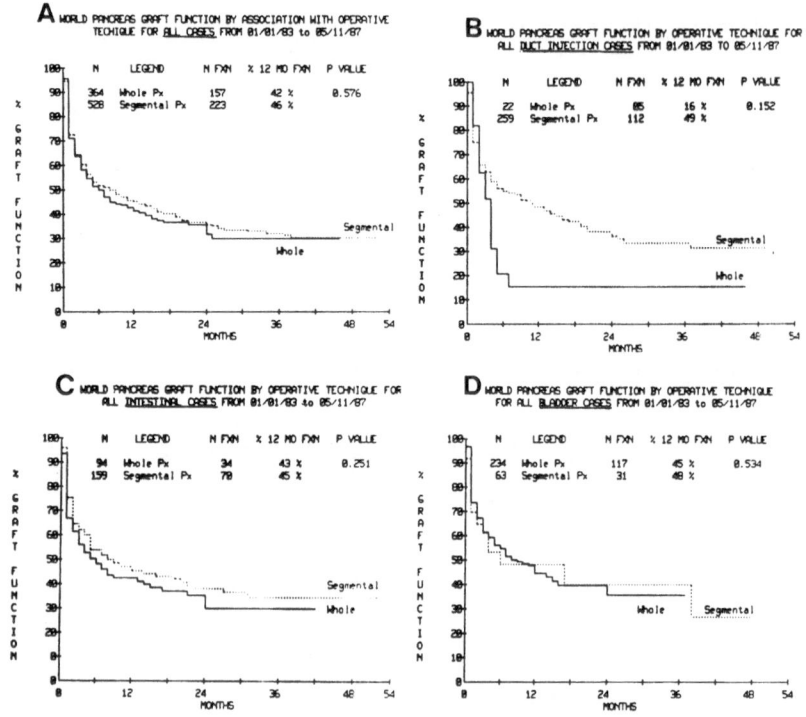

Figure 7. Functional survival rates for 1983–87 recipients of whole versus segmental pancreas transplants in (A) all cases, (B) duct-injected grafts, (C) small intestine-drained grafts, and (D) bladder-drained grafts.

grafts was made for intestinal drainage, and, one year survival rates were nearly identical (Figure 7C). In the bladder drainage cases, functional survival rates year were also similar for segmental and of whole grafts (Figure 7D). There also was no difference in functional survival rates for ureter drained segmental (n = 8) and whole (n = 10) grafts (13% versus 20% at one year).

Table 2 shows that whole pancreas transplants were performed in a higher percentage of North American than European cases (72% versus 18%). Both within and between continents, the functional survival rates according to type of graft were not significantly different (p>0.1).

Results of pancreas-spleen transplants

Since 1982, the spleen has been included with 27 of the 363 whole pancreas transplants (7%), but with none of 529 segmental grafts. The grafts survival rates were insignificantly (p≥0.3) lower for the 27 whole pancreas-spleen transplants than for the 865 pancreas transplants that did not include the spleen (32% versus 44% at one year). The same relative differences were seen in an analysis of whole pancreas-spleen grafts versus whole or segmental grafts that did not include the spleen both for all (Figure 8A) and for technically successful cases (Figure 8B).

The incidence of technical failures was 26% for whole pancreas-spleen grafts and 25% and 26% for whole and segmental pancreas grafts without the spleen (p>0.8). The incidence of thrombosis was actually higher for whole pancreas-spleen grafts (14.8%) than for whole or segmental pancreas grafts without the spleen (12.5% and 12.4%).

Although graft survival rates did not differ significantly, patient survival rates were significantly lower in recipients of composite whole pancreas-spleen transplants than in recipients of whole or segmental pancreas transplants without the spleen (Figure 8C). The detrimental effect of including the spleen on patient survival was also seen in the analysis of technically successful cases (Figure 8D).

Pancreas transplant results according to duration of graft preservation

The duration of hypothermic storage between removal of the graft and transplantation in the recipient were reported on 799 cadaveric pancreas grafts in the 1983–87 era. The functional survival rates for recipients of grafts stored <6 hours was significantly higher than for recipients of grafts stored from 6 to 12 hours, but there was not a significant difference in insulin-independent rates for recipients of grafts those stored <6 hours versus ≥12 hours (Figure 9A). The difference in functional survival rates for grafts stored 6 to 12 versus ≥12 hours also was not significant. Patient survival rates did not differ significantly according to graft preservation time (Figure 9B).

The proportions of cadaveric grafts preserved longer than 6 hours was higher in North America (36%) than in Europe (24%), but very few grafts were preserved >12 hours in Europe (2%), while 16% were preserved for this length of time in North America (Table 2). On both continents preservation times <6 hours were associated with higher graft survival rates than were preservation times of 6–12 hours, but the difference was significant only in Europe. Between continents, the functional survival rates for grafts stored <6 hours was significantly higher in Europe than in North America, while that of grafts stored >12 hours was significantly higher in North America than in Europe.

The incidence of technical failures was significantly lower for grafts stored <6 hours versus those stored 6–12 hours (p = 0.003) but the differences between those stored for <6 hours or 6–12 hours vs those stored >12 hours were not significant (Table 3). The lower functional survival rate for grafts stored 6 to 12 hours than those stored <6 hours may relate to a higher

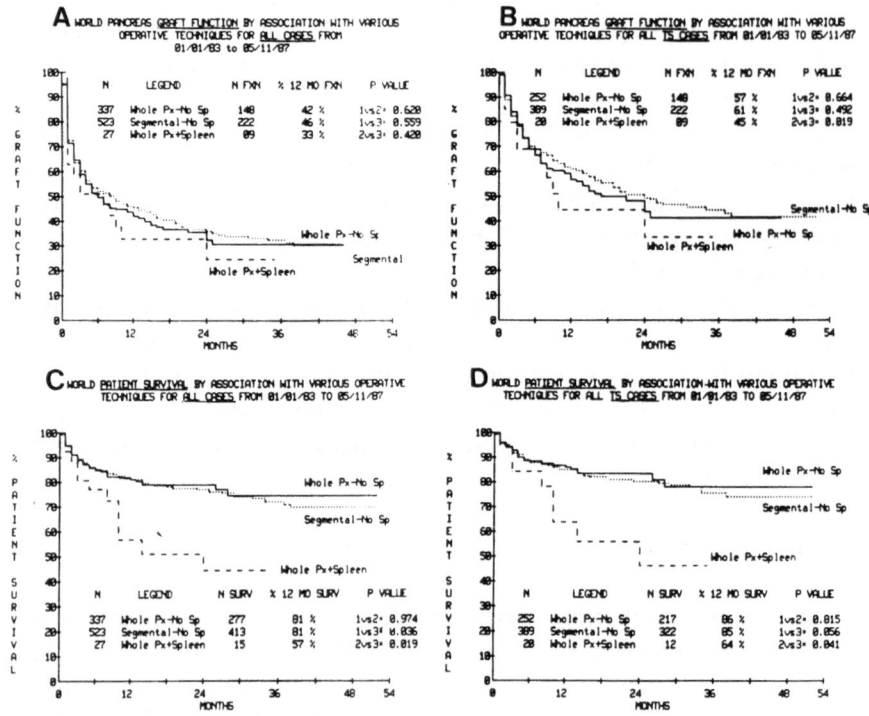

Figure 8. (A and B) Graft and (C and D) patient survival rates for 1983–87 recipients of whole pancreas-spleen transplants versus recipients of whole or segmental pancreas transplants without the spleen in (A and C) all cases and (B and D) technically successful cases.

incidence of technical failures in the 6–12 hour group that was independent of preservation time; otherwise, a higher incidence of technical failures would be expected in the ≥12 hour preservation group, and such was not the case.

Pancreas results according to immunosuppressive treatment of the recipients

Several different immunosuppressive regimens have been used to treat pancreas transplant recipients. The regimens were classified into six groups:
1. Cyclosporin (CSA) alone,
2. CSA and Prednisone (Pred) only,
3. CSA plus Azathioprine (AZA) plus Pred,
4. CSA and AZA only,
5. AZA and Pred initially with CSA added later in the posttransplant course,
6. AZA and Pred only.
The graft and patient survival rates in each group were calculated for all cases and for recipients of technically successful transplants (Table 4). In addition,

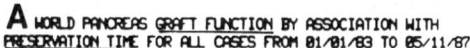

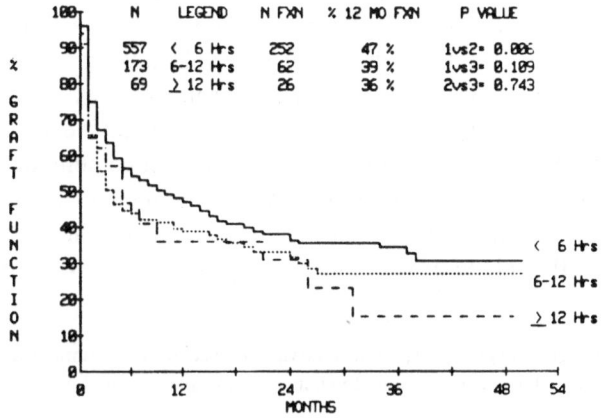

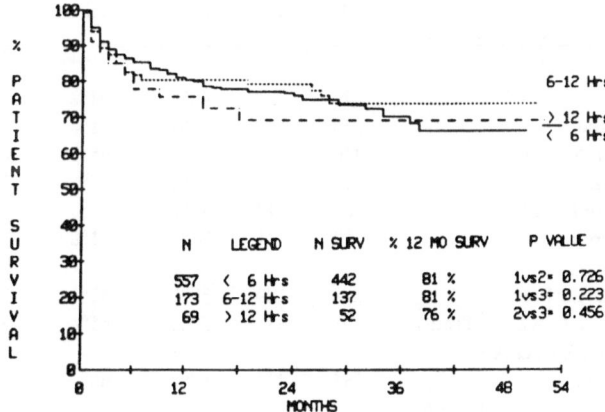

Figure 9. (A) Graft and (B) patient survival rates for 1983–87 recipients of cadaver pancreas transplants according to duration of preservation prior to transplantation.

graft and patient survival rates were calculated for all and for technically successful cases in categories of various combined the groups:

I.   (1 + 2), CSA + Pred,
II. (3 + 4), CSA + AZA ± Pred,
III. (3 + 4 + 5), (All AZA + CSA) ± Pred,
IV. (1 + 2 + 3 + 4 + 5), (All CSA) ± AZA ± Pred.

The regimen employing triple therapy from the time of transplant (Group 3,

CSA + AZA + Pred) was associated with significantly higher graft survival rates than the CSA + Pred (Group 2) or AZA + Pred (Group 6) regimens, whether all or technically successful cases only were analyzed.

In the analysis of technically successful cases, both triple therapy regimens (Group 3 and Group 5, AZA + Pred initially with CsA added later) were associated with significantly higher graft survival rates than the Group 2 or Group 6 regimens, as was the regimen of Group 4 (CsA + AZA without prednisone) vs Group 6 (p = 0.05). The Category (II) that included the groups in which cyclosporin and azathioprine were given in combination for initial immunosuppression was also associated with a significantly higher graft survival rate than the Category (I) that included the groups in which CSA was administered either alone or with prednisone only or the group that received

Table 4. One year actuarial graft and patient survival rates according to immunosuppression in all and in recipients of technically successful (TS) pancreas transplants from January 1, 1983 to April 24, 1987.

		No cases		Graft survival rates		Pt surv rate	
		All	TS	All	TS	All	TS
	Group						
1	CSA	32	23	46%	64%	67%	78%
2	CSA + Pred	236	166	37%	51%	78%	81%
3	CSA + AZA + Pred	476	369	49%	65%	86%	91%
4	CSA + AZA	15	12	67%	83%	79%	83%
5	AZA + Pred + CSA	64	42	47%	70%	83%	90%
6	AZA + Pred	59	44	31%	41%	58%	66%
	Category						
I	(1 + 2) CSA ± Pred	268	189	38%	53%	77%	80%
II	(3 + 4) CSA + AZA ± Pred	491	381	50%	65%	86%	90%
III	(3 + 4 + 5) (All AZA + CSA) ± Pred	555	423	50%	66%	85%	90%
IV	(1 + 2 + 3 + 4 + 5) (All CSA) ± AZA ± Pred	823	612	45%	61%	82%	87%
	P values <0.05						
	Insulin-independence						
	All cases	2 vs 3, 4 vs 6,					
		I vs II, I vs III, II vs 6, III vs 6, IV vs 6					
	TS cases	2 vs 3, 2 vs 5, 3 vs 6, 4 vs 6, 5 vs 6					
		I vs II, I vs III, 1 vs 5, II vs 6, III vs I, III vs 6, IV vs 6					
	Patient survival						
	All cases	1 vs 3, 2 vs 6, 3 vs 6, 5 vs 6,					
		I vs II, I vs III, I vs 6, II vs 6 , III vs 6, IV vs 6					
	TS cases	I vs 3, 2 vs 3, 2 vs 6, 3 vs 6, 5 vs 6					
		I vs II, I vs III, I vs 6, II vs 6, III vs 6, IV vs 6					

azathioprine without cyclosporin (Group 6), whether all or technically successful cases were analyzed.

The graft survival rate curves for recipients in immunosuppressive Categories I (CSA ± Pred) versus III (all groups in which CSA and AZA were given in combination for initial or maintenance immunosuppression) versus Group 6 (AZA + Pred) are shown for all cases (Figure 10A) and for technically successful cases (Figure 10B). The graft survival rate in patients treated with both AZA and CSA was significantly higher than in the patients who received either CSA without azathioprine or AZA without cyclosporin, but the graft survival rates (for all and for technically successful cases) in patients treated with CSA ± Pred were not significantly better than in those treated with AZA and prednisone.

Only 59 (7%) of the 882 recipients classified as to immunosuppressive regimen did not receive cyclosporin during the 1893–87 era. When the recipients who were not treated with cyclosporin (Category IV) were compared to the patients who did not receive cyclosporin (Group 6), the differences in insulin-independent rates were significant for the analysis of all cases as well as for the analysis of technically successful cases (Table 4).

No apparent penalty was paid for giving cyclosporin in combination with azathioprine or prednisone or both drugs (Table 4), since the patient survival rates were higher for Groups 2 (CsA + Pred), 3 (CSA + AZA + Pred), 4 (CsA + AZA) and 5 (AZA + Pred + CSA) versus Group 1 (CsA alone), and the differences were significant for Group 3 vs 1. The triple drug regimen (Groups 3 and 5) were also associated with higher recipient survival rates than the double drug regimens, differences that were significant for Group 3 and 5 versus 6 (AZA + Pred).

The patient survival rate curves for immunosuppressive Category I (CSA ± Pred) versus Category III (CSA and AZA in combination) versus Group 6 (AZA + Pred) are shown for all cases (Figure 10C) and for technically successful cases (Figure 10D). The CSA-AZA combination was associated with significantly higher patient survival rates then the use of CSA without azathioprine or AZA without cyclosporin. The recipient survival rates in the CSA ± Pred category were also significantly higher than in the AZA + Pred group. Indeed the recipient survival rates were significantly higher for all patients who received cyclosporin (Category IV) versus those who never received cyclosporin (Table 4).

Azathioprine and cyclosporin were combined more commonly in North America than in Europe (Table 2). In both continents, the combination of azathioprine and cyclosporin was associated with significantly higher graft survival rates than the regimens using cyclosporin without azathioprine or azathioprine without cyclosporin. The differences in graft survival rates between the latter two regimens were significant only in Europe. Between

308

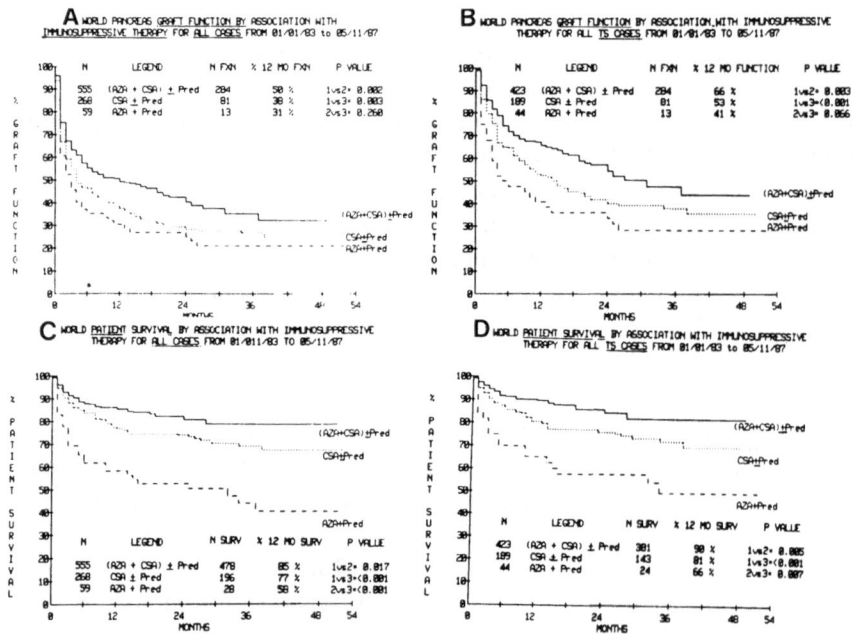

Figure 10. (A and B) Graft and (C and D) patient survival rates according to immunosuppression for 1983–87 pancreas transplant recipients in (A and C) all cases and (B and D) technically successful (TS) cases. CSA ± Pred includes 32 patients (23 TS) treated with cyclosporin alone and 236 patients (166 TS) treated with cyclosporin and prednisone; (AZA ± CSA) ± Pred includes 15 patients (12 TS) treated with cyclosporin and azathioprine alone, 476 patients (369 TS) treated with cyclosporin plus azathioprine plus prednisone beginning in the immediate posttransplant period, and 64 patients (42 TS) treated with azathioprine and prednisone initially followed by addition of cyclosporin in the posttransplant period; AZA ± Pred includes patients who received only azathioprine and prednisone for immnosuppression.

continents graft survival rates were significantly higher in Europe than in North America for patients treated with azathioprine and cyclosporin in combination, the differences between the continents were not significant for the other regimens.

Pancreas transplant results according to HLA matching

HLA typing data on the recipients and donors of cadaver pancreas transplants was available on 682 of cases for the A and B loci, 527 for the DR loci and 524 for all three loci (Table 3).

The functional survival rate was higher for pancreas grafts mismatched for ≤3 than for ≥4 A, B and DR antigens (Table 3), but the difference was not significant (p = 0.078). The functional survival rates were also higher for grafts mismatched for ≤2 than for ≥3 A and B antigens (51% vs 41% at 1 year, p = 0.056), or for 0 than for 1 or 2 DR antigens (54% vs 38% and 40% at 1 year, p = 0.034 and 0.168, respectively). The beneficial effect of minimizing the number of HLA mismatches on graft survival was most apparent in the analysis of technically successful grafts (Figure 11). The functional survival rate for recipients of technically successful grafts mismatched for ≤3 A, B, and DR antigens was significantly higher than for recipients grafts mismatched for ≥4 antigens (Figure 11A). The favorable effect of minimizing the number of HLA antigen mismatches was seen at the A and B (Figure 11B) as well as the DR (Figure 11C) loci, and was statistically significant in the latter analysis.

The results were also analyzed according to the number of HLA antigens matched at the A, B and DR loci. For all cases with typing data, the functional survival rates were significantly (p = 0.027) higher (63% vs 40% at one year) for grafts matched for ≥4 than for ≤3 antigens at all three loci, an effect that was more due to matching at the DR loci, 64% versus 41% and 39% at one year for 2 versus 1 and 0 antigen matches (p>0.17), than at the A and B loci, 53% versus 45% at one year for ≥3 than ≤2 antigens (p = 0.25). In the corresponding analysis of technically successful grafts functional survival rates were also higher for recipient grafts matched for ≥4 than for ≤3 antigens at all three loci (Figure 10D). Again, the difference in functional survival rates between well and poorly matched technically successful grafts was due to the DR loci (80% versus 57% and 54% at one year for 2 versus 1 and 0 antigen matches, p>0.08) and not the A and B loci (62% versus 61% at one year for ≥3 and ≤2 antigen matches).

Histocompatibility differences between cadaver donors and pancreas transplant recipients appear to affect graft outcome. Maximizing the number of matches or minimizing the number of mismatches is associated with higher graft survival rates when antigens of all three loci are considered for matches and when all three loci or only the DR loci are considered for mismatches in technically successful cases.

Pancreas transplant results according to donor source

Of the pancreas transplants reported to the Registry since 1982, 37 (41%) were from living related donors. The functional survival rates were higher (p = 0.272) in recipients of related than of cadaver donor grafts (53% vs 43% at 1 year), and the difference (77% vs 58% at 1 year) was statistically significant (p = 0.024) in the analysis of technically successful cases. Patient survival rates were significantly (p = 0.032) higher (94% vs 80% at 1 year) for recipients of related than of cadaver donor grafts in the analysis of all cases, and were insignificantly (p = 0.154) higher (96% vs 84% at 1 year) in the analysis of technically successful cases. The higher graft survival rate for pancreas trans-

310

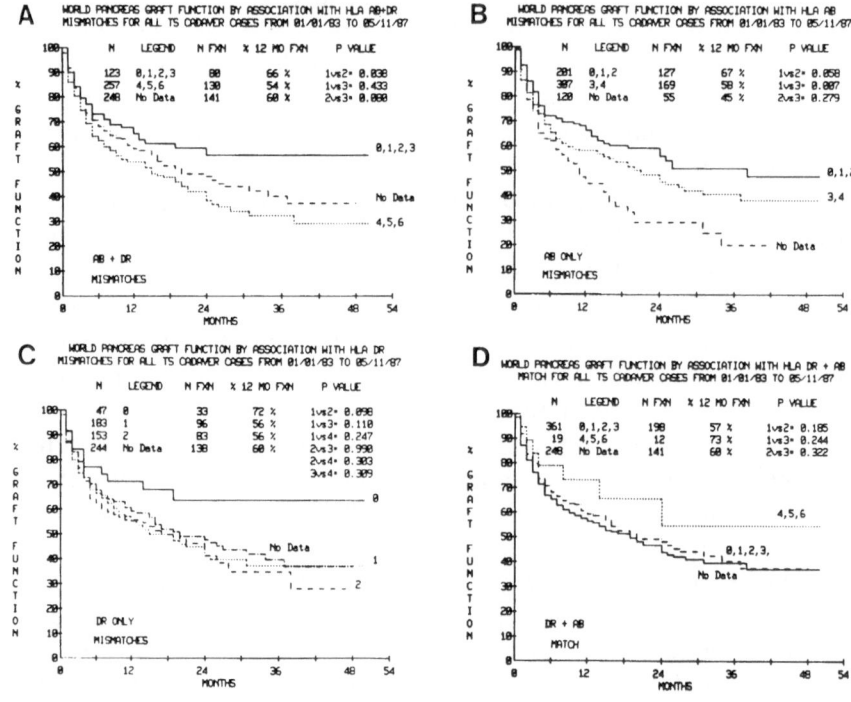

Figure 11. Graft survival rates in 1983–87 recipients of technically successful cadaveric pancreas transplants according to number of HLA mismatches at (A) and A, B and DR loci, (B) the A and B loci and (C) the DR loci.

plants from related donors is consistent with the beneficial effect of matching for transplants.

Pancreas transplant results according to presence or absence of End Stage Diabetic Nephropathy (ESDN) in the recipients

Of the 892 pancreas transplants in the 1983–87 cases, 735 (82%) were in recipients with ESDN. In an analysis performed without regard to the timing of the pancreas and kidney transplants relative to each other (Figure 12A), graft survival rates were significantly higher in recipients with than in those without ESDN. Patient survival rates, however, were significantly higher in those without than in those with ESDN (Figure 12B).

The graft survival rate was significantly higher in recipients of a pancreas transplanted simultaneous with a kidney than in recipients of a pancreas after a kidney, and was also significantly higher than that in nonuremic, nonkidney transplant recipients of a pancreas alone (Figure 13A). The difference be-

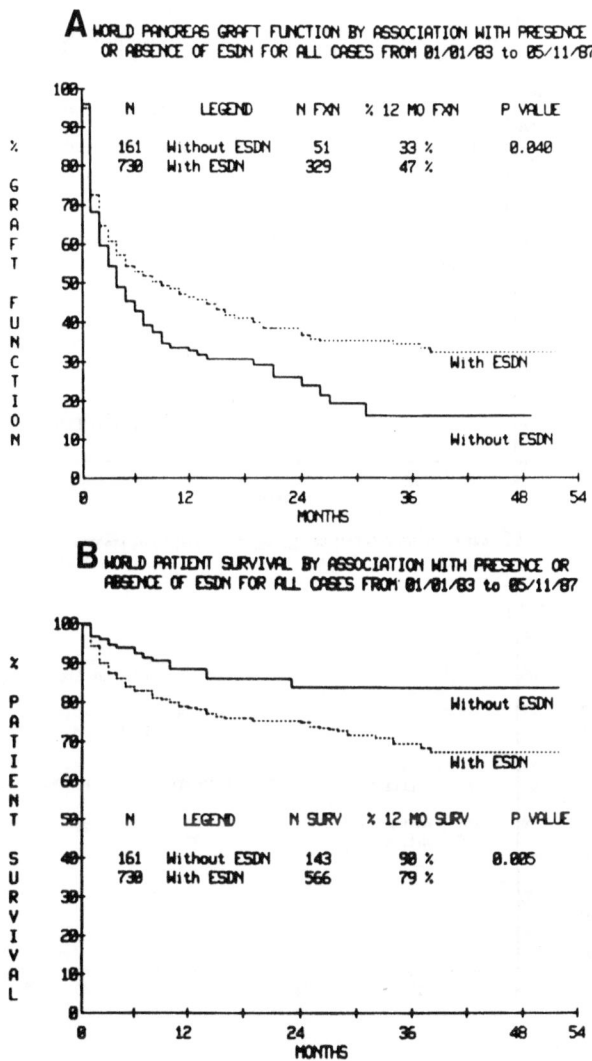

Figure 12. (A) Pancreas graft and (B) patient survival rates for 1983–87 transplant recipients with or without end stage diabetic nephropathy (ESDN).

tween the latter two groups, however, was not significant.

The patient survival rate (Figure 13B) was significantly higher in non-uremic, non-kidney transplant recipients of pancreas grafts alone than in uremic recipients of simultaneous pancreas and kidney transplants. The survival of recipients of pancreas grafts after kidney transplants was not significantly different from that of recipients of a pancreas alone or of recipients of a simultaneous kidney.

312

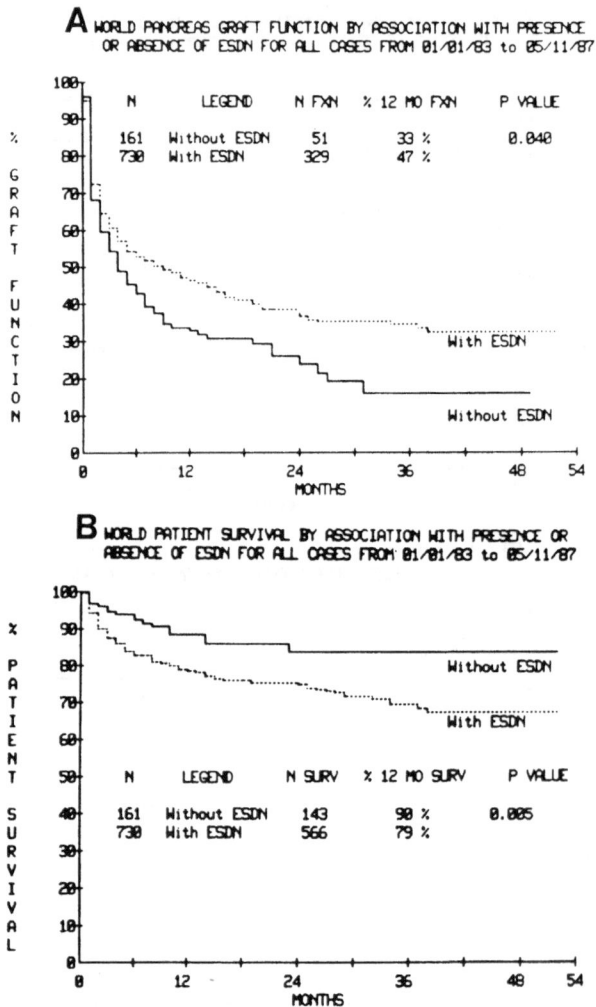

Figure 13. (A) Pancreas graft and (B) patient survival rates for 1983–87 transplant recipients according to whether they did or did not receive a kidney transplant and if they did according to wether the kidney was transplanted simultaneously with or after the pancreas.

An analysis by continent (Table 2) showed most pancreas transplants were performed in combination with kidney transplants in Europe (83%), while less than half of the pancreas transplants in North America were synchronous with a kidney (44%). Conversely, the proportion of pancreas transplants alone was higher in North America (23%) than in Europe (11% of cases). In both continents, pancreas graft survival rates were higher in recipients of simultaneous pancreas and kidney transplants than in recipients of pancreas transplants after a kidney or recipients of pancreas transplants alone. Within North America the differences were not significant, while in Europe the difference was significant for the pancreas alone versus the pancreas plus kidney group. Between continents the survival rate of pancreas transplants alone was significantly higher in North America than in Europe.

Cadaver pancreas transplant results according to technique and association with kidney transplants

The pancreas graft survival rates were significantly higher in recipients of simultaneous kidney transplants from the same donor than in the other categories (Figure 13A). In such recipients both plasma glucose and serum creatinine as indicators of rejection could be monitored. A rise of creatinine would indicate rejection of the kidney, and if it preceded a rise in glucose, lead to earlier diagnosis and treatment of rejection of the pancreas. The only other situation where a parameter of graft function other than plasma glucose can be monitored indefinitely is in the recipient of a graft managed by urinary drainage, where urine amylase activity can be used. Thus, the insulin-independent rates in recipients of bladder drained grafts versus intestinal drained and duct injected grafts without a kidney from the same donor (pancreas transplants alone or after a kidney from a different donor) were compared, as were the insulin-independent rates in recipients of simultaneous pancreas and kidney transplants versus recipients of pancreas transplants alone and after a kidney within the various duct management categories (Table 5).

Table 5. Pancreas graft survival rates in 1983–87 recipients of transplants from cadaver donors according to duct management technique and association with kidney transplants.

	Bladder		Intestine		Duct injection	
	No Cases	1 Yr Fxn	No Cases	1 Yr Fxn	No Cases	1 Yr Fxn
All cases						
Px + Kid (SD)	157	50%	133	51%[a]	223	52%[b, c]
Px after Kid (DD)	98	40%	35	37%	17	15%[b]
Px alone	37	38%	49	24%[a]	39	28%[c]
Tech suc cases						
Px + Kid (SD)	124	64%	97	69%[d]	178	65%[e, f]
Px after Kid (DD)	71	56%	23	56%	12	21%[e]
Px alone	27	52%	33	35[d]	33	33%[f]

P values <0.05 between groups are indicated by letter superscripts.
SD = Same Donor for each organ, DD = Different Donor for each organ, Px = Pancreas, Kid = Kidney, Tech = Technical, Suc = Successful, Fxn = Function (Recipient insulin-independent).

In all duct management categories, graft survival rates were higher in recipients of simultaneous kidney transplants than in recipients of pancreas transplants alone or pancreas transplants after a kidney from a different donor. Within the bladder drainage category the differences were not significant. Within the duct injection and intestinal drainage categories, however, functional survival rates were significantly higher in SPK recipients than in recipients of pancreas grafts alone, and in the duct injection category the graft survival rate for SPK recipients was also significantly higher than that of a pancreas performed after a kidney from a different donor.

Thus, for recipients of pancreas transplants simultaneous with a kidney from the same donor, graft survival rates are similar no matter which of the three most common duct management techniques are used. For recipients of pancreas transplants alone or pancreas transplants after a kidney from a different donor, the graft survival rates are higher with the bladder drainage than with the other techniques.

The beneficial effect of transplanting pancreas grafts by approaches that provide a permanent parameter other than plasma glucose levels to monitor for rejection is additive with that of HLA matching (Figure 14). In a group that

Table 6. Functional status listed in the registry for both organs in 565 recipients of simultaneous pancreas and kidney transplants between January 1, 1983 and April 24, 1987.

Category (N)	No of cases at interval		
	<6 mo	6–12 mo	>12 mo
Pancreas & kidney both functioning (255)			
Mos post-Tx	79	60	116
Pancreas & kidney both failed (178)			
Mos post-Tx Px failed	149	13	16
Mos post-Tx Kid failed	132	25	21
Interval between losses	155	12	11
Px failed before Kid (75)	57	10	8
Kid failed before Px (41)	36	2	3
Simultaneous [± 1 mos] (62)	62	–	–
Kidney Fxn, pancreas failed (117)			
Mos Kid Fxn since Px failed	31	17	69
Mos Kid Fxn since Tx	21	18	78
Mos post-Tx Px failed	92	11	14
Pancreas Fxn, kidney failed (15)			
Mos Px Fxn since Kid failed	4	2	9
Mos Px Fxn since Tx	2	1	12
Mos post-Tx Kid failed	8	3	4

Fxn = functioning (recipient insulin-independent for pancreas, dialysis free for kidney), Px = pancreas, Kid = kidney, Tx = transplant.

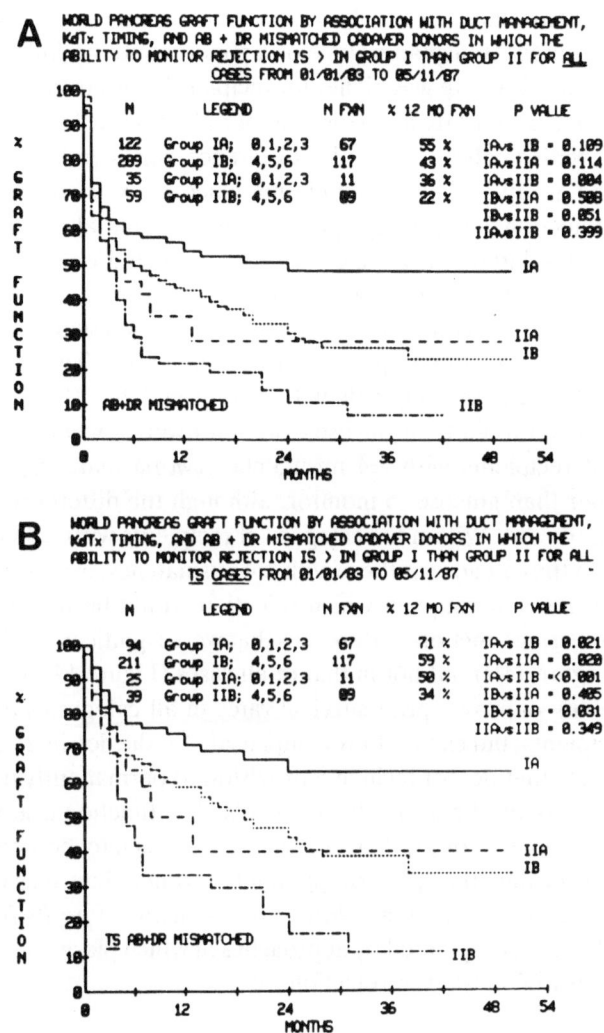

Figure 14. Functional survival rates for 1983–87 cadaveric pancreas transplant recipients according to number of HLA antigens mismatched at the A, B and DR loci and according to whether there is (Group I, simultaneous kidney transplants for all pancreas graft duct management techniques and bladder drainage for pancreas transplants alone or after a previous kidney) or is not (Group II, enteric drainage or duct injection of a pancreas transplant alone or a pancreas transplant after a previous kidney) a parameter other than plasma glucose to permanently monitor for rejection. Group I A mismatched ≤3 and B for ≥4 HLA antigens in whom monitoring other than glucose is possible and Group II A mismatched for ≤3 and B for ≥4 HLA antigen in whom only glucose can be monitored.

included SPK transplants in all duct management categories and urinary drainage for pancreas transplants alone or a pancreas after a kidney, the one year functional survival rate was higher for recipients of grafts mismatched for ≤3 versus ≥4 A, B and DR antigens whether all (Figure 14A) or TS cases (Figure 14B) were analyzed, and the difference was significant for latter analysis. In the group in which only plasma glucose levels could be used to monitor for rejection indefinitely (pancreas transplants alone or pancreas transplants after a kidney in recipients of duct injected or enteric drained grafts), graft survival rates were also higher in recipients of grafts mismatched for ≤3 than ≥4 HLA antigens, but the differences were not significant whether all (Figure 14A) or TS cases (Figure 14B) were analyzed. The graft survival rates in the subgroups of recipients with ≤3 mismatches (best match) but without a parameter other than glucose to monitor were lower than that of the subcategory of recipients with ≥4 mismatches (worst matches) but with a parameter other than glucose to monitor, although the differences were not statistically significant. Within the category of recipients with ≤3 mismatches as well as within the category of those with ≥4 mismatches, graft survival rates were higher in the subgroups in which rejection would be monitored independent of endocrine function, differences that were significant in the analysis of TS cases (Figure 14B) but not in that of all cases (Figure 14A).

HLA matching improves graft survival rates in all categories of pancreas transplant recipients, but cannot fully compensate for the detrimental effect of using approaches that do not include a provision to permanently monitor for rejection independent of plasma glucose levels. The functional survival rates are highest in recipients of grafts from minimally mismatched donors transplanted by approaches that provide parameters other than plasma glucose levels to monitor for rejection, and lowest in recipients of grafts from highly mismatched donors transplanted by approaches in which plasma glucose is the only easily measured marker of rejection.

Results of primary kidney transplant outcome in pancreas transplant recipients

The renal graft functional survival rates in the 1983–87 recipients of pancreas transplants in the 1983–87 era who also received kidney transplants was 72% at one year (Figure 3A). The functional survival rates of kidneys transplanted before a pancreas transplant was high (Figure 15), since the patients had to survive with a functioning kidney to receive the pancreas transplant, most of which were performed more than one year after the kidney transplant. For recipients of simultaneous kidney and pancreas transplants, the renal graft function survival rate was much lower, but most losses occurred early, and after one year the curve paralleled that for kidneys transplanted prior to a pancreas (Figure 16).

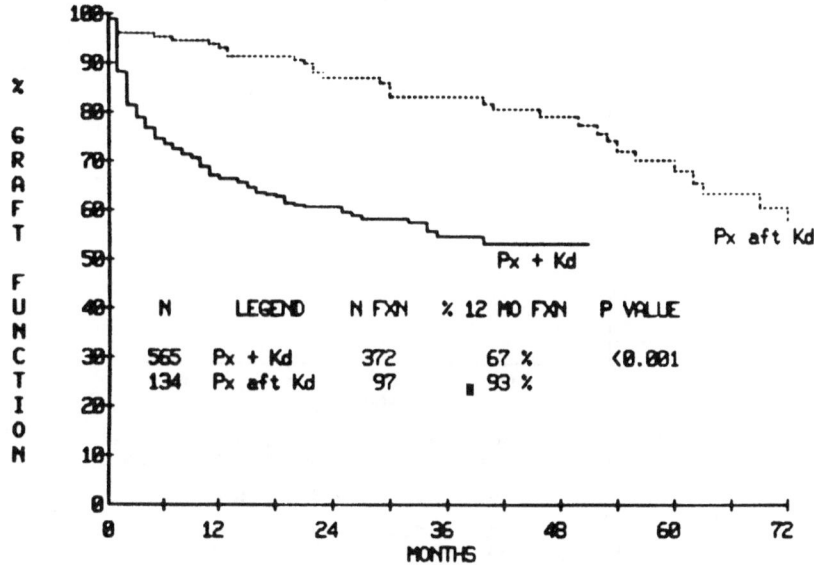

Figure 15. Renal graft functional survival rates in 1983–87 recipients of pancreas transplants according to timing of the kidney transplant relative to the pancreas.

Pancreas and kidney graft outcome in recipients of synchronous transplants

The one year actuarial recipient, kidney and pancreas survival rates in simultaneous pancreas-kidney (SPK) transplant cases for 1983–87 are shown in Figure 15. Of 133 SPK cases where the pancreas failed for a technical reason (90% of occurred within the first 2 months posttransplant), the one year recipient and kidney survival rates were 61% and 51%, respectively, significantly less (p<0.001) than the corresponding figures (81% and 71%) for the TS pancreas transplant cases.

The outcomes for SPK cases can be classified into four categories:
a) both grafts functioning,
b) both grafts failed,
c) kidney functioning, pancreas failed,
d) pancreas functioning, kidney failed.

The number of cases in each category is given in Table 6. In most cases the outcome is similar for both grafts, but failure of the pancreas with continued functioning of the kidney (Figure 17A) is a much more likely outcome than the reverse situation (Figure 17B).

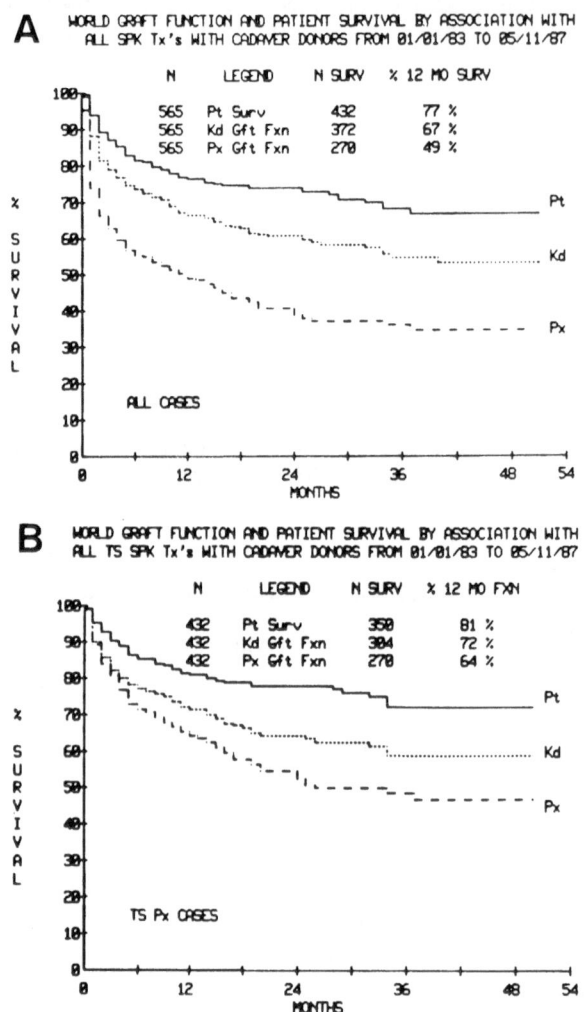

Figure 16. Patient, kidney and pancreas functional survival rates for 1983–87 recipients of simultaneous pancreas and kidney cadaveric transplants (SPK) in (A) all and (B) technically successful cases.

Summary and comments

The pancreas transplant registry data shows a progressive improvement in both patient and graft functional survival rates. The results have been similar for the commonly used duct management techniques (polymer injection, intestinal drainage, bladder drainage), and there has been no difference in the outcome for segmental or whole organ grafts. Inclusion of the spleen has a

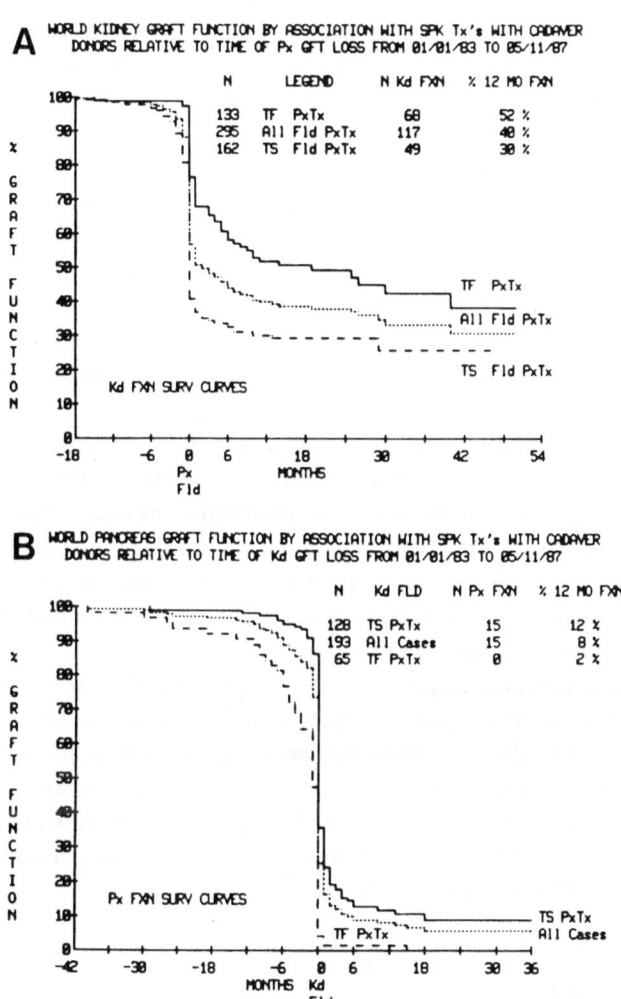

Figure 17. Kidney graft functional survival rates for 1983–87 recipients of simultaneous pancreas transplants relative to time of pancreas graft loss in all failed (fld) pancreas (Px) transplant (Tx) cases and in pancreas transplant cases which failed for technical (TF) versus other reasons (TS). Most kidneys that failed did so simultaneous or nearly simultaneous with the pancreas. A few failed before or after the pancreas. Kidney failure was not inevitable, however, and nearly one-third continued to function long-term after loss of the pancreas, including more than half of the kidneys in TF pancreas transplant cases.

detrimental effect on patient survival without influencing pancreas graft survival rates. Short preservation times (<6 hours) are associated with the highest functional survival rates than long times, but the difference was not statistically significant compared to the results for grafts stored >12 hours.

Graft and patient survival rates were higher in patients who received cyclosporin and azathioprine in combination than in those who received either drug alone or in combination with agents other than each other. HLA matching appears to have a favorable effect on pancreas graft functional survival rates.

Pancreas graft survival rates are higher in recipients with than without end stage diabetic nephropathy, and are highest in recipients of simultaneous kidney transplants. Patient survival rates, however, are highest in those without end stage diabetic nephropathy who receive pancreas transplants alone. Pancreas transplant approaches in which rejection can be monitored independent of plasma glucose levels (kidney transplant from some donor, bladder drainage) in any category are associated with higher graft survival rates than those which do not.

Recipients of simultaneous pancreas and kidney transplants had kidney graft functional survival rates similar to those reported by the UCLA Kidney Transplant Registry for diabetic recipients of cadaver kidney transplants alone [12], suggesting that pancreas transplantation does not adversely effect outcome in renal allograft recipients. In SPK cases when one organ fails the other organ may continue to function. Retention of kidney function after loss of the pancreas is more common than the reverse situation.

Nearly all pancreas transplants have been performed in North America and Europe, the number being nearly equal on both continents. The frequency by which various techniques of regimens were employed differ in each continent, and there are also differences in outcome in some categories. The methods used most frequently tended to have the highest success rates in each of the continents, but overall there were no differences in patient and graft survival rates between North America and Europe.

Acknowledgements

The institutions that have reported cases to the Pancreas Registry are: University of Austria; University of Barcelona; Barcelona General Hospital; Baviere Hospital, Liege, Belgium; University of Berlin, GDR; University of British Columbia, Vancouver General Hospital, Canada; Buenos Aires National Hospital; University of California, Irvine; University of California at Los Angeles (UCLA); Cardiff Royal Infirmary Hospital, Wales; Case Western Reserve University Hospital, Cleveland; University of Chicago; Chung Yung Hospital, Taiwan; University of Cincinnati; Cleveland Clinic; University of Cologne, Germany; University of Colorado; University of East Carolina, Greenville, NC; Erasme hospital, Brussels; University of Erlangen, Germany; University of Florida, Gainesville; University of Genoa, Italy;

Froedtert Memorial Lutheran Hospital, Medical College of Wisconsin, Milwaukee; Good Samaritan Hospital, Phoenix; University of Gothenberg; University of Groningen; Guy's Hospital, University of London; University of Helsinki; Henan Medical University, China; Herriot Hospital, Lyon; Johns Hopkins Hospital, Baltimore; Karolinska Institute, Huddinge Hospital, Stockholm; Kuwait University; Latter Day Saints Hospital, Salt Lake City; University of Leeds, England; University of Leiden, Holland; Baviere Hospital, Liege, Belgium; Liverpool Royal Hospital, England; Louisiana State University, Shreveport; University of Louisville; University of Louvain, Belgium; University of Lubeck, Germany; University of Lund, Sweden; University of Maastricht, Holland; University of Maryland; Massachusetts General Hospital, Boston; Melbourne Prince Henry Hospital, Australia; Methodist Hospital, Dallas; University of Miami; Milan San Raffaele Institute, Italy; University of Minnesota, Minneapolis; University of Montepelier, France; University of Montreal, Canada; Mount Carmel Hospital, Detroit; University of Munich; University of Iowa, Iowa City; University of Cambridge, England; University of Innsbruck; University of Miami; University of Michigan, Ann Arbor; Montefiore Hospital, New York; National Institute, Mexico; University of Nebraska, Omaha; New England Deaconess Hospital, Boston; University of Newcastle Upon Tyne, England; Northwestern University, Chicago; Ohio State University of Columbus; University of Oslo; University of Oxford, England; Pacific Medical College, San Franciso; University of Pennsylvania, Philadelphia; University of Pittsburgh; Prague Institute Clinical Medicine, Czechoslovakia; Queen Elizabeth Hospital, Birmingham, England; University de Rio de Janeiro; University of Rome; Rush Medical School, Chicago; St. Barnabas Hospital, New Jersey; St. Francis Hospital, Kansas City; St. Louis University; St. Lukes Hospital, Phoenix; University of Sao Paulo, Brazil; University of Stellenbosch, South Africa; Strausbourg Hospital Civil, France; University of Texas Southwestern, Parkland Hospital, Dallas; University of Texas, Houston; University of Tsukuba, Japan; University of Tubingen, Germany; University of Utah, Salt Lake City; Vanderbilt University, Nashville; Victoria General Hospital, Nova Scotia; University of Vienna; University of Western Ontario, London, Canada; University of Wisconsin, Madison; Wuhan Medical College, China; and University of Zurich. The Pancreas Transplant Registry is supported by grants from the National Institutes of Health (DK13083 and RR-400), the Diabetes Research Education Foundation and the Diabetes Treatment Centers of America.

References

1. Sutherland DER: International human pancreas and islet transplant registry. Transpl Proc 12 (No 4, Suppl 2): 229–236, 1980.

2. Gerrish EW: Final newsletter. American college of surgeons/national institutes of health organ transplant registry, Chicago, Illinois, pp 1–4, June 30, 1977.
3. Sutherland DER: Report of international human pancreas and islet transplant registry cases through 1981. Diabetes 31 (Suppl 4): 112–116, 1982.
4. Sutherland DER: The current status of pancreas transplantation: registry statistics. Transpl Proc 15: 1301–1307, 1983.
5. Sutherland DER: Pancreas and islet transplant registry data. World J Surg 8: 270–271, 1984.
6. Sutherland DER, Kendall D: Clinical pancreas and islet transplant registry report. Transpl proc 17: 307–311, 1985.
7. Sutherland DER, Moudry KC: Report of the pancreas transplant registry. In: Terasaki PI (ed) Clinical transplants; pp 7–15. UCLA Press, Los Angeles, 1986.
8. Sutherland DER, Moudry KC: Pancreas transplant registry report – 1986. Clin Transpl 1: 3–17, 1987.
9. Sutherland DER, Moudry KC: Pancreas transplant registry: history and analysis of cases 1966 to October 1986. Pancreas 2: 473–488, 1987.
10. Sutherland DER, Moudry KC: Pancreas transplantation: North American versus European experience. Transpl Proc 19: 3867–3869, 1987.
11. Gehan E: A generalized Wilcoxin test for comparing arbitrarily singly censored samples. Biometrika 52: 203–221, 1965.
12. Cats S, Gallon J: Effect of original disease on kidney transplant outcome. In: Terasaki PI (ed) Clinical kidney transplantation; p 35. UCLA Press, Los Angeles, 1985.

15. Pancreas transplant experience of individual institutions

Experience of the University of Michigan Medical School, Ann Arbor, Michigan, USA

D.C. DAFOE, D.A. CAMPBELL Jr, R.M. MERION, L. ROSENBERG, L.L. ROCHER, A.I. VINIK and J.G. TURCOTTE

At the University of Michigan, 18 pancreas transplants have been carried out between March 1984 and October 1986. At our Center and other centers, the surgical technique, immunosuppressive regimen and candidate criteria have continued to evolve during this period. The impetus for constant re-evaluation and change has been dissatisfaction with historically low graft survival rates and the significant morbidity and mortality associated with pancreatic transplantation [1]. However, this process has produced several incremental advances which have resulted in improved success rates.

Evolution of Technique

In our experience, technical advances have been foremost in achieving success in pancreatic transplantation. The use of the whole organ pancreas graft to maximize islet mass has been applied from the inception of our program. To facilitate drainage of pancreatic exocrine secretions and preserve blood flow through the pancreaticoduodenal arcade, a segment or periampullary 'button' of donor duodenum has been included in the graft. Work accomplished in dogs in our transplantation laboratory in 1975 suggested that a defunctionalized loop of small bowel offered a physiological site for the drainage of exocrine secretions [2]. Placement of the loop in the extraperitoneal iliac fossa was thought to be advantageous allowing for simple open wound drainage if anastomotic leaks occurred. Therefore, we initially created such a loop during a first stage procedure. At the time of pancreatic transplantation, the second stage, a side-to-side anastomosis was constructed between the apex of the loop and the donor duodenum. Despite the apparent soundness of the approach, four of five recipients developed subfascial wound infections. In all cases, post-operative ultrasound evaluation demonstrated a peritransplant fluid collection. It is plausible that opening the bowel loop introduced an innoculum which developed into an abscess. After one patient developed an infection of

323

J.M. Dubernard and D.E.R. Sutherland (eds.), International Handbook of Pancreas Transplantation, 323–328.
© *1989 by Kluwer Academic Publishers.*

the vascular anastomosis requiring external iliac artery ligation, we began to anastomose the celiac axis alone (instead of a Carrell patch of aorta including the celiac axis and superior mesenteric artery) end-to-end to the internal iliac artery. As expected, no ischemia to the graft was encountered using this technique due to the rich collateral circulation.

Because of the occurrence of venous thromboses, we began to include the donor spleen in the pancreaticoduodenal graft to maintain blood flow as advocated by Starzl [3]. Interestingly, we documented chimerism in a female recipient of a male donor graft by karyotypic analysis demonstrating a Y chromosome in some of the peripheral white blood cells. During a period of graft acceptance, 12% of peripheral white blood cells carried the Y chromosome. This percentage fell progressively with the onset of rejection until no chimerism could be detected coincident with irreversible graft failure [4]. Inclusion of donor spleen in the pancreaticoduodenal graft was purported to be of possible immunological benefit [5]. Our laboratory studies, using a porcine pancreaticoduodenal allograft model, showed that inclusion of the donor spleen was associated with an increased incidence of graft rejection [6]. In addition, the development of lethal graft versus host disease in a recipient of a pancreas graft that included the donor spleen led us to discontinue the technique [7].

Our first long-term successful pancreas transplant followed several technical alterations based on lessons from our earlier experience. One major change was the drainage of the pancreas graft into the urinary bladder – a technique pioneered by Sollinger and Belzer [8]. We lengthened the portal vein with donor iliac vein as described by Corry [9]. We also began to place the pancreas grafts intraperitoneally and cold stored pancreas grafts in silica gel filtered plasma rather than EuroCollins' solution. In the subsequent seven consecutive pancreas transplant recipients, graft function was excellent for at least two months after transplantation. When anastomotic leaks at the duodenocystostomy and intra-abdominal abscesses occurred with the periampullary duodenal 'button' we began to employ a segment of donor duodenum. A side-to-side anastomosis to the large, thick-walled bladder of the diabetic recipient has obviated the problem of anastomotic leaks. A drawback of the urinary bladder drainage technique is systemic acidosis resulting from bicarbonate loss which must be replaced.

Thromboses, unrelated to venous malpositioning or arterial occlusion, continue to claim pancreas grafts. Our most recent technical innovation to address the problem was based on laboratory work in a porcine pancreaticoduodenal model. Ex vivo irradiation of the spleen was found to abrogate the detrimental effect of donor spleen inclusion on graft survival due to rejection [10]. Currently, the donor spleen is included in pancreaticoduodenal graft but the spleen is irradiated to eliminate sensitizing lymphoid cells and avoid the risk of graft versus host disease.

Immunosuppression

Our primary immunosuppressive regimen has consisted of cyclosporin and prednisone. Since pancreas transplant recipients develop a post-operative ileus, cyclosporin (Sandimmune, Sandoz Pharmaceuticals, New Hanover, NJ, 6 mg/kg/day) has been administered by the intravenous route in the early post-operative period then orally (16 mg/kg/day). Ten days of antithymocyte globulin (ATGAM, Upjohn Company, Kalamazoo, MI, 15 mg/kg/day) treatment has been given to provide coverage against rejection until adequate cyclosporin levels (150–250 ng/ml by whole blood high performance liquid chromatography) are established via the oral route. More recently, we have added azathioprine (Imuran, Burroughs Wellcome Co., Research Triangle Park, NC, 2 mg/kg/day) to the regimen upon completion of the course of prophylactic antithymocyte globulin.

In simultaneous renal/pancreas graft recipients, the best correlate of pancreatic rejection has been serum creatinine elevation. Acute rejection of the pancreas has been indicated by fasting hyperglycemia (>150 mg/dl), fever, mild hyperamylasemia, leukocytosis, decreased urinary amylase and decreased urinary protein. Anti-rejection treatment has consisted of three doses of methylprednisolone (20 mg/kg/day) followed by 10–14 days of antithymocyte globulin if needed. In 18 pancreas graft recipients, only two patients have had intractable acute rejection episodes which necessitated graft removal.

Recipient criteria

Our initial candidates were late-stage diabetics with advanced complications. In 1984 the International Registry statistics showed a one year graft survival of 38% and a 23% one year mortality [1]. Pancreatic transplantation in the diabetic patient who was 'doing well' was controversial. Our initial candidate criteria dictated that potential pancreas transplant recipients were recipients of a renal transplant which provided stable function (serum creatinine <2 mg/dl) for a minimum of six months. It was reasoned that these patients were selected for the ability to accept an allograft, tolerate immunosuppression and survive transplant surgery.

Subsequently we accepted candidates for simultaneous renal/pancreas transplantation. This decision was based on a reported >50% one year pancreas graft survival in this group (without jeopardizing renal transplant success rates) [9, 11, 12]. Since the five year mortality of the diabetic patient who develops chronic renal failure has been found to be as high as 55–88% [13], a potentially high risk procedure such as pancreatic transplantation was justifiable. The biological basis for changing the candidate criteria included the immunosuppressive effect of uremia and the observation that the familiar signs of kidney transplant rejection usually preceded hyperglycemia – a late sign of pancreatic rejection. On the other hand, end stage diabetic nephropathy is usually accompanied by advanced retinopathy and neuropathy. Therefore, any benefit of a successful pancreas transplant on these neurovascular complications would be difficult to quantitate. Furthermore, the ability of such patients to tolerate a surgical or infectious complication was considerably reduced. In an effort to carefully select the optimal candidate with end stage diabetic nephropathy, we have adhered to a policy of careful evaluation of cardiac status using non-invasive cardiac function studies (e.g. exercise thallium test) and angiographic studies of the coronary arteries of patients with minimal criteria for ischemia. With improved technical success, we have recently expanded our candidate criteria to include non-uremic diabetes. Candidates must exhibit signs of progressive diabetic complications such as proliferative retinopathy, proteinuria or mild serum creatinine elevation. All candidates must be approved by our multidisciplinary Pancreas Transplant Evaluation Committee.

Results

None of our first five pancreas transplant recipients had graft survival for longer than three and one-half months. Four were technical failures due to thrombosis and/or peri-transplant abscess. After several modifications in technique, 11 of the next 13 consecutive pancreas transplants were technically successful. The two technical failures were due to thrombosis. Currently, only 4 pancreas grafts are fuctioning well 27, 29, 31 and 31 months following transplantation (all 4 simultaneous with renal graft).

Of six recipients of a pancreas transplant sequential to a functioning renal transplant, renal transplant function was unimpaired in the five survivors. In the 11 simultaneous renal/pancreas recipients renal grafts functioned initially in ten patients. Two renal grafts were rejected after complications of the pancreas transplant mandated reduction of immunosuppression. One patient lost both grafts to severe acute rejection 13 months after transplantation. Currently, 5 simultaneously transplanted *renal* grafts continue to function 27, 29, 31, 31 and 37 months after transplantation.

In the year following transplantation, 5 patients died. The cause of death was sepsis in 3 cases. Sepsis was often related to technical complications of the pancreas transplant (e.g., peri-transplant abscess, anastomotic leak) or over-immunosuppression (e.g., cytomegalovirus erosive gastritis requiring total gastrectomy). One patient died secondary to status epilepticus 13 months after transplantation; one patient died due to diabetic ketoacidosis 5 months after transplantation.

Endocrine function of the pancreas graft has been excellent. Diurnal glucose profiles and responses to intravenous glucose have become normal. For example, in five pancreas transplant recipients studied 2–9 months after transplantation, the mean blood glucose 120 minutes after intravenous glucose challenge (18 grams) was 100 mg/dl. As an index of glucose control, glycosylated hemaglobin levels have been determined. The mean glycosylated hemoglobin level decreased from 9.2% prior to pancreatic transplantation to 6.5% (normal range 5.5–8.5%) in six patients studied from 1–11 months after successful transplantation. Elevated fasting triglyceride levels were normalized in five of six recipients but serum cholesterol was not significantly lower following successful pancreatic transplantation. Retinopathy has stabilized in three of four patients evaluated six months after transplantation. Nerve conduction velocity has uniformly improved in patients studied. However, because these patients also received a successful simultaneous renal transplant, correction of the uremic component of the neuropathy may have been responsible for the improvement.

Refinement of surgical technique, evolution of immunosuppressive medications and development of optimal candidate selection criteria will allow pancreatic transplantation to be practiced more safely and successfully. Sufficient numbers of pancreas transplant recipients may then be studied over many years to determine the validity of the underlying rationale for pancreatic transplantation – stabilization or reversal of micro-vascular and macro-vascular and neurologic complications. The assessment of quality of life and rehabilitation rates for the successful pancreas transplant recipient will also be forthcoming.

References

1. Sutherland DER, Kendall D: Clinical pancreas and islet transplant registry report. Transplant Proc 17 (1): 307–311, 1985.
2. Dickerman RM, Twiest MW, Crudup JW, Turcotte JG: Transplantation of the pancreas into a retroperitoneal jejunal loop. Am J Surg 129: 48–54, 1975.
3. Starzl TE, Iwatsuki S, Shaw BW Jr, Greene DA, Van Thiel GH, Nalesnik MA, Nusbacher J, Diliz-Perez H, Hakala TR: Pancreaticoduodenal transplantation in humans. Surg Gynecol Obstet 159: 265–272, 1984.
4. Dafoe DC, Campbell DA Jr, Marks WH, Wilson GN, Turcotte JG: Karyotypic chimerism and rejection in a pancreaticoduodenosplenic transplant. Transplantation 40(5): 572–574, 1985.
5. Bitter-Suermann H, Save-Soderbergh J: The course of pancreas allografts in rats conditioned by spleen allografts. Transplantation 26(1): 28–34, 1978.
6. Dafoe DC, Campbell DA Jr, Marks WH, Borgstrom A, Lloyd RV, Turcotte JG: Association of inclusion of the donor spleen in pancreaticoduodenal transplantation with rejection. Transplantation 40(6): 579–584, 1985.

328

7. Deierhoi MH, Sollinger HW, Bozdeck MJ, Belzer FO: Lethal graft versus host disease in a recipient of a pancreas-spleen transplant. Transplantation 41(4): 544–546, 1986.

8. Sollinger HW, Kalayoglu M, Hoffman RM, Belzer FO: Results of segmental and pancreaticosplenic transplantation with pancreaticocystostomy. Transplant Proc 17 (1): 360–362, 1985.

9. Corry RJ, Nghiem DD, Schulak JA, Bentel WD, Gonwa TA: Surgical treatment of diabetic nephropathy with simultaneous pancreatic duodenal and renal transplantation. Surg Gynecol Obstet 162(6): 547–555, 1986.

10. Dafoe DC, Campbell DA, Marks WH, Borgstrom A, Lichter AS, Turcotte JG: The effect of irradiation of the donor spleen on rejection of porcine pancreaticoduodenosplenic allografts. Transplantation (in press).

11. Land W, Landgraf R, Illner WD, Wirsching R, Jensen N, Gokel M, Castro LA, Fornara P, Burg F, Kampik A: Improved results in combined segmental pancreatic and renal transplantation in diabetic patients under cyclosporin therapy. Transplant Proc 17 (1): 317–324, 1985.

12. Traeger J, Dubernard JM, Piatti PM, Bosi E, Al Yafi S, Lefrancois N, Contarovich D, Secchi A, Gelet A, Kamel G, Monti LD, Touraine JL, Pozza G: Cyclosporin in double simultaneous pancreas plus kidney transplantation. Transplant Proc 17 (1): 336–339, 1985.

13. Khauli RB, Steinmuller DR, Novick AC, Buszta C, Goormastic M, Nakamoto S, Vidt DG, Magnusson M, Paganine E, Schreiber MJ: A critical look at survival of diabetics with end-stage renal disease. Transplantation 41(5): 598–605, 1986.

Experience of the University of Barcelona

L. FERNÁNDEZ-CRUZ, J.Mª. GIL-VERNET, J. ANDREU,
E. ESMATGES and E.M. TARGARONA

Pancreas transplantation for the treatment of diabetes mellitus has proven increasingly successful in recent years. The handling of the exocrine pancreatic secretion has been a subject of controversy. Satisfactory results have been achieved with diversion to the stomach and the intestine [1, 2]. However, one of the main problems of clinical pancreas transplantation is the lack of a reliable technique for early diagnosis of rejection, particularly in non-simultaneous pancreas and kidney transplants where the only valid parameter has been an increase in the plasma glucose concentrations. A rise in plasma glucose levels has been demonstrated to be a late indicator of pancreas allograft rejection, both experimentally and clinically [3]. Conversely, simultaneous kidney and pancreas transplantation from the same donor has the advantage of allowing the pancreas to be indirectly monitored for possible rejection by assessing kidney function through serum creatinine levels or renal biopsy.

Gliedman et al. [4] reported in 1973 their experience with five patients who underwent pancreatic grafting with ureter-pancreatic duct anastomosis for exocrine drainages. Sollinger et al. [5] published the preliminary results with the technique of pancreatico-cystostomy. Our group described [6] in 1985 the feasability of using the renal pelvis as a drainage conduit placing the graft in a paratopic position providing portal venous drainage. At the same period [7] we also described the pancreatico-ureterostomy technique in which the whole organ preserving the ampulla of Vater was anastomosed to the ureter. Recently Nghiem et al. [8] prefer the duodenocystostomy in which 10 cm long segment of duodenum is stapled at both ends and pancreatico-cystostomy is performed by making an opening at the antemesenteric border and performing a two layer anastomosis to the bladder (Table 1).

Urinary tract diversion (UTD) of the graft exocrine secretions either by pancreatico-pyelostomy (PPy), pancreatico-ureterostomy (PUr) or pancreatico-cystostomy (PCys) has the advantage of allowing exocrine pancreatic function to be assessed directly by measurement of pancreatic enzymes in the

329

J.M. Dubernard and D.E.R. Sutherland (eds.), International Handbook of Pancreas Transplantation, 329–340.
© *1989 by Kluwer Academic Publishers.*

urine [9]. Experimental studies and clinical pathological observations suggest that the acinar tissue is more sensitive than endocrine cells to rejection effector mechanisms [10]. In these pages we present the results of our clinical experience with urinary drainage and with the injection of a polymer into the ductal system.

Material and methods

Our total experience between February 1983 and November 1987 comprises 20 transplants, 16 whom were combined cadaveric renal and pancreatic transplantations, with both of the organs provided by the same donor. Four patients were non-uremic non kidney transplant diabetic patients with mild renal disease and retinopathy. The recipients were sixteen men and four women, all of whom suffered from juvenile diabetes of long standing (14 to 32 years); their age range was 29 to 54 years.

One patient underwent segmental pancreatic grafting, with the pancreatic duct injected with 4 ml of prolamine and the vessels anastomosed to the patient's iliac vessels.

In four patients, a retroperitoneal method by removal of the 12th rib was used, which permits exposure of the left kidney with its corresponding vascular pedicle. This is followed by a side peritoneal incision to expose the spleen and its vascular pedicle. Splenectomy was performed and the distal splenic artery and vein were preserved for anastomosis.

Nephrectomy had to be performed in order to use the pelvis as a drainage conduit. Pancreas graft placement involved situating the resected side at the level of the uncinate process cranially (with the main pancreatic duct and bleeding vessels on the cut surface of the pancreas oversewn) and the tail of the pancreas caudaly for pancreaticopyelostomy. Direct end-to-end vascular anastomoses between the splenic artery and vein of the graft and the splenic vessels of the recipient were performed in two cases using 6-0 Prolene (Ethicon, Scotland). In one case, end-to-end vascular anastomoses with the left renal artery and vein was performed. In another case, the splenic artery and

Table 1. History of the urinary tract diversion in clinical pancreas transplantation.

Author	Year	Technique
Gliedman et al.	1973	Segmental urether-pancreatic duct anastomosis
Sollinger et al.	1983	Segmental pancreaticocystostomy
Gil-Vernet & Fernandez-Cruz	1985	Segmental pancreaticopyelostomy
Gil-Vernet & Fernandez-Cruz	1985	Whole organ pancreaticoureterostomy
Nghiem and Corry	1987	Whole organ duodenocystostomy

the renal vein of the recipient were used for anastomosis. Following nephrectomy, exocrine secretion drainage was accomplished through the left renal pelvis, managed by preserving the retropyelic vessels. Approximately 1 cm of the tail of the pancreas was resected in order to allow exposure of the Wirsung duct. Pancreaticopyelostomy was accomplished by suturing the wall of the duct and the pancreatic capsule with the renal pelvis, using 6-0 prolene (Figure 1). A suction drain was left in place.

In five patients, the whole pancreas was transplanted without the duodenum, but preserving the sphincter of Oddi, with a circular layer of duodenal wall (Figure 2).

There are several important features in the preparation of the graft prior to transplantation. The duodenum is separated from the uncinate process and pancreatic head leaving an attachment of approximately 3 to 4 cm surrounding the ampulla of Vater. To identify the ampulla of Vater a catheter is introduced through the common bile duct into the duodenum. Then, the duodenum is opened longitudinally at the antimesenteric border and the duodenal button is tailored. The whole organ included celiac artery, intact splenic artery, common hepatic artery distal to the origin of the gastroduodenal artery, distal end of mesenteric vein, and portal vein. The whole organ graft vessels (celiac artery and portal vein) were anastomosed to the patient's right iliac artery and vena cava. Pancreaticoureterostomy was accomplished by telescoping the papilla of Vater into the ureter by means of one-layer anastomoses with interrupted 6-0 Prolene between the duodenal wall, 0.5 cm away from the edge of the papilla, and the ureter (WOPUr). The renal graft was then anastomosed to the left illiac vessels extraperitoneally. In ten patients the whole organ without the duodenum, but preserving 3 to 4 cm of duodenal wall surrounding the ampulla of Vater, was anastomosed to the anterior wall of the bladder, pancreatico-cystostomy (WOPCys). A cystostomy catheter is left in place during two weeks (Figure 3). Immunosuppression consisted of azathioprine 2.5 mg/kg/d in the group of polymer injection and PPy patients and cyclosporin 8 mg/kg/d in the WOPUr and WOPCys patients. In the group of patients with simultaneous kidney transplants, the increase in the serum creatinine level, morphological (echography), and functional studies (isotope) were used as an early determinant of rejection initiating immunosuppressive therapy. Rejection was treated with 0.25 to 1 g doses of methylprednisolone given intravenously (IV) over several days. In all patients urine amylase (U/24 h) was measured daily until the patient was discharged and monthly thereafter. Only in six patients urine lipase (U/24 h) was also measured. Renal function was monitored at frequent intervals.

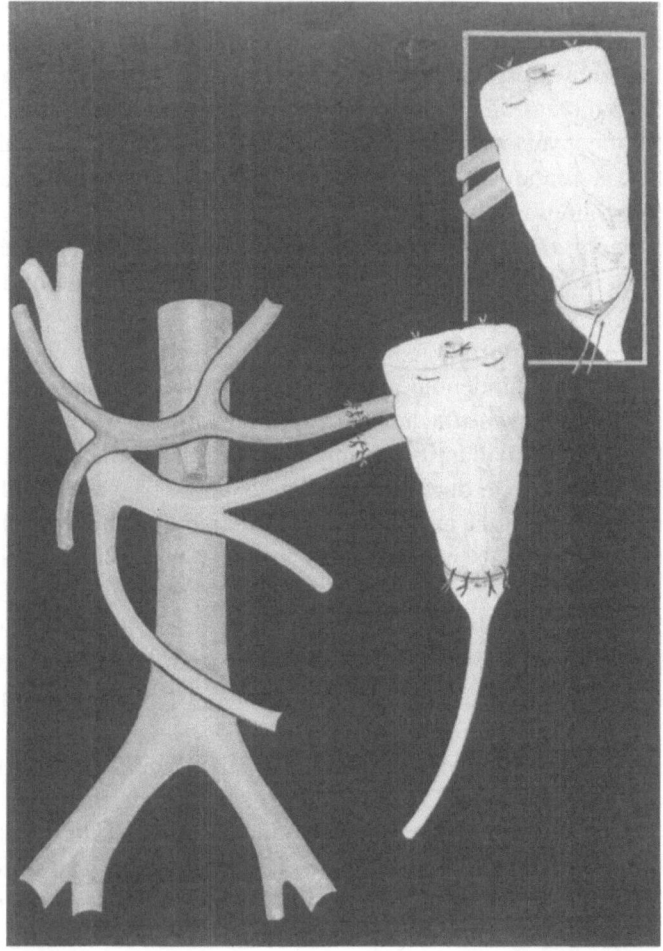

Figure 1. Pancretico-pyelostomy, vascular anastomoses between the splenic vessels of the graft with the splenic vessels of the recipient providing portal venous drainage.

Results

Endocrine function

All grafts demonstrated immediate initial function, with cessation of exogenous insulin administration. In an intravenous glucose tolerance test (25 g) performed 24 hours after transplantation, all patients had normal K values. Blood glucose fasting and postprandial levels were higher in those patients with PPy and portal venous drainage although not statistically significant compared with those drained into the systemic circulation.

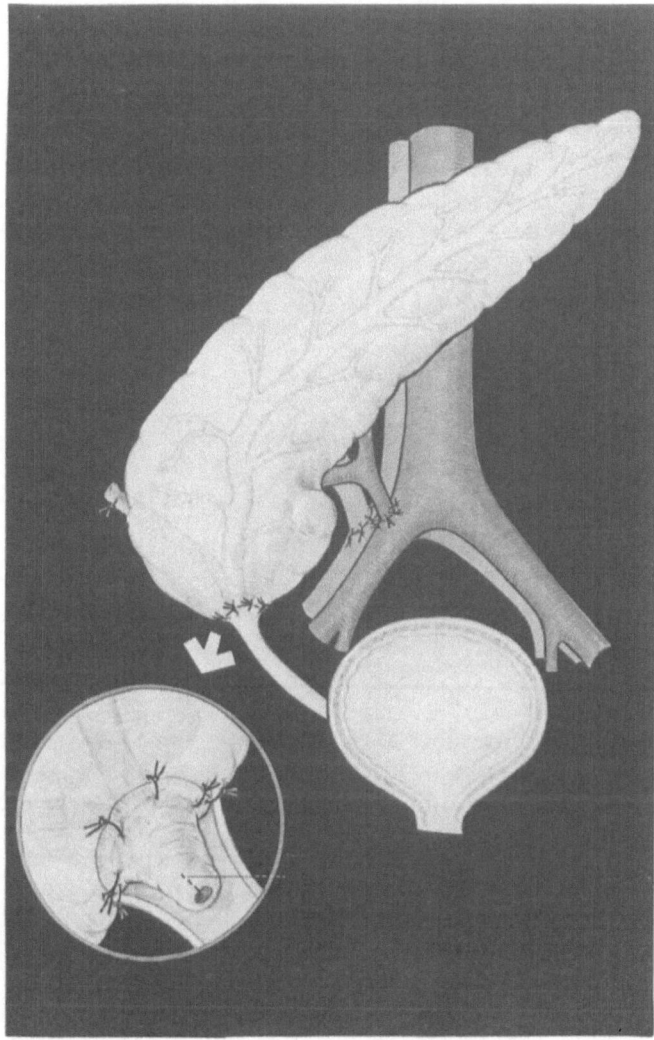

Figure 2. Whole organ and pancreatico-ureterostomy.

All techniques demonstrated long-term survival. The patient with segmental pancreas and the polymer injection is with both grafts kidney and
pancreas currently functioning for more than 5 years and four months. Patients
with segmental pancreas and PPy had the grafts functioning for a variable
period of time. One patient (54 years old) had graft vascular occlusion 1 week
after transplantation. Another patient after more than 4 months with good
functioning of kidney and pancreas grafts had a fulminant and irreversible
kidney rejection related to the patient's failure to continue the immunosuppressive drugs. Forty-one days later, the pancreas was rejected. One

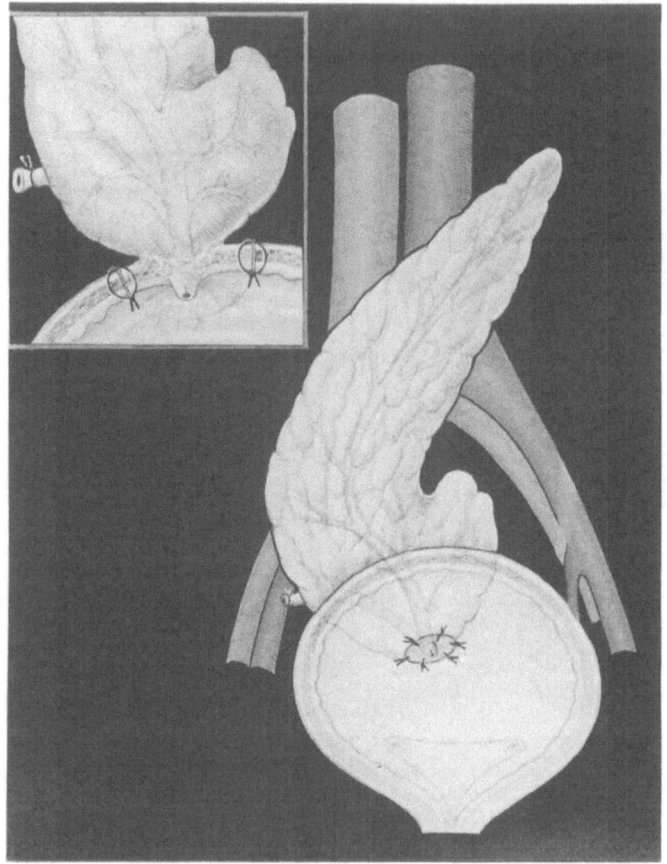

Figure 3. Whole organ and pancreatico-cystostomy.

patient died of sepsis of unknown origin with kidney and pancreas functioning 9 months after transplantation. One patient with portal venous drainage is currently with both kidney and pancreas functioning for more than 5 years and two months after transplantation.

Two death were found in the group of WOPUr patients. One patient died following an acute myocardial infarct 72 hours after transplantation. Another patient died 3 weeks after transplantation of septic shock after reoperation of partial pancreatic necrosis and ascitis. Two patients had graft failure 5 and 7 months after transplantation for immunologic reasons. A clinical picture of late graft rejection is illustrated in this example.

Patient AM had graft stabilization four weeks until 29 weeks after transplantation with a mean of UA 193,939 ± 83,665 U/24 h. He was readmitted to the hospital 30 weeks after transplantation with abdominal pain and distension and rebound tenderness. Serum amylase and lipase were clearly elevated 1,940 U (NV<200) and 507 U (NV<70), respectively. An exploratory laparotomy was indicated and the only clinical finding was an enlarged pancreatic graft with dark discoloration in the tail of the pancreas. Blood glucose remained normal and stable in spite of a significant decrease of UA (39,927 ± 23,307) and renal function was also normal. However, four weeks later the patient suffered of episodes of abdominal pain and elevations of serum pancreatic enzymes and hyperglycemia was detected requiring the reasumption of insulin (20 to 30 U). This clinical picture led to indicate pancreas transplantectomy at 46 weeks after transplantation.

In ten patients whole organ and pancreatico-cystostomy was performed. Two patients non uremic non kidney transplants patients had venous graft thrombosis. In this group of patients two had irreversible rejection 6 and 8 weeks after transplantation.

One patient had a disruption and leakage of the pancreatico-cystostomy anastomosis 3 weeks after transplantation due to severe bladder distension and dysfunction. In three patients, pancreatic graft failed for immunological reasons for periods of 1, 1, 3 months after transplantation. Two patients are currently functioning and insulin independent 28 and 42 months after transplantation.

Exocrine function

The exocrine function could be only measured in the group of patients with urinary diversion. The levels of urinary amylase into the urine each 24 hours was determined at regular intervals after transplantation ranging at the early postoperative period between 1028 and 21.683 U/24 h. A significant drop of the UA concentration occurred in 10 patients at the same time that rejection was diagnosed by means of an increase of serum creatinine levels and other morphological studies of the kidney graft. In eight patients postrejection urinary amylase reached higher values than the initial levels. The gradual increase of the urinary amylase after antirejection therapy could be the result of healing of an ischemic injury. A progressive increase and higher levels were reached after stabilization.

However, one patient with simultaneous kidney and pancreas transplantation, hyperglycemia occurred with concomitant elevated levels of urinary amylase and normal serum creatinine 3 months after transplantation. A marked decrease in urinary amylase was noted only as a late manifestation of irreversible rejection (Table 2).

Comments

Although it has been said the potential advantages of occlusion of the ductal system eliminating the exocrine part of the graft over other methods, however a high incidence of early postoperative local complications were observed [11]. In our patient with segmental graft has had 9 months, 3 and 5 years after transplantation a pancreatic pseudocyst treated successfully by percutaneous needle aspiration. This patient is currently without insulin administration for more than 5 years and 4 months after grafting. Metabolic profile showed a clear diminution of insulin levels at 5 years after transplantation. We could speculate that may be the result of progressive fibrosis induced by prolamine injection involving the islet of Langerhans (Table 3). We believe that duct injection is safe but may lead to loss of the graft in the long term as a result of severe fibrosis.

Rejection and technical complications are the leading causes of failure in clinical PTx. UTD provides an advantage for monitoring graft function and treating rejection. Animal experiments and clinical experience have shown that an increase in plasma glucose is a late indication of pancreatic rejection while a decline in urinary amylase in UTD grafts is an early indicator of

Table 2. Patient ER, 32 Yr. old (kidney and pancreas transplantation with whole organ pancreatico-cystostomy).

	Weeks after Tx	Glucose (mg/dl)	Amylase (U/day)	Creatinine (mg/dl)
Before rejection	1	105	252,207	1.4
Rejection	4	78	84,614	2.7
Graft stabilization	5–12	93	284,080 ± 62000	1.1
Rejection	13	> 400[a]	121,342	1.3[b]

[a] Resume insulin treatment.
[b] Currently functioning 9 months after Tx.

Table 3. Patient NR, 38 Yr. old (kidney and pancreas transplantation with prolamine injection). Insulin levels after OGTT-75 g glucose.

OGTT-75 g glucose	Insulin (μU/ml) (NV = $12.4 \pm 3.8 \mu$U/ml)			
	6 m	2 yrs	3 yrs	>5 yrs
0 min	24	20	19	10
60 min	63	42	155	47
90 min	87	70	113	63
120 min	155	77	104	51

rejection. Pancreatico-pyelostomy is a feasible alternative technique for the management of exocrine pancreatic secretion only in patients with end stage renal failure. The disadvantage of this method is that nephrectomy has to be performed in order to use the pelvis as a drainage conduit. The advantage is that the pancreas can be placed in a paratopic position anastomosing the splenic vessels of the graft with the splenic vessels of the recipient providing physiological portal venous drainage.

In normal individuals insulin is secreted directly into the portal vein circulation so the liver is exposed to relatively high concentration of pancreatic hormones. In the majority of clinical pancreas transplants, the venous effluent has been drained into the inferior vena cava or one of its tributaries and normoglycemia with absolutely normal glucose tolerance test results has been demonstrated in several patients with long-term functioning grafts. Systemic drainage is associated with higher blood insulin levels and the pancreas graft may have to secrete more insulin than would otherwise be required to maintain the same degree of control of carbohydrate metabolism that can be accomplished by direct discharge into the portal circulation. On the other hand it is not known the possible consequence of hyperinsulinemia in promoting or avoiding the beneficial effect of pancreas grafting in the clinical manifestations of atherosclerosis. The use of the portal circulation for venous drainage of the graft has the potential benefit to obtain normoglycemia with normal insulin levels. Portal venous drainage has been performed using the splenic vein [1, 6]

Table 4. Fasting glucose and glucose profile in patients with portal (PVD) and systemic venous drainage (SVD).

Fasting glucose (MG %)			Postprandial glucose (MG %)	
Cases	PVD	SVD	PVD	SVD
1[a]	–	109 ± 20	–	111 ± 29
2[b]	–	89 ± 21	–	149 ± 29
3[a]	–	99 ± 28	–	113 ± 10
4[a]	99,2 ± 20	–	150 ± 42	–
5	119 ± 24	–	209 ± 15	–
6[c]	–	62 ± 19	–	–
7	–	75 ± 13	–	136 ± 29
8	–	115 ± 34	–	137 ± 19
Mean ± SD	106 ± 23	96,9 ± 28	184 ± 42	96.9 ± 28
		p : NS		p : NS

[a] Number of determinations 14.

[b] Number of determinations 10.

[c] Number of determinations 2.

the superior mesenteric vein [12] and the inferior mesenteric vein [13].

In regard to metabolic studies, fasting blood glucose levels 24 hours metabolic profile and K values on IVGTT, the differences were not significant between systemic and portal drained patients (Tables 4 and 5).

The preservation of the normal anatomic and physiologic relationship between acinar and islet cell component is clearly demonstrated in one patient with a segmental graft drained into the portal venous drainage currently functioning for more than 5 years (Table 6).

Pancreaticoureterostomy has the potential advantage to avoid urine reflux into the pancreas and to keep the graft far away from the bladder usually with dysfunction and prone to bacterial contamination. Pancreaticocystostomy is less complex than the other techniques above discussed and is associated with very low morbidity.

The major disadvantage of UTD is the obligatory loss of bicarbonate from

Table 5. K-values on IVGTT in patient with portal and systemic venous drainage.

Cases	Portal venous drainage (K values)	Systemic venous drainage) (K values)
1	–	1,75
2	–	1,50
3	–	1,61
4	1,12	–
5	1,05	–
6	–	1,26
7	–	1,30
8	–	1,65
Mean ± SD	1,08 ± 0,04	1,50 ± 0,19
	$p < 0,05$	

Table 6. Patient CC, 30 Yr. old. Urinary amylase values until 5 years after transplantation.

	Weeks after Tx	Amylasa (U/24 hs)
Before rejection	1	3375 ± 1634
Rejection	1	973
After rejection	2–3	3880 ± 2723
	Years after Tx	
	1	76817 ± 10900
	2	86665 ± 20927
	3	100018 ± 19645
	4	97106 ± 20114
	5	88228 ± 15720

Table 7. Metabolic profile of pancreatic transplants recipients with urinary tract diversion.

	Patients		
	1	2	3
Period of renal dysfunction (weeks after Tx)	5–20	2–6	1–4
Mean S. creatinine (mg/dl)	2,55	1,98	1,73
Mean HCO_3 (mEq/l)	15,4	16,43	20,46
Mean pH	7,35	7,20	7,28
Mean S. glucose (mg/dl)	70 ± 15	85 ± 11	98 ± 4
Mean U. amylase (U/day)	$293,328 \pm 120,412$	$139,313 \pm 64,000$	$199,750 \pm 78,310$
Oral bicarbonate (daily)	9–21 gr	3–9 gr	3–9 gr

the pancreas graft resulting in a metabolic acidosis particularly during periods of renal dysfunction from allograft rejection as we have seen in three of our patients (Table 7).

References

1. Brons IGM, Calne RY, Rolles K, Olczak S, Evans DB: Paratopic segmental pancreas with simultaneous kidney transplantation in man: a 1 year follow-up study. Transplant Proc 18: 1129, 1986.
2. Tyden G, Mellgren A, Brattström C, Ost L, Gunnarsson R, Ostman J, Groth CG: Stockholm experience with 32 combined renal and segmental pancreatic transplants. Transplant Proc 18: 1114, 1986.
3. Prieto M, Sutherland DER, Fernández-Cruz L, Heil J, Najarian J: Urinary amylase monitoring for early diagnosis of pancreas allograft rejection in dogs. J Surg Res 40: 597–604, 1986.
4. Gliedman M.L., Gold M, Whittacker J, Rifkin H, Soberman R, Selwyn F, Tellis V, Veith F: Clinical segmental pancreatic transplantation with ureter-pancreatic duct anastomosis for exocrine drainage. Surgery 74: 171, 1973.
5. Sollinger HW, Kamps D, Cook K, Warner T, Belzer FO: Results of segmental and pancreatico-splenic transplantation with pancreatico-cystostomy. Transplant Proc 15: 2997, 1983.
6. Gil-Vernet JM, Fernández-Cruz L, Andreu J, Figuerola D, Caralps A: Clinical experience with pancreaticopyelostomy for exocrine pancreatic drainage and portal venous drainage in pancreas transplantation. Transplant Proc 17: 342, 1985.
7. Gil-Vernet JM, Fernández-Cruz L, Caralps A, Andreu J, Figuerola D: Whole organ and pancreaticoureterostomy in clinical pancreas transplantation. Transplant Proc 17: 2019, 1985.
8. Nghiem DD, Gouwa TA, Corry RJ: Metabolic effects of urinary diversion of exocrine secretions in pancreas transplantation. Transplantation 43: 70, 1987.
9. Gil-Vernet JM, Fernández-Cruz L, Andreu J, Figuerola D, Caralps A: Urinary tract diversion in clinical pancreas transplantation. Transplant Proc 18: 1132, 1986.
10. Prieto M, Sutherland DER, Fernández-Cruz L, Heil J, Najarian J: Experimental and clinical experience with urine amylase monitoring for early diagnosis of rejection in pancreas transplantation. Transplantation 43: 73, 1987.

11. Tyden G, Wilczek H, Lundren G, Ostman J: Experience with 21 intraperitoneal segmental pancreatic transplants with enteric or gastric exocrine diversion in humans. Transplant Proc 17: 331, 1985.
12. Landgraf R, Landgraf-Leurs MMC, Burg D, Kampik A, Castro LA, Abendroth A, Illner WD, Land W: Long-term follow-up of segmental pancreas transplantation in type I diabetics. Transplant Proc 18: 1118, 1986.
13. Sutherland DER, Goetz FC, Mondry KC, Abouna GM, Najarian JS: Use of recipient mesenteric vessels for revascularization of segmental pancreatic grafts: technical and metabolic considerations. Transplant Proc 19: 2300, 1987.

Experience of the University of Birmingham, Queen Elizabeth Hospital, Edgbaston, Birmingham, UK

B.K. GUNSON and P. McMASTER

Pancreas transplantation in Birmingham

In Birmingham the policy has been to consider all uraemic diabetics in the renal failure programme for combined pancreas and kidney transplantation. A detailed evaluation is made of each patient before accepting them onto the transplant waiting list. This includes cardiovascular, autonomic function and social assessments. The patients selected for transplantation have all suffered from various diabetic complications such as retinopathy, neuropathy and cardiovascular problems.

Techniques

Eighteen combined pancreas and kidney transplants have been performed since 1981 in 10 males and 8 females aged between 13 and 52 (mean 35 years) who had been diabetic for between 3 and 29 years (mean 18 years) and who all had various complications of their disease (Table 1). The organs were harvested from the same donor, the kidneys usually being removed prior to a detailed dissection of the pancreas whilst the circulation was still intact. Sixteen of the 18 grafts were segmental, and two whole pancreatic grafts were implanted incorporating the head of the pancreas, with revascularisation of the coeliac

Table 1. Diabetic complications.

18 transplant patients	
Hypertension	94%
Myocardial	78%
Retinal	83%
Peripheral vascular	61%
Neuropathic	50%
Dialysis	100%

341

J.M. Dubernard and D.E.R. Sutherland (eds.), International Handbook of Pancreas Transplantation, 341–344.
© 1989 by Kluwer Academic Publishers.

axis and supermesenteric artery. A distal arteriovenous fistula was created in the last 8 patients in order to reduce the incidence of vascular thrombosis.

The highly purified latex polymer Polyisoprene was injected to occlude the ducts, 4 to 6 cc being introduced at a low pressure. The cold ischaemic time of the pancreas graft was less than six hours in all cases.

The recipient operation commenced immediately after the renal transplant. In 13 patients the pancreas was placed intraperitoneally, in the rest it was placed extraperitoneally. Postoperative monitoring included hourly blood glucose measurements with insulin injections if necessary. Constant infusions of heparin (5000 units/8 hours) and Trasylol (200.000 units/8 hours) were given. Daily monitoring of rejection in the first few weeks was based on fasting and post-prandial blood glucoses, serum C-peptide levels and Indium-111 labelled platelet accumulation. This last technique, which was developed in Birmingham, utilises radioactively tagged autologous platelets to monitor the development of rejection and/or thrombosis in the transplanted organs by both qualitative and quantitative methods [1]. Immunosuppression was based on cyclosporin A in conjunction with low dose steroids (20 mg prednisolone/ day). The cyclosporin was given in a tapering dose starting with 15 mg/kg/day orally, with either reductions or increments depending upon drug levels in the blood. These were monitored by a whole blood radioimmunoassay (Sandoz).

Results

The one year patient survival following combined grafting is 78%. Ten patients are currently alive. The causes of death in the other 8 patients are outlined in Table 2. In 5 cases the pancreas was functioning up until the time of death. The patient dying of undiagnosed malignant lymphoma at 2 years had good pancreatic and renal function, and the patient dying of an acute subdural haemorrhage at 5 years still had good pancreas function although the kidney had been rejected at 4 years.

Graft survival

The one year pancreatic graft survival is 39% with seven grafts functioning for more than one year, five of these for more than two years. The longest

Table 2. Causes of death in 8 patients receiving combined kidney and pancreas transplants.

2	Infection (3 and 10 months)
5	Cardiovascular (1 and 5 months, 2, $2^{1}/_{2}$ and 5 years)
1	Lymphoma (2 years)

surviving graft lasted for more than 5 years in the patient who died from an acute subdural haemorrhage.

Two pancreases are currently functioning, both at $3^1/_2$ years. One patient has excellent renal and pancreatic function and leads a normal life, the other patient has a functioning pancreatic graft, but her kidney failed at 3 years. Three further renal grafts are still working at 4,6 and $6^1/_2$ years. Two patients who lost both grafts have each received another kidney which are functioning well. The causes of pancreatic graft failure are summarised in Table 3.

Primary vascular thrombosis of the pancreas grafts occurred in 4 of the first 10 grafts despite the administration of intravenous heparin. In an effort to increase perfusion a distal arteriovenous fistula has been created in the last 8 patients via the donor portal vein and the recipient coeliac access. None of these patients have had a vascular thrombosis.

Graft losses from presumed rejection have occurred in three cases presenting with features of rising blood glucose and a diffuse accumulation of radiolabelled platelets in the graft. One patient had a transplant nephrectomy for his severely rejected graft and had the pancreatic graft removed at the same time despite the fact it was still functioning moderately well because it was felt that he would fare better without immunosuppression. In 3 patients the most likely cause of their late graft failure was progressive sclerosis. In animals it has been shown that the technique of direct ductal injection leads to progressive fibrosis and reduction in the endocrine function of the pancreatic graft [2].

Morbidity

The most serious concern has been the possibility of peritoneal leakage arising from incomplete occlusion of the pancreatic duct (Table 4). Minor seepages of

Table 3. Causes of pancreatic graft failure.

4	Thrombosis	4, 7, 7, 14 days
3	Rejection	4 weeks, 3 and 4 months
3	Fibrosis	14, 14 and 40 months
5	Death	1, 3 and 10 months, 2 and 5 years
1	Other	6 weeks

Table 4. Post-operative morbidity.

4	Wound infection
4	Haemorrhage
5	Peritoneal leak
6	Peritoneal infection

amylase rich fluid have occurred in a number of patients but this has only created significant problems in three. In one patient a persistent peritoneal leak was associated with other infective complications leading ultimately to death. In several cases peritoneal infection followed implantation of the pancreas into the peritoneal cavity. Seventeen patients were on CAPD prior to transplantation, and significant infection occurred in the one patient who required peritoneal dialysis following the operation. Following this, it is no longer the policy to carry out peritoneal dialysis posttransplantation and haemodialysis is performed if necessary.

Carbohydrate control

In patients with functioning pancreas grafts, good carbohydrate control was achieved and insulin was not required although the response to oral glucose tolerance tests remained somewhat delayed and flattened compared with normal. This is probably partly due to the position and dernevation of the pancreas grafts with the resulting delay in insulin response to the glucose stimulus.

Conclusions

These results partly relect the quality of patients coming to combined kidney and pancreas grafting, many being blind or suffering from other complications such as cardiac and peripheral vascular disease. Perhaps the trend should now move towards earlier pancreas grafting of diabetics before the full-house of diabetic complications sets in. Thanks to improved techniques in grafting and better handling of immunosuppressive drugs and their side effects, this now looks more feasible. For the uraemic diabetic with poor cardiovascular function, a kidney transplant alone might be a more realistic proposition.

References

1. Jurewicz WA, Buckels JAC, Dykes JGA, Chandler ST, Gunson BK, Hawker RJ, McCollum CN, McMaster P: Brit J Surg 72: 228–231, 1985.
2. Gooszen HG, Bosman FT, van Schilfgaarde R: Transplant Proc 16 (3): 776–777, 1984.

Experience of the University of Louvain Medical School, Brussels, Belgium

J.P. SQUIFFLET

Since March 1982, any patient with Type I diabetes and pre or end-stage renal failure (creatinine clearance less than 20 ml/min), severe retinopathy and neuropathy, and not having a living (un)related kidney donor was considered as a potential candidate for pancreas and kidney cadaver transplantation [1]. A negative T-cell cross-match with the donor cells was an absolute prerequisit for transplantation; the HLA-Matching was not taken in consideration but usual ABO-compatibility was requested. The pancreatic graft was segmental (body and tail) in all patients except in the last five patients who received a whole pancreatico-duodenal graft. All grafts were preserved by Euro-Collins' solution or Silica Gel Filtered Plasma (SGF – Minneapolis) and implanted through a midline incision in the peritoneal cavity [2].

The exocrine secretion was diverted into either the bowel by performing and end-to-end pancreaticojejunostomy in a Roux-en-Y loop for the segmental grafts (Figure 1) or the bladder, with a side-to-side duodenocystostomy for the whole grafts (Figure 2). In the jejunal diversion recipients the duct was stented with a catheter which was brought outside through the intestine and the abdominal wall, allowing external collection of the pancreatic graft secretions during the period of anastomosis healing. A renal graft coming from the same donor was implanted simultaneously in the pelvis – the heterolateral iliac fossa – through a flanc incision in all cases. Cyclosporin was used in combination with azathioprine, prednisolone and antilymphocyte globulins (Pressimum, Behring, Marburg, West-Germany), or rabbit antithymocyte globulins (ATG, Fresenius, West-Germany). Monoclonal antibodies (OKT3, Orthoclone, Cilag, New-Jersey) were used for the treatment of rejection crises episodes in three cases. The postoperative management was identical in all recipients and reported elsewhere [3]; briefly, it included low doses of heparin and rheo-macrodex® for ten days, total parenteral nutrition with insulin therapy in order to avoid any stimulation of the pancreatic graft and to maintain the plasma glucose levels lower than 160 mg/dl.

Between November 20th, 1982, and December 1986, ten patients (mean

345

J.M. Dubernard and D.E.R. Sutherland (eds.), International Handbook of Pancreas Transplantation, 345–351.
© *1989 by Kluwer Academic Publishers.*

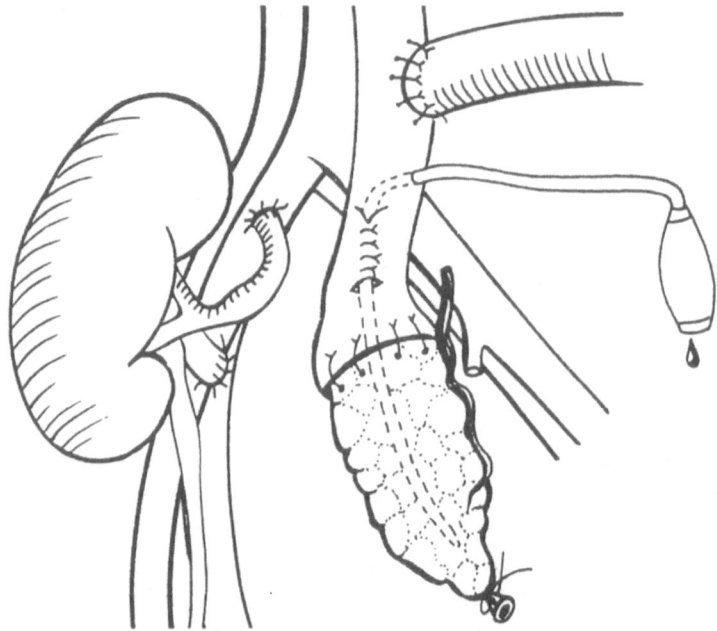

Figure 1. First technique of simultaneous kidney and pancreas transplantation at the university of Louvain. The enteric drainage (pancreaticojejunostomy on a Roux-en-Y loop) of the segmental pancreatic graft is performed through a midline incision.

age ± S.D.: 36.3 ± 6.9 years) underwent a simultaneous renal and pancreas transplantation with enteric diversion of the segmental graft; one patient (case no 2) received two successive pancreatic grafts (Table 1). Seven patients were on chronic hemodialysis at the time of transplantation and 3 in pre-end-stage renal failure (cases no 2, 3, 5). Three patients died (cases no 2, 6, 9) during the postoperative course: the first one, 38 years old, died on day 12 after his second pancreas transplantation from metabolic disorders following ischemic bowel disease; the second one, 51 years old, died on day 38 from a gram negative septic shock; finally, the third one, 42 years old, died on day 56 from a CMV encephalitis. The pancreas and kidney grafts of these 3 patients were functioning at the time of death.

Currently, 6 patients (cases no 1, 3, 4, 5, 7, 8) are alive with a functioning renal graft in all of them (mean serum creatinine ± S.D.: 1.47 ± 0.75 mg/dl); rejection at 2 months of both organs led to a double transplantectomy in one patient (case no 10) who died from a myocardial infarct two months after dialysis was resumed. Four patients (cases no 3, 5, 7, 8) were insulin independent on May 1988 (follow-up: 54, 38, 28 and 27 months) (Table 1 and Figure 3). Another patient (case no 1) was insulin independent during 2 years; progressive deterioration of pancreas endocrine function necessitated resumption of

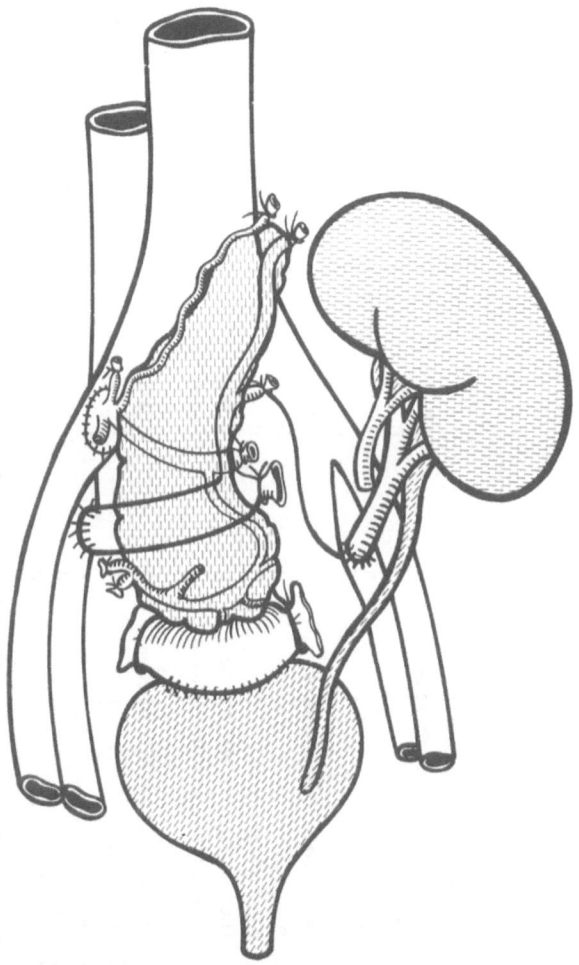

Figure 2. Second technique of simultaneous kidney and pancreas transplantation at the university of Louvain. The bladder drainage (duodenocystostomy) of the whole pancreatic graft is performed through a midline incision.

insulin therapy (20 units per day) although renal graft function has remained normal (follow-up: 65 months). The last patient (case no 4) was never off insulin therapy after transplantation (follow-up: 50 months). Patient no 8 underwent a successful pregnancy and delivered a normal baby girl 19 months after transplantation [4].

Since January 1987, the technique of pancreas grafting was modified: five patients received simultaneously a kidney and a whole pancreaticoduodenal graft with a duodenocystostomy (Figure 2). Unfortunately, the first one died from a CMV pulmonary infection on day 52; both grafts were functioning at

Table 1. Recipient's data and outcome – pancreas and kidney current function.

Case	Diabetes duration (yrs)	Transplantation			Follow-up (months)	Outcome			
		Date	Age	Type of graft		Pancreas rejection	Insulin	Kidney rejection	Creatinine
1	26	11/82	29	P + K S PJ	Alive (65)	0	20 U/d	1	1.2 mg/dl
2a	26	2/83	37	P S	Immediate transplantectomy				
2b	27	7/83	38	P + K S PJ	Died on day 12 (metabolic disorder)	0	DWGF	1	DWFG
3	16	10/83	30	P + K S PJ	Alive (54)	0	0	1	1.22 mg/dl
4	19	2/84	39	P + K S PJ	Alive (50)	0	14 U/d since Tx	1	0.96 mg/dl
5	31	2/85	34	P + K S PJ	Alive (38)	0	0	3	3 mg/dl
6	47	5/85	51	P + K S PJ	Died on day 38 (septic shock)	0	DWFG	1	DWGF
7	13	12/85	36	P + K S PJ	Alive (28)	0	0	1	1.23 mg/dl
8	23	1/86	28	P + K S PJ	Alive (pregnancy) (27)	0	0	1	1.23 mg/dl
9	28	5/86	42	P + K S PJ	Died on day 56 (CMV infection)	0	DWGF	0	DWGF
10	24	7/86	37	P + K S PJ	Double transplantectomy on day 65	1	32 U/d	3	died on dialysis on day 126
11	24	1/87	36	P + K W DC	Died on day 52 (CMV infection)	0	DWGF	2	DWGF
12	28	5/87	37	P + K W DC	Alive (12)	0	0	1	1.42 mg/dl
13	25	6/87	36	P + K W DC	Alive (11)	1	0	2	1.08 mg/dl
14	21	4/88	28	P + K W DC	Alive (1)	0	0	2	1.3 mg/dl
15	26	5/88	42	P + K W DC	Alive (2 weeks)	0	0	0	1.1 mg/dl

P = Pancreas, K = Kidney, S = Segmental Graft, W = Whole pancreas graft, PJ = Pancreaticojejunostomy, DC = Duodenocystostomy, DWFG = Died with functioning graft, Tx = Transplantectomy, CMV = Cytomegalovirus.

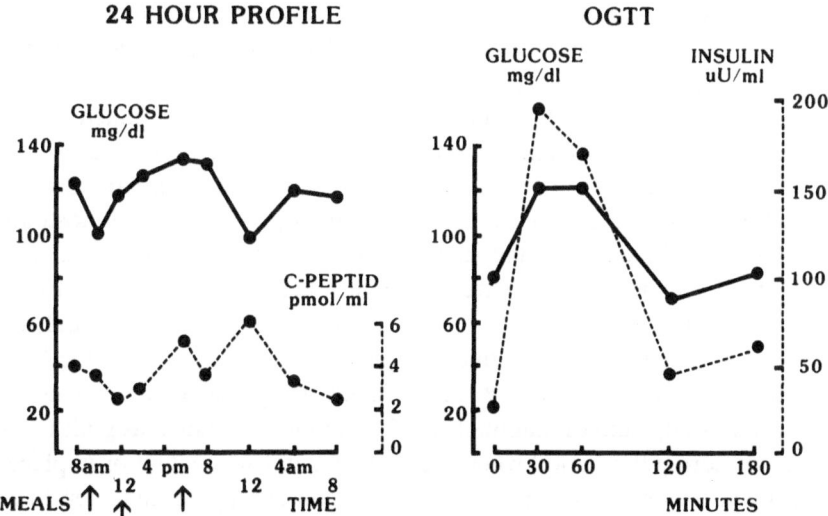

Figure 3. Results of (A) 24 hour metabolic profile and (B) oral glucose tolerance test in a patient who has been insulin independent for 4 years since pancreas transplantation.

the time of death (no insulin and 1 mg/dl of creatinine level) although the immunosuppressive therapy had been withdrawn 3 weeks before death. Four patients are currently alive (12, 11, 1 months and 2 weeks) with both functioning grafts (cases 12, 13, 14, and 15). Patient no 13 presented an isolated pancreas rejection crises which was diagnosed based upon a significant fall in urine amylases without any sign of renal rejection.

Comments

The results encountered at a single Institution with a starting program in pancreas transplantation are moreless similar to those of the corresponding groups from the Registry data [5]. This experience however allows us to bring some further informations.

The first one is concerning the donor selection: during the first pancreas transplantation in case no 2, it happened that the graft remained poorly vascularized due to an interstitial hemorragic pancreatitis which was unnoticed in the donor. That observation suggests that pretransplant histological examination might be usefull to detect subclinical graft pancreatitis in the donor [6]. The second information is concerning the implantation technique in the recipient. The more physiologic approach of diverting the pancreatic juice into the jejunum does not offer only advantages. Firstly, it activates the pancreatic enzymes and leads to partial leakage of the pancreaticojejunostomy in some of our patients: a peripancreatic infected fluid collection was drained through the rectum in patient no 4 while surgical reoperations – with a second look on the suture line – were necessary in patients no 6, 9 and 10. That happened few days after the catheter stented the pancreatic duct of Wirsung was pulled out or concommittently to a rejection treatment. Perhaps undergoing pancreatic rejection, which is often a vascular type [7] leads to partial pancreatic vascular thrombosis, necrosis and than leakage. Secondly, the pancreaticojejunostomy offers long term risk of endocrine function loss: indeed, in patient no 1, insulin therapy was resumed 2 years after combined kidney and pancreas transplantation, with no sign of chronic rejection of the renal graft. This partial loss of pancreatic function might be due to a progressive obstruction of the Wirsung duct leading to fibrosis of the gland. Finally, the pancreaticojejunostomy does not allow any kind of immunological monitoring of pancreas graft function except during the period when the duct catheter was patent or in place. Surprisingly, only renal rejection crises were seen during the same period of time with no striking modifications in the pancreas fluid content. By contrast, the exocrine secretion diversion into the bladder avoids some of the pancreaticojejunostomy disadvantages. Our experience with the last five patients consolidates that hypothesis. Even if our results are preliminary, we noticed that this technique is simplier – at least for the recipient's operation – and safer.

All five pancreases implanted according to that technique had well functioned, although patient no 11 died from a CMV pulmonary infection. The most interesting advantage is the possible detection of rejection by the dosage of the amylases content in the urine. A significant drop in amylasuria signes a rejection crises and allows effective therapy with complete recover of the pancreatic graft [7]. With that type of monitoring, we feel more confident to consider pancreas transplantation alone in absence of chronic renal failure.

Acknowledgements

To Dr. G.P.J. Alexandre (Chairman of the Department of Transplantation), Dr. M. Carlier, Dr. F. Veyckmanns (Department of Anaesthesiology), Dr. P. Mahieu, Dr. M. Reynaert (Intensive Care Units), Dr. J. Rahier (Department of Pathology), Dr. B. Vandeleene (Department of Diabetology), and Dr. Y. Pirson (Department of Nephrology) who participated in the patients' management.
To Miss B. François for secretarial assistance.

References

1. Squifflet JP, Gianello P, Pirson Y et al: Nine human pancreas transplants: results and management. Digestive Surg 9: 77, 1986.
2. Squifflet JP, Vandeleene B, Rahier J et al: In situ rather than ex-vivo euro-collins perfusion of cadaveric segmental pancreatic graft? Transplant Proc 16: 130, 1984.
3. Squifflet JP, Carlier M, Pirson Y et al: Six human pancreas transplants: Results and perioperative management. Acta Anaesth Belg 37: 107, 1986.
4. Tyden G, Brattstrom C, Bjorkman U et al: Pregnancy following combined renal and pancreatic transplantation: 4 successful cases at 4 different centers. Diabetes: in press, 1988.
5. Sutherland DER, Moudry K: Pancreas transplant registry report – 1986. Clinical Transplantation 1: 3, 1987.
6. Squifflet JP, Rahier J, Vandeleene B et al: The need of pretransplant pathologic examination in cadaver donor segmental pancreas transplantation. Transplant Proc 16: 677, 1984.
7. Prieto M, Sutherland DER, Fernandez-Cruz L et al: Rejection in pancreas transplantation. Transplant Proc 19: 2348, 1987.

Experience of the University of Cambridge Clinical School, Department of Surgery, Addenbrooke's hospital, Cambridge, England

I.G.M. BRONS and R.Y. CALNE

The introduction of the powerful immunosuppressive drug cyclosporin A (CyA) [1] as well as a new surgical technique to deal with the exocrine secretion [2] renewed interest in pancreatic transplantation. Since then several new or modified techniques of transplanting whole or segmental pancreatic tissue have been employed worldwide. In our Unit in Cambridge five different surgical techniques have been used over the last nine years, results of which are reported here (Table 1 and 2).

The ablation of exocrine secretion by the injection of neoprene into the pancreatic duct of the donor pancreas results in atrophy and fibrosis of the acinar tissue but preserves the endocrine part of the pancreas [2]. In view of the encouraging results in kidney transplantation with CyA as a steroid sparing and effective immunosuppressant and the technique of duct injection a pancreas transplantation program was started. Ten insulin-dependent diabetic patients were transplanted with segmental pancreata placed in the groin using the iliac vessels for revascularisation. The donor pancreata were injected with 1–2 ml of latex, polyisoprene, or Ethibloc. Seven patients in renal failure also

Table 1. Cambridge experience of segmental pancreas transplantation. August 1979 to May 1988.

	Patients	Re-transpl.	Pancreatic function		Additional allografts			
			Part	Full	Kidney function		Liver function	
Heterotopic								
Duct occlusion	10	1	–	1	7	–	1	1
Roux-loop	6	1	1	1	5	2	–	–
Bladder	2	–	–	–	2	–	–	–
Paratopic								
Stomach	20	–	2	6	18	8	1	1
Roux-loop	1	–		1	1	1	–	–
Total number	39	2	3	9	33	11	2	2

J.M. Dubernard and D.E.R. Sutherland (eds.), International Handbook of Pancreas Transplantation, 353–357.
© 1989 by Kluwer Academic Publishers.

received kidney grafts and one patient with cirrhosis was given a liver graft from the same donor. CyA was the sole immunosuppressant [3].

Of ten patients transplanted one has not required exogenous insulin for nearly 9 years although her kidney graft was rejected after $2^1/_2$ years. The pancreas of the patient with an additional liver allograft ceased to function after 11 months for no apparent reason, no rejection signs were seen in the liver, which is still functioning well after 9 years. The pancreatic graft function of the other patients ranged from 6 weeks to 20 months. The very sudden loss of function in some patients, without any evidence of rejection in coexisting kidney or liver grafts suggested that severe fibrosis induced by the duct occlusion technique may have led to the deterioration of islet cell function.

We therefore attempted a different approach to deal with the exocrine secretory function of the gland by drainage of pancreatic juice into a Roux-y-loop of small intestine, a technique pioneered by Groth et al. [4]. This technique preserves the architecture of the pancreas but can lead to infections since the Roux loop lies like a sump with gravity acting against drainage of exocrine fluid.

Of seven insulin-dependent diabetic patients who were transplanted by this method, one has good function in both his pancreatic and renal allografts for over almost 5 years being well rehabilitated and leading a normal life. Another patient had good pancreatic function for $3^1/_2$ years but then acutely required some supplementary exogenous insulin treatment. His renal function is excellent and fasting c-peptide levels are between 1 and 2 nmol/l. The other patients had good pancreatic function for 1–8 months.

A different technique for exocrine drainage was employed in two insulin-dependent diabetic patients in renal failure. The pancreatic segment and the kidney from the same donor were transplanted heterotopically into the groin on either side and revascularised from the iliac vessels. The exocrine system was drained into the bladder. Due to severe CMV infection and local haemorrhage the still functioning pancreas was removed one month later in the first

Table 2. Paratopic segmental pancreas transplantation in man. January 1984 to June 1988.

Outcome	Number of cases	Duration of function
Thrombosis	6	for up to 14 days
Sepsis	3	10 days, 6 months, 9 months
Rejection	2	$3^1/_2$ years, 16 months
Brainhaemorrhage	1	3 years
Part function	2	reduced exogenous insulin for >4 years
Full function	7	>4 years, >$3^1/_2$ years, >3 years, >$2^1/_2$ years, >1 year, >6 weeks, >5 weeks
Total number	21	

patient but he died from generalised CMV infection 2 weeks later. There was a question whether the cytomegalo virus was transfered from the donor tissue. We now try to match patients for their CMV status so that CMV negative patients will not receive CMV positive donor tissue.

The other patient was transplanted according to the Gothenburg technique [5]. She rejected her kidney graft 2 months later but despite high dose steroid treatment her pancreatic segment functioned well for over 7 months. The graft thrombosed after a second kidney transplant was grafted. Histological sections showed a freshly infarcted graft with both endocrine and exocrine tissue in excellent condition with no signs of rejection.

In January 1984 a new technique of transplanting the pancreas was developed in our Unit [6]. Usually the endocrine secretion is drained into the systemic circulation when the pancreas is transplanted heterotopically rather than physiologically into the portal system. In the new surgical procedure the pancreatic segment consisting of the tail, body and part of the neck, is transplanted between the stomach and the spleen, close to the patients own pancreas in the 'so-called' paratopic position. The segment is vascularized by the recipients splenic vessels. This physiological approach allows portal venous drainage of the endocrine secretion. The pancreatic duct is anastomosed to the mucosa of the stomach. This viscus provides a low bacterial background and the digestive pancreatic enzymes are not activated by the low pH of the gastric fluid [7]. In contrast to the urinary drainage technique chronic metabolic acidosis does not occur.

Twentyone insulin-dependent diabetic patients with severe microangiopathy have been transplanted with this new technique; nineteen patients were in renal failure and a kidney from the same donor was transplanted simultaneously. One patient with chronic liver disease received simultaneously a liver from the same donor. Immunosuppression was CyA intravenously for 2 to 4 days at 4 mg/kg/day and then orally at 17 mg/kg/day reducing the dose to achieve a blood level of 400 to 800 ng/ml. A new monoclonal antibody, Campath 1 [8], was given intravenously during the first 10 days in the first 14 patients. This complement fixing antibody is active against human mature T and B lymphocytes. The other patients received triple therapy consisting of prednisolone, azathioprene and CyA. As it is too hazardous to biopsy the pancreatic graft in the paratopic position in order to assess rejection, the additional grafts served as a monitor. On the basis of deteriorating function in the accompanying grafts and subsequent biopsy results rejection episodes were treated with bolus doses of steroids. No attempt was made to match for histocompatibility and therefore in all but one case with a 'full house match' the degree of matching was poor.

Postoperatively all patients recovered well and did not require exogenous insulin. Six patients lost their initial function due to postoperative thrombosis around day 10 and their pancreatic grafts were removed. The kidney graft survival in five of these patients ranged from 5, 9, 12, 15 to 24 months. Three patients died with functioning allografts: one from peritonitis due to leakage of pancreatic and gastric juice 10 days postoperatively; two patients died at 6 and 9 months from sepsis and pneumocystis pneumonia respectively.

Partial loss of pancreatic function was seen in two patients at 8 and 14 months post transplant. Renal function was good in both patients with normal creatinine levels and no other diseases were apparent. Postprandial serum c-peptide levels were shown to be reduced by about 60% when compared with previous post transplant levels. Exogenous insulin treatment was reinstituted but at a lower dosage than pretransplantation. Both these patients have good renal function at over 4 years. The reason for this reduced pancreatic function is not known but the possibility of recurrence of the original diabetic disease can not be excluded.

One patient rejected her kidney graft at 17 months after several severe rejection episodes, which were treated with high dose steroids and finally her pancreatic graft ceased effective function. A second kidney graft is functioning well under conventional immunosuppressive treatment. Rejection of the kidney occurred in another patient after $2^1/_2$ years of good function. The pancreas functioned well throughout. The rejected kidney graft was removed one year later and within 3 weeks the pancreatic function deteriorated. The patient is now back on exogenous insulin treatment after $3^1/_2$ years of independence and normoglycemia.

Of nineteen patients transplanted with pancreas and kidney grafts, seven have full function in both their pancreatic and renal allografts at over 4, $3^1/_2$, 3, $2^1/_2$ and one year. Two patients were transplanted 3 and 2 weeks ago. The patients are well rehabilitated, on normal diets and enjoying life to the full. One patient became pregnant 27 months post transplantation and delivered a healthy baby girl at 35 weeks gestation. Both allografts responded well and in a physiological way to the added stress of the pregnancy [9].

The clinical post transplant follow up of metabolic function showed normal day to day fasting blood glucose values and 24 hour metabolic profiles with virtually normal glucose control. HbA1 values returned to normal shortly after transplantation. Oral glucose tolerance tests (OGTT) showed near normal glucose tolerance in most patients and were similar to non-diabetic patients with partial pancreatico-duodenectomy (identical amount of pancreatic tissue and exocrine drainage). Fasting serum c-peptide levels were increased in all patients with a co-existing kidney allograft when compared with healthy volunteers. Similarly elevated levels were found in non-diabetic kidney-transplanted patients with slightly impaired renal function with raised serum creatinine values. Serum insulin levels fasting and during oral glucose tolerance tests were found to range within the values of healthy volunteers. Thus, in contrast to heterotopic pancreas transplantation or conventional insulin therapy, peripheral hyperinsulinaemia was not seen. The rapid first pass hepatic metabolism of insulin drained into the portal circulation by the paratopic procedure contributes to the more physiological peripheral insulin levels.

The progression of secondary lesions of diabetes mellitus like retinopathy and neuropathy and the improvement of some of the reversible damages awaits assessment in patients with longer-term functioning pancreas transplants in the paratopic position. This technique has improved our previous results of segmental pancreas transplantation and we will continue our programme with this technique.

References

1. Calne RY, Rolles K, White DJG et al: Cyclosporin A initially as the only immunosuppressant in 34 recipients of cadaveric organs: 32 kidneys, 2 pancreases and 2 livers. Lancet ii: 1033–1036, 1979.
2. Dubernard JM, Traeger J, Neyra P, Touraine JL, Tranchant D, Blanc-Brunat N: A new method of preparation of segmental pancreatic grafts for transplantation: trials in dogs and in man. Surgery 84: 633–639, 1978.
3. Brons IGM, Calne RY: Transplantation of the pancreas in man. Hormone and Metabolic Research 13: 81–84, 1983.
4. Groth CG, Collste H, Lundgren G et al: Successful outcome of segmental human pancreatic transplantation with enteric exocrine diversion after modification in technique. Lancet ii: 522–524, 1982.
5. Frisk B, Hedman L, Brynger H: Pancreaticocystostomy with a two layer anastomosis technique in human segmental pancreas transplantation. Transplantation 44, 6: 836–837, 1987.
6. Calne RY: Paratopic segmental pancreas grafting: a technique with portal venous drainage. Lancet i: 595–597, 1984.
7. Brons IGM, Calne RY, Rolles K, Williams PF, Fishwick NG, Evans DB: Glucose control after segmental pancreas with simultaneous kidney transplantation. Trans Proc 19, 3: 2288–2289, 1987.
8. Hale G, Bright S, Chumbley G, Hoang T, Metcalfe D, Munro AJ, Waldmann H: Removal of T-cells from bone marrow for transplantation. A monoclonal antilymphocyte antibody with fixed human complement. Blood 62: 873–882, 1983.
9. Calne RY, Brons IGM, Williams PF et al: Successful pregnancy after paratopic segmental pancreas and kidney transplantation. BMJ Vol 296: 1709, 1988.

University of Cincinnati Medical Center, Cincinnati, Ohio, USA

R. MUNDA and J.W. ALEXANDER

The first kidney-pancreas transplant at the University of Cincinnati was performed on February 1, 1970. This was a composite pancreas-duodenal graft where the duodenum had been anastomosed to the jejunum. This patient died one month after transplantation due to septic complications following the performation of an ulcer in the transplanted duodenal segment, both grafts were functional at the time of his demise. Following that experience, there was a moratorium in our program until June 1979, when stimulated by a report from the Lyon group [1] this continuous present series was initiated.

Patients

From June 1979 until February 1988, 23 recipients received 27 cadaveric pancreas transplants at the University of Cincinnati Medical Center. Four patients underwent two consecutive pancreas transplants. Fourteen were male and seven were female. Their ages were from 24 to 50 years (average 33 years) all of them insulin dependent diabetics.

Donors

All organs were retrieved from local heart beating cadavers. Donor age ranged from 20 months to 39 years. After removal, the pancreas was immediately flushed and preserved in Euro-Collins solution at 4°C from 3 to 16 hours. Average preservation time was 7.4 hours. Eleven pancreases were retrieved as segmental grafts (body and tail) and sixteen as whole pancreas grafts.

J.M. Dubernard and D.E.R. Sutherland (eds.), International Handbook of Pancreas Transplantation, 359–364.
© *1989 by Kluwer Academic Publishers.*

Transplantation techniques

All recipients were ABO compatible and all pretransplant crossmatches were negative. Except in one patient where a 3-HLA and 1 DR antigens were matched, no donor-recipient combination showed more than 1-HLA or 1 DR antigens. Five patients received six segmental pancreas transplants, one patient receiving two, where the pancreatic duct had been obliterated with neoprene, four of these were located in a subcutaneous pocket and anastomized to the femoral vessels while two were placed in the iliac fossa anastomosed to the iliac vessels, artery and vein. Twenty one of the allografts were drained into the urinary tract, nine by means of a duct to ureter anastomosis following ipsilateral nephrectomy, [2] and twelve were drained directly into the urinary bladder [3]. In one patient, conversion from bladder to enteral drainage (jejunal loop) was performed six months after transplantation. Three whole pancreas grafts were transplanted as complete grafts including the donor spleen. In all of the pancreatic transplants, the celiac or splenic artery and portal vein were anastomosed to the host vessels. For those grafts located in the iliac fossa, a wide peritoneal window was created. In this series, a total of 14 pancreases were transplanted synchronously with the donor kidney. Eight were transplanted into recipients of well established kidney grafts and five into three nonuremic diabetic recipients.

Immunosuppression

Three different immunosuppression schedules were used. Schedule one from June 1979 to July 1983 consisted of azathioprine 1–2 mg/kg/day adjusted for renal function and/or leukopenia and prednisone given at an initial dose of 4 mg/kg/day and tapered down to 0.5 mg/kg/day by posttransplant day 30. Schedule two, after July 1983, consisted of a triple immunosuppressive protocol which included cyclosporin, prednisone and azathioprine. Dosages were as follows: Cyclosporin was given per os initially at 10 mg/kg/day for 8 days then reduced to 8 mg/kg/day at the time of discharge. Prednisone was started at 2 mg/kg/day and then reduced to 0.5 mg/kg/day by posttransplant day 15. Azathioprine 1.5 mg/kg/day was adjusted for renal function and/or leukopenia. Schedule three; after July, 1986: Same as schedule two but ATG (AT-GAM, The Upjohn Company) at a dose of 10 mg/kg/day was given for 10 days following transplantation.

Rejection episodes (diagnosed by hyperglycemia) were treated with intravenous methylprednisolone 'pulses' using 250 mg/kg or the anti-T cell monoclonal antibody (OKT3 Ortho Pharmaceutical Corporation, Raritan, New Jersey).

Results

Neoprene injected grafts (6)

One of these, a segmental graft of iliac location, remains functional now 78 months following transplantation. Others have been lost due to various causes: technical – a graft from neoprene extravasation into the splenic vein; two deaths, both grafts with functional grafts due to cardiovascular events, 1 and 4 months following transplantation, rejection of one graft and one (20 months old donor) either from fibrosis or graft thrombosis. Complications of neoprene treated grafts in groin location (2) included peripancreatitis and wound infection, and cutaneous fistula formation.

Grafts drained to the ureter (9)

In this group there were five segmental and four whole pancreas transplants. Two of these remain functional at 70 and 54 months, one segmental and another whole graft, respectively. Three grafts were lost because of the death of the recipient following sepsis, in two instances were associated with anastomotic leaks of the duct to the ureter suture line. One segmental graft was lost due to arterial thrombosis, which occurred despite the creation of an arteriovenous fistula between the distal splenic vessels.

Grafts drained to the bladder (12)

All of these were whole organ grafts. Three of these grafts remain functional at 6, 24 and 37 months posttransplantation. Eight other grafts were rejected anywhere from 1 to 11 months posttransplantation. One graft was lost due to arterial thrombosis 12 days following transplantation. With this technique, there were no associated anastomotic leaks. Surgical complications in 5 patients were related to graft pancreatitis. All but one of the infectious complications, which resulted in the recipient's death, were resolved with systemic antibiotics and local wound care. Another patient died one month after removal of a rejected pancreas graft due to arterial bleeding following infection of a suture line. One patient was converted to enteric drainage due to an acute balanitis urethritis.

Pancreas graft survival in relations to kidney transplantation

Fourteen pancreas transplants were performed synchronously with kidney transplants from the same donor, eight following kidney transplantation (dysynchronous) and five in three preuremic diabetic patients. When excluding technical complications (four patients), pancreas graft survival 50% one year was achieved in the synchronously transplanted group. In the dysynchronous transplant group, the average survival for the pancreas grafts was 3 to 5 months. One of five non-uremic transplant recipients one graft is functional 24 months following transplantation.

Graft function

Immediate graft function defined as normoglycemia with no insulin supplementation was observed within 2 hours after revascularization of 25 pancreas grafts. Two early failures, both in neoprene treated group, were due to technical complications. Observations of glucose homeostasis and systemic manifestations of diabetes on long term functioning pancreas graft recipients can be seen in (Table 1).

Physiologic observations of pancreas allograft drainage into the urinary tract

Chronic metabolic acidosis was noted in eight functioning grafts which had been drained into the urinary tract. This acidosis was due to bicarbonate losses in relation to the pancreatic urinary fistula and accentuated during periods of renal dysfunction presumably due to loss of compensatory mechanisms. Metabolic acidosis occurred irrespective of the etiology of renal dysfunction, either due to tubular necrosis, graft rejection or cyclosporin toxicity. This syndrome was treated successfully with intravenous and/or oral bicarbonate supplementation and bicarbonate dialysis for uremic patients.

In addition, in one patient a severe balanitis urethritis occurred four months posttransplantation. Urinary assay documented a 10^{2-3} increase in activated trypsin and chymotrypsin when compared to other asymptomatic similarly drained allograft recipients. This activation occurred presumably due to recurrent episodes of urinary tract infection. Conversion to ductal enteric drainage led to resolution of both balanitis and bicarbonate wasting. In our experience, measurement of urinary amylase levels for the diagnosis of rejection were gross indicators of graft function since no precise correlation could be found between those levels, onset of hyperglycemia and eventual graft rejection [4].

Conclusions

Long term graft survival, with normalization of glucose homeostasis, can be

Table 1. Long term effects of successful graft function.

	Hb A1c 5.5–8.5%	Transplant renal function	Peripheral vascular disease	Retinopathy	Peripheral neuropathy	Pancreas graft function
#6	6.3	S. Cr. 1.2	No change	Stable	Normal EMG	78 months
#7	7.0	S. Cr. 2.0	No change	Stable	EMG and clinical improvement	70 months
#12	6.7	1st kidney Tx acute rejection 2nd kidney Tx S. Cr. 1.2	Hemodynamic deterioration clinically no change	Stable	EMG + clinically	54 months
#14	7.0	Chronic rejection	No change	–	no change	lost at 24 months (chronic rejection)
#16	6.1	Chronic rejection	No change	–	EMG + clinically worse	lost at (chronic rejection)
#18	6.5	S. Cr. 2.3	No change	Stable	EMG + clinically no change	37 months
#24	6.3	Non-ESRD patient	No change	Developed proliferative retinopathy after Tx	Improvement EMG	24 months

EMG: electromyogram, Tx: Transplantation.

achieved by pancreas transplantation. Drainage of the pancreas grafts to the urinary tract is well tolerated in most patients if precautions are taken to recognize and/or treat metabolic acidosis. Activation of pancreatic enzymes in the urine is possible; this complication can be manifested clinically by inflammatory changes in the urinary tract and can be confirmed by detection of activated trypsin and chymotrypsin in the recipients' urine. With increasing experience, technical complications following this procedure have been reduced while rejection continues to take a toll in many of the technically successful grafts. When considering pancreas transplantation, there is the need to develop a sensitive method to diagnose early graft rejection since hyperglycemia is usually a late and terminal event. At the present, time, synchronous transplantation of kidney pancreas graft can improve pancreas graft survival (since the function and biopsy of the kidney graft being a marker for immunological events).

Although there is some suggestion of stabilization of retinopathy and improvement of peripheral neuropathy, the long term effect of normoglycemia brought about by pancreas transplantation upon the secondary diabetic complications has yet to be proven in the human experience.

References

1. Dubernard JM, Traeger J, Neyra P: A new method of preparation of segmental pancreatic grafts for transplantation trials in dogs and in man. Surgery 84: 633–639, 1978.
2. Gliedman ML, Gold M, Whittaker J, Rifkin H: Pancreatic duct to ureter anastomosis for exocrine drainage in pancreatic transplantation. Am J Surg 125: 245–252, 1973.
3. Sollinger HW, Kalayoglu M, Hoffman RM, Deierhoi MH, Belzer FO: Experience with pancreaticystostomy in 24 consecutive pancreas transplants. Transplant Proc 17 (Suppl 2): 141–143, 1985.
4. Munda R, Tom WW, First MR, Alexander JW: Pancreatic allograft exocrine urinary tract diversion: pathophysiology. Transplantation 43: 95–99, 1987.

Experience of the Mount Carmel Mercy Hospital, Detroit, Michigan, USA

L.H. TOLEDO-PEREYRA, V.K. MITTAL and D.A. GORDON

Through January, 1988, 41 diabetic patients have received pancreas transplants at our center. Seventeen patients received segmental pancreas allografts (eight with simultaneous kidney grafts), and 24 patients received combined kidney and whole pancreas grafts. This manuscript will briefly review our techniques for procurement and preservation, surgery, postoperative management, immunosuppression, and diagnosis and management of rejection. The results of pancreas transplantation at our center will also be presented.

Donor criteria

The criteria used for pancreas donation are similar to that for kidney donation [1]. Donors should be brain-dead, have stable cardiovascular function, be apneic, and on ventilatory support. The donor history should be free of diabetes mellitus in the donor or the donor's immediate family. A history of pancreatic disease of previous duodenal of pancreatic surgery is also a contraindication to donation. Hyperglycemia secondary to trauma is not considered a contraindication to pancreas donation. Amylase levels above 100 U/L and/or lipase levels greater than 1.0 U/L are relative contraindications, however, each case must be individually evaluated. Ideal donor age is between 8 and 40 years old, however, these are not strict limits.

Donor operation

The pancreas is procured in multiple organ harvesting settings in one of two ways [2, 3]. If the liver is not simultaneously procured, we prefer to remove the whole pancreas and bloc with the kidneys. If a donor hepatectomy is also done, the pancreas is taken as a segmental graft. Bench surgery is performed in cases

365

J.M. Dubernard and D.E.R. Sutherland (eds.), International Handbook of Pancreas Transplantation, 365–370.
© *1989 by Kluwer Academic Publishers.*

where the superior mesenteric artery and celiac axis are very short, by anastomosis of the celiac artery to the proximal end of the superior mesenteric artery [4].

Pancreas preservation

In 40 of 41 cases, pancreases were preserved by hypothermic storage. The first pancreas graft in our series was unsuccessfully preserved by combined hypothermic storage (3 hours) followed by hypothermic pulsatile perfusion (13 hours). Preservation time for the hypothermically stored pancreases ranged between 3 hours 48 minutes to 43 hours 45 minutes (mean $\pm$ SD = 15.1 $\pm$ 7.5 hrs.). Two types of preservation solutions have been utilized: albumin-augmented crystalloid solutions and hyperosmolar silica gel-based solutions [5]. Thirty-six of the 40 pancreases preserved by hypothermic storage have had complete or partial immediate function. The four pancreases not functioning in the immediate postoperative period never recovered function and were stored for 15 hr 35 min, 20 hrs, 28 hrs, 43 hrs, 45 min, respectively.

Recipient surgical techniques

Several methods have been used in our series for management of the exocrine secretions of the pancreas allografts. In the segmental pancreas grafts, duct occlusion (n = 12) and duct ligation with graft irradiation (2000 rad) (n = 5) were used. In the whole pancreas transplants, free drainage (n = 1), ductocystostomy (n = 6), pancreaticocutaneous fistula with delayed occlusion (n = 8) and duodenocystostomy (n = 9) were used (6).

Postoperative management

In the first three postoperative days, the patient is given dextran (40,000 molecular weight) (500 ml/24 hr). No heparin is administered. Dextrose (10%) in water with normal saline and 10 mEq of sodium bicarbonate are given to replace urinary output on a ml-per-ml basis, in an attempt to keep 30 ml ahead every hour. The plasma glucose concentration is measured every 6 hours. Regular insulin coverage is given for blood glucose levels above 250 mg/dl. Urinary amylase and glycosylated hemoglobin concentrations are measured daily. Serum insulin, glucagon, and human C-peptide levels are measured twice weekly. Pancreatic scans are performed once a week and at discharge. Cefotaxime (1 g intravenously $\times$ 3) is given prophylactically before and during surgery. Further use of antibiotics depends on the demonstration of specific infections. Hyperalimentation is given if the initial hospitalization is greater than 3 weeks. A liquid diet is instituted on the third to fifth postoperative day. A soft diet is begun on the fourth to sixth day after surgery, and a regular (2000 cal) diet is started on the seventh day. The Foley catheter is generally maintained for three weeks, and at that time a cystogram is performed before removal.

Immunosuppression

Initially, for the segmental transplants in our series, our immunosuppressive protocol consisted of azathioprine, low-dose steroids, and antilymphocyte globulin/antithymocyte globulin. Rejection was treated with ALG/ATG without a concomittant increase in steroids (Table 1).

A quadruple drug therapy approach was used for all of the combined whole pancreas and kidney transplant cases, consisting of imuran, prednisolone, cyclosporin, and ALG/ATG. Rejection was first treated with bolus Solumedrol (250 mg × 3 days). If this was not effective in reversing rejection, a course of ALG or ATG was given (5–12 g/kg × 10–14 days). OKT3 (5 mg/day × 10–14 days) was given if the ALG/ATG approach was unsuccessful (Table 2).

Diagnosis of acute pancreatic allograft rejection

The criteria used to diagnose rejection in pancreas transplant recipients varied depending in the type of transplant. In combined kidney and pancreas grafts from the same donor, changes in kidney function indicative of renal rejection, were closely monitored to assist in diagnosis of potential simultaneous pan-

Table 1. Immunosuppression regimen (ALG/ATG era).

	Initial	Maintenance
1. Prednisolone	1 mg/kg/day for 3–4 weeks	20–25 mg/day[a]
2. Azathioprine	5 mg/kg on first day	1.0–2.5 mg/kg/day[a]
3. ALG/ATG	15–20 mg/kg for 14 days[a]	
Antirejection protocol		
ALG/ATG 10–20 mg/kg/day up to 10 days for 1st, 2nd, 3rd rejection		
10–20 mg/kg/day every 4th–5th day for subsequent rejections		

[a] Dosage adjusted depending on WBC and platelet counts.

creatic rejection. With respect to changes in pancreatic function, rejection was diagnosed by the following criteria: an increase in plasma glucose levels $\geqq 200$ mg/dl, the need for exogenous insulin to maintain normoglycemia, a decrease in human C-peptide levels <0.7 ng/ml, a decrease in urinary amylase (for bladder drained pancreases), an increase in graft size as demonstrated by ultrasonography, and decreased graft uptake demonstrated by a radionuclide scan.

In patients receiving segmental pancreas allografts alone, it was often very difficult to diagnose rejection early enough to reverse it and prevent graft loss. Whereas, in combined pancreas and kidney transplants, changes in renal function could be used as indicators of rejection and antirejection therapy could be instituted earlier to prevent graft loss. Of the nine segmental pancreas grafts, transplanted alone, seven were lost to rejection or technical complications in the first three months posttransplant. In comparison, in the eight patients that received a simultaneous segmental pancreas and kidney transplant, only two pancreas grafts were lost to rejection in the first three months. In the segmental pancreas transplant group, pancreatitis also frequently compromised graft function and made it hard to differentiate it from rejection. In the whole pancreas group, all with simultaneous kidneys, eight of 24 kidneys were lost to rejection in the first three months posttransplantation.

Table 2. Immunosuppression regimen (cyclosporin era).

1. Solumedrol:	1 g/day on days 0, 1, and 2	
2. Azathioprine:	2–5 mg/kg on first day, maintenance 1.0–2.5 mg/kg/day[a]	
3. Prednisolone:	1 mg/kg/day on days 1, 2, and 3	
	0.8 mg/kg/day on day 4 and 5	
	0.6 mg/kg/day on day 6	
	0.5 mg/kg/day thereafter	
4. Cyclosporin[a]:	4 mg/kg/day IV over 24 hours on day 0, 1, 2, and 3	
	4 mg/kg/day PO in 2 doses thereafter	
5. ALG/ATG[a]:	0.5 g IV on day 1, 0.7 g IV on day 2, 0.9 g IV on day 3, 1.2 g IV on day 4,	
	1.5 g IV thereafter (Dose adjusted to WBC and platelet count)	

Antirejection protocol
Option 1: Solumedrol 250 mg every 8 hours for 3 days
Option 2: ALG/ATG 7–12 mg/kg/day for 10 days
Option 3: OKT3 5 mg/day for 10–14 days

[a] During OKT3 therapy, the dosages of steroids and azathioprine are reduced markedly and resumed at prerejection treatment dosages 3 days prior to cessation of OKT3.

Graft and patient survival

The overall 1-year actuarial graft and patient survival for our entire experience was 28.5% and 67.4%, respectively. When the survival results of segmental and whole pancreas transplantation are compared, whole pancreas grafts had significantly better 1-year actuarial survival (42.1% vs 11.8%, p<.05). The use of whole pancreas grafts in our series coincided with the implementation of the quadruple immunosuppressive regimen which included cyclosporin. Although, patient survival in the cyclosporin era was compromised by the use of the pancreaticocutaneous fistula technique with delayed ductal occlusion, no patients were lost in whole pancreas allograft groups using either the ductocystostomy or the pancreaticoduodenocystostomy techniques (Table 3). The effects of ductal technique on graft and patient survival are shown in Table III. Based on these results we currently recommend the use of either ductocystostomy or duodenocystostomy techniques together with quadruple immunosuppression (Table 2).

Surgical complications

Postoperative surgical complications were mostly related to the choice of technique for management of the pancreatic duct. Only a few grafts were lost due to ischemic or preservation injury. Complications of the segmental pancreas grafts included peripancreatic fluid collections, and wound infections. In whole pancreas grafts with the ductocystostomy, postoperative complications included peripancreatic fluid collections, wound infections, cystitis/urethritis, and bladder leakage. When pancreaticocutaneous fistulas were used for initial exocrine drainage, with delayed ductal occlusion, postoperative peripancreat-

Table 3. Effect of ductal technique on pancreas graft and patient survival rates.

Type of transplant/technique	N	1-Year actuarial survival (%)	
		Graft	Patient
Segmental pancreas transplantation			
Duct occlusion	12	16.7	82
Irradiation and duct ligation	5	0	50
Whole pancreas transplantation			
Free drainage	1	0	0
Ductocystostomy	6	50	100
Pancreaticocutaneous fistula with delayed occlusion	8	25	33
Duodenocystostomy	9	64.7	100

370

ic fluid collections, wound infections, multiple bleeding episodes, and septicemia were encountered. The use of the pancreaticoduodenocystostomy technique, used in the last nine cases, has been the most satisfactory procedure
with fewer complications.

Discussion

Through our clinical pancreas transplantation experience, improved techniques for procurement and preservation, pancreatic transplant surgery, postoperative management, immunosuppression, and diagnosis and management
of rejection have evolved. Improved graft function has especially been obtained, in our program, through the use of cyclosporin as part of the immunosuppressive regimen and the use of the duodenocystostomy technique. We
continue to search for new approaches to safely extend the length of pancreas
preservation so that it may be comparable with kidney preservation.

References

1. Toledo-Pereyra LH: Organ harvesting. In: Toledo-Pereyra LH (ed) Basic concepts of organ
   procurement, perfusion and preservation for transplantation; p 57. Academic Press Inc., New
   York, 1982.
2. Toledo-Pereyra LH, Mittal VK: Clinical segmental pancreatic transplantation. American
   Surgeon 48: 584, 1982.
3. Mittal VK, Chiu C, Toledo-Pereyra LH: Cadaver en-bloc bilateral nephrectomy and pancreat-
   icoduodenectomy for transplantation. Dialysis and Transplantation 16: 316, 1987.
4. Mittal VK, Toledo-Pereyra LH: Bench surgery under hypothermia for pancreatic allografts
   prior to transplantation. Transplant Proc, (in press).
5. Toledo-Pereyra LH, Mittal VK, Gordon DA: Albumin augmented crystalloid or hyperosmolar
   colloid solutions for clinical pancreas preservation. Transplant. Proc., in press.
6. Mittal VK, Toledo-Pereyra LH: Surgical techniques. In: Toledo-Pereyra LH (ed) Pancreas
   transplantation. Kluwer Academic Publishers, Boston, 1988 (in press).

Experience of the University of Genoa, Transplant Unit, Genoa, Italy

U. VALENTE

Our experience with pancreas transplantation in man from 1978 to 1986 is represented by 3 segmental autotransplantations and 14 segmental and whole pancreas transplantations. In the same time we have developed the islet isolation technique carrying out 24 autotransplantations, 16 adult islet transplantations in diffusion chambers, 13 fetal pancreas transplantations and 5 adult islet transplantations after treatment with monoclonal antibodies. The 3 segmental autotransplantations were performed between 1978 and 1979 after 95% pancreatectomy for chronic pancreatitis using the injected duct technique by Neoprene sec. Dubernard. In all cases the graft was anastomozed to femoral vessels in the inguinal region. In all cases we observed a pancreatic fistula lasting respectively 60-14-10 days and in 1 case there was a hemorrage on the 5th day. The endocrine function of the graft was assessed with O.G.T.T., I.V.G.T.T., Arginine test, Glucagon test, with simultaneous sampling for glycemia, insulinemia and C-peptide. After a follow-up of 8 years, 2 of the 3 patients are still functioning with a satisfactory response as above. The third patient began the insulin therapy after 2 years of normal function.

In the last 6 years we performed 14 allotransplantations. All of the patients were affected by Type I Diabetes with complications: retinopathy in 100%, nephropathy in 85%, neuropathy in 57.1%. The average age was 32 years (ranging from 21 to 51), the average duration of the disease before transplantation was 16 years (ranging from 8 to 25). In 13 cases we performed a segmental pancreatic graft and in 1 case we transplanted the whole organ; in two cases we have associated a kidney transplant. In 13 cases the graft was extraperitoneal and intraperitoneal, in 1 case with anastomosis to the iliac vessels. We utilized the injected duct technique in all cases using Neoprene in 4 cases and Prolamine in 10 cases. One patient died on the 45th day (7.14%) because of myocardial infarction with a functioning graft. In the post-operative period we observed a pancreatic fistula in 21.42% of the patients and sepsis in 7.14%. We used 2 immunosuppressive protocols: Azathioprine 1.5 mg/kg/day, Prednisone 20 mg/day, ALG for 3 weeks and Azathioprine

J.M. Dubernard and D.E.R. Sutherland (eds.), International Handbook of Pancreas Transplantation, 371–374.
© *1989 by Kluwer Academic Publishers.*

2.5 mg/kg/day, Prednisone 20 mg/day, cyclosporin 8 mg/kg/day. Rejection episodes have been treated with methyl-prednisolone 10 mg/kg/day for 3 days. The first protocol has been used in 10 cases and the second in 4 cases. In 71.4% of cases the graft began to function immediately; in 14.3% the function was lost during the first three months respectively on the 64th and 96th day because of rejection with histologic diagnosis in both cases; in 14.3% the graft was lost after a period of function because of fibrosis (histologic diagnosis with open biopsy); in 28.3% we have not seen a resumption of function and we removed the graft: in these cases the failure was owing to vascular complications. One case is to be considered still functioning even if it needs, after a period of complete recovery of 31 months, a small amount of insulin (12 IU/day). 4 patients have had a functioning graft with a follow-up of 26-23-18-7 months with good response to above mentioned test. The actual survival rate of this series is given in Figure 1.

Discussion

Segmental pancreatic autotransplantation was an ideal model for studying the technical problems of transplantation without the uncertainty caused by rejection. The pancreatic fistula that complicated these three cases is undoubtedly a sign of an incomplete suppression of exocrine function. As a result of improvement of this technique, the incidence of this complication was radically reduced in the transplant series. The analysis of our casuistic shows the fibrosis induced by Neoprene had caused the loss of the function in 14.3%. Thrombosis of the vessels was the most frequent cause of loss of the graft that was seen even after anticoagulant therapy. There were no significant differences between the patients treated with the first or the second protocol. The low incidence of sepsis, fistula and hemorrage shows that the suppression of exocrine function with injected duct is good and that in general, the surgical technique employed is safe and sufficient for the patient. The first observation from our experience is that the greatest care must be given in selection of the patient. From the analysis of greater casuistics other than ours emerge in fact that one of the most frequent causes of loss is the death of the patient usually as a result of a heart or brain vascular accident. We have included in the selection criteria, an accurate cardiovascular screening with regard to heart vascularization and to iliac and carotid vessels, first with Doppler echo and then with digital arteriography (Figure 2). The second observation is that the more frequent cause of failure is vascular thrombosis. We think that the basis of this phenomenon is the vascular characteristic of the organ (high intraparenchimal resistance) and the flow variation in iliac vessels of the patients due to atherosclerosis. These alterations should be identified and if is not possible to correct,

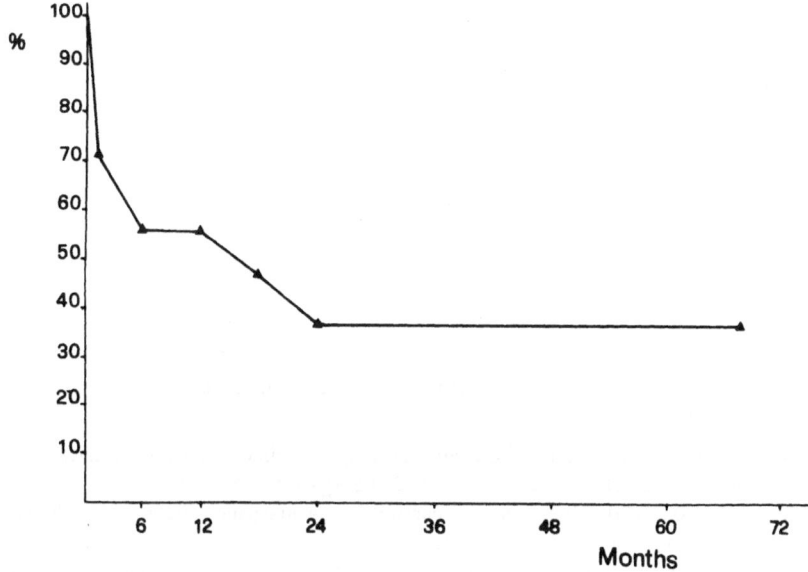

Figure 1. Actuarial survival rate of our series.

it should be cause of exclusion from the transplant list. It is true that technical difficulties often exist for the anastomoses (short vessels submitted to traction) so the technique of extending vascular axis, using donor vessels, as used by other authors, can be undoubtedly useful. We think that the whole pancreas technique should be taken in consideration and this, with some variation, does not prevent the liver removal from the same donor. Recent studies show a potential diabetogenic effect of cyclosporin, but otherwise according to other authors the better results of the last two years are due to this drug. Waiting for further confirmation we utilize cyclosporin at low doses in association to conventional therapy. In relation to the injected duct technique this seems still present and above all secure because it is not burdened with the risk of sepsis or fistulas connected to enteric diversion even if more or less later complicated by fibrosis. The urinary diversion with the bladder already employed by some teams, is also very promising. It allows the utilization of dosage of amylasuria as early marker of rejection. In the next months we want to begin our clinical experience with this technique, finalizing the research of a better method of pancreatic transplantation.

References

1. Baumgartner D, Largiader F: Simultaneous renal and intraperitoneal segmental pancreatic transplantation. World J Surg 8: 267, 1984.

374

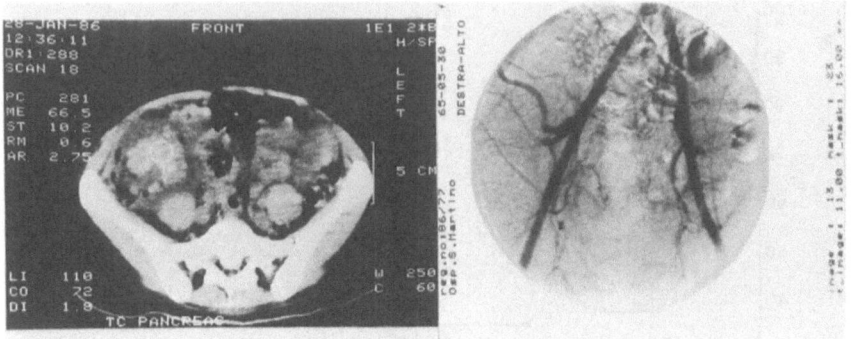

Figure 2. Angio-TAC and digital arteriography of one case of our series.

2. Bjorken C, Lundgren G, Ringden O et al: A technique for rapid harvesting of cadaveric renal and pancreatic graft after circulating arrest. Br J Surg 63: 517–519, 1976.
3. Calne RY, Brons IGM: Observations on paratopic segmental pancreatic grafting with splenic venous drainage. Transplant Proc 17: 340, 1985.
4. Dubernard JM, Traeger J, Piatti PM et al: Report of 54 segmental pancreatic allograft prepared by duct obstruction with Neoprene. Transplant Proc 17, 312, 1986.
5. Gil-Vernet JM, Fernandez-Cruz L, Andreu D et al: Clinical experience with pancreaticopyelodtomy for exocrine pancreatic drainage and portal venous drainage in pancreas transplantation. Transplant Proc 17: 342, 1985.
6. Land W, Landgraf R, Illner WD et al: Improved results in combined segmental pancreatic and renal transplantation in diabetic patients under cyclosporin therapy using ethibloc for duct obliteration. Transplant Proc 17: 317, 1985.
7. Munda R, First MR, Joffe SN et al: Experience with pancreatic allograft in renal transplant recipients with segmental pancreatic allograft. Transplant Proc 17: 353, 1986.
8. Sollinger H, Kalayoglu M, Hoffman RM et al: Result of segmental and pancreaticosplenic transplantation with pancreaticocystomy. Transplant Proc 17: 360, 1985.
9. Sutherland DER, Goetz FC, Kendall DM et al: Effect of donor source, technique, immunosuppression and presence or absence of end stage diabetic nephropathy on outcome in pancreas transplantation recipients. Transplant Proc 17: 325, 1985.
10. Sutherland DER, Goetz FC, Kendall DM et al: One institution's experience with pancreas transplantation. West J Med 143: 838, 1985.
11. Sutherland DER, Kendall D: Clinical pancreas and islet transplant reistry report. Transplant Proc 17: 307, 1985.
12. Toledo-Pereyra LH: Pancreas transplantation. Surg Gynecol Obstet 157: 49, 1983.
13. Traeger J, Bosi E, Dubernard JM et al: Thirthy months experience with cyclosporin in human pancreatic transplantation. Diabetologia 27: 154–156, 1984.
14. Tyden G, Wilczek H, Lundgren G et al: Experience with 21 intraperitoneal segmental pancreatic transplants with enteric or gastric exocrine diversion in human. Transplant Proc 17: 331, 1985.
15. Valente U, Barabino C, Barocci S et al: Segmental pancreatic transplantation in diabetics: follow-up in eight patients. Transplant Proc 17: 349, 1985.

Experience of the Sahlgren's Hospital, Göteborg, Sweden

B.A. FRISK, L.A. HEDMAN and H.A. BRYNGER

Pancreas transplantation to diabetic patients was first performed in 1966 [1]. The development of the technique to an accepted surgical treatment was very slow, with less than 100 transplants being performed during the subsequent 12 year period [2]. During this early period, two segmental duct-ligated pancreatic grafts were performed in Gothenburg. Both grafts were lost due to thrombosis [3]. The improvement of the outcome after pancreas transplantation reported during recent years [2] motivated us to restart a pancreas transplant program in 1985. Drainage of the exocrine secretion to the urinary bladder has been reported to be a successful method in transplantation of the whole pancreas [4, 5]. However, we have used in our series segmental pancreatic grafts with drainage of the exocrine secretion to the bladder. This surgical technique is a modification of earlier described method [6].

Technique

Donor operation: The pancreas segment distal to the right border of the portal vein is removed en bloc with the spleen. The graft vessels to be anastomosed consist of the splenic vessels, preferably with a segment of the coeliac artery and a patch of the portal vein. Collins solution (4–8°C) is used for perfusion and preservation. Bench surgery is commenced with removal of the spleen and ligation of the distal ends of the splenic vessels. The pancreatic duct is dissected for a length of 5 to 8 mm and a slice of parenchyma of corresponding thickness is resected. The transsected surface is closed by two running sutures, leaving the duct protruding from the gland.

Recipient operation: The abdominal cavity is opened by a low, rightsided paramedial incision. The graft is placed intraperitoneally, and the graft vessels are anastomosed end-to-side to the right external iliac vessels. The pancreaticocystostomy is performed with a two-layer anastomosis technique (Figure 1). Bladder muscular flaps are dissected off the mucosa, and the posterior flap

J.M. Dubernard and D.E.R. Sutherland (eds.), International Handbook of Pancreas Transplantation, 375–378.
© *1989 by Kluwer Academic Publishers.*

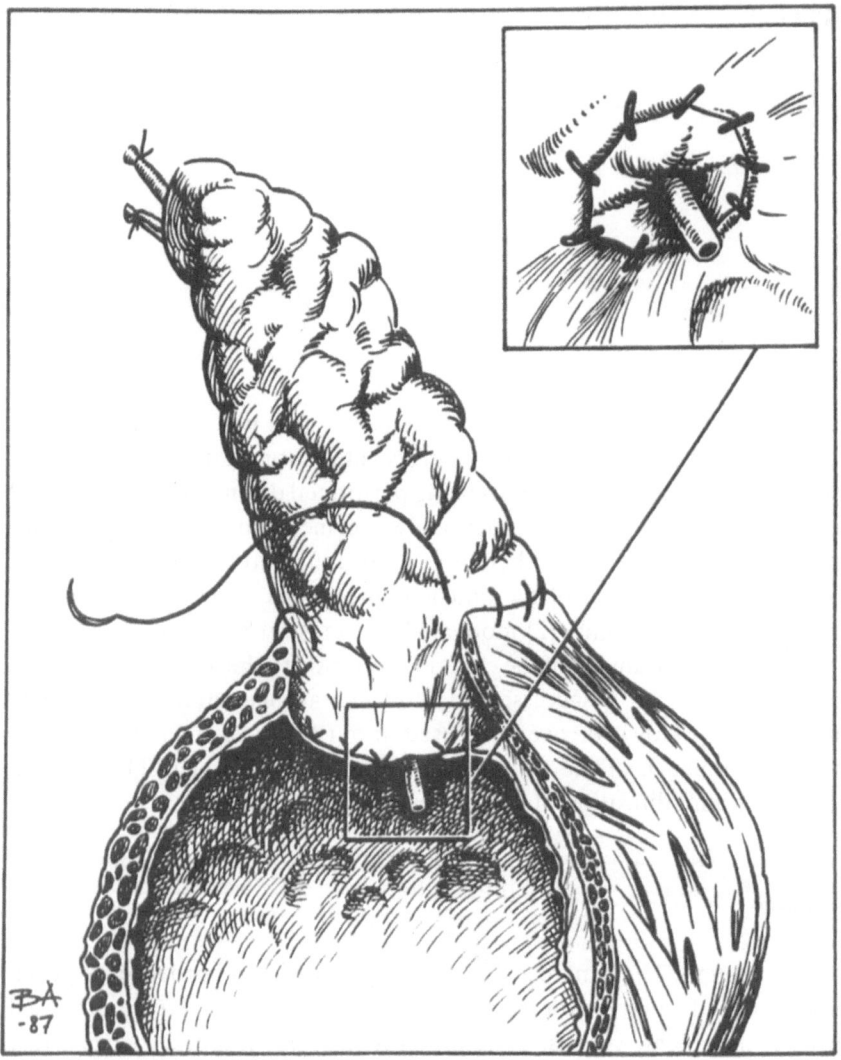

Figure 1. The pancreaticocystostomy is performed with a two-layer running suture technique. The bladder muscular layer is sutured to the pancreatic surface and the mucosa to the paraductal pancreatic tissue.

is sutured to the posterior pancreatic surface. The pancreatic duct is then pulled into the bladder cavity through a puncture hole in the bladder mucosa, and the mucosal edge is sutured to the paraductal pancreatic tissue. Finally, the anterior muscular flap is sutured to the anterior pancreatic surface. Both suturlines are performed with a running technique using absorbable sutures. When the anastomosis is completed, a collar of bladder muscle surrounds the proximal end of the graft, the bladder mucosa covers the closed surface, and the pancreatic duct drains freely into the bladder cavity (Figure 1).

Outcome

Twenty-five patients aged 25–49, with insulin-dependent diabetes mellitus and end-stage diabetic nephropathy, simultaneously received cadaveric kidney and segmental pancreatic grafts. Seventeen were on dialysis while eight were in a predialytic state. All had diabetic retinopathy of varying degrees. The cold ischemia time ranged between 2 and $7^{1}/_{2}$ hours. A combination of cyclosporin, azathioprine and prednisolone was used for immunosuppression, with addition of rabbit antithymocyteglobulin (Fresenius) in 19 cases. An indwelling bladder catheter was used for 10–14 days and all patients received prophylactic anticoagulation treatment for the first 6 months.

Actuarial survival at 3 months for patient, pancreas graft and kidney graft were 92%, 79% and 74%, and at one year 86%, 63% and 64%, respectively. All patients had normal fasting blood glucose and decreased glucosylated hemoglobin and had no need for exogenous insulin. Nine grafts were lost. Two patients died with functioning grafts, four grafts were lost due to rejection and three due to vascular complications. No graft was lost due to complications of the pancreaticocystostomy. Three patients had, however, complications of the pancreaticocystostomy, but all were successfully treated – three urinary leakage of which one developed a temporary pancreatic fistula.

The 24 hour amylase output from the graft was about 2,000 ukat after one week and doubled within three months in those patients with enough observation time. High excretion of sodium bicarbonate kept the pH of the urine between 7 and 8. Most patients were substituted orally with sodium bicarbonate to prevent acidosis.

Summary

Twentyfive insulin-dependent diabetic patients with end-stage diabetic nephropathy received simultaneously cadaveric kidney and segmental pancreatic grafts. Pancreaticocystostomy with a two-layer technique was used for drainage of the exocrine secretion. Actuarial one year pancreas graft survival was 63%, all patients without insulin need. A constant high amylase output and pH of the urine gave evidence of pancreatic duct patulence and good exocrine function of the graft. No graft was lost due to complications related to the technique of the pancreaticocystostomy.

References

1. Kelly WD, Lilehei RC, Merkel FK, Idezuki Y, Goetz FC: Allotransplantation of the pancreas

378

and duodenum along with the kidney in diabetic nephropathy. Surgery 61: 827–837, 1967.

2. Sutherland DER, Moudry K: Pancreas transplant registry report. Transplant Proc 18: 1739–1746, 1986.

3. Brynger H, Gelin L-E: Clinical experience in transplantation in the duct-ligated pancreas segment. Transplant Proc 12: 91–92, 1980.

4. Sollinger HW, Kalayoglu M, Hoffman RM, Belzer FO: Results of segmental and pancreatico-splenic transplantation with pancreaticocystostomy. Transplant Proc 17: 360–362, 1985.

5. Nghiem DD, Beutel WD, Correy RJ: Duodenocystostomy for exocrine pancreatic drainage in experimental and clinical pancreaticoduodenal transplantation. Transplant Proc 18: 1762–1764, 1986.

6. Cook K, Sollinger HW, Warner T, Kamps D, Belzer FO: Pancreaticocystostomy: an alternative method for exocrine drainage of segmental pancreatic allografts. Transplantation 35: 634–636, 1983.

Experience of University Hospital, Innsbruck, Austria

R. MARGREITER, E. STEINER, A. KÖNIGSRAINER, F. AIGNER,
M. SPIELBERGER and C. BÖSMÜLLER

Between December 1979 and November 1986 a total of 32 pancreas transplants were performed at our center. Twenty-six pancreases were transplanted together with a kidney from the same donor in patients with end-stage diabetic nephropathy, three pancreases sometime after a successful renal transplantation and three in two nonuremic patients for progressive proliferative retinopathy.

In our first patient we used the technique originally described by Dubernard [1]: the pancreatic duct was occluded with an alcoholic prolamine solution and the graft placed in the right iliac fossa. After excellent initial function of the renal and pancreatic graft both organs were lost for immunological reasons. Immunosuppression in this and the next patient consisted of steroids and azathioprine, in the following 14 recipients of cyclosporin and steroids. Thereafter, all patients were treated with cyclosporin, steroids and azathioprine.

Because of severe tryptic lesions at the site of the pancreatic graft, we changed our surgical technique: the pancreas was put in the Douglas pouch, where it was sufficiently fixed but not compressed by surrounding tissue particularly in case of acute rejection. Furthermore, it was easy to palpate from the rectum and to examine by sonography through the optical window of the full urinary bladder. Leakage from the graft was thought to be absorbed by the peritoneum [2]. In this first series consisting of five patients only one pancreas graft functioned at one year. In two of the grafts it was felt that loss of endocrine function was due to severe fibrosis after duct occlusion. We therefore abandoned this technique, and in the next eleven cases the pancreatic juice was drained into a Roux-en-Y loop of proximal jejunum. The graft-gut anastomosis was carried out in two layers and a small catheter was inserted in the pancreatic duct and brought out through the gut and the abdominal wall for drainage of pancreatic juice to the exterior for two weeks. In most of the patients in this series, the graft comprised not only body and tail of the gland but also major parts of the head of the pancreas and was therefore called subtotal [3]. Pancreas graft survival at one year was 30%, renal graft survival

J.M. Dubernard and D.E.R. Sutherland (eds.), International Handbook of Pancreas Transplantation, 379–381.
© *1989 by Kluwer Academic Publishers.*

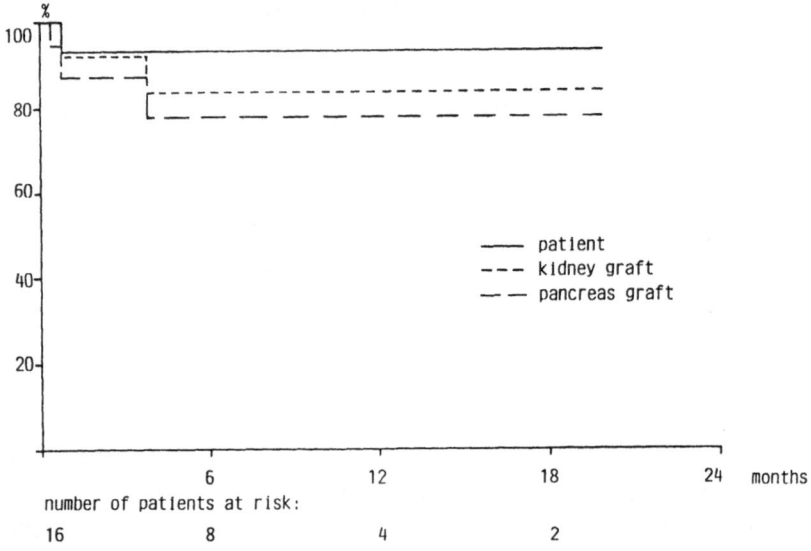

Figure 1. Combined kidney-pancreas transplants. Delayed duct occlusion. 5/4/1985–1/12/1986.

75% and patient survival 80%. However, two patients became septicemic after having rejected their pancreas graft. Enteric bacteria were cultured from the blood in these patients and were thought to have penetrated the partly necrotic graft into the bloodstream. We felt that these patients represented an extremely high-risk population: they are highly immunosuppressed, again diabetic and septic. Because of this negative experience, in the following series of 16 patients the pancreas graft was placed in the Douglas pouch again, the transected area oversown and extraperitonealized in the right lower abdomen. Pancreatic juice was drained to the exterior until graft function stabilized and was used for monitoring of the exocrine graft function, which correlated well with rejection episodes diagnosed on the basis of renal allograft histology [4]. In 9 patients the pancreatic duct was occluded after a mean of 53 days, or in three cases of pancreatic juice infection anastomosed to a jejunum loop. This technique was associated with a relatively high local complication rate such as paravasation or abscess formation. However, all these problems were managed by surgical means. Pancreas graft survival at one year was calculated at 78% and kidney graft survival at 83%. In this group only one patient died from an extensive myocardial infarction with two normally functioning grafts (Figure 1).

The advantages of this technique are the following: The procedure is relatively simple, fast and does the least harm to the graft. Furthermore, it facilitates exact monitoring of the exocrine graft function, and the graft can easily be removed in case of irreversible rejection.

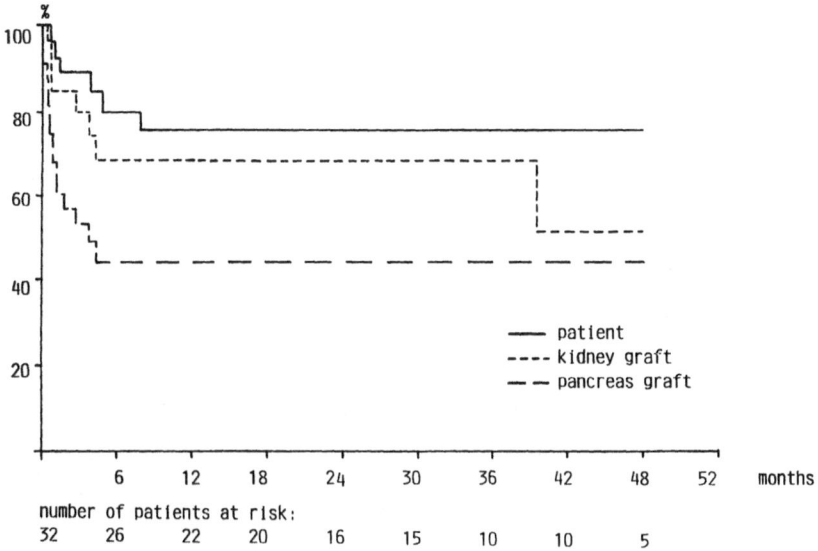

Figure 2. Combined kidney-pancreas transplants. 15/12/1979–1/12/1986.

However, the major drawback associated with this delayed duct occlusion technique turned out to be the extremely long hospitalization time, and we therefore will probably change our technique again.

Our overall results are summarized in Figure 2. Considering the poor results in our first patients, we feel that the results achieved in our latest series are quite favourable.

References

1. Dubernard JM, Traeger J, Neyra P et al: Surgery 84: 633, 1978.
2. Margreiter R, Steiner E, Spielberger M et al: Hormone and Metabol, Research Suppl 13: 86, 1983.
3. Margreiter R, Steiner E, Aigner F et al: Transplant Proc 16 (Suppl 5): 1277. 1984.
4. Steiner E, Klima G, Niederwieser D et al: Transplant Proc 19: 2336, 1987.

Experience of the University of Iowa College of Medicine, Iowa City, Iowa, USA

R.J. CORRY, F.H. WRIGHT and J.L. SMITH

Between March 29, 1984 and March 31, 1988, 68 pancreaticoduodenal transplants from cadaver donors were performed on 61 patients. 42 (62%) were simultaneous renal-pancreas transplants, 21 (31%) were sequential post-renal transplants, and 5 (8%) were pre-uremic transplants. In 5 early cases, the spleen was transplanted with the pancreas. The arterial supply of the transplanted organ was based on the celiac and superior mesenteric arteries, sharing a common aortic patch. Arterial anastomosis was accomplished by joining the aortic patch to the external iliac artery, with the venous drainage accomplished by a portal vein-to-external iliac vein anastomosis. In a few cases, a portal vein extension was fashioned by joining a segment of donor external iliac vein to the portal vein of the graft. Drainage of the pancreatic exocrine system was carried out by a side-to-side duodenojejunostomy in 31 cases, and by a side-to-side duodenocystostomy in 37 cases. Details of the donor and recipient operations have been described previously [1].

All organs were procured from heart-beating cadaver donors, from whom the kidneys were removed and utilized in all cases, and the hearts in the majority of cases [2]. Simultaneous procurement of the liver and pancreas has been performed in several cases using grafts from the donor iliac artery and vein to reconstruct the vasculature of the pancreas [3]. In all cases, in situ cooling was accomplished with an aortic flush with cold Ringer's lactate or Collins solution. Following removal of the organs, the pancreas was flushed at a separate table using a preservation solution. In the first part of the series, Collins solution was used for preservation, followed by the use of silica gel-filtered plasma. Currently, University of Wisconsin solution is being used for preservation and cold storage of the pancreas. Iliac artery and vein grafts are taken in all cases. The spleen is left intact and attached to the pancreas for removal after revascularization of the organ.

J.M. Dubernard and D.E.R. Sutherland (eds.), International Handbook of Pancreas Transplantation, 383–388.
© *1989 by Kluwer Academic Publishers.*

Complications

Graft thrombosis

The major cause of pancreas graft loss was thrombosis, which occurred in 14 of 66 cases, including 6 of 20 post-renal pancreas transplants, 7 of 40 simultaneous renal-pancreas transplants, and 1 of 5 pre-uremic transplants. Thrombosis appears to arise from an intra-glandular process involving the small intra-pancreatic vessels and appears to be related to graft pancreatitis and to preservation and reperfusion factors.

The current incidence of graft thrombosis is 10%. The decreased incidence of thrombosis is most probably related to an improved donor pancreatectomy technique stressing limited manipulation during the recovery procedure and a low-pressure, low-volume flush to avoid intravascular damage to the gland and to improved preservation techniques. Additionally, an anticoagulant protocol employing low molecular weight dextran, subcutaneous heparin, and aspirin is now employed in all post-renal and pre-uremic graft recipients.

Infection

Wound infections occurred in 13 of 68 cases. The most serious wound complications occurred after removal of the pancreas for graft thrombosis. Three patients developed infections of the external iliac artery suture line, and arterial disruption following graft removal. These patients all required resection and ligation of the external iliac artery, and one patient required a femoral bypass to maintain lower extremity viability. All of these arterial fistulas occurred in patients who had bowel anastomoses. Since adopting the bladder anastomosis as the procedure of choice, we have noted a decreased incidence of wound infection following graft removal for thrombosis and no major wound infections resulting in arterial disruption. The bladder drainage technique appears significantly safer should the pancreas graft require removal for graft thrombosis.

There have been three deaths related to infection. One occurred in a patient with peritoneal sepsis related to a previous peritoneal dialysis catheter and infection. Two deaths occurred as a result of cytomegalovirus infection following the use of monoclonal antibody preparations to treat rejection episodes.

Patient survival and graft function

Actuarial patient survival and renal graft and pancreatic graft survival curves are shown for all patients in Figure 1 and for simultaneous renal-pancreas

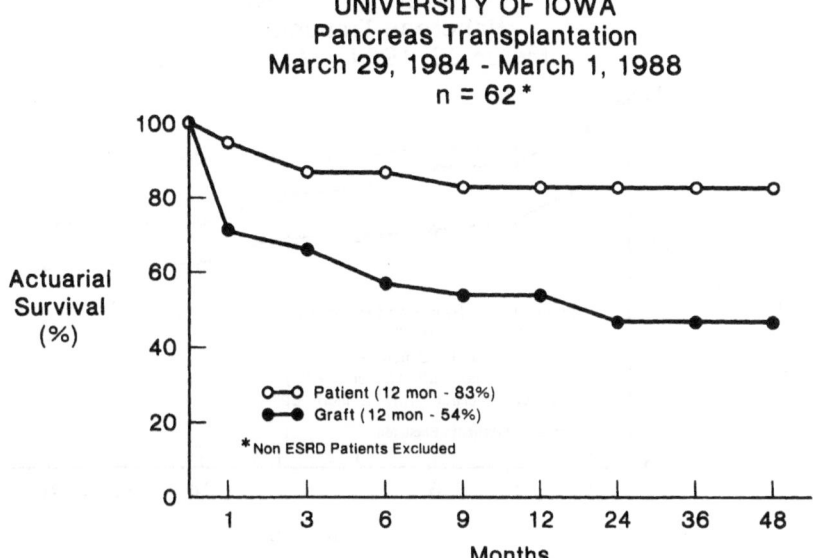

Figure 1. Actuarial survival showing patient and graft survival curves of all patients receiving pancreas transplants.

recipients in Figure 2. The majority of deaths occurred early in the series and were the result of pre-existing coronary artery disease. This experience led to the initiation of a thorough pre-operative cardiac evaluation before acceptance of the patient for simultaneous renal-pancreas transplantation. The current evaluation includes an isotope ventriculogram, thalium stress test, and coronary angiography in all cases. If significant coronary artery disease is identified, it is treated appropriately prior to kidney transplantation. Pancreas transplantation is then held as a sequential option. An analysis of the early mortality of the series and of strategies for improving patient and graft survival are reported elsewhere [4, 5].

Diagnosis and treatment of rejection

The diagnosis of rejection of the transplanted pancreas, particularly insidious late rejection, remains a major problem contributing to graft loss. The ability to monitor rejection activity in the kidney is a major factor contributing to the improved success rates for simultaneous renal-pancreas transplantation. However, there have been instances of loss of the kidney to rejection with maintenance of pancreas function, and loss of the pancreas with maintenance of renal function. The bladder drainage technique also allows determinations of uri-

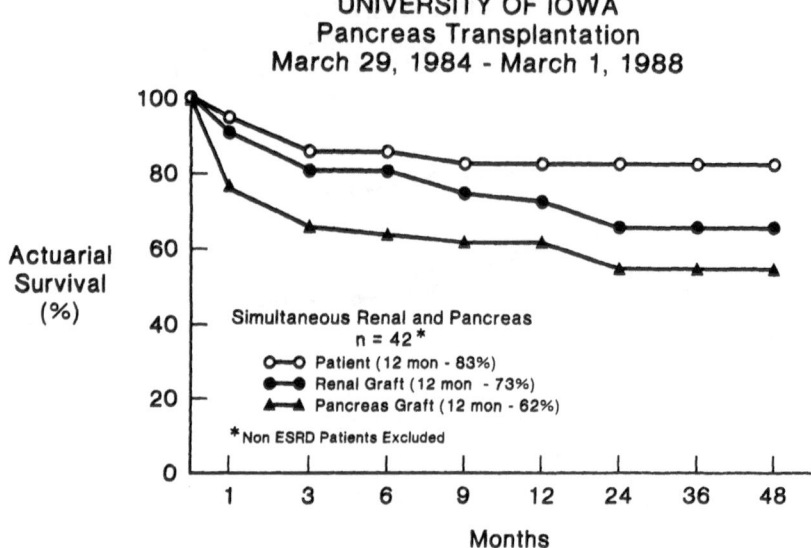

Figure 2. Actuarial survival showing patient and graft survival curves of the simultaneous renal-pancreas transplant group.

nary amylase and pH values, which may be helpful in the diagnosis of rejection. Decreases in these values have been shown to occur earlier than blood sugar elevation with pancreas rejection [6]. However, the ability to follow urinary amylase levels in the post-renal pancreas recipient with a bladder anastomosis has not led to the same level of graft survival that has been achieved in the simultaneous renal-pancreas recipient.

Recent experience has shown that magnetic resonance imaging may be helpful in the diagnosis of pancreatic graft rejection and this has been reported in more detail elsewhere [7]. Additional techniques being evaluated for possible utility in the diagnosis of rejection include urinary interleukin-2 levels and fine-needle aspiration biopsies of the pancreas.

Rejection is now being treated by a combination of intravenous pulses of methylprednisolone and the use of monoclonal antibody (OKT3) preparations. There is a tendency toward early use of monoclonal antibody preparations because the rejection process in the pancreas may be relatively advanced by the time the diagnosis is made. Improved graft survival may result from more vigorous treatment of the rejection process.

It is anticipated that new immunosuppressive techniques and the possibility of histocompatibility matching may result in improved pancreatic graft survival. It now appears that utilization of University of Wisconsin solution for organ preservation may allow time for tissue typing and for increased sharing of organs among centers.

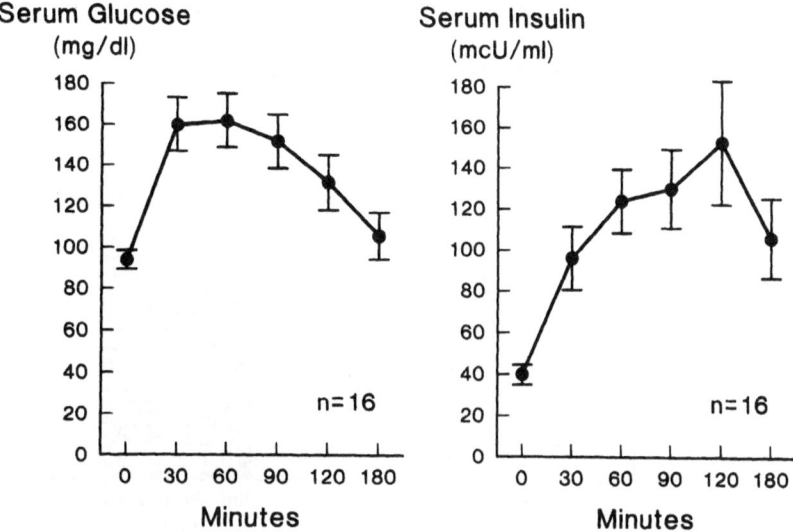

Figure 3A. Oral glucose tolerance test results after 100 grams of glucose for patients who underwent pancreas transplantation. Left, mean plus or minus the standard error of the mean of serum glucose, and right, of serum insulin.

Summary

Our four-year experience with pancreas transplantation has led to the conclusion that the operation can be performed safely and with a graft survival rate which has shown consistent improvement. It has become apparent that a functioning pancreas graft is capable of maintaining glycosylated hemoglobin levels in the normal range and is the only available method for the long-term normalization of carbohydrate metabolism in the diabetic (Figures 3a and 3b). It now must be demonstrated that this normalization of carbohydrate metabolism will result in prevention or regression of the vascular complications of diabetes. There are reports from a number of centers, including our own, that demonstrate subjective improvements in the patients' symptoms of gastroenteropathy, neuropathy, fatigue, and quality of life. Careful clinical studies are now in progress to evaluate the impact of successful pancreatic transplantation on the progressive complications of diabetes. Our improving experience and success rate makes us optimistic for the future, and we feel there is every reason to continue with pancreatic transplantation in selected centers and in selected patients.

388

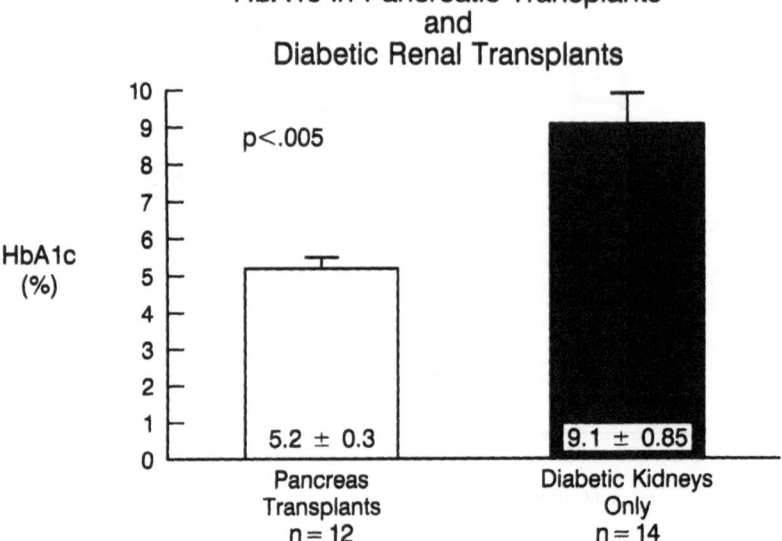

Figure 3B. Glycosylated hemoglobin (HbA1C) levels for renal-pancreas transplant recipients and levels for diabetic renal recipients only.

References

1. Corry RJ, Nghiem DD, Schulak JA et al: Surgical treatment of diabetic nephropathy with simultaneous pancreatic duodenal and renal transplantation. Surg Gynecol Obstet 162: 547–555, 1986.
2. Nghiem DD, Schulak JA, Beutel WD et al: Function of organs obtained from pancreas donors. Transplant Proc 18: 538–539, 1986.
3. Corry RJ: Pancreatic-duodenal transplantation with urinary tract drainage. In: Groth C (ed) Pancreatic transplantation. Grune & Stratton Ltd, London, 1988.
4. Corry RJ, Nghiem DD, Gonwa TA: Critical analysis of mortality and graft loss following simultaneous renal-pancreatic duodenal transplantation. Transplant Proc, in press.
5. Corry RJ, Nghiem DD: Evolution of technique and results of pancreas transplantation at the University of Iowa. Clinical Transplantation 1(1): 52–56, 1987.
6. Nghiem DD, Gonwa TA, Corry RJ: Metabolic effects of urinary diversion of exocrine secretions in pancreas transplantation. Transplantation 43(1): 70–73, 1987.
7. Yuh WTC, Wiese JA, Abu-Yousef MM et al: Pancreatic transplant imaging. Radiology, in press.
8. Wright FH, Zehr P, Schanbacher BA et al: Improved functional status of patients following successful pancreatic transplantation. Poster at First International Congress on Pancreatic and Islet Transplantation, Stockholm, Sweden, March 27–29, 1988; Abstract: Diabetes, in press.

Experience of the Hôpital Edouard Herriot, University of Lyon I, Lyon, France

J.M. DUBERNARD, J. TRAEGER, E. LA ROCCA, M. MELANDRI, R. SANSEVERINO, N. LEFRANÇOIS, X. MARTIN, A. GELET and J.L. TOURAINE

Introduction

In September 1987, a total of 90 pancreatic transplantations had been performed in our center.

In most cases we have used the technique of segmental transplantation prepared by duct obstruction by neoprene. As demonstrated by our experimental series including in situ injection, auto and allotransplantation in dogs, as well as iso or allotransplantation in rats, we observed that the suppression of the pancreatic exocrine function by injection of a synthetic rubber (neoprene) into the ductal system of the pancreas, was immediate and permanent [1]. An extensive fibrosis replaced the exocrine parenchyma, and B cell function was preserved at long term (18 months in rats, up to 8 years in dogs). Metabolic investigations showed a normal endocrine function of duct injected pancreas [2]. Neither acute pancreatitis nor lysis of the gland were observed with this technique.

From January 1985 to September 1987 we carried out a prospective comparative study between segmental pancreatic transplantation with duct obstruction by intraductal neoprene injection and pancreatico-duodenal transplantation with enteric diversion of pancreatic juice.

Material and methods

Patient selection

All recipients were non selected insulin-dependent diabetic patients (I.D.D.) frequently in poor physical conditions and with evidence of diabetic compatibilities (Table 1).

Donors were heart-beating cadavers selected for ABO complications and negative cross matches. HLA and DR typing were routinely performed, but not considered for recipient selection.

389

J.M. Dubernard and D.E.R. Sutherland (eds.), International Handbook of Pancreas Transplantation, 389–398.
© *1989 by Kluwer Academic Publishers.*

Technical details of our method for pancreas and kidney removal from cadavers, were described in another chapter of this book. The grafts were reflushed ex situ and ice packed in chilled Collins solution.

Cold ischemia was less than 5 hours in 83 cases, between 5 and 6 hours in 5 cases and more than 6 hours in 2 cases.

At the beginning of our experience we have performed 12 transplantations of the pancreas alone. Then double simultaneous kidney and pancreas transplantation became our preferred approach.

From November 1976 to September 1987, 90 pancreatic transplantations were performed in 86 I.D.D. uremic patients: in 72 cases pancreas and kidney were grafted simultaneously, both organs being harvested from the same donor. In 2 cases pancreatic transplantation was performed before kidney transplantation and in 4 other cases the pancreas was transplanted after the kidney. In 12 cases pancreas was transplanted alone. In 4 instances a pancreas retransplantation was performed after failure of a previous pancreatic graft: 1 patient had received a pancreas alone and 3 patients a double kidney and pancreas transplantation.

Surgical technique

In 76 cases a segmental graft was used, including the body and the tail of the donor pancreas; just after harvesting pancreatic duct was injected with Neoprene to control exocrine secretion. Graft revascularization was obtained via an end to side anastomosis of the donor celiac axis and portal vein to the recipient iliac vessels.

In 14 cases a whole pancreas with a segment of donor duodenum was harvested. Vascular anastomoses were realized in the same fashion, but aortic patch included the superior mesenteric artery to ensure viable vascular supply

Table 1. Clinical data.

Patients population	86 (56M − 30F)
Mean age[a]	36,05 +/− 1,1
Mean duration of diabetes[a]	22,3 +/− 0,6
Dialysis	74 (86%)
Months of dialysis[a]	22,9 +/− 1,3
Retinopathy	83 (96%)
Blind	14 (16%)
Peripheral macroangiopathy	66 (77%)
Cardiopathy	46 (53%)
Amputation	10 (12%)
Neuropathy	86 (100%)

[a] = +/− SEM.

to donor duodenum and pancreatic head. Drainage of exocrine juice was obtained performing a side to side duodeno-ileal anastomosis in a Roux-en-Y defunctionalized intestinal loop. Graft placement was in 10 cases extraperitoneal, in 43 cases extraperitoneal with the graft wrapped with omentum attracted into the iliac fossa via a peritoneal window, and in 37 cases (including all pancreaticoduodenal grafts) intraperitoneal).

Immunosuppressive treatment

All patients were submitted to a preoperative program of blood transfusions.

Different immunosuppressive treatments have been employed in our series. In the first 20 recipients immunosuppression consisted in a combination of azathioprine (AZA) steroids and antilymphocyte globulins (ALG) (protocol A, conventional treatment).

Since 1982 all patients have been treated by cyclosporin (CYA) according to different protocols (protocols B, C, D, E): 9 patients were treated by CYA from the day of transplantation and ALG for 4–12 weeks (protocol B), 28 patients were treated by CYA subsequent to an initial course of conventional treatment (protocol C) and in 33 others CYA, AZA and prednisone were used from the day of transplantation and ALG was employed only for treatment of rejection (protocol D). In the last four patients a quadruple association was used adding to protocol D, ALG or OKT3 during two weeks after transplantation (protocol E).

Post-operative management and graft monitoring

In the immediate post-transplant period parenteral nutrition was usually administered for 10 days and intravenous therapies were performed. Even though pancreatic graft were functioning, during this period high glycemic levels were often observed. In order to avoid an islet stress, insulin treatment was restored if glycemia was higher than 8 mmol/l.

Endocrine function was evaluated by plasmatic and urinary C-peptide, glycemia and glycosuria. High glycemic values may be of difficult interpretation and due to different causes: glucose infusion, steroid pulse in case of renal graft rejection, vascular thrombosis, infection.

An increase in blood glucose, appearance of glycosuria and decrease in plasmatic and urinary C-peptide levels, were considered as patterns of possible pancreatic graft rejection.

In recipients of simultaneous kidney plus pancreas transplantation, kidney rejection was evaluated according to Williams' classification [3].

Isolated pancreatic functional changes, or simultaneous to kidney functional changes, but occurring before steroid treatment, was interpreted as pancreatic rejection. Pancreas endocrine functional changes occurring during a kidney rejection were considered as consecutive to steroid treatment or to pancreatic rejection.

Metabolic function and degenerative complications

In some patients of our series, blood glucose control was achieved during surgery, using a feed-back glucose controlled insulin infusion by means of an artificial pancreas [4]. The function of the pancreatic graft was evaluated measuring serum free insulin, C-Peptide and glucagon starting from the peroperative period.

When the patient was insulin-independent with good metabolic control, and steroid treatment was lower than 20 mg/day, endocrine function was evaluated by several tests (after pancreas transplantation endocrine and metabolic evaluation, 24 hours metabolic profile on glucose, free insulin, C-Peptide, B-OH-Butyrate, lactate and glucagon, oral glucose tolerance test (OGTT), intravenous glucose tolerance test (IVGTT), arginine test, Tolbutamide test, Insulin induced hypoglycemia test, glycosylated hemoglobin (HbA$_1$). Furthermore the endocrine pancreatic function and metabolic control was studied every six months, by a 24 hour metabolic profile (including glycemia, insulinemia, lactate, B-OH butyrate and serum glycerol), OGTT and HbA1.

In all patients neuropathy and retinopathy was studied by electromyography and fluoresceine angiography before and every 6 months after transplantation.

Results

Overall patients and graft survival rates

In September 1987, 33 of the 90 pancreatic grafts (36,7%) were still functioning from 1 to 72 months. The overall 6 years actuarial patient and graft survivals were 52% and 17% respectively. In recipients of a simultaneous kidney and pancreas transplantation, patients, pancreas, and kidney overall survivals were respectively: 64%, 40% and 50% at 2 years and 56%, 20% and 34% at 6 years. Results were evaluated according to time, to type of immunosuppression and to different surgical techniques.

Outcome according to immunosuppressive treatment and time. The overall actuarial survival of patients, kidney and pancreas improved with amelioration of immunosuppressive treatments. The advantage of triple therapy including CYA is clearly shown in Figures 1 and 2.

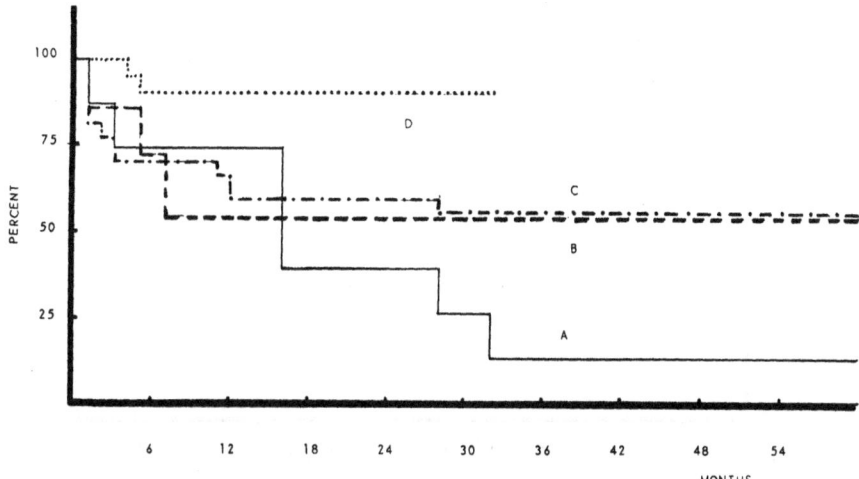

Figure 1. Patient survival according to different therapeutical approaches. A = Conventional therapy, B = CsA from beginning, C = CsA after conventional therapy, D = CsA + AZA + prednisone.

Outcome according to 2 different surgical techniques in patients receiving the same immunosuppressive treatment (protocol D). At present there are not statistically significant difference in patients and pancreas survival between the 17 cases of segmental pancreas transplantation with neoprene duct obstruction and the 14 cases of whole pancreas transplantation with enteric diversion.

Figure 3 and Figure 4 show patients and pancreas overall survival during a 30 month follow up period [5–6].

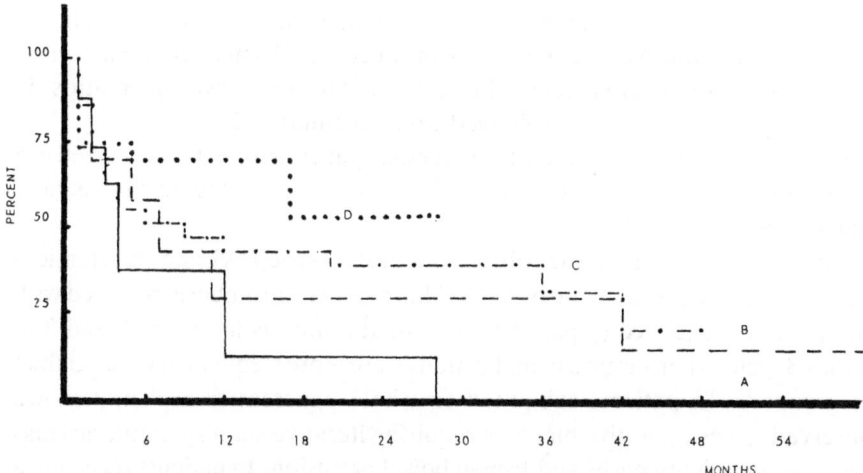

Figure 2. Pancreas survival according to different therapeutical approaches. A = Conventional therapy, B = CsA from beginning, C = CsA after conventional therapy, D = CsA + AZA + prednisone.

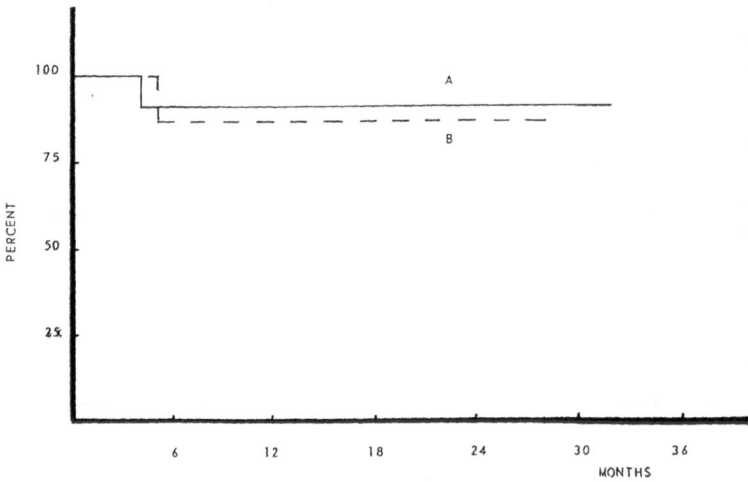

Figure 3. Enteric diversion (A) versus duct obstruction (B). Overall patient survival. A = 14 pts, B = 16 pts.

Causes of graft failure and surgical complications

57 of the 90 transplantations performed at our institution failed between 1 day and 2 years after surgery. 15 patients died with functioning graft without technical complications: 2 were recipients of a pancreatic graft alone and 13 were recipients of double kidney and pancreas transplantation. Causes of death are summarized in Table 2.

Vascular thrombosis was observed in 5 recipients of a pancreatic graft alone and in 11 recipients of a simultaneous kidney and pancreas transplantation.

Functional grafts were removed in 4 instances: for local infection in 1 case, for major postoperative bleeding in 1 case, and for extensive pancreatitis (in one case probably due to a prolonged cold ischemia) in 2 cases.

Late graft failure, considered as irreversible pancreas rejection occurred in 5 patients receiving a pancreas alone and in 17 receiving a double pancreatico-renal transplant.

Comparing segmental duct obstructed grafts (group A) and pancreatico-duodenal grafts (group B) we observed that vascular thrombosis occurred with comparable frequence (2 pancreas lost for thrombosis in group A and 3 in group B), but other surgical complications were more frequent in group B than in group A. In patients submitted to whole pancreas transplantation we observed: 1 postoperative bleeding requiring iterative surgery, 1 enteric leakage, 2 wound dehiscences and 1 small bowel occlusion. In patients receiving a segmental graft, only one wound dehiscence and one postoperative bleeding occurred. The relatively high incidence of wound dehiscences may be due to

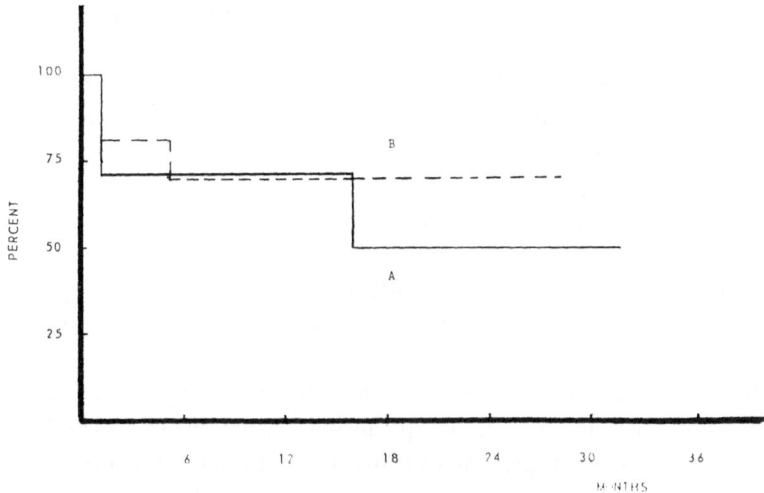

Figure 4. Enteric diversion (A) versus duct obstruction (B). Overall pancreas survival. A = 14 pts, B = 17 pts.

poor healing in immunosuppressed diabetic patients and the use of adsorbable sutures, that was further abandoned.

Pancreas and kidney rejection

In recipients of a pancreas alone, without surgical complications, irreversible acute graft failure occurred in 5 cases and insulin treatment had to be resumed.

In patients receiving double renal and pancreas allografts 106 episodes of renal failure were observed. Rejection affected the kidney alone in 46 episodes (2R, 25R2, 3R3, 16R5); functional changes of both organs occurred in 60 cases. In 54 instances steroid treatment for renal rejection was followed by pancreatic functional changes (5R, 33R2, 8R3, 1R4, 7R5) pancreatic function returned to normal in 49 cases of them (4R1, 33R2, 8R3, 1R4, 3R5) and loss of

Table 2. Causes of death in patients with functioning grat.

Patients	15
Vascular causes	7
Chronic hepatitis	1
Pulmonary embolism	1
D.I.C. after irreversible kidney rejection	2
Septicemia	1
Necrotising enteritis	1
Lymphoproliferative syndrome	2

pancreatic function, with restorement of insulin therapy was observed in 5 other cases.

Simultaneous functional changes of both organs was noted in 4 episodes (3R2, 1R3); steroids pulses were followed by a return to normal of both creatinine and glycemia.

In 2 episodes pancreatic functional changes preceeded kidney rejection (1R1, 1R2): steroid treatment induced normal serum creatinine and blood glucose.

Diagnosis of pancreas rejection is difficult to establish: even though different methods have been used in order to prevent a pancreatic failure: at present there is no marker of early rejection episodes.

An helpful method to detect early pancreatic graft failure, is to stop both parenteral nutrition and insulin therapy during a two hours period in the early morning. An increase of glycemia in this time lag, may be considered as a possible impairement in endocrine function.

In the grafts of the pancreas alone, rejection appeared as on 'all ore none' phenomenon. Changes of metabolic function were irreversible despite the rejection therapy.

Results of other series, as well as our results confirmed that in terms of pancreas survival, better results were achieved in recipients of simultaneous kidney transplants, than in recipients of a pancreas alone, or in recipients of a pancreas after a kidney. The better results achieved, suggest that it is easier to treat rejection episodes in patients receiving both organs from the same donors, and it is easier to prevent or to treat rejection of the pancreas in recipients of simultaneous renal and pancreas transplantation.

Metabolic function and degenerative complications

The details of the metabolic function and results have been described in another chapter of this issue.

Similar results were achieved in patients submitted to different immuno-suppressive regimens, however a better metabolic function was achieved in patients treated with CyA.

Glycemic control was similar in patients receiving a whole pancreas with enteric diversion or a segmental duct obstructed pancreas, whole pancreas having a slightly better response to provocative tests and a more evident hyperinsulinemia in comparison to segmental grafts.

In a great number of cases, secondary lesions of diabetes mellitus, were so far advanced before surgery, that it was difficult to evaluate the effect of transplantation on them. However, in all patients with a graft functioning more than 3 months, subjective symptoms of neuropathy improved, and an increase in muscular mass was observed [7].

In 5 patients with grafts functioning more than 2 years, electromyographical examinations showed an amelioration in 4 cases and a constant degradation in another. Ophtalmological investigations performed in 6 patients with grafts functioning more than 2 years, showed a stabilization of proliferative retinopathy in 5 cases and a progression of lesions in one.

Stabilization of retinopathy and neuropathy observed in our series, are difficult to correlate to graft function: in fact most of our patients undergo panphotocoagulation and it is hard to discriminate whether improvement or stabilization of retinal lesions were due to laser treatment or to normalization of glycemic control.

Furthermore, in uremic diabetic patients receiving a simultaneous kidney and pancreas graft it was difficult to discriminate whether improvement of peripheral neuropathy should be related to correction of diabetes or to reversal of uremia.

Discussion and conclusion

Pancreas and patients survival rate have progressively increased between 1976 and 1987 at our institution. Overall patient and graft survival is 74% and 43% respectively at one year.

In patients transplanted during 1985, 1986 and 1987, a great improvement of results was observed, due to larger experience, better physical conditions of recipients and better immunosuppression.

Early post-operative graft loss and pancreas rejection in our experience is comparable to that of other authors. Incidence of venous thrombosis remain high despite prophylactic anticoagulant treatment.

Even though Sollinger, reported a good correlation between dosage of amylasuria and marker of pancreatic rejection, in recipients of pancreaticoduodenal transplantation with urinary drainage of exocrine secretion [8], at present no marker of early pancreas rejection is available: definite diagnosis is only possible by pancreatic biopsy. According to the experience of most authors, simultaneous kidney and pancreas transplantation, seems to be the best method, for prevention or early treatment of pancreas rejection.

Improvement of degenerative complications of diabetes mellitus is still to be demonstrated. The new immunosuppressive treatments, including CyA allowed to lower steroids and to improve overall results [9].

After a two year follow up, the comparison between segmental Neoprene and whole pancreas transplantation does not show any difference in terms of overall patients and pancreas survival. Equally satisfactory results were achieved using both surgical techniques. Transplantation performed using graft prepared by duct obstruction with Neoprene, seems to be the easiest and safest surgical approach. The metabolic control achieved in patients receiving an injected segmental graft, is as satisfactory as that achieved with pancreatico-duodenal transplantation, whole pancreas showing a better response to induced hyperglycemia but a more marked hyperinsulinemia.

Diabetic end stage renal failure, clearly seems to be the best indication for simultaneous kidney and pancreas transplantation.

References

1. Dubernard JM, Traeger J, Neyra P et al: New method of a segmental pancreatic graft for transplantation. Trials in dogs and in man. Surgery 84: 634, 1978.
2. Dubernard JM, Traeger J, Neyra P et al: Long term effect of Neoprene injection in the canine pancreatic duct. Transpl Proc 11, 1979.
3. Williams GM, White HJ, Hame DM: Transplantation 5: 837, 1967.
4. Piatti PM, Traeger J, Dubernard JM et al: Hormonal evaluation of immediate pancreatic function in simultaneous kidney plus pancreas transplantation during artificial pancreas monitoring. Transpl Proc 17: 346, 1985.
5. Cantarovich D, Traeger J, La Rocca E et al: Evaluation of metabolic and endocrine function in the neoprene injected segmental pancreas allografts at three months after transplantation versus preliminary results in nine whole pancreas allografts with enteric diversion. Transplant Proc 19: 2310, 1987.
6. Dubernard JM, La Rocca E, Faure JL et al: Simultaneous pancreas and kidney transplantation: long term results and comparison of 2 surgical techniques, Transpl Proc in press.
7. Traeger J, Dubernard JM, Monti D et al: Clinical experience with long-term studies of degenerative complications in man after pancreas transplantation. Transpl Proc 17: 1740, 1986.
8. Sollinger HW, Cook K, Kamps D et al: Transplant Proc 16: 749, 1984.
9. Pozza G, Secchi A, Pontiroli AE et al: Segmental neoprene injected pancreas allotransplantation: influence on the endocrine function of different immunosuppressive treatments. Pozza G et al (eds) Diet, diabetes and atherosclerosis. Raven Press, New York, 1984.

Experience of the University of Minnesota, Minneapolis, Minnesota, USA

D.E.R. SUTHERLAND, F.C. GOETZ, K.C. MOUDRY and
J.S. NAGARIAN

The University of Minnesota Pancreas Transplant Program began in 1966 [1] and by January 1988 included 224 cases [2]. Several changes in recipient selection immunosuppression, and surgical technique have occurred over the years [3–12]. Our past and current results and protocols are briefly summarized here.

Historical results

Fourteen pancreas transplants were performed between 1966 and 1973. Ten were simultaneous with a kidney [3]. Only one recipient had both grafts function for more than one year [4].

One hundred pancreas transplants were performed from July 1978 through October 1984 [9]. Twenty-seven grafts (27%) functioned (recipients euglycemic and insulin independent) for ≧ one year with one currently functioning for >9 years. The actual recipient survival rate at one year was 88%. More than half (fifty-two) of the recipients had had previous kidney transplants. Most recipients were immunosuppressed with double drug therapy.

Current results

In November 1984, we began to compare the bladder and enteric drainage techniques for graft duct management, used triple drug immunosuppressive therapy (cyclosporin, prednisone, azathioprine) in all patients, and expanded the acceptance criteria to include three categories of recipients [11]. Since this time 110 pancreas transplants have been performed, 64 with bladder and 43 with enteric drainage. The categories (with number of recipients as of January, 1988 given in parentheses), are as follows:

a)   Non-uremic, non-kidney transplant patients (n = 62);

J.M. Dubernard and D.E.R. Sutherland (eds.), International Handbook of Pancreas Transplantation, 399–404.
© *1989 by Kluwer Academic Publishers.*

b) Recipients of previous kidney transplants with functioning grafts (n = 28);
c) Uremic (n = 13) or pre-uremic (n = 7) patients undergoing simultaneous pancreas and kidney transplants (n = 20).

Actuarial graft and patient survival rates were calculated in February, 1988 [11]. The overall one year patient survival was 91%, and was identical for recipients of enteric and bladder drained grafts. The one year graft survival rate was 49% overall and 70% for 77 technically successful cases.

The one year actuarial graft survival rate was higher for bladder (60%) than for enteric (40%) drained transplants. For technically successful cases the one year graft survivals for bladder (n = 48) and enteric (n = 28) drained cases were 80% and 60%, respectively. The higher one year graft survival rates with bladder drainage are a reflection of the enhanced ability to diagnose and treat allograft rejection episodes early based on changes in urine amylase activity [13].

The actuarial one year pancreatic graft function rate within the three recipient categories are as follows:
a) 48% for 62 non-uremic, non-kidney transplant patients (58% for 30 bladder and 40% for 32 enteric drained cases);
b) 32% for 28 recipients of previous kidney transplants (47% for 15 bladder and 36% for 11 enteric drained cases);
c) 73% for 20 uremic (n = 13) or pre-uremic (n = 7) patients undergoing simultaneous pancreas and kidney transplants (all bladder drained).

The one year graft function rates in recipients of technically successful operations were 63% for 47 pancreas transplants alone (75% for 24 bladder and 56% for 23 enteric drained cases), 75% for 13 pancreas transplants after a kidney (86% for 7 bladder and 80% for 5 enteric cases), and 86% for 17 pancreas transplants received simultaneously with a kidney.

Pancreas grafts from living related donors [14] have been used during this period. Related donor grafts appear to have a decreased propensity for rejection as compared to cadaveric grafts. The actuarial one year patient and graft survival rates for grafts from living related donors (n = 25) were 92% and 50% versus 92% and 49% for cadaver cases (n = 85). The one year function rates for technically successful living related (n = 15) and cadaver (n = 62) donor transplants were 85% and 67%. Currently, we are using bladder drainage for pancreas grafts obtained from cadaver donors and enteric or bladder drainage for transplants from related donors [2]. The results of transplants performed since November 1984 by the techniques currently exclusively used are summarized in Table 1.

Technical aspects

In regard to procurement and preservation of grafts from cadaveric donors we routinely obtained the pancreas from liver donors, the type of graft, whole or segmental, being dependent on the vascular anatomy of the donor [10]. If the blood supply to the head of the pancreas and duodenum can be maintained without compromise to the hepatic vasculature, a whole pancreas graft is obtained.

Preservation times of over 24 hours are possible with a hyperosmolar silica gel filtered plasma (SGF) solution [15]. Our mean ($\pm$ S.D.) average preservation time since November 1984 has been 13.7 ± 6.5 hours. The results of oral and intravenous glucose tolerance and metabolic profiles have been similar in recipients of grafts stored for <6, 6–12, or 12–24 hours [16, 17].

Metabolic studies and course of secondary complications

Detailed studies on the earliest successful pancreas transplants clearly showed the ability of a functioning graft to restore an euglycemic, insulin-independent state, with most metabolic parameters being normalized [18]. Virtually all recipients maintain normal glycosolated hemoglobin levels, even though glucose tolerance test results are not entirely normal in about half of the recipients [8, 9].

Table 1. Patient and graft functional survival rates at one year for pancreas transplants performed from November 1984 to January 1988 at the University of Minnesota by techniques in current use.

Category	No Txs	No TS	Patient survival	Graft survival	
				All	TS
Px alone	45	34	95%	56%[a]	76%
Cad bladder	30	24	96%	58%[b]	75%
Rel enteric	15	10	93%	51%	77%
Px after kidney	22	10	86%	45%[a]	90%
Cad bladder	13	5	85%	38%[b, c]	80%
Rel bladder	2	2	100%	100%	100%
Rel enteric	7	3	83%	43%	100%
Px + kidney[d]					
Cad bladder	19	17	88%	77%[b]	86%
Total	86	61	91%	57%	80%

[a, b, c] p values ≤0.05.

[d] 13 uremic and 6 pre-uremic patients. For the pre-uremic patients, the patient survival rate at 1 year was 100% and the pancreas graft survival rate 92%.

The course of pre-existing secondary complications of the kidneys, nerves and eyes have been studied in detail in our recipients [18]. Biopsies of native kidney in nonuremic patients followed for >2 years have shown significant decreases in glomerular mesangial volume from pretransplant values [19], indicating an amelioration of a lesion specific for diabetic nephropathy, but serum creatinine levels have increased and creatinine clearance values have decreased from cyclosporin nephrotoxicity [20]. The decrease in creatinine clearance occurs in the immediate posttransplant period, but so far has not been progressive [20]. Nevertheless, the long-term effect of cyclosporin on renal pathology remains to be determined.

Retinopathy, at least during the first year post-transplant, continue to progress in some patients in spite of a functioning graft [21]. After 2 years, however, retinopathy appears to stabilize in virtually all patients with functioning grafts.

Neuropathy improves with significant increases in nerve conduction velocities occur during the first year after pancreas transplantation to nonuremic recipients [22]. Deterioration of evoked muscle action potentials is also halted by a successful pancreas transplant [11].

Discussion

The University of Minnesota results show that pancreas transplantation is applicable to selected diabetic patients with early but emerging complications that would otherwise predictably progress to a stage more serious than that of potential side effects of chronic immunosuppression. Other groups have largely confined pancreas transplants to recipients of kidney transplants [24–26]. Such a selection process is reflected in the International Pancreas Transplant Registry statistics, where more than 60% of the transplants have been simultaneous with a kidney transplant and nearly 20% after a kidney transplant; less than 20% have been in patients without end stage diabetic nephropathy (see chapter on registry). There also are no differences in graft survival rates according to Registry analysis of the three major duct management techniques (polymer injection, bladder drainage and enteric drainage).

Our results are dissimilar to the Registry results. We show a superior outcome with bladder drainage for transplants from cadaver donors. Other institutions [24], including the one where it was first employed [25], have also had excellent results with this technique. For related donor grafts, enteric drainage has had a relatively high success rate because rejection episodes are less likely to occur for transplants from this source. Another group has had excellent results with enteric drainage from cadaver donors, perhaps because the graft duct secretions are collected via catheter in the early post transplant period allowing monitoring of exocrine function for early diagnosis of rejection [26].

In summary, we currently use bladder drainage for cadaver donor and enteric drainage for related donor transplants [2], preserve grafts in SGF made hyperosmolar with mannitol for whatever period up to 30 hours is necessary to solve the logistical problems associated with transplantation from cadaver donors [16], and use quadruple immunosuppressive therapy [8]. We perform pancreas transplants in patients who have complications of diabetes more serious than the side effects of anti-rejection treatment. For pancreas transplantation to be applicable to a wider range of patients less toxic immunosuppression is needed. If anti-rejection treatment becomes safer, pancreas transplantation could have a prophylactic as well as a therapeutic role for treatment of diabetes and its complications.

References

1. Kelly WD, Lillehei RC, Merkel FK, Idezuki Y, Goetz FC: Allotransplantation of the pancreas and duodenum along with the kidney in diabetic nephropathy. Surgery 61: 827, 1967.
2. Sutherland DER, Moudry KC, Elick BA, Goetz FC, Najarian JS: Pancreas transplant protocols at the university of Minnesota: recipient and donor selection, operation and postoperative management and outcome. In: Terasaki PI (ed) Clinical transplants; pp 109–126. Los Angeles, 1987.
3. Lillehei RC, Simmons RL, Najarian JS et al: Pancreaticoduodenal allotransplantation: experimental and clinical experience. Ann Surg 172: 405–436, 1970.
4. Lillehei RC, Ruiz JO, Acquino C, Goetz FC: Transplantation of the pancreas. Acta Endocrinol 83 (Suppl 205): 303, 1976.
5. Sutherland DER, Goetz FC, Najarian JS: Intraperitoneal transplantation of immediately vascularized segmental pancreatic grafts without duct ligation: a clinical trial. Transplantation 28: 485–491, 1971.
6. Sutherland DER, Goetz FC, Rynasiewicz JJ, Baumgartner D, White DC, Elick BA, Najarian JS: Segmental pancreas transplantation from living related and cadaver donors: a clinical experience. Surgery 90: 159–169, 1981.
7. Sutherland DER, Goetz FC, Elick BA, Najarian JS: Experience with 49 segmental pancreas transplants in 45 diabetic patients. Transplantation 34: 330–338, 1982.
8. Sutherland DER, Goetz FC, Najarian JS: One hundred pancreas transplants at a single institution. Ann Surg 200: 414–440, 1984.
9. Sutherland DER, Goetz FC, Kendall DM, Najarian JS: One institutions experience with pancreas transplantation. West J Med 143: 838–844, 1985.
10. Prieto M, Sutherland DER, Goetz FC, Rosenberg ME, Najarian JS: Pancreas transplant results according to technique of duct management: bladder versus enteric drainage. Surgery 102: 680–691, 1987.
11. Sutherland DER, Goetz FC, Moudry KC, Najarian JS: Pancreatic transplantation – a single institution's experience. Diab Nut Metabol 1: 57–64, 1988.
12. Sutherland DER, Kendall DM, Moudry KC: Pancreas transplantation in nonuremic type I diabetic recipients. Surgery 104: 453–464, 1988.

404

13. Prieto M, Sutherland DER, Fernandez-Cruz L, Heil J, Najarian JS: Experimental and clinical experience with urine amylase monitoring for early diagnosis of rejection in pancreas transplantation. Transplantation 43: 71–79, 1987.
14. Sutherland DER, Goetz FC, Najarian JS: Pancreas transplants from related donors. Transplantation 38: 625–633, 1984.
15. Florack G, Sutherland DER, Heil J, Squifflet JP, Najarian JS: Preservation of canine segmental pancreatic autografts: cold storage versus pulsatile machine perfusion. J Surg Res 34: 493–504, 1983.
16. Florack G, Sutherland DER, Heise J, Najarian JS: Successful preservation of human pancreas grafts for up to 28 hours. Transpl Proc 19: 3882–3885, 1987.
17. Abouna GM, Sutherland DER, Florack G, Najarian JS: Function of transplanted human pancreatic allografts after preservation in cold storage for 6 to 26 hours. Transplantation 43: 630–636, 1987.
18. Sutherland DER, Najarian JS, Greenberg BZ, Senske BJ, Anderson GE, Francis RS, Goetz FC: Vascularized segmental transplantation on the pancreas in insulin-dependent patients: hormonal and metabolic effects of an endocrine graft. Ann Int Med 95: 537–541, 1981.
19. Bilous RW, Mauer SM, Sutherland DER, Steffes MW: Glomerular structure and function following successful pancreas transplantation for insulin- dependent diabetes mellitus. Diabetes 36: 43A, 1987.
20. De Francisco A, Mauer SM, Steffes MW, Goetz FC, Najarian JS, Sutherland DER: The effect of cyclosporin on native renal function in nonuremic diabetic recipients of pancreas transplants. J Diab Complications 1: 128–131, 1987.
21. Ramsay RC, Goetz FC, Sutherland DER, Mauer SM, Robinson LL, Cantrill HL, Knobloch WH, Najarian JS: Progression of diabetic retinopathy after pancreas transplantation for insulin-dependent diabetes mellitus. New Engl J Med 318: 208–214, 1988.
22. van der Vliet D, Navarro X, Kennedy WR, Goetz FC, Sutherland DER, Najarian JS: Effect of pancreas transplantation on diabetic polyneuropathy. Transplantation 45: 368–370, 1988.
23. Sutherland DER, Moudry KC: Pancreas transplant registry report. In: Terasaki PI (ed) Clinical transplants; UCLA Press, pp 63–101, 1987.
24. Corry RJ, Nghiem DD: Evolution of technique and results of pancreas transplantation at the university of Iowa. Clin Transpl 1: 52–56, 1987.
25. Sollinger HW, Cook K, Kamps D, Glass NR, Belzer FO: Clinical and experimental experience with pancreaticocystostomy for exocrine pancreatic drainage in pancreas transplantation. Transpl Proc 16: 749, 1984.
26. Groth GC, Collste H, Lundgren G et al: Successful outcome of segmental human pancreatic transplantation with enteric exocrine diversion after modifications in technique. Lancet 2: 522–524, 1982.

Experience of the University of Munich, Klinikum Grosshadern, Munich, FRG

W. LAND, R. LANDGRAF, W.-D. ILLNER, D. ABENDROTH,
A. KAMPIK, F.P. LENHART, D. BURG, G. HILLEBRAND,
L.A. CASTRO (†), M.M.C. LANDGRAF-LEURS, M. GOKEL,
St. SCHLEIBNER, J. NUSSER and M. ULBIG

The first pancreatic transplant at the University of Munich was performed in August 1979. Since then, 91 pancreatic transplants have been performed: combined pancreas and kidney transplantation (n = 80), pancreas transplantation alone (n = 7), and pancreas retransplantation (n = 4). In all cases, duct obliteration with prolamine in a segmental pancreatic graft was used as the standard procedure. Patient selection criteria, surgical technique of recipients' operations, postoperative management, and immunosuppressive protocols were modified several times, however, during the past 7 years. Recently, assessment of a potentially beneficial effect on secondary complications was studied more intensively.

In this paper, our experience with the current immunosuppressive protocol, recent results, metabolic studies, and in particular, the effect of successful transplantation on the secondary complications of diabetes will be described. Since our results of pancreas transplantation alone in nonuremic patients are still extremely poor (no successful case in 7 patients so far), we concentrate here on the clinical observations obtained in cyclosporin-treated patients who have undergone combined (simultaneous) transplantation of the pancreas and kidney (n = 85).

This report summarizes some of our experiences during the past 7 years, which has been published in part elsewhere (1–28).

Current immunosuppressive protocol

Basic immunosuppressive regimen for induction treatment

1. Cyclosporin initially administered intravenously (24-hour infusion) at a starting dose of 1 to 2 mg/kg bodyweight (BW) and day (desired cyclosporin target levels in whole blood RIA-tests using polyclonal antibody assay SANDOZ: 100 to 250 ng/ml); this regimen is switched to oral adminis-

405

J.M. Dubernard and D.E.R. Sutherland (eds.), International Handbook of Pancreas Transplantation, 405–411.
© *1989 by Kluwer Academic Publishers.*

tration by the tenth day postoperatively (doses of 6 to 12 mg/kg BW and day, adjusted to trough levels of 300 to 500 ng/ml).

2. Azathioprine is given at a dose of 1 to 2 mg/kg BW and day (formerly discontinued at 3 weeks but now reduced to 1 mg/kg BW and day for maintenance treatment);
3. Methylprednisolone is rapidly tapered from 250 mg/d to 30 mg and day.
4. Either ATG (Fresenius, Bad Homburg, FRG) or ALG (Behring, Marburg, FRG) are administered from day 1 to day 10 at a dose of 4 mg/kg BW and day or 20 mg/kg BW and day, respectively.

Maintenance treatment is as follows: cyclosporin in given orally at doses of 4 to 6 mg/kg BW and day (keeping trough levels at 300 ng/ml), azathioprine at a dose of 1 mg/kg BW and day, and methylprednisolone at a dose of 5 to 10 mg/d over a period of 6 months. From month 7 double drug maintenance treatment consisting of cyclosporin and azathioprine is continued.

Antirejection treatment

Methylprednisolone is given by intravenous bolus injection at a dose of 250 mg/d for three days. More recently, we administer ALG or ATG in conjunction with steroids, 125 to 250 mg/d methylprednisolone from the first day of antirejection therapy for a period of seven days. To avoid secondary venous thrombosis due to immunologically induced inflammatory edema, we combine this treatment with anticoagulation (low-dose heparin for a period of seven days).

Results

Simultaneous pancreas and kidney transplantation has been performed in 80 cyclosporin-treated type I diabetes recipients. In autumn 1984, four major modifications were introduced:

1. restrictive recipient selection (exclusion criteria: coronary heart disease),
2. intraperitoneal positioning of the graft,
3. multiple-drug induction treatment, and
4. anticoagulation protocol using dextran 40 plus low-dose heparin. Since this time, a subgroup of 43 patients underwent combined pancreas and kidney transplantation.

The current 4-year survival probability rate is 100% for patients; 78% for kidney grafts and 55% for pancreatic grafts. The causes of loss of pancreatic grafts were 1 acute rejection; 4 chronic rejection; 6 venous thrombosis; 4 infected fistulas; 1 bleeding.

Long-term follow-up of secondary complications of diabetes

Metabolic control

Because our definition of successful pancreatic transplantation is no further requirement for exogenous insulin for glucose control, all of our patients with functioning grafts are free of insulin. 27 long-term patients so far studied (all combined kidney and pancreatic transplant recipients) have functioning grafts at 3 months to 5 years posttransplant, with normal fasting blood glucose levels (89 ± 3 mg/dl) and normal HbA$_1$ values (7.0% ± 0.2%); but a slightly elevated basal insulin value (26 ± 2 μU/ml; range, 9 to 46 μU/ml; normal, 17 μU/ml). This may be due to decreased insulin clearance by the transplanted but not always normally functioning kidney graft (serum creatinine level, 2.6 ± 0.5 mg/dl; range, 0.8 to 9.1 mg/dl). The oral glucose tolerance with 100 g glucose is normal in 63% (n = 17) and impaired in 37% (n = 10) of the patients. Insulin and C-peptide secretion analysis after glucose load and intravenous arginine stimulation showed no significant differences in patients with or without normal glucose tolerance. Glucagon suppressibility after glucose and the stimulatory action of arginine are similar in both groups of pancreatic transplant recipients. In 19 patients followed for a mean of 27 ± 6 months (mean ± SEM), there has been no gradual impairment of glucose tolerance or insulin release.

Other important parameters associated with the development or progression of angiopathy were improved after transplantation: uric acid, 6.3 ± 0.3 mg/dl; triglycerides, 137 ± 15 mg/dl; total cholesterol, 214 ± 8 mg/dl; and high-density lipoprotein-cholesterol, 62 ± 7 mg/dl. Hypertension, which was present in 27 patients with functioning grafts before transplantation, disappeared in 11 patients (41%); the mean BP values fell to 130/83 ± 8/2 mm Hg) and could be controlled by antihypertensive treatment in the other patients (151/92 ± 6/2 mm Hg).

Neuropathy

Twenty-two patients were studied for a mean time of 24 months for peripheral sensory and motor polyneuropathy. Before transplantation 17 patients complained of neuropathic symptoms such as paraesthesia, sensory loss, or gait disturbances. At the first examination 19 patients had clinical signs of neuropathy, and all had pathological electrophysiological test results. After transplantation paraesthesias and painful sensations improved or disappeared in 16 patients within the first 3 to 6 months. Clinical signs of neuropathy improved in 11 patients and stabilized in the others. Peroneal, sural, and median nerve conduction velocities increased significantly (p<0.5) during follow-up. Five patients developed symptoms of carpal tunnel syndrome; in one patient, distal latencies of median nerve conduction increased with no clinical symptoms. Surgery was necessary for the carpal tunnel syndrome in one patient. Seven patients developed trophic ulcers despite the improvements in neuropathy and peripheral microcirculation. Surgery was necessary in five of these patients. After renal graft loss with continuing pancreatic transplant function, there was a decrease in nerve conduction velocity in two patients and no changes in the other two. There was no correlation between kidney function and nerve conduction velocity. Exact analysis of autonomic neuropathy is difficult. However, subjective and objective clinical signs of autonomic neuropathy such as beat-to-beat variations are resistant to the effects of normalization of glucose metabolism and kidney function.

Retinopathy

As series of 34 patients was followed for 1 to 58 months (mean, 21 months) after successful combined pancreatic and renal transplantation. Follow-up data included visual acuity, slit-lamp examination, fundus photographs, and if possible, fluorescein angiography and computerized perimetry. Funduscopy and fundus photographs were analyzed independently by the same two ophthalmologists. Visual acuity improved in 56%, stabilized in 32%, and deteriorated in 12% (n = 4). Two of the latter patients developed a cataract, which was responsible for the change. The incidence of vitreous hemorrhages pretransplant was 69%, and early posttransplant (10 months), it was 24%, and thereafter fell to 12%. The hemorrhages cleared more quickly after grafting. The proliferative process in the retina increased in only two eyes of all the patients. During the follow-up period, additional laser treatment was performed in three eyes. The fundus photographs revealed obliteration of neovascular strands in the vitreous body and their change into fibrocellular remnants. Ten patients staged as preproliferative retinopathy with nonperfusion areas seen on fluorescein angiography have not progressed to proliferative retinopathy.

Peripheral microcirculation

To evaluate the effect of pancreas transplantation on the microcirculation, we have introduced the noninvasive combination of transcutaneous oxygen pressure measurements ($tcpO_2$) and telethermography. With $tcpO_2$ electrodes, the skin is locally warmed to 44° C so that maximum intradermal and subdermal vessel dilation is achieved and the maximum dilation reserve capacity can be measured. The thermocamera allows examination of the whole extremity, and detection of the peripheral perfusion border. Quatity and quality of perfusion at this borderline are of the utmost importance for attachment of the $tcpO_2$

electrode and study of microcirculatory behavior. Data from 15 patients over a follow-up period of 17 months (range, 6 to 30 months) show a significant change in the microcirculatory pattern within 12 weeks after pancreas transplantation, which indicates improvement. The tcpO$_2$ values increased from 44 ± 4 mm Hg preoperatively to 62 ± 3 mm Hg, a nearly normal value. Control groups (single-kidney transplantation in type I diabetics ($n = 5$) and in nondiabetics ($n = 8$) did not show any changes. We conclude from these preliminary data that successful pancreas transplantation has a beneficial effect on peripheral diabetic microangiopathy.

Conclusions

In summary, at the University of Munich we have performed 91 transplants using duct-occluded segmental pancreatic allografts. With this technique and after some modifications in the protocol 4 years ago (concerning recipient selection criteria, recipient operation, immunosuppressive protocol, anticoagulation protocol) a 4-year graft survival probability rate in uremic patients (receiving a pancreatic and renal graft) has been achieved by 55%. Moreover, 63% of all successfully transplanted recipients show a completely normal glucose tolerance. There is growing clinical evidence suggesting that successful pancreatic transplantation can exert a beneficial effect on late secondary complications. In our experience, progession of diabetic polyneuropathy, retinopathy, and peripheral microangiopathy could at least been stopped in a vast majority of patients sometimes even reversed. Evaluation of the potential benefits of pancreas transplantation still remains a problem for the following reasons:

(1) So far, only secondary intervention and no primary prevention trials of secondary complications in diabetics have been conducted;
(2) Only about 10% of all transplanted diabetics have received a single pancreatic graft;
(3) Most of the diabetics have received a combined kidney/pancreas graft due to end-stage renal failure and for other advanced diabetic lesions: Uremia and diabetes are eliminated at the same time;
(4) Patients with pancreatic grafts survival longer than 5 years are still exceptions.

We remain aware, of the fact that the technique of duct occlusion is not physiological for the graft and is still associated with a high incidence of pancreatic fistulas. However, it has proven to be safe in the recent series of patients. Thus far, there is no clinical or metabolic evidence that occlusion-induced fibrosis can lead to a steadily decreasing endocrine function of the graft secondary to a disturbance in the microcirculation of the islets (maximal observation period; 6 years).

In addition, it has to be mentioned that the process of occlusion-induced fibrosis takes about 6 months. From that time post transplant onwards only islet in surrounding fibrous tissue are existing within the previous pancreatic graft. Therefore this type of pancreatic transplantation looses its character of an active-gland-transplantation over a period of 6 months, but then, can be regarded as transplantation of vascularized islets. This implies that there is no potential long-term risk neither to the graft nor to the patient when compared to the other techniques performing transplantation of an active gland with maintained exocrine function.

In our opinion, this is the main advantage of the technique of duct occlusion in pancreatic transplantation. Consequently, our main research in clinical pancreatic transplantation will concentrate on further optimization of that technique.

References

1. Land W, Weitz H: Lancet 2: 1131, 1979.
2. Land W, von Liebe S, Kuhlmann H et al: Transpl Proc 12: (suppl 2) 76, 1980.
3. Land W, Eberhard K, Weitz H et al: In: Gebhardt Ch, Stolte M (eds) Pankreasgang-okklusion; p 103. Verlag G. Witzstrock, Köln, 1980.
4. Land W, Gebhardt ChH, Gall FP et al: Transpl Proc 12: (suppl 2) 72, 1980.
5. Land W, von Liebe S, Höpp H et al: Chir Praxis 27: 15, 1980.
6. Hahn D, Büll U, Unertl R et al: Münch Med Woch 123: 1262, 1981.
7. Landgraf R, Abendroth D, Land W et al: Somatostatin. Athens, Greece, Second International Symposium 1981.
8. Abendroth D, Landgraf R, Land W: Langenbecks Arch Chir 358: 1982.
9. Abendroth D, Steiner E, Illner W-D et al: V Nied Westf Chir 149: 12, 1982.
10. Gruner P, Schneeberger H, Stangl M et al: International symposium on organ transplantation in diabetics. The Hague, Netherlands (abstr 44) 1983.
11. Hahn D, Büll U, Land W: Horm Metab Res 13: (Suppl) 78, 1983.
12. Illner W-D, Land W, Abendroth D et al: Internation symposium on organ transplantation in diabetics. The Hague, Netherlands (abstr 10) 1983.
13. Land W, Landgraf R, Illner W-D et al: Langenbecks Arch Chir 361: 752, 1983.
14. Land W, Landgraf R, Heberer G: 30. Congress of the societe internationale de chirurgie, Hamburg, FRG (abstr p 219).
15. Landgraf R, Abendroth D, Land W: Horm Metab Res 13: (Suppl) 67, 1983.
16. Landgraf R, Landgraf-Leurs MMC, Kampik A et al: Second symposium study group of the european association for study of diabetes, Austria (abstr) 1983.
17. Landgraf R, Landgraf-Leurs MMC, Kampik A et al: International symposium on organ transplantation in diabetics. The Hague, Netherlands (abstr 18) 1983.
18. Landgraf R, Abendroth D, Land W: Horm Metab Res 13: (Suppl) 67, 1983.
19. Landgraf R, Land W: Bayer Internist 5: 5, 1983.
20. Lenhart FP, Unertl K, Jensen U et al: International symposium on organ transplantation in diabetics. The Hague, Netherlands, (abstr 23) 1983.
21. Steiner E, Landgraf R, Gruner P et al: International symposium on organ transplantation in diabetics. The Hague, Netherlands, (abstr 58) 1983.

22. Landgraf R, Landgraf-Leurs MMC, Burg D et al: Transpl Proc 16 (3): 687, 1984.
23. Land W, Landgraf R, Illner W-D et al: Niere u. Hochdruck 1987.
24. Landgraf R, Landgraf-Leurs MMC, Burg D et al: Intensivmedizin. Gg. Thieme Verlag 44, Stuttgart, 1985.
25. Land W, Landgraf R, Illner W-D et al: Bayer. Internist 7: 28, 1985.
26. Jensen U, Lenhart FP, Militzer H et al: In: Lawin P, Peter K, von Ackern H (eds) Sixth international symposium. Gg. Thieme Verlag 41, Stuttgart, 1985.
27. Landgraf T, Land W: Internist (Berlin) 26: 557, 1985.
28. Land W, Landgraf R. et al: Transpl Proc 19: (Suppl 4), 75–83, 1987.

Experience of the National Hospital, Oslo, Norway

I.B. BREKKE

A pancreas transplant programme was initiated in Norway in 1983 and so far (March 1988) a total of 53 diabetic patients have been treated with duct occluded segmental grafts. In 46 uremic patients the pancreas was transplanted simultaneously with a renal graft. The one year pancreas graft survival (insulin independent recipient) in this group was 66%. The 94% patient and 85% kidney graft survival rates over three years were identical with the results achieved in diabetic recipients of kidney grafts from living related donors. Of 7 non-uremic patients who received pancreatic grafts only, two have been insulin independent for more than one year. Next to rejection, late graft artery thrombosis was the most frequent known cause of graft loss in both groups. With the intention of increasing arterial blood flow and thus preventing thrombus formation, a new technique for graft revascularisation was developed, consisting of interposition of the graft artery between the common iliac and the inferior epigastric artery. This technique has been applied in 17 patients.

It is concluded that the combined pancreas/kidney transplantation will continue to be the standard treatment for uremic diabetic patients in Norway, while in non-uremic diabetics, pancreas transplantation will be performed in selected patients only.

Introduction

In Norway with a population of 4 million, all organ transplant activity is located to a single center, the Rikshospital in Oslo, where a programme for pancreas transplantation was initiated in June 1983. Our experience with 46 recipients of combined pancreas and kidney transplants and 7 non-uremic recipients of pancreatic transplants is reported.

J.M. Dubernard and D.E.R. Sutherland (eds.), International Handbook of Pancreas Transplantation, 413–419.
© *1989 by Kluwer Academic Publishers.*

Patients and methods

Since 1983, all diabetic patients with end stage renal disease who do not have a living related kidney donor, have been offered the simultaneous transplantation of pancreas and kidney grafts from a cadaveric donor (Figure 1). Only 3 patients have actually been excluded from the combined transplantation because of high age and extremely advanced and generalized atherosclerosis. Blindness (10 patients), symptomatic coronary heart disease (3 patients), previous myocardial infarction (2 patients) or even sequelae of cerebro-vascular insults (6 patients), did not preclude the transplantation. So far (March 1988), a total of 46 patients have received combined transplants. Twentynine patients (63%) were on dialysis treatment at the time of transplantation, and 17 (37%) were predialytic.

In addition to the 46 recipients of combined grafts, 7 non-uremic diabetic patients underwent pancreas transplantation because of extremely unstable diabetes with frequent hypoglycemic episodes.

Sex distribution, mean age, and duration of diabetes at the time of transplantation are shown in Table 1.

Donors were heart-beating cadavers aged 5–55 years. A standardized multiorgan harvesting technique was used with in situ perfusion with Ringer acetate. The left segment of the pancreas together with the splenic vessels was removed. Neoprene was injected into the pancreatic duct and the pancreas was stored for 3 to 8 hours in chilled Euro-Collins solution until transplanted.

Surgical technique

The first 34 transplantations were performed by a previously described technique [1] which included extraperitoneally located vascular anastomoses and partial intraperitoneal placement of the pancreas. The occurence of wound fistulation in about 30% of the recipients, and graft artery thrombosis occuring in some patients several months after transplantation, led us to change the technique. In the following 17 recipients, the pancreatic graft was placed entirely intraperitoneally and dual arterial anastomoses were constructed by

Table 1. Recipients of pancreatic transplants. June 1983 – March 1988.

Category	Sex (M/F)	Age mean (range)	Diabetes duration mean (range)
A	34/12	39 (24–52)	24 (7–37)
B	2/5	35 (18–52)	15 (9–19)

A = uremic recipients of combined renal/pancreatic transplants.
B = non-uremic recipients of pancreatic transplants.

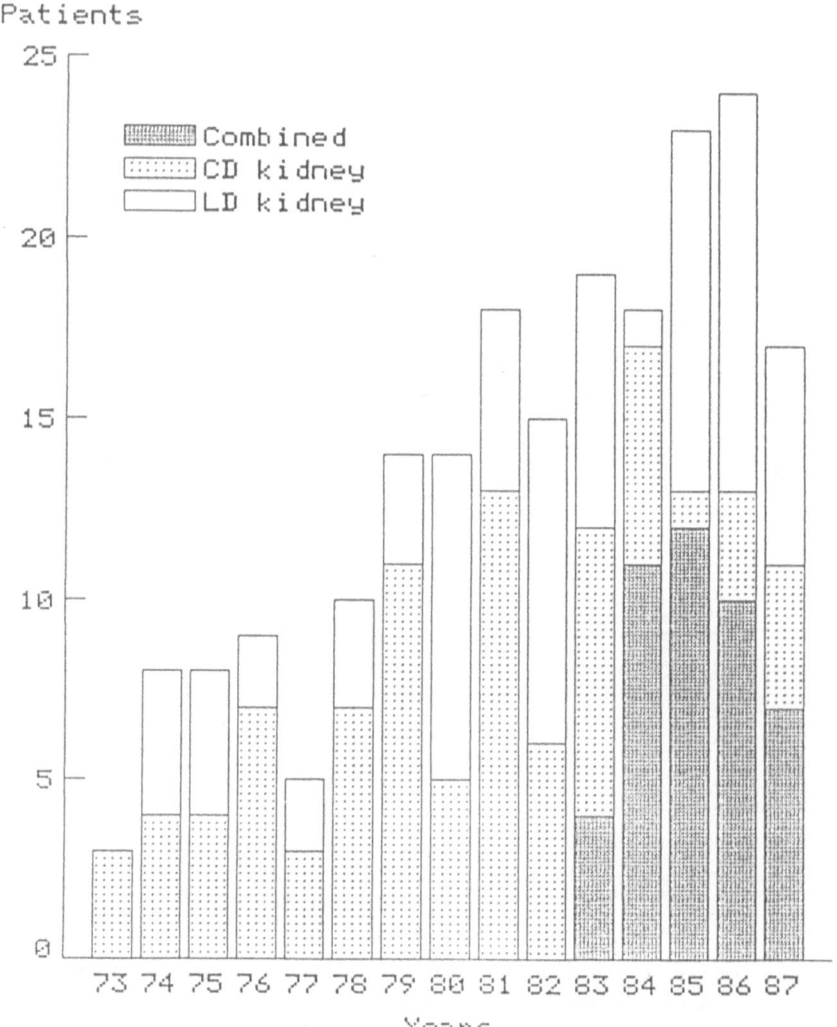

Figure 1. Annual number of diabetic recipients of renal transplants from cadaveric (dotted) and living related donors (open), and recipients of combined renal and pancreatic grafts (shaded parts of columns).

interposing the splenic artery between the common iliac and inferior epigastric artery (Figure 2).

Post operative treatment

The post operative regime has been the same as for renal transplant recipients,

416

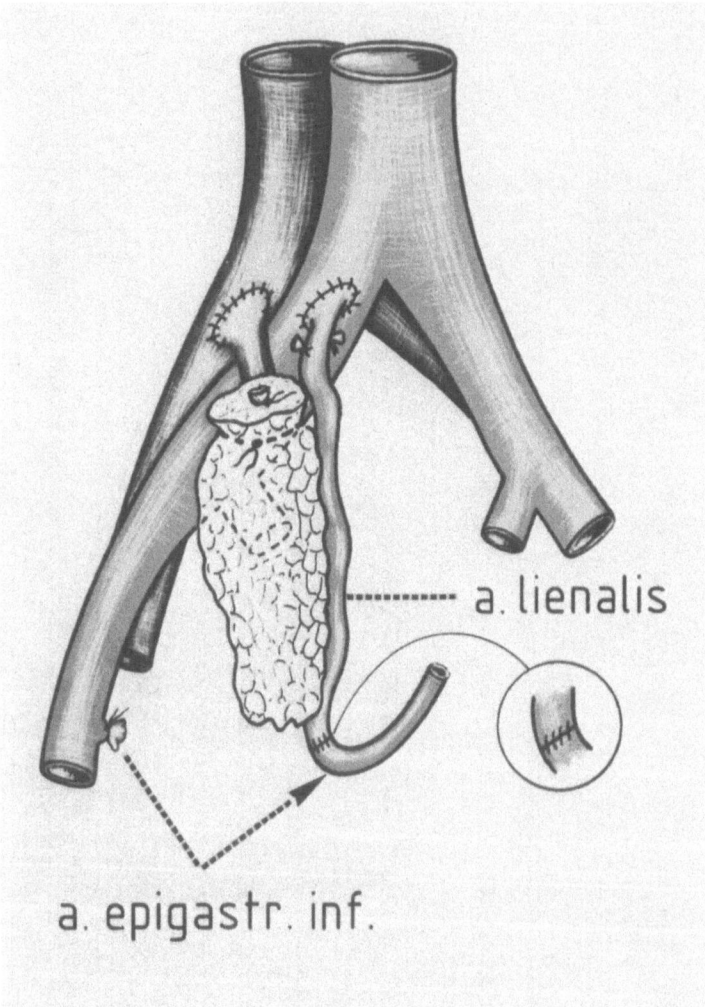

Figure 2. Technique of segmental pancreas transplantation with interposition of splenic artery between common iliac and inferior epigastric artery.

except that parenteral nutrition is given during the first week, and dextran 70, 500 ml, every second day, for 1–2 weeks. Dextran is then replaced with acetylsalicylic acid, 500 mg, on alternate days.

Immunosuppression

Currently triple immunosuppressive therapy consisting of low dose prednisolone, azathioprine and cyclosporin is given. Rejection episodes are treated with methylprednisolone in repeated bolus doses.

Results

Initial good function was achieved in all pancreas transplants so that insulin treatment could be stopped.

Surgical intervention was required in 4 of the initial recipients because of postoperative hemorrhage. Wound secretion occurred during the first post-operative weeks in about 30% of the patients.

Three recipients of combined grafts died with functioning pancreas transplant within two years of transplantation, two of myocardial infarction at 1 and 3 weeks respectively, and one of an accidental bleeding from a Scribner arteriovenous shunt at 11 months. One patient who rejected both grafts at 14 days, later died of septicemia caused by an infected lower extremity gangrene. The actuarial one year patient, kidney and pancreas graft survival rates were; 94%, 85%, and 66% respectively. (Pancreatic graft function meaning insulin independent patient).

In Table 2, the patient and renal graft survival rates are compared with those of recipients of kidneys from living related donors and with those who received a kidney but not a pancreas from a cadaveric donor.

Currently, 44 pancreas transplant recipients are alive, 20 are insulin independent, while an additional 9 patients have impaired pancreatic graft function as judged by insulin dependency and C-peptide values.

Of the 7 non-uremic recipients of pancreas transplants, only two are currently insulin independent, at $1^{1}/_{2}$ and $2^{1}/_{2}$ years after the transplantation.

Causes of 24 graft losses were rejection in 8, graft vascular thrombosis in 5, death of patient in 3, bleeding in 2, local infection in one, and unknown in 5 cases.

The long term effects of pancreas transplantation on diabetic neuropathy and retinopathy registered in our patients have been published previously [2].

Table 2. Actuarial patient and renal graft survival according to type of transplant and donor source in 85 diabetic patients transplanted between January 1983 and April 1987 (Figures are percentage survival).

	Patient		Kidney	
	1 year	3 years	1 year	3 years
Kidney from LRD (n = 29)	92	92	92	92
Kidney from CD (n = 19)	88	88	78	78
Kidney and pancreas from CD (n = 37)	94	94	85	85

LRD = one haplotype mismatched living related donor.
CD = cadaveric donor.

Discussion

Even though the functional survival of the pancreas transplant has greatly improved during the last few years, it still is inferior to that of the renal transplant. This difference does not seem to reflect differences in susceptability to immunological damage. Next to graft rejection, graft vascular thrombosis was the most important cause of pancreatic graft loss in this series. Slow blood flow in the relatively wide splenic artery is supposed to play an important role in thrombus formation. The reported new surgical technique developed to increase the arterial blood flow, was applied in 17 patients with promising results so far.

Several factors may be implicated in the development of impaired pancreas graft function over time, as manifested in some patients by hyperglycemia and need of exogeneous insulin. Both chronic rejection and fibrosis caused by the exocrine atrophy following duct occlusion may be responsible for this. However, in 2 patients, insulin independency could be reestablished by dilating a stenosed graft artery.

Our main indication for pancreas transplantation has been end-stage diabetic renal disease. Our policy of accepting practically all diabetic uremic patients for the combined pancreas and kidney transplantation may be questioned. However, this policy has not resulted in increased postoperative morbidity or mortality even when compared with the results in diabetic recipients of renal transplants from living related donors (Table 2). In contrast to some centres, we have felt that blindness may in fact serve as a special indication for pancreas transplantation because independence of insulin injections is particularly important to this category of patients.

It is shown that the simultaneous transplantation of kidney and duct occluded pancreas segment has not in any way jeopardized the life of the patient or the functional survival of the renal transplant. The improved well-being and improved quality of life experienced by the patient with a functioning pancreatic transplant justifies this treatment when immunosuppressive therapy is required anyway as part of a renal transplant procedure. The simultaneous transplantation of pancreas and kidney will therefore continue to be the standard treatment for uremic diabetic patients in Norway.

Because of the potential side effects of the currently used immunosuppressive drugs, pancreas transplantation in non-uremic diabetic patients seems indicated only when acceptable blood sugar control is not obtainable by the existing methods of insulin administration. The extraordinary low pancreas graft survival rates achieved in these patients, in which graft vascular thrombosis obviously plays a major role, may hopefully be improved by new surgical techniques aiming at increasing blood flow through the graft artery.

Acknowledgement

The pancreas transplant program has been supported by Norges Diabetes-forbund (Norwegian Diabetes Association).

References

1. Brekke IB, Dyrbekk D, Jakobsen A, Jervell J, Sådal G, Flatmark A: Combined pancreas and kidney transplantation for diabetic nephropathy. Transplant Proc 18: 63–64, 1986.
2. Dyrbekk D, Brekke IB, Jervell J et al: Long term effects of pancreas transplantation on blood glucose control and diabetic complications. In: Brunetti P, Waldhäusl WK (eds). Advanced models for the therapy of insulin-dependent diabetes; pp 371–376. Raven press, New York, 1987.

Experience of the University of Pittsburgh, Pittsburgh, Pennsylvania, USA

A.G. TZAKIS, P.B. CARROLL, V. KAMP-NIELSEN, T. FRIBERG and T.E. STARZL

Between March 1983 and July, 1986 a modest clinical trial of whole pancreas transplantation was undertaken at the University of Pittsburgh. Followups were to 12 May 1988.

Number of patients:	15
Mean age (years):	30
Number of grafts:	16
Previous kidney transplantation:	7
Simultaneous kidney transplantation:	5
Subsequent kidney transplantation:	1
Deaths less than one year:	3
Deaths greater than one year:	1
One year pancreas survival (actual):	50%
Pancreas lost after one year:	4
Pancreas functioning (3 to 5 years):	4

Composite pancreaticoduodenal grafts were used preferentially in our series, because they allowed transplantation of all the available pancreatic islets, using large vascular and conventional intestinal anastomoses [1, 2]. The blood supply was through the donor celiac axis and the superior mesenteric artery of the donor which were anastomosed using a common Carrel patch of the donor aorta to either the common or external iliac artery of the recipient. Venous drainage was through the donor portal vein which was anastomosed to an iliac vein of the recipient. The pancreatic secretions were drained into the intestinal tract, through a duodenojejunostomy. In 7 of our early cases, the spleen was included in the graft: 3 of these patients required allograft splenectomies due to the development of graft versus host disease, which manifested itself as severe hemolysis, thrombocytopenia and leucopenia (one case each).

Four of our patients developed mycotic aneurysms of the iliac artery, at the site of the Carrel patch. These ruptured, 3 of them into the retroperitoneum and one into the jejunum, at the site of the pancreatic graft drainage. The ruptures occurred a few days to more than a year after the failed pancreatic

J.M. Dubernard and D.E.R. Sutherland (eds.), International Handbook of Pancreas Transplantation, 421–422.
© *1989 by Kluwer Academic Publishers.*

grafts had been removed. Surgical treatment required emergency ligation of the illiac artery and extraanatomical femorofemoral bypass in all but one. The exceptional patient maintained sufficient blood supply to her lower extremity after the common iliac artery was ligated.

Immunosuppression was with cyclosporin and prednisone. Azathioprine and antilymphocyte globulin were used as necessary.

Although in our series the livers of the pancreas donors were not used for transplantation, we have since performed combined liver-pancreas donor operations. This is fairly simple in case of segmental pancreatic transplantation, provided, there is a single hepatic artery; the splenic artery and vein remain with the segment of pancreas and the hepatic artery anatomy remains intact.

When the total pancreas and liver are harvested together, part of the portal vein can be left with the pancreas. The celiac axis can be left with the pancreas and the common hepatic or proper hepatic artery can be used for the arterial revascularization of the liver. Arterial or venous grafts can be used as needed for either the liver or the pancreas. It has been our experience that handling of the structures may be equally important as the anatomical considerations if inadvertent ischemic injury of either organ is to be avoided. We have been sent two dead livers from well meaning members of 2 pancreas teams in other cities. Not only were the livers ruined, but both pancreas were discarded eventually. A collegeal interaction among the interested teams can usually resolve the dilemma of using the one organ in preference to the other, especially as the demand for both grafts grows. Technical and judgement matters of the kind are discussed elsewhere [2].

All of our pancreas recipients except one who had a technical failure, had non diabetic glucose tolerance tests after transplantation and were able to discontinue exogenous insulin treatment. They had high peripheral fasting insulin and C-peptide levels. Stimulated values to oral, intravenous and mixed meals were normal.

Retinopathy as evaluated with fundoscopic photos and visual acuity measurements did not improve or became worse during the study period despite achievement of a euglycemic state. In contrast, peripheral neuropathy as evaluated with nerve conduction studies showed a persistent trend to improvement. Large vessel disease, manifested by myocardial infarctions or by complications of peripheral vascular disease continued to progress.

References

1. Starzl TE, Iwatsuki S, Shaw BW Jr, Greene DA, Van Thiel DH, Nalesnik MA, Nusbacher J, Diliz-Perez H, Hakala TR: Pancreaticoduodenal transplantation in humans. Surg Gynecol Obstet 159: 265–272,1984.
2. Starzl TE, Tzakis AG: Pancreatic-duodenal transplantation with enteric exocrine drainage. In: Groth CG (ed) Pancreatic transplantation; pp 113–129. W.B. Saunders Co, Philadelphia, 1988.

Experience of the Institute for Clinical and Experimental Medicine, Prague, Czechoslovakia

V. BARTOŠ and I. VANĚK

A systematic approach to a clinical programme of pancreas transplantation (PTx) requires that three prerequisites have been met before it gets under way:
1. own experimental studies to develop a safe surgical technique,
2. comprehensive methods of examination for diabetes and its complications to define the indications and,
3. experience with kidney transplantation (KTx) and with haemodialysis to control renal failure.

Our experiments were aimed at evaluating different methods of segmental PTx to find the best technique of vascular anastomosis and a simple technique of handling exocrine secretion [1]. Comparing three modalities of vascular reconstruction in segmental PTx in the dog, we found that interposition of the splenic artery into the iliac artery results in optimal haemodynamics. This technique of vascular anastomosis can be regarded as the best one to minimize the genesis of vascular thrombosis. In another study [2] we proved that occlusion of the canine pancreatic duct results, within four to six weeks, in destruction of the exocrine tissue and maintenance of a viable endocrine tissue. Functional islets survive in a fibrous pancreas for at least two years as documented by fasting normoglycaemia and a near-normal glucose tolerance test and insulin secretion. These experiments were the basis for clinical PTx.

The programme of combined PTx + KTx in Prague was started in June 1983. Up to April 1988, 26 transplantations have been performed.

Methods

The organs were all retrieved from heart-beating cadaver donors aged 12 to 50 years. Donor criteria are the same as in renal transplantation while pancreas diseases, previous splenectomy and abnormal blood supply to the left pancreatic segment represent a contraindication. In each donor, arteriography of the pancreas is performed to determine whether the pancreatic segment is

J.M. Dubernard and D.E.R. Sutherland (eds.), International Handbook of Pancreas Transplantation, 423–427.
© 1989 by Kluwer Academic Publishers.

perfused from the splenic artery only. In 15% of cases, pancreatic segment removal was not carried out because of an abnormal blood supply. After in situ Euro-Collins perfusion, the pancreatic segment including the spleen is removed, followed by kidney retrieval. Organ preservation consists of cold storage at 4° C for a maximum of 6 hours.

Simultaneous PTx + KTx is performed with the use of a pancreatic segment occluded by prolamine. Pancreatic duct obliteration is carried out once the graft has been revascularised. Next, splenic artery interposition into the recipient iliac arteries is accomplished. After transplantation of the pancreatic segment, oriented with the cut surface cephalad to the right side, the renal graft is transplanted to the left side. In 6 recipients, the pancreatic graft was located extraperitoneally, and intraperitoneally in 20 recipients. No anticoagulants were administered. The patency of both splenic artery anastomoses in a recipient 3 months after PTx is demonstrated in Figure 1.

With the exception of the first 5 cases where a combination of azathioprine and low doses of steroids was used, the immunosuppressive protocol is based on the combination of cyclosporin A, azathioprine and low doses of steroids. For 2 to 3 postoperative days, cyclosporin A is administered in continuous intravenous infusion and, later, orally. The policy is to maintain trough blood levels of 600 ng/ml for the first 4 weeks to decrease gradually later to a level of 200–300 ng/ml in the second semester postoperatively. Prednisone is tapered to 10 mg daily.

Selection of recipients is limited by the age of 50 years in type I diabetics (a near 0 serum C-peptide level) suffering from renal insufficiency and progression of retinopathy. Patients with a serum creatinine level between 200 and 600 μmol/l are classified as potential, and those over 600 μmol/l as urgent, candidates for transplantation. The contraindications are as follows: severe heart disease, severe iliac atherosclerosis and high titres of lymphocytotoxic antibodies. Patients with one or more of these signs are put on the waiting list for kidney transplantation solely.

All patients indicated for PTx + KTx were uraemic diabetics with preproliferative or proliferative retinopathy and neuropathy. Their age range was 25 to 50 years and duration of type I diabetes 17 to 31 years.

Results

Five of the 26 recipients died during the postoperative period. In two of them, sudden cardiac death due to arrhythmia they had developed during haemodialysis was established as the cause of death. Both deceased had severe autonomic neuropathy. One patient died of heart failure accompanied by coronary atherosclerosis as confirmed by autopsy and two of purulent peritonitis. In 3

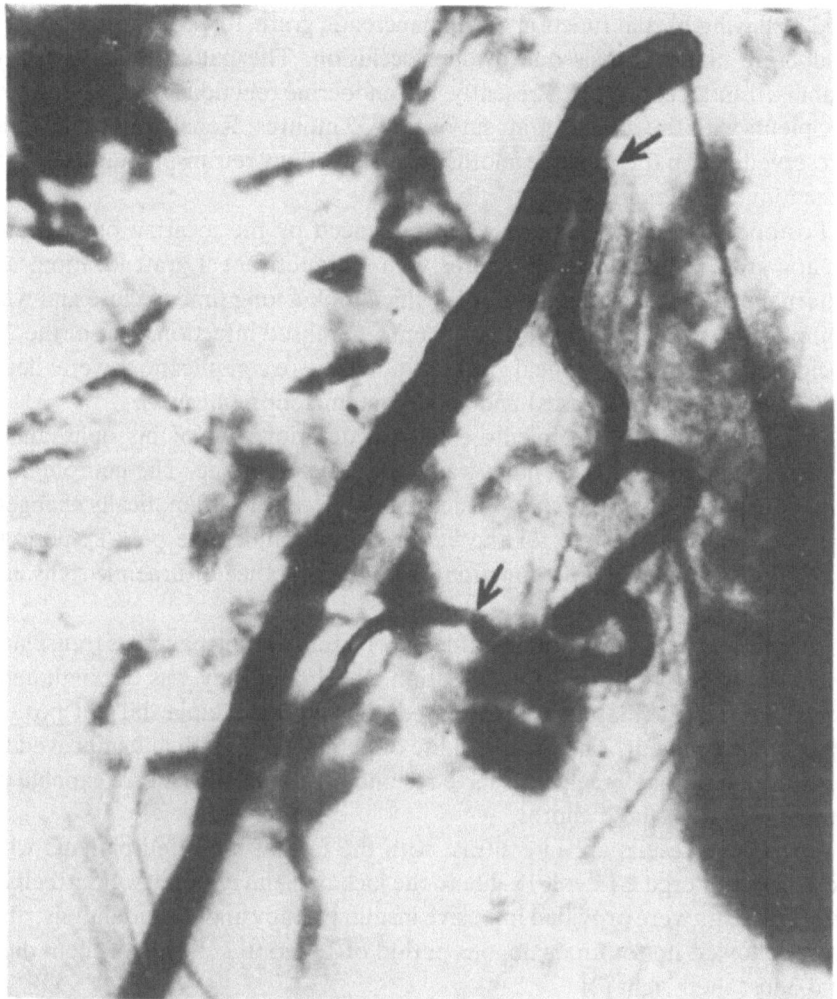

Figure 1. Arteriography of interposition of the pancreatic graft splenic artery into the recipient iliac arteries. Arrows show the patency of both anastomoses.

cases, PTx was not successful: in one recipient, the graft had to be removed for ischaemic necrosis, the other two had an afunctional graft as a result of primary ischaemic lesion.

Hence, pancreatic graft function developed in 18, and renal graft function in 21 recipients. In 3 cases, function of the pancreatic graft disappeared, most likely due to rejection, after 4, 20 and 22 months of full function. In 4 recipients, a decrease in pancreatic graft function appeared, requiring a limited dose of insulin to achieve normoglycaemia 2, 2, 3, and 20 months post-Tx. These patients maintain a serum C-peptide level over 0.5 ng/ml and are classified as having partial function of the pancreatic graft. Its probable cause was endocrine tissue fibrosis due to duct occlusion. The patients are perfectly stabilised and feel healthy. Presently, full endocrine function is maintained in 9 recipients with the longest graft survival of 37 months. Renal graft function is preserved in 17 patients while another one had kidney retransplantation with a functioning pancreatic graft.

Postoperative complications were influenced by the location of the pancreatic graft [3]. In 4 of the 6 cases with extraperitoneal graft location, an external pancreatic fistula developed which took a long time to close and was complicated by wound infection or even generalised infection. Out of the 20 recipients with intraperitoneal graft location, severe complications were: ileus requiring operation (2 cases) and abdominal infection (4 cases).

While none of the recipients exhibited deterioration of his ophthalmic finding, significant improvement was demonstrated in one. The neurological finding improved in 6 patients. A successful PTx + KTx dramatically changed the patient's overall state for the better. In the immediate post-Tx period, development of renal graft function and disappearance of uraemic signs are most important.

The first sign of a favourable influence of a functioning pancreas transplant was intermediary metabolic stabilisation. Insulin therapy was discontinued. No glycaemic fluctuation was observed and hypoglycaemia did not pose a threat to the patient. The quality of life of patients has gradually improved to such an extent that 9 recipients have resumed work and others are capable of performing household chores.

The above results are in contrast with the fate of indicated patients who could not undergo PTx + KTx due to the lack of cadaver donors. Fourteen of these patients were provided intensive insulin therapy and haemodialysis, and were followed up for an analogous period of 18 months. Seven of them died and 3 lost their sight [4].

Conclusion

Advances in surgical techniques and immunosuppression, using cyclosporin, make PTx increasingly more reliable and safer. A combined PTx + KTx does not increase the risk of KTx which should be performed in all diabetic recipients with renal failure. The risk factors include cardiac disease, autonomic neuropathy and long-term treatment by haemodialysis. It would therefore be appropriate to perform PTx + KTx prior to the onset of renal failure. However, the lack of cadaver donors restricts the development of such a programme. Compared with conventional treatment, PTx + KTx offers the best prognosis for diabetic patients with advanced organ complications. In patients with a good graft function, insulin therapy can be discontinued, dietary measures can be relaxed, metabolism is stabilised, progression of organ complications is hindered and both the physical and mental state is improved.

References

1. Vaněk I, Bartoš V, Kočandrle V: Prognosis of experimental pancreatic transplantation in relation to vascular reconstructive procedure. Transplant Proc 16: 764–765, 1984.
2. Bartoš V, Kolc J, Nožičková M, Málek P: Indications and experimental preparatory studies for pancreas transplantation. Czechoslovak Med 8: 158–162, 1985.
3. Bartoš V, Vaněk I, Pavel P, Saudek F, Kočandrle V, Vondra K: Complications of simultaneous segmental pancreatic and renal transplantation in diabetics. Transplant Proc 18: 1131, 1986.
4. Bartoš V, Vaněk I, Saudek F, Kočandrle V, Pavel P, Vondra K: Comparison of the effect of pancreas and kidney transplantation with conventional treatment in diabetics. Transplant Proc 18: 1768–1769, 1986.

Experience of the St. Louis University School of Medicine, Saint Louis, Missouri, USA

P.J. GARVIN, M. CASTANEDA, K. CARNEY, D. ARIDGE and J. HOFF

Although the theoretical advantages of pancreatic transplantation in select Type I diabetic patients have been realized for several years, the benefit/risk ratio of earlier published series seemed too narrow to apply to our diabetic population. This bias was confirmed in our initial small series of pancreatic transplantation following successful renal transplantation. As a result, our initial emphasis was to investigate, in the laboratory setting, techniques to minimize the frequently reported technical problems of pancreatic transplantation. Towards the end, we evaluated, in the canine model, the problems of ductal management [1], vascular thrombosis of the splenic vessels [2], pancreatic preservation [3] and predictors of viability during pancreatic preservation [3]. With this information, and technical experience gained in the laboratory, a protocol was designed to initiate a clinical trial of combined renal and pancreatic transplantation in select Type I diabetics. This approach seemed optimal in that these patients were already candidates for renal transplantation, and would, thus, require immunosuppression, with its associated risks. In addition, only one operative procedure was required, as opposed to the staged approach, in a diabetic patient with a functioning allograft. Lastly, the combined approach allowed for utilization of parameters of renal allograft rejection; both to institute anti-rejection therapy, and to help identify a marker(s) of pancreatic allograft rejection. We felt than once technical complications were minimized, and, a predictive index of early pancreatic rejection was established, then application of isolated pancreatic transplantation to select pre-uremic diabetics, and diabetics with functioning transplants, would be indicated. In this report, our experience with 36 consecutive dual renal and pancreatic allografts performed between February 1985 and December 1987, is described. An emphasis on evolution of our protocol, and parameters to assess pancreatic allograft function, will be accomplished to indicate the progress, as well as the problems to be resolved, at our center.

J.M. Dubernard and D.E.R. Sutherland (eds.), International Handbook of Pancreas Transplantation, 429–437.
© *1989 by Kluwer Academic Publishers.*

Patient and methods

Since institution of this protocol, 85 patients have completed evaluation for combined renal and segmental pancreatic transplantation. An indication of the high risk nature of this population is evident by the fact that 14 patients have died awaiting transplantation, and nine patients have been temporarily (or permanently) withdrawn from the waiting list, secondary to symptomatic progression of cerebrovascular disease (2), cardiac disease (4), and/or peripheral vascular disease (3). To date, 36 patients (24 males, 12 females), ranging in age from 20 to 52 years (mean = 35.2 years), have received dual allografts. The duration of insulin dependent diabetes was 15 to 35 years (mean =23.6 years). Thirty-three patients had end-stage renal disease secondary to diabetic nephropathy and were on maintenance hemodialysis (25) or continuous ambulatory peritoneal dialysis (8) from 1 to 96 months (mean = 8.9 months). The remaining three patients received dual allografts prior to requiring dialytic therapy. In these 36 patients, other secondary complications were frequent and included: neuropathy (mild = 24, moderate = 12), retinopathy (mild = 13, severe = 23, with 10 patients being totally blind), and overt cardiac disease (4).

All patients received at least one random third party blood transfusion within 6 months of transplantation as part of our routine preparation for transplantation. Recipients were selected on the basis of a negative lymphocytotoxicity cross match, utilizing current serum, with a minor emphasis on HLA, A, B and DR matching. In each case, both organs came from the same donor. The organs underwent cold storage preservation after Collin's C-4 flush. The pancreatic grafts consisted of the body and tail. The spleen was left attached to utilize as a 'handle' during engraftment. The graft vessels were the splenic artery and vein, or the celiac artery and portal vein. Interposition of donor iliac artery and vein was utilized in five cases for increased vessel length. All pancreatic grafts were placed extraperitoneally, utilizing end to side anastomosis to the left external iliac vessels. After restoring pancreatic blood flow, the renal allograft was placed in the opposite iliac fossa in a standard fashion and a ureteroneocystostomy was accomplished. A donor splenectomy was then performed followed by a pancreaticocystostomy utilizing a stent. Prior to June 1986, this stent was internal. Due to a high incidence of local complications (urinary and/or pancreatic fistulae), we now utilize a temporary (6 weeks) external stent for complete exocrine diversion. Bilateral closed drainage systems were utilized in all cases.

All patients received cyclosporin immunosuppression. Prior to May 1986, our protocol consisted of cyclosporin (12.5 mg/kg/day) and prednisone (0.75 mg/kg/day). Since that time, all patients received triple therapy consisting of cyclosporin (6 mg/kg/day), azathioprine (1.5 mg/kg/day) and prednisone

(0.75 mg/kg/day). At seven days post transplant, the steroid dosage was tapered to achieve a dosage of 15–20 mg daily at one month. Azathioprine dosage reductions were accomplished only if leukopenia (WBC<5,000) developed. The cyclosporin dosage was tapered in patients with suspected toxicity, and/or elevated trough levels of cyclosporin.

Rejection episodes were treated with local irradiation (600 rads in 4 divided doses for each graft), and a doubling of the steroid dose. Systemic cephalosporins were administered preoperatively, and continued postoperatively for 5–7 days. Beginning in November 1985, postoperative anticoagulation with subcutaneous heparin (5,000 units every 12 hours) was utilized until graft failure, or discharge.

Techniques to assess pancreatic graft function included: fasting blood sugars, urinary and serum amylase levels, and radioimmunoassays for insulin, C-peptide, and glucagon. Patients with an external stent, or evidence of a pancreatic fistula from the drainage catheters, had serial measurements of this drainage for amylase and creatinine. Radiologic assessment included: sequential perfusion scanning with technetium – 99 glucoheptonate and sulfur colloid, ultrasonography and computerized tomography. The effect of successful pancreatic transplantation on the secondary complications of diabetes was evaluated by serial nerve conduction tests, retinal photography/function tests, and radionuclide gastric emptying studies.

Immediate function of the kidney was defined as not requiring dialysis in the first post transplant week. Immediate pancreatic allograft function was defined as insulin independence within 6 hours of operation. The diagnosis of rejection was made on the basis of our standard clinical and diagnostic criteria of renal allograft rejection. An analysis of pancreatic functional parameters at the onset of renal allograft rejection was accomplished, in an attempt to established criteria for pancreatic allograft rejection.

Results

Graft and patient survival

Pancreatic allograft warm ischemia time ranged from 0 to 4 minutes and preservation time from 2.9 to 10.25 hours (mean = 5.2 hours). One patient died in the immediate postoperative period from a myocardial infarction. In 30 of the remaining 35 patients, the kidney functioned immediately. All of the pancreatic grafts functioned immediately. Pancreatic graft failure occurred within the first week in eight patients. The etiology of graft failure was vascular thrombosis (5), hemorrhagic pancreatitis (1), acute rejection (1) and rupture of a splenic artery aneurysm requiring graft removal (1). Excluding the patient with acute rejection, early pancreatic allograft failure was not associated with loss of renal allograft function. In addition to the perioperative cardiac death, four patients died from 1–6 weeks postoperatively (3 sepsis, 1 technical), and one patient died at eight months post transplant (complications of peripheral vascular disease). At the time of death, four renal and three pancreatic grafts were functioning.

Currently, 23 renal and 14 pancreata are functioning from 2 to 36 months (mean = 15.6 months) post transplant. In the patient with functioning pancreata, metabolic profiles (C-peptide, insulin levels, and glucose tolerance tests) demonstrate reversal of the metabolic abnormalities of Type 1 diabetes. In ten patients with functioning pancreata for greater than one year, nerve conduction tests, retinal photography/function tests and radionuclide gastric emptying studies demonstrate stabilization, or an improvement, in the secondary complications of diabetes.

As our experience increased, three factors were identified as reducing pancreatic allograft, and/or patient survival:
1. splenic artery or vein thrombosis,
2. inadequate control of pancreatic secretions,
3. coronary artery disease.
In an attempt to minimize the morbidity and mortality of this procedure, we have continued to modify our protocol. Postoperative mini-dose heparin has been utilized since November 1985, in an attempt to prevent vascular thrombosis. With this modification, the incidence of this complication has been reduced from 37.5% (3/8) to 6.1% (2/28). Our initial technique of pancreaticocystostomy with an internal stent was associated with a high incidence of severe wound sepsis secondary to poorly controlled pancreatic secretions, leading to technical graft loss, and/or death. Beginning in June 1986, our technique was modified to provede six weeks of external stenting of the pancreatic duct (Figure 1). With this modification, the incidence of graft loss, and/or death, secondary to local complications has been reduced from 36% (5/14) to 14% (3/22). Severe cardiovascular disease is a frequent occurrence in this patient population as evidenced by nine patients, referred for dual allografting, who died of myocardial infarction before transplantation. This fact, in addition to the patient death from a perioperative cardiac event, resulted in our pretransplant protocol being adjusted, in May 1986, to screen for coronary artery disease by stress and/or intravenous dipyridamole thallium testing and, if positive, coronary angiograms. Since this modification, nine patients have been excluded from transplantation, due to severe cardiac and/or peripheral vascular disease, and 24 patients have undergone dual allografting with only one, nonfatal, cardiac event. As our protocol for dual allografting has evolved, a progressive reduction in morbidity has occurred in our last twenty patients, with a resultant increase in six month graft (75% renal, 60% pancreatic), and patient (95%) survival.

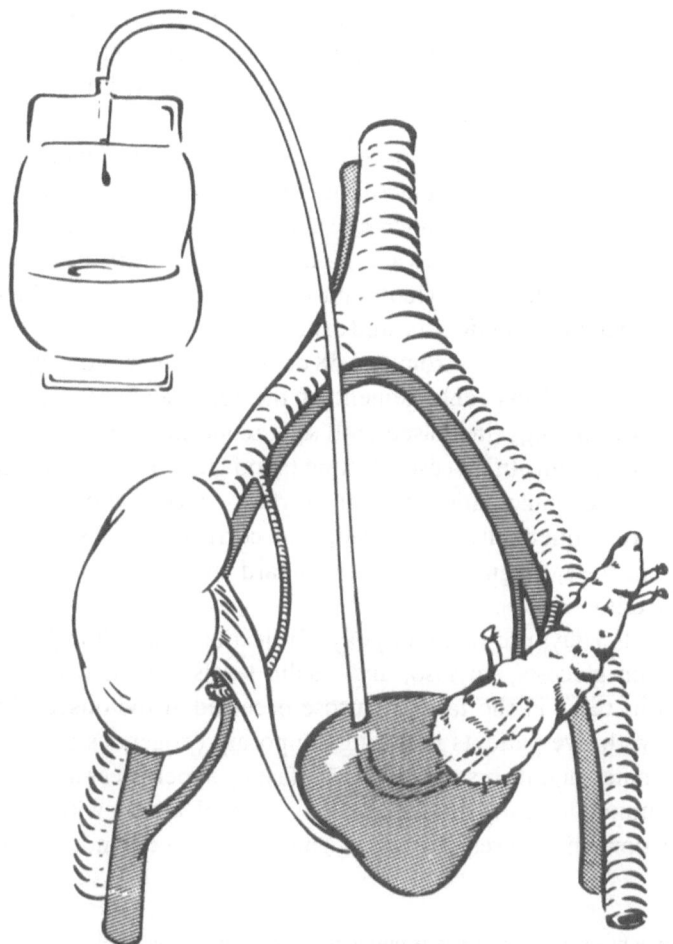

Figure 1. Diagram illustrating dual renal-pancreatic allografts with external stenting of the pancreaticocystostomy.

Assessment of the pancreatic allograft

Excluding the patient requiring graft removal for bleeding, the remaining seven patients with early pancreatic allograft failure (<1 week) demonstrated a dramatic increase in the fasting serum glucose, and urgent nuclide scanning demonstrated absence of graft blood flow. Three patients with graft failure secondary to splenic artery thrombosis, had no local symptoms. The other four patients (splenic vein thrombosis – 2; hemorrhagic pancreatitis – 1; acute rejection – 1) developed local symptoms and an enlarged, tender, pancreatic allograft. The serum amylase was elevated for 12 hours prior to the onset of hyperglycemia only in the patient with pancreatitis. In all seven patients, the urinary amylase concentration (5 patients), or external stent volume, and amylase output (2 patients), decreased precipitously, with the onset of hyperglycemia.

Since one of our objectives in performing dual renal – pancreatic transplantation was to identify a predictive index of pancreatic allograft rejection, an analysis of parameters of pancreatic allograft function, during acute renal allograft rejection episodes, was accomplished. Only reversible rejection episodes (N = 20) in which sufficient data was available to assess the effect of rejection on pancreatic endocrine and exocrine function were analyzed. These rejection episodes occurred from 6 to 58 days (mean = 16.9 days) post transplant. In these patients, enlargement of the renal allograft was frequent, however, local findings (increased graft size, tenderness) over the pancreatic allograft were absent. In all cases, fasting blood glucose, amylase and insulin levels, as well as pancreatic allograft amylase concentrations, and rate of release, were sequentially monitored, and correlated with renal allograft rejection episodes, diagnosed by our standard clinical, biochemical and radiographic criteria.

Baseline (1–3 days pre-rejection) day of rejection, and 7 days post rejection fasting serum glucose, amylase, and insulin levels are listed in Table 1. A significant increase in the fasting glucose occurred at the onset of rejection ($p<0.01$), with five patients requiring temporary exogenous insulin, and an additional nine patients manifesting mild, fasting hyperglycemia. This finding suggests immunologically mediated islet cell involvement with the onset of renal rejection. In all cases, the fasting glucose returned to normal, although,

Table 1. Serum biochemical parameters during reversible renal allograft rejection in dual renal-pancreas recipients.

All rejection episodes (n = 20)	Fasting glucose (mg%)	Fasting amylase (U/L)	Fasting insulin (μU/ml)
Baseline	73–214 (114.1 ± 8.2)	27–182 (71.1 ± 10.5)	12–387 (76.2 ± 22.0)
Day of rejection	73–288 (139.8 ± 11.9)	38–162 (81.4 ± 11.2)	14–390 (70.9 ± 20.6)
Post-treatment	71–450 (129.9 ± 19.2)	20–157 (71.6 ± 10.2)	12–341 (60.1 ± 17.5)
Rejection episodes not requiring insulin (n = 15)			
Baseline	73–148 (106.9 ± 5.6)	27–173 (60.9 ± 9.7)	12–246 (62.4 ± 17.2)
Day of rejection	73–175 (121.5 ± 8.7)	36–122 (68.0 ± 9.1)	14–164 (54.7 ± 10.2)
Post-treatment	71–199 (101.3 ± 9.4)	23–158 (77.1 ± 11.8)	12–112 (45.2 ± 7.2)
Rejection episodes requiring insulin (n = 5)			
Baseline	78–214 (135.4 ± 28.1)	32–182 (99.6 ± 27.5)	
Day of rejection	117–288 (194.4 ± 30.2)	38–162 (111.0 ± 27.1)	On insulin
Post-treatment	98–450 (215.4 ± 60.6)	28–134 (56.4 ± 20.9)	

in several patients, this occurred one to four weeks after the serum creatinine had returned to baseline. This delayed resolution of hyperglycemia may represent a response to the increased steroids, cyclosporin toxicity to the islet cells, or rejection induced graft pancreatitis. Serum amylase levels remained in the normal range during all 20 rejection episodes.

At the onset of renal rejection, fasting serum insulin levels, in the 15 patients not requiring exogenous insulin, either decreased (N = 5), increased (N = 9) or were unchanged (N = 1). The poor correlation of insulin levels with rejection in dual allografts recipients probably reflects the decreased insulin clearance associated with rejection induced renal dysfunction. The allograft amylase concentration, and rate of release, during rejection are listed in Table 2. It is evident that these parameters varied widely among individual patients, and for each patient over time. There were no significant differences in allograft amylase concentrations, or rate of amylase release, when the day of rejection, and post rejection values, were compared to the baseline values. When individual rejection episodes are examined, however, 14 of 20 cases were associated with a 1.2–81.3 fold increase in the rate of amylase release at the onset of renal rejection, which was sustained over ten days after the diagnosis of rejection. In no instance was there a dramatic decrease in allograft amylase release during the course of reversible renal allograft rejection, even in the patients requiring exogenous insulin.

Sequential radionuclide assessment utilizing ^{99M}Tc sulfur colloid as an in-

Table 2. Pancreatic allograft amylase concentration and rate of release during reversible renal allograft rejection in dual renal-pancreas recipients.

	Baseline	Day of rejection	1–3 days post treatment	7–10 days post treatment
All rejection episodes (n = 20)				
Amylase concentration	395–100232	2601–58885	3816–72815	59–95344
(U/L)	(35800 ± 13020)	(24309 ± 3957)	(24553 ± 4925)	(35086 ± 7145)
Rate of release (U/Hr)	35–8148	183–5305	178–6210	103–8032
	(1114.8 ± 394.9)	(1352.8 ± 272.2)	(1487.2 ± 363.8)	(2063.8 ± 413.0)
Rejection episodes not requiring insulin (n = 15)				
Amylase concentration	395–100232	2601–58883	3816–72815	59–91560
(U/L)	(43200 ± 17045)	(25766 ± 5098)	(23387 ± 5853)	(37939 ± 7785)
Rate of release (U/Hr)	35–8148	183–5305	178–5552	642–8032
	(1222.5 ± 521.8)	(1333.0 ± 341.9)	(1225.2 ± 348.3)	(2121.8 ± 495.3)
Rejection episodes requiring insulin (n = 5)				
Amylase concentrations	6300–17962	9020–34255	9978–64260	1097–95344
(U/L)	(13601 ± 2426)	(19943 ± 4273)	(28060 ± 9858)	(27099 ± 17316)
Rate of release (U/Hr)	180–1676	216–2383	458–6210	103–4030
	(791.8 ± 264.5)	(1411.9 ± 423.8)	(2273.4 ± 1017.5)	(1901.6 ± 821.9)

dicator of thrombotic, vasculitis, and ^{99M} glucoheptonate to monitor pancreatic perfusion, and blood pool parameters, has been used for several years as a method of surveillance of our renal allograft recipients. In dual allograft recipients, scintigraphic changes, at the onset of rejection, occur simultaneously in both organs and consist of an increased sulfur colloid thrombotic index and decreased glucoheptonate perfusion, when compared to baseline. Renal time and pulsed Doppler evaluation of the pancreatic allograft, at the onset of rejection, have demonstrated mild enlargement of the organ with foci of anechogenicity and an increased resistive index.

Discussion

The ultimate goal of pancreatic transplantation is to apply this technique to select Type I diabetics and prevent the development of secondary complications. Despite significant progress, in both the laboratory and clinical setting, several obstacles prevent widespread application of this procedure to this patient population. Technical problems (vascular thrombosis, control of exocrine secretions), and the inability to identify a predictive index of early pancreatic rejection, contribute significantly to pancreatic allograft failure. After extensive background work in the laboratory, we initiated a clinical trial of pancreatic transplantation. We restricted our patient population to Type I diabetics with end stage renal disease who were candidates for cadaver renal transplantation. All pancreatic transplants would be performed synchronously with cyclosporin immunosuppression, and the technique of ductal management would be consistent – i.e., – pancreaticocystostomy. At the onset, several objectives were established for this clinical trial. Critical to the success of pancreatic transplantation is the identification of technical factors contributing to pancreatic allograft failure, and/or patient morbidity and mortality. Once identified, then modifications in the protocol can be accomplished to minimize these complications. To date, three complications that alter allograft, and/or patient, survival have been identified – i.e., vascular thrombosis, inadequate control of exocrine secretions, and post transplant cardiac events. Alterations in our pre-transplant protocol (routine cardiac evaluation), our operative technique (external stenting of the pancreatic duct) and our post transplant protocol (postoperative heparin) have dramatically reduced these complications, with a resultant increase in early allograft and patient survival.

Another major objective was to identify a predictive index of early pancreatic allograft rejection, by monitoring various parameters of pancreatic function, and observing if changes in these parameters occur in association with renal allograft rejection. A major assumption with this approach is that the onset of rejection is similar in both organs. Our findings of mild to moderate hyperglycemia, as well as radionuclide and ultrasound abnormalities of the pancreatic allograft, at the onset of renal rejection, make this assumption plausible. In our experience, serum amylase and insulin levels did not correlate with the onset of renal rejection. Pancreatic allograft amylase output increased with the onset of rejection in 70% of our patients, and this increase was sustained for ten or more days. Unlike other reports, in no case of reversible rejection was there a profound decrease in amylase secretion.

In conclusion, dual renal-pancreatic transplantation has evolved to the point that it should now be considered a therapeutic option for Type I diabetics with end stage renal disease. With more rigid pretransplant screening for coronary artery disease, and continued refinements in operative technique, and postoperative management, a continued improvement in results can be anticipated.

References

1. Garvin PJ, Castaneda MA, Niehoff ML, Mauller KE, Brems JJ: An in situ evaluation of a distal splenic arteriovenous fistula on pancreas function in an isolated pancreas segment. Arch Surg 120: 1148–1151, 1985.
2. Garvin PJ, Castaneda MA, Codd J, Pennell R, Niehoff M, Tumulty D: A comparison of ductal management techniques in an in situ canine pancreas model. Arch Surg 119: 829–832, 1984.
3. Garvin PJ, Castaneda MA, Niehoff ML: In search of an in vitro index of viability during pancreatic preservation. Journal Surg Res 40: 455–461, 1986.

Experience of the Huddinge Hospital, Karolinska Institute, Stockholm, Sweden

C.G. GROTH, G. TYDÉN and J. ÖSTMAN

Introduction

This chapter will describe the Stockholm experience with 103 pancreatic transplantations in diabetic patients. When the program was initiated in 1974, it was decided to use segmental pancreatic grafts and since then this type of graft has been used in all but four instances where whole organ grafts were used. Originally, the reason for using the segmental graft was that it did away with the duodenum, an organ which was then believed to be dangerous to transplant. More recently, the chief reason for using such a graft is that it makes possible the harvesting of the liver as well as the pancreas from a cadaveric donor without creating a conflict over the arterial trunks that lead to both organs. Also from the beginning, we chose to drain the exocrine secretion of the graft to the patients bowel. One reason for this was that it is physiological. Furthermore, a considerable experience with pancreatico-enteric anastomosis was available from general surgery where such techniques are used routinely after pancreatic resections. In a few exceptional Stockholm cases, pancreatic duct ligature or exocrine diversion to the patients stomach was used instead.

Patients and donors

Since April 1974 and through 1987, 103 pancreatic transplantations have been performed at Huddinge Hospital (Figure 1).

Grafts with pancreatico-enterostomy

In 92 transplantations, pancreatico-enterostomy was used [1, 2]. In 88 instances segmental grafts were used, while in 2 cases whole organ pancreatic grafts and in 2 cases pancreatico-duodenal grafts were utilized. In 89 instances

439

J.M. Dubernard and D.E.R. Sutherland (eds.), International Handbook of Pancreas Transplantation, 439–447.
© *1989 by Kluwer Academic Publishers.*

440

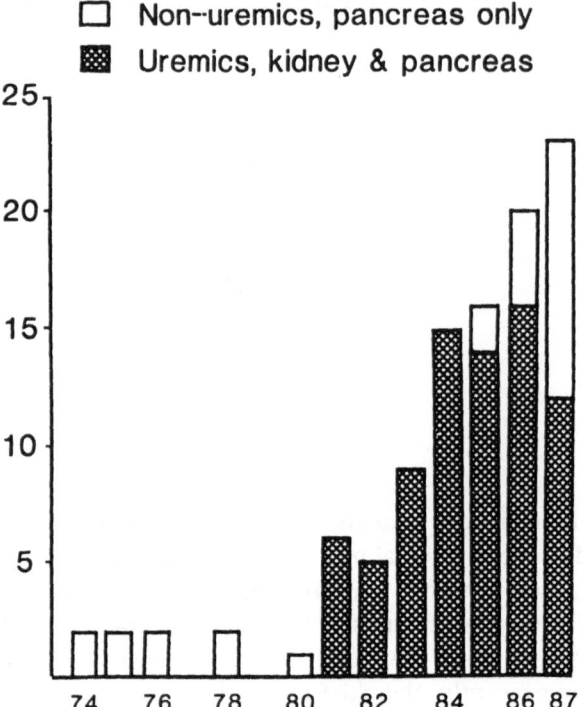

Figure 1. The number of pancreatic transplantations performed in Stockholm per year. Also indicated is the number of patients that were uremics and received kidney and pancreas grafts and those that were not uremics and received a pancreas only.

the grafts were from ABO-compatible cadaveric donors and in 3 cases segmental grafts were obtained from the patients mother. There were 83 diabetic recipients, 9 of them underwent a second transplantation after the first had failed. All recipients suffered from type-1 diabetes of longstanding. Most of the transplantations were performed on uremic diabetics; in 58 instances a combined renal and pancreatic transplantation was performed and in 6 instances the pancreatic transplantation was performed in a patient already carrying a renal graft. The first few transplantations were, however, to non-uremic diabetics [3] and recently we have again treated such patients (Figure 1). The indications for 25 single pancreatic transplantations in 20 non-uremic diabetic patients included hyperlabile diabetes (2 patients), severe progressive angiopathy (1 patient), rapidly progressing retinopathy (2 patients), severe neuropathy (2 patients) and pre-uremic nephropathy (13 patients).

Duct ligated grafts and grafts with gastric diversion

Before November 1981 duct ligated grafts were used in 4 instances [1, 4]. In

1983 – 1984, 7 transplantations were performed with gastric exocrine diversion: the cut end of the segmental pancreatic graft was telescoped into the recipients stomach near the major curvature [5]. In all instances segmental cadaveric grafts were used. One patient had hyperlabile diabetes, all the others were uremic diabetics.

Preservation of the cadaveric graft

With a few exceptions, the technique for graft preservation has been intraarterial perfusion with cold Ringer-type electrolyte solution followed by simple cold storage [6]. Since organs can be harvested only after cardiac arrest in Sweden, the grafts were also exposed to warm ischemia for a mean of 7 min (range 1–18 min).

In the beginning of the Stockholm programme, the graft cold ischemia time was kept below 6 hours, but subsequently the criteria were relaxed and a CIT for as long as 12 hours was accepted. With this policy, severe graft pancreatitis occurred in several patients and many of these grafts were lost [5]. It then again became our policy to avoid cold ischemia time beyond 6 hours.

The technique for transplantation with pancreatico-enterostomy

The details of the recipient operation have developed over the years. In the first five cases and end-to-end pancreatico-Roux-loop enterostomy was created [1]. In many of these patients, a pancreatic fistula developed in the anastomosis and in the following five transplantations a ducto-enterostomy was performed instead: the ductal anastomosis was either to a jejunal Roux-loop or to an ileal U-loop [7]. Again, however, pancreatic fistulas occurred in many of the patients. In 1981, end-to-end pancreatico-enterostomy was reintroduced but with some important modifications [2].

A pancreatic duct catheter was used to temporarily exteriorize the pancreatic juice, thus allowing the anastomosis to heal without being exposed to the digestive forces of the pancreatic exocrine secretion. Also the graft was placed intra- instead of extraperitoneally with the assumption that the conditions for anastomotic healing would thereby be improved. Originally the graft was placed obliquely in the iliac fossa, but since 1984 it has been placed in the midst of the abdomen thereby avoiding a bend in the Roux-loop at the site of the anastomosis (Figure 2). Also, a midline incision is now used instead of an oblique incision over the iliac fossa.

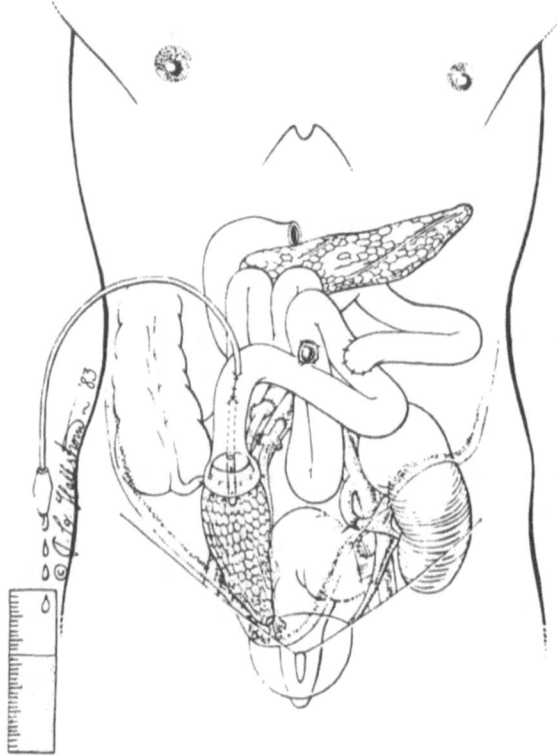

Figure 2. Technique used for segmental pancreatic transplantation with pancreatico-enterostomy to a Roux-loop. Temporary exteriorization of the pancreatic juice is accomplished by the use of a pancreatic duct catheter, which is brought out through the abdominal wall. This catheter is removed after approximately 4 weeks. When a combined procedure is performed, the kidney is anastomosed to the contralateral iliac vessels and placed extraperitoneally

Immunosuppression and anticoagulation therapy

Until 1981, the immunosuppression consisted of azathioprine, prednisolone and horse-antilymphocyte globulin [1]. Since 1982, cyclosporin has been used. Initially, the patients were still started on a conventional drug regimen, 2 to 4 weeks after transplantation a switch was made from azathioprine to cyclosporin [2]. Since 1984 cyclosporin has been given from the outset in combination with prednisolone or azathioprine plus prednisolone. Since 1986, a quadruple drug regimen which also included rabbit-antithymocyte globulin has been used.

After one of the first cases had suffered a venous graft thrombosis only hours after transplantation, dextran-70 and warfarin were introduced as prophylaxis for thrombosis. In 1982, the use of warfarin was abandoned but in 1984 it became our practice to give the drug to all patients, the dose being adjusted to give a prothrombin time between 10 and 20 per cent. During the 3–4 days it takes before warfarin exerts its full effect, heparin is given subcutaneously (8).

Results

Duct ligated grafts and grafts with gastric diversion

When duct ligature was used there was exocrine leakage from all the 4 grafts this leading to a fistula to the exterior (2 cases), a pancreatic pseudocyst (1 case) or pancreatic ascites (1 case). All grafts were lost within a few months with rejection or thrombosis but the fistula contributed to the unsuccessful course. Of the 7 transplantations with gastric exocrine diversion 6 were unsuccessful because of posttransplantation pancreatitis (3 cases) anastomotic leak, (1 case) and thrombosis (2 cases). One graft remains functioning more than 4 years after transplantation with excellent blood glucose control.

Grafts with pancreatico-enterostomy

This series was divided into 4 groups based on the time period when the patient was treated (1974–81, 1981–83, 1984–85, 1986–87). It was then found that there had occurred a marked improvement in overall results with time (Table 1).

When the series was divided into different groups according to patient categories, it was found that the most favourable results had been obtained in the uremic diabetic patients receiving combined kidney and pancreatic grafts from one donor, Table 1 and Figure 3. In the most recent series of combined transplantations, the 1-year patient and pancreatic survival rates were 100% and 77%, respectively. The renal graft 1-year success rate was 82%. With single pancreatic transplantation in non-uremic diabetic patients the results were also improved, but only from poor to intermediary (Table 1). In our small series of pancreatic transplantations after a previous kidney transplantation the 1-year pancreatic graft success rate is poor (Table 1).

Several factors explain the improvement in results which has occurred with time. Thus, it has been possible to reduce the incidence of graft failure due to thrombosis by the use of anticoagulation therapy [1]. In the first two series (1974–81, 1981–83), 25% of the grafts were lost due to thrombosis while in the latter two series (1984–85, 1986–87), the figure has been reduced to 12%. Also we have achieved a marked reduction in posttransplantation pancreatitis simply by avoiding excessive ischemic injury to the graft. With the preservation technique used, cold storage times beyond 6 hours must then be avoided [8]. With this precaution, the number of grafts lost due to early pancreatitis has been reduced from 12% in the first two series to 3% in the latter two series. In addition, the number of grafts lost because of pancreatic fistulas dropped from 13% to 1%, this probably being due to avoidance of pancreatitis and the temporary exteriorization of the pancreatic juice by means of a pancreatic duct catheter [2]. Also there have been important improvements related to graft rejection. Thus, the rejection frequency appears to have been reduced since cyclosporine was introduced in 1982. Probably even more important is the application of new methods for prompt diagnosis of rejection, namely the monitoring of amylase and of inflammatory cells in the exteriorized pancreatic juice [9].

Comments and conclusion

Our results with duct ligated graft were discouraging with exocrine pancreatic leakage occurring in all patients. Similar negative results have been reported by others and this technique is presently not to be recommended for clinical use.

Gastric exocrine diversion would seem to have some potential advantages. The exocrine secretion would be to the gastrointestinal tract but the risk for

Table 1. Results with pancreatic transplantation with enteric exocrine drainage in Stockholm 1974–87.

	(n)	1 year actuar patient survival rate	(n)	1 year actuar graft success rate
All cases[a]				
1974–81	(7)	71%	(10)	0%
1981–83	(14)	85%	(14)	29%
1984–85	(24)	83%	(25)	52%
1986–87	(38)	97%	(43)	56%
Combined pancreas and kidney				
1974–81	(2)	50%	(2)	0%
1981–83	(13)	85%	(13)	31%
1984–85	(20)	90%	(20)	65%
1986–87	(22)	100%	(23)	77%
Single pancreas				
1974–85	(7)	71%	(10)	0%
1986–87	(13)	92%	(15)	34%
Pancreas after kidney				
1974–87	(6)	83%	(6)	17%

[a] The analysis of all cases included 3 grafts have been classified as preservation injuries. These grafts did not perfuse after revascularization and were removed after a few hours.

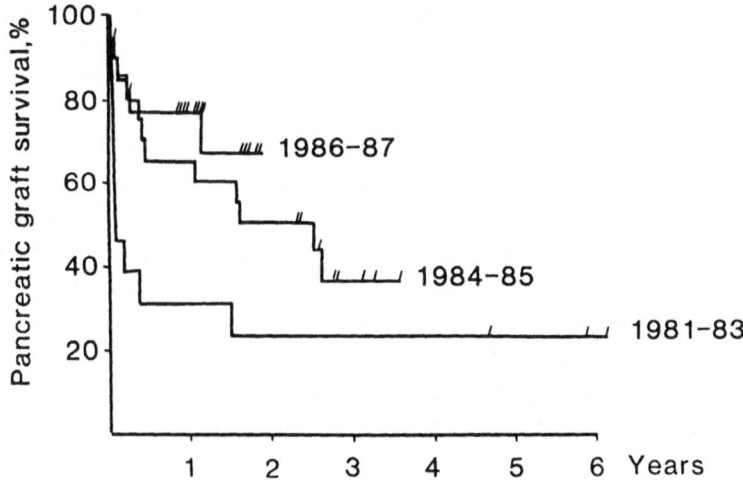

Figure 3. Actuarial pancreatic graft survival rates in the three most recent series of patients given combined pancreatic and renal grafts. Each notch denotes a patient with a functioning graft.

bacterial contamination should be reduced. The telescoping technique should make possible graft biopsies by means of gastroscopy [10]. The position of the graft behind the transverse mesocolon was found, however, to be dangerous. If pancreatitis occurred the patients developed bacterial peritonitis, the bacteria probably emenating from the transverse colon which was in direct contact with the inflammed pancreas.

Pancreatico-enterostomy offers the most physiological way to handle the exocrine secretion. Initially the results with this technique were poor, but more recently there was been a marked improvement. The key factors in this evolution has been the avoidance of exocrine leakage, posttransplantation pancreatitis and graft thrombosis. Also improved prevention and diagnosis of rejection have played a substantial role.

Most groups, including our own, have mostly performed pancreatic transplantation as an ancillary procedure to renal transplantation in diabetic patients with end-stage renal disease. By so doing the question of whether it is justifiable to expose the diabetic patient to a surgical procedure which is to be followed by chronic immunosuppression has been largely circumvented. The recent marked improvement in results with combined pancreatic and renal transplantation has, however, made us decide to offer pancreatic transplantation also to non-uremic diabetics. Further support for this change in policy has been provided by the finding that the vascular lesions in the diabetic patients with end-stage renal disease are not reversed and perhaps not even halted following pancreatic transplantation [11, 12], a finding that probably has its explanation in the fact that the secondary lesions in these patients are too far advanced to be affected.

446

At this time, the results with single pancreatic transplantation are similar to what we had with the combined transplantation some years back. Grafts have been lost due to a variety of causes, including some of the well known technical complications. Chronic rejection which has been uncommon in our recipients of combined grafts, has destroyed 20% of the single pancreatic grafts. Apparently, a learning phase has to be passed also with this procedure.

All patients with functioning grafts have normal or near normal fasting blood glucose levels [13]. The glycosylated-hemoglobin levels and the oral glucose tolerance are normal in most of the patients. The IVGTT is normal in approximately two-thirds of the patients but abnormal in the remainder, probably as a consequence of the immunosuppressive therapy with cyclosporine and prednisolone [14]. Also there is evidence that with the superior blood glucose control achieved, the secondary lesions of diabetes can indeed be prevented [15].

References

1. Groth CG, Lundgren G, Arner P, Collste H et al: Rejection of isolated pancreatic allografts in patients with diabetes. Surg Gynecol & Obstet 143: 933, 1976.
2. Groth CG, Collste H, Lundgren G, Wilczek H et al: Successful outcome of segmental human pancreatic transplantation with enteric exocrine diversion after modifications in technique. Lancet ii: 533, 1982.
3. Groth CG, Lundgen G, Östman J, Gunnarsson R: Experience with nine segmental pancreatic transplantations in pre-uremic diabetic patients in Stockholm Transplant Proc 16: 681, 1980.
4. Groth CG, Collste H, Lundgren G, Ringdén O et al: Surgical techniques for pancreatic transplantation: a critical appraisal of methods used and a suggested new modification. Horm Metab Res 13: 37, 1983.
5. Tydén G, Wilczek H, Lundgren G, Östman J et al: Experience with 21 intraperitoneal segmental pancreatic transplantations with enteric or gastric diversion in man. Transplant Proc 17: 331, 1985.
6. Lundgren G, Wilczek H, Klintmalm G, Tydén G et al: Procurement and preservation of human pancreatic grafts. Transplant Proc 16: 681, 1984.
7. Groth CG, Lundgren G, Wilczek H, Klintmalm G et al: Segmental pancreatic transplantation with duct ligature or enteric diversion: technical aspects. Transplant Proc 16: 724, 1984.
8. Tydén G, Brattström C, Lundgren G, Östman J et al: Improved results in pancreatic transplantation by avoidance of non-immunological graft failures. Transplantation 43: 674, 1987.
9. Brattström C, Tydén G, Reinholt F, Bohman S-O et al: Markers for pancreatic graft rejection in man. Diabetes, (in press) 1988.
10. Tydén G, Lundgren G, Östman J, Gunnarsson R, Groth CG: Grafted pancreas with portal venous drainage. Lancet i: 964, 1981.
11. Solders G, Gunnarsson R, Persson A et al: Effects of combined pancreatic and renal transplantation on diabetic neuropathy: A two-year follow-up study. Lancet ii: 1232, 1987.
12. Ramsay RC, Goetz FC, Sutherland DER et al: Progression of diabetic retinopathy after pancreas transplantation for insulin dependent diabetes mellitus. N Engl J Med 318: 208, 1988.

13. Tydén G, Brattström C, Gunnarsson R, Lundgren G et al: Metabolic control 2 months to 4.5 years after pancreatic transplantation with special reference to the role of cyclosporin. Transplant Proc 19: 2294, 1987.
14. Gunnarsson R, Klintmalm G, Lundgren G, Tydén G et al: Deterioration in glucose metabolism in pancreatic transplant recipients after conversion from azathioprine to cyclosporin. Transplant Proc 16: 709, 1984.
15. Bohman S-O, Tydén G, Wilczek H, Lundgren G et al: Prevention of kidney graft diabetic nephropathy by pancreas transplantation in man. Diabetes 34: 306, 1985.

Experience of the University Hospital Zurich, Zurich, Switzerland

R. SCHLUMPF and F. LARGIADÈR

In Zurich between December 1973 and December 1987 50 pancreatic transplantations had been carried out, 49 times simultaneously with a kidney.

In the first two patients (1973–74) a whole pancreatico-duododenal graft, in the following two (1975–76) a pancreatic segment was transplanted extraperitoneally into the left iliac fossa. Each time enteric exocrine drainage was established by a jejunal Roux-en-Y loop. In all these cases despite good transplant function local complications, i.e. infections in the retroperitoneal space, caused by transcapsular secretion in spite of exocrine drainage led to a fatal outcome [1]. In the light of these disappointing experiences pancreatic organ transplantation was abandoned in favour of an islet transplantation programme started in 1977. Up to 1979 seven patients were treated with intraportal (4 patients) or intrasplenic (3 patients) injection of pancreatic microfragments [2]. This method proved to be safe but rather ineffective as only one of these patients became insulin independent for a prolonged period of time [3]. The results showed that it was much harder to achieve success in patients than in experimental animals, the main problem being the poor yield and purity of the available isolation technique and the rapid intractable rejection.

In a next step henceforth, pancreatic organ transplantation was resumed.

Table 1. Pancreas transplantation (Dec 87).

I.	1973–76	4	extraperitoneal organ/segment-TPL + enteric drainage
II.	1977–79	7	islet cell transplantation
		39	intraperitoneal segment-TPL
III.	1980–83		14 + primary duct occlusion
IV	1983–87		25 + delayed duct occlusion
Total		50	

J.M. Dubernard and D.E.R. Sutherland (eds.), International Handbook of Pancreas Transplantation, 449–453.

The planned new surgical technique had to fulfill the following criteria: the pancreas graft should be segmental, the implantation site intraperitoneal, the surgical procedure an uncomplicated minor one with the optimal management of exocrine secretion known at that time. With these considerations in mind it was decided to choose intraperitoneal segmental pancreatic transplantation with primary Prolamine duct obliteration as technique for the subsequent patients.

Since 1980 this method was used in 14 consecutive cases and hence turned to more encouraging results [4]. However 6 out of these 14 grafts showed loss of function in the first week (4 never worked, 1 was lost due to venous thrombosis, 1 patient died from myocardial infarction). Further 3 grafts were lost after $1\frac{1}{2}$ months (2 due to rejection, 1 patient died from myocardial infarction). Of the only 5 with graft function longer than 2 months, 4 developed a fistula treated with a total of 10 reoperations. This high incidence of early function loss and exocrine fistulae caused a rethink and a change in technique and timing of our procedure in 1983.

Consequently primary duct occlusion was discontinued but a silicon rubber tube was placed in the main pancreatic duct at operation, draining the exocrine secretions percutaneously until delayed duct obliteration was performed [5, 6]. In a study 1987 [7] the results of 21 patients operated with the new technique since 1983 were compared with the outcome of the previous method. In the new series 5 out of 21 had loss of graft function in the first week (for unknown reasons in 1, due to rejection in 1 and due to venous thrombosis in 3 cases respectively). Thereafter 4 transplants were lost, in 2 cases due to transplant-thrombosis after $1\frac{1}{2}$ months, in 1 case for unknown reasons after 2 months; 1 patient died after 2 months from pulmonary embolism. In the 12 patients with transplant function longer than 2 months, 4 fistulae arose, necessitating a total of 7 reoperations. The comparison of the results either with the primary of the delayed duct obliteration technique is depicted in Figure 1. The number of early function loss and incidence of fistulae were clearly reduced by the new duct management. Moreover, the two-months success rates increased, and the frequency of reoperation decreased from two per patient to one in every second patient. The comparison of the 1-year pancreas graft function rates (Figure 2) shows an improvement from 14% by the primary occlusion technique to more than 40% by the delayed duct obliteration method.

Since 1983 our immunosuppressive protocol is a triple therapy regimen with cyclosporine, azathioprine and prednisone. Azathioprine was given in a dose of 1 mg/kg/day continuously, whereas prednison, started in the same dose, was then tapered to a minimum maintenance dose of 5 to 10 mg/day. Experience showed, that the use the cyclosporin in the immediate postoperative phase impaired graft function [8]. Therefore, since 1986, no cyclosporin was given during the first 2 weeks after transplantation. It was replaced by treatment

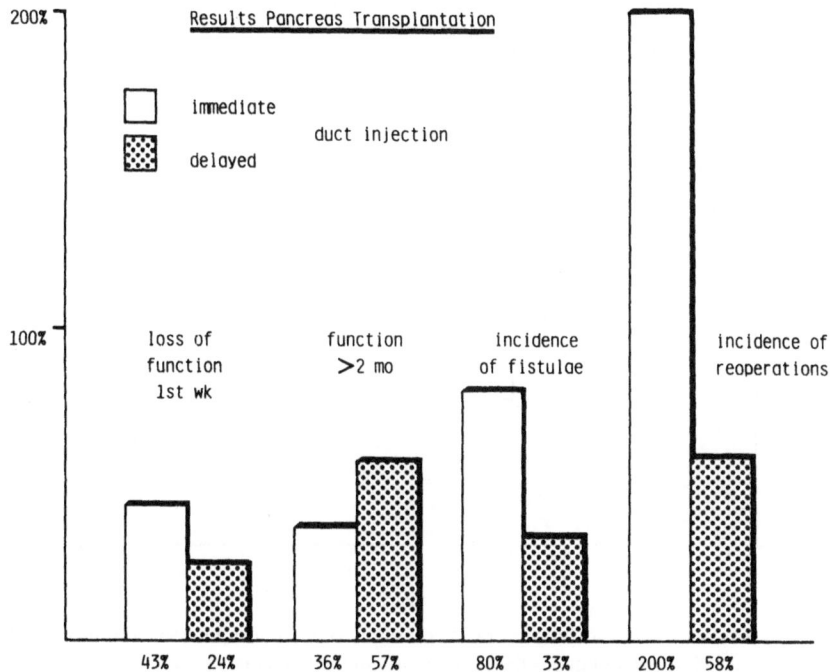

Figure 1. Results of pancreatic segment transplantation with primary or delayed duct occlusion.

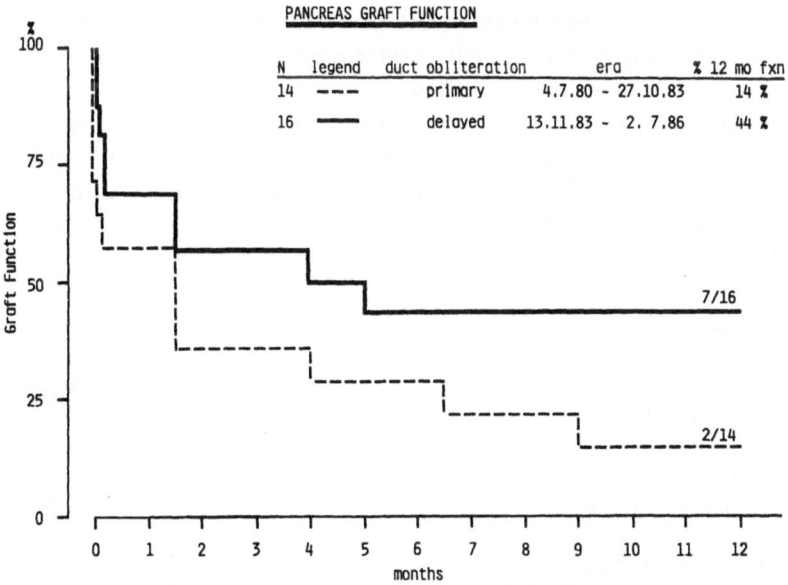

Figure 2. Comparison of the 1-year pancreas graft function rates after primary (broken line) versus delayed (continuous line) duct occlusion technique (only grafts with an observation period of at least 12 months up to July 1987).

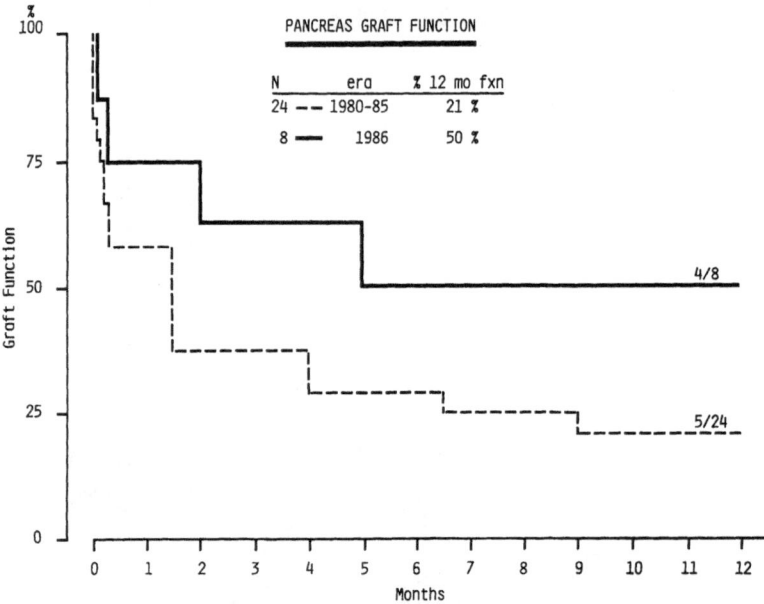

Figure 3. 1-year pancreas graft function rates according to immunosuppressive protocol. With (broken line) or without (continuous line) cyclosporin in the immediate postoperative phase (s. also text).

with antithymocyte globulin in a dose of 3 mg/kg/day. If after 14 days the transplant was functioning normally, cyclosporin therapy was resumed (serum levels desirably ranging between 400 and 600 ng/ml). The 1-year graft function rates of all pancreatic transplants prior to 1986 compared to the group of 1986, having the new immunosuppressive regimen, shows a marked improvement (Figure 3). However, this is not definitely conclusive, as also technical modifications separate the two groups.

Table 2. Graft and patient survival (Dec 87).

Graft		> 1 yr
– Never showed function	4	
– Lost due to thrombosis	9	
– Rejected	4	
– Lost for unknown reason	9	2
Patients		
– Died with functioning graft	5	
– Have functioning graft at 79, 49, 36, 21, 20, 20, 15, 11 months	8	7
Total	39	9

Table 2 shows the overall results of the 39 intraperitoneal segmental pancreatic transplantations since 1980 to the end of 1987. 4 of them never showed graft function. 9 transplants were lost due to venous or arterial thrombosis, 4 by rejection and 9 due to unknown reasons, two of the latter after more than one year. 5 patients died with good functioning grafts. 8 patients have functioning grafts, are insulin independent and free from dialysis, seven of them for more than one year, the longest to date $6^{1}/_{2}$ years.

References

1. Largiadèr F: Farewell to pancreatic organ transplantation? Eur Surg Res 9: 399–402, 1977.
2. Kolb E, Largiadèr F: Clinical islet transplantation. Transplant Proc 12: 205–207, 1980.
3. Largiadèr F, Kolb E, Binswanger U: A long term functioning human pancreatic islet allotransplant. Transplantation 29: 76–77, 1980.
4. Baumgartner D, Largiadèr F: Simultaneous renal and intraperitoneal segmental pancreatic transplantation: the Zürich experience. World J Surg 8: 267–269, 1984.
5. Baumgartner D, Brühlmann W, Largiadèr F: Technique and timing of pancreatic duct occlusion with prolamine in recipients of simultaneous renal and intraperitoneal segmental pancreas allotransplants. Transplant Proc 18: 1134–1135, 1986.
6. Schlumpf R, Largiadèr F, Decurtins M: Experience in clinical pancreas transplantation – university of Zürich. Transplant Proc 19 (Suppl 4): 92–95, 1987.
7. Decurtins M, Schlumpf R, Baumgartner D, Largiadèr F: Three-year experience with delayed duct occlusion in intraperitoneal pancreas transplantation. Transplant Proc 19: 3939–3940, 1987.
8. Baumgartner D, Schlumpf R, Largiadèr F: Cyclosporin A interferes with postoperative blood glucose control after clinical pancreas transplantation. Transplant Proc 19: 4009–1010, 1987.

16. Islet transplantation a review of the objective, the concepts, the problems, the progress and the future

D.W. SCHARP and P.E. LACY

The objective

If one examines the impact in the world today that results from the complications of diabetes mellitus, one recognizes the need to find an alternative therapy to the standard use of exogenous insulin injections. The total impact of this disease in the USA has been estimated to be $ 14 billion affecting some 2 million patients with Type I, Insulin Dependent Diabetes Mellitus (IDDM), and some 8–10 million patients with Type II, non-IDDM [1]. It is the microvascular complications that make this disease the third leading cause of death, the leading cause of new blindness, the cause of kidney failure resulting in 30% of the kidney transplants done in this country, a major contributor to myocardial infarction and stroke, a major cause of gangrene and amputation, and a important cause of male impotence. The use of exogenous insulin therapy has not prevented these complications to date. New efforts with insulin monitoring and treatment have certainly changed the way patients with Type I disease care for themselves. Yet, definitive proof of this aggressive control significantly reducing the risk of complications is still not available. While research into the pathophysiology of the complications and their prevention and treatment are imperative to answer the basic question, research into the transplantation of islet tissue is also important in the development of clinical trials that may provide new answers.

The concept of transplanting islet tissue is certainly not new. The earliest documented case of transplanting slices of sheep pancreas into the thight of a child dying of diabetes took place in 1893 [2], before the discovery of insulin in 1922 [3] with these early transplant studies demonstrating feasibility [4]. Such an enormous change resulted in the care of diabetic patients by the use of insulin injections that the marked reduction in the primary cause of death from hyperglycemic, ketoacidosis made many at the time consider this disease to have been cured by insulin. Interest in transplantation waned until more recent years when it has become apparent that the secondary complications of

J.M. Dubernard and D.E.R. Sutherland (eds.), International Handbook of Pancreas Transplantation, 455–478.
© 1989 by Kluwer Academic Publishers.

the disease are now the primary cause of morbidity and mortality and are not prevented by modern insulin therapy.

Two events took place between 1965 and 1970 that set the stage for reconsidering the transplantation of insulin producing tissue:
a) Moskalewski [5] published his preliminary work followed by modifications by Lacy [6] in the collagenase digestion of the pancreas to liberate isolated islets;
b) Lillehei [7] published his first trials of the clinical transplantation of the human pancreas.

These two areas, the use of isolated islets, and the use of the pancreas, have developed in a parallel fashion up to the present time as a potential alternate form of therapy to insulin for treatment of this disease. This chapter will focus on the use of islet tissue for transplantation. Another chapter is focussed on pancreas transplantation which has advanced at a faster rate than islets in terms of clinical transplantation. Given this historical perspective, both proposed treatments have a common objective:

The objective is the successful transplantation of normal insulin producing, islet tissue into patients with diabetes that can be accomplished early enough in the course of the disease to either prevent or at least stabilize the microvascular complications of diabetes.

With the objective defined, this chapter will focus on four concepts needed to achieve this objective, defining them, their problems, their progress, and their future. These four concepts are presented in Table 1. Discussion of each of these concepts follows.

The concepts

The first concept:

Sufficient insulin producing islet tissue can be isolated and purified from the

Table 1. The concepts for successful islet transplantation.

---

1. Sufficient insulin producing islet tissue can be isolated and purified from the pancreas to result in successful clinical transplantation, eliminating the insulin requirement of the recipients.
2. Sufficient transplanted islet function can be achieved to prevent or stabilize the microvascular complications in patients with diabetes.
3. The rejection of islet tissue can be prevented by one of three methods: a) immunosuppression, b) immuno-alteration, c) immuno-isolation.
4. The prevention of auto-immune recurrence of Type I, IDDM, can be accomplished by one of the methods used to prevent rejection.

---

pancreas to result in successful clinical transplantation, eliminating the insulin requirement for diabetic recipients.

The problems

Available islet tissue for clinical transplantation

If one assumes that the methods of islet isolation and purification that are being applied to non-human pancreas can be successfully applied to the human pancreas sufficient to result in successful clinical trials, then one is faced with an immediate dilemma. With 2 million Type I, IDDM patients currently at risk for the complications, with an additional 10,000 to 20,000 new cases each year, and with only 4,000 cadaver organ donors last year, where will one obtain sufficient human pancreas for islet isolation to solve this disease by transplantation? Possible solutions are:
1. to increase the yield of isolated islets from the human pancreas,
2. to increase the number of cadaver donors each year,
3. to find a way to cause adult islets to reproduce themselves,
4. to use fetal islet tissue,
5. to use non-human islet tissue.

While each of these have different times for their possible achievement, they all may have long term potential of success. Staying with the proposed use of human tissue, one can prepare the use of human fetal islet tissue with its main advantages of availability in terms of the number of human abortions done in this country each year and the demonstration of the human fetal islet tissue to reproduce itself some 10–20 fold. Yet, disadvantages of proposing human fetal islet tissue may be the apparent requirement of second trimester abortions to retrieve sufficient islet tissue with their genetic abnormality risks and the potential ethical considerations. In addition, it is not clear that fetal islet tissue can be sufficiently treated prior to transplantation to prevent its rejection as has been proven with adult islet tissue. The use of non-human islet tissue for transplantation into patients with diabetes is a definite possibility with many advantages. Yet, to be practical, the problem of xenograft acceptance in terms of the potential of rejection and destruction by pre-formed antibodies must be overcome. Thus, as effective clinical trials are developing in patients, the answer to the availability of sufficient quantities of islet tissue remains to be solved.

The mass isolation of islet tissue

All reported methods of islet isolation currently being investigated are modifications of the original collagenase digestion method [5, 6]. To date, no patient has received sufficient numbers of isolated islets to be able to come off insulin therapy completely. The primary remaining problem is the development of technological methods of large scale human islet isolation. Simple modifications of rodent and dog islet isolations have not solved this isolation barrier. While the exact requirement of the amount of islet tissue needed to eliminate the insulin requirement in man has not been reported, calculations would suggest the minimal numbers of islets needed would be approximately 500,000 islets in a pure form containing over 100 units of insulin. While these levels of human islet isolation are just being reached [8], there are a number of specific problems limiting this success.

A review of the variables involved in processing the human pancreas is available [9]. The first variables are the donor pancreas itself. The pancreas is removed from cadaver multiple organ donors in competition with the requirements for liver transplantation and whole pancreas transplantation. There appears to be direct damage due from both warm and cold pancreatic ischemia that results from pancreas removal and distribution to islet isolation centers. The damage seems to be much worse than that observed for whole pancreas transplantation [10]. The second variables involve the reagents which are not standardized. This is especially true for collagenase which is a mixture of enzymes produced by bacterial fermentation of *Clostridia perfringins*. Standardization of this reagent is a critical factor for the future success of clinical trials. Another set of variables involves the digestion process itself which is difficult to control once initiating the digestion of the pancreas with the potential activation of the endogenous pancreatic enzymes as well. Controlling this digestion so that the islets can be removed once released while continuing the digestion of the pancreas seems to be an important concept which is called digestion-filtration [11, 12]. Another major problem plaguing investigators is the accurate documentation of islet yield and function of the islets. Standardization is critically needed in this effort in order for investigators to accurately compare their methods and the results of future trials [9, 13, 14]. Table 2 presents a proposed way of classifying and confirming the results of islet isolation methods. A final problem with isolation of human islet tissue is that most all reported methods are essentially still bench top curiousities with limited ability to establish a standardized method to date. Major effort needs to be made in standardizing human islet isolation as the scale up needed to accomplish multi-center, nationwide clinical islet transplantation begins.

The mass purification of islet tissue

The variables involved in islet purification have also been presented [9]. Many patients have been transplanted with unpurified human islet tissue referred to as islet transplantation [15]. There are two primary requirements that justify the need for purified islet tissue for human transplantation. The first is the need to optimize the number of islets that can achieve succesful engraftment in the transplant site. Activation of non-islet, acinar cells with their enzymatic content of digestive enzymes in a questionable state of viability is certainly not an ideal tissue preparation to maximize transplanted islet survival. A second requirement is that successful immuno-alteration results in rodents requires purified islet tissue. The optimal purification method for islets is not determined at this point. The use of density gradients have problems relating to their efficiency and the maintenance of different densities between islets and aciner cells which can be changed by events in pancreas procurement. The use of specific tags to islet tissue such as monoclonal antibodies or lectins have not demonstrated efficiency or practical usage at this point. The fluorescent activated cell sorter (FACS) should be efficient but at present has not been demonstrated to be able to process the large particle size that would be needed for intact islets. There also remain the problems of scale up for mass purification for each of these methods. Thus, numerous problems remain for this critical step of isolated islet purification.

The progress

There have been a number of reviews published that adequately describe the

Table 2. Documentation of isolated islets for human transplantation.

1. Islet yield
   a) Counting islets by size
   b) Calculating islet volume
   c) Confirmation by insulin content
   d) Confirmation by histology
   e) Determination of islet purity
2. Islet viability
   a) Demonstrated insulin release
      1. Response to glucose challenge
      2. Return to basal release after challenge
   b) Calculation of stimulation index
3. Islet sterility
   a) Donor screening for viral antibodies
   b) Bacteriologic testing
      1. Donor pancreas
      2. Islet processing
      3. Islet culture
4. Islet transplantability
   a) Transplantation into diabetic nude mouse
   b) Demonstrate graft function
   c) Removal of graft to prove dependency

progress in islet transplantation [4, 15–23] over the last few years. This section will not attempt to duplicate their reports but rather highlight significant achievements. Since the first demonstrations of the feasibility of islet transplantation in the rat in 1972–3 [24–26], the objective has been to take this approach to the patient with Type 1, IDDM. Yet, the techniques involving collagenase digestion of the pancreas and Ficoll partial purification of the islets that worked for the rat had little effect on isolating human islets. It soon became obvious that the isolation and purification of islets from the human pancreas was going to be a major impediment to testing this approach in man.

With failure using the human pancreas, attention turned to the dog and other larger animal pancreas to develop isolation methods that might be more effective on the human pancreas. Mirkovitch [27] described successful islet transplantation in dogs after collagenase digestion by eliminating the purification step. While others demonstrated the reversal of the hyperglycemia in dogs following transplantation of unpurified islets into the spleen [27–29], it became apparent that the metabolic response to glucose stimulation was not normal in these dogs [30, 31]. Attempts at placing the unpurified islet tissue into other sites have demonstrated damage from the contaminating exocrine tissue as seen when using the renal, subcapsular space [32]. Transplanting the unpurified islet tissue directly into the portal vein can also have harmful results [33, 34]. Yet, others have shown success with impure islet preparations in this site [35]. The problem with purification steps has been the increasing loss of yield of islets associated with improving the purity.

Intraductal delivery of collagenase into the pancreas has improved yields of isolated islets from the dog [36] and has led to improved islet preparations for transplant studies [37–39]. More recently, these improved islet preparations also seem more easily purified leading to better post transplant results in the dog [40]. Examination of the pig [41] and the beef [42] pancreas as models for human islet isolation have also been productive.

The problem of human islet isolation remains but marked improvements have been noted most recently. Early attempts at isolating islet tissue from the human pancreas [15, 20, 22] and even transplanting it [23] had little success. More recent success has been coming slowly but progressively with new approaches being described from several centers [43–45]. As noted above, one of the problems with these studies in human islet isolation is to be able to document the yields appropriately. Efforts to do this are being developed [46, 47]. While studies of human islet isolation from our own laboratory and others have led to a preliminary trials of human islet transplantation [48, 49], to date no one has been able to come off insulin therapy. Our latest improvements in human islet isolation and purification [50] have sufficiently increased the yields to permit new trials of human islet transplantation. Hopefully, the objective of achieving insulin independence after islet transplantation can be reached in the near future.

The second concept:

Sufficient transplanted islet function can be achieved to prevent or stabilize the microvascular complications in patients

The problems

Unknown etiology of diabetic complications

If one is proposing to eliminate the complications of a disease for which the cause of the complications are not clearly known by providing a new treatment, then it will be difficult to understand the mechanism of this treatment. This makes it difficult to precisely propose the treatment and to evaluate results. A recent example may clarify this point. The results of pancreas transplantation were evaluated regarding their effect on diabetic retinopathy [51]. It was observed that the retinopathy in none of the patients improved while it stabilized in many and worsened in others following pancreas transplantation. Since the basic mechanisms of diabetic retinopathy are unknown as well as their natural history, a definite conclusion is impossible. It is possible to conclude that pancreas transplantation does not effect diabetic complications. Yet, there may be a point in retinopathy beyond which restoration of normal metabolism provides no benefit and the process continues. Some of the recipients of pancreas transplants in this study may have been beyond this point and others may not have been. Thus, interpretation of post-transplant results is compromised by the lack of understanding of the pathophysiologic events that lead to the complications and their natural progression.

Inability to predict which patients with diabetes will develop severe complications

At present, it seems that 40% of patients with Type I, IDDM at the time of clinical diagnosis will eventually develop the life treatening complications. Unfortunately, there is no way to predict which of these patients will be involved until many years have passed and their complications are documented. If one now proposed a treatment to prevent complications prior to their development, one would have to potentially treat all the patients since there is no current way to identify who is at risk. If one does not know whether the transplant will prevent the complications, one will have great difficulty in deciding the validity of the transplant results on preventing the complications since 60% of those transplanted would not have developed the complications anyway. Thus, the dilemma will be the choice of transplanting sufficiently early to prevent the complications and accepting transplanting patients who may not need the procedure versus waiting until the complications have developed and hoping the transplants will stabilize the complications so that they cannot continue to progress.

This argument ignores the quality of life, risk-benefit analysis, and the cost involved in elimination of this insulin requirement. A potential advantage of islet transplantation over pancreas transplantation is the possibility of transplanting patients in the early stages of their disease since the risks involved with islets would be less than those involved in pancreas transplantation. Thus, if the identification of patients at risk for the complications is not possible, then islet transplantation may be offered early after diagnosis if its risks are minimal. Hopefully, the patients at risk for the complications can be identified.

Difficulty in documenting diabetic complications

Each of the organ systems affected by diabetic complications manifest their specific damage differently and at different times. Currently, methods of documenting this damage are either not very sophisticated or hampered by treatments of the affected organ designed to retard their progression. Certainly, nerve conduction times and signal amplitude can be measured. But, reduction of pain and neurologic function is predominantly a subjective determination. Progression of renal change by decreasing glomerular filtration rate (GFR) and biopsy are measurable. But, methods of reducing investigator bias in reading damaged glomeruli and interpretation of histologic data remains a problem. Visual acuity can be measured. But the effect of laser treatments, scarring, and stimulation of neovascularization make these retinal changes difficult to understand in terms of their natural history and in terms of proposed treatment such as pancreas or islet transplantation. When examining the effect of autonomic neuropathy, objective measurements are even more difficult with reliance on subjective determinations. When trying to evaluate the complications from diabetes on coronary artery disease and cerebral vascular disease, it is difficult to isolate the primary damage from diabetes from additional factors such as smoking, hypertension, or when a self-perpetuating type of damage may be involved. Thus, improvements in documentation of diabetic complications must be pursued in order to more effectively understand the potential results of the transplant.

Lack of standardization of transplant results

There has not been an accepted method of analyzing the results of transplanting islet tissue into diabetic animals or man. Many have suggested that successful transplantation equals the cure of this disease. As mentioned, this was erroneously thought about the discovery of insulin. Transplantation of islet tissue is a proposed alternative therapy to insulin that has the potential in preventing the complications (see objective). The cure for this disease will happen when its cause is understood and eliminated.

Many investigators report success as a normal fasting blood glucose. This can also be achieved by starvation. What must be understood is that a fasting normal blood glucose in a transplanted animal is only the first level of a result. With a marginal islet transplant, one can easily achieve a normal fasting blood glucose and a very abnormal insulin response to glucose challenge. Again, since the mechanisms causing the complications are unknown, the degree of normalcy required in terms of glucose tolerance test results required to prevent the complications is also unknown. Expectations are that a relatively 'normal' glucose tolerance test will be required to prevent the complications.

Standardized and accepted criteria for islet transplant success need to be determined. Table 3 presents a recommended proposal for this standardization. Adequacy of pretransplant documentation of the diabetic state has been lacking in many studies. Popular claims of success have been made without these critically important pretransplant measurements. Some patients with renal transplants for diabetic nephropathy have been observed to have residual C-peptide function. Peri-transplant documentation includes the proposed standardization of the islet preparation as given in Table 2. In addition, information about the donor and the pancreas as well as the type of transplant

Table 3. Criteria for successful islet transplantation.

Pretransplant documentation	*Post-transplant documentation*
C-peptide levels	Prevention of rejection
fasting and post-stimulation	Immunosuppression regimen
Average insulin requirement	Immuno-alteration regimen
Glycosylated hemoglobin	Immuno-isolation regimen
Average glucose	Document rejection and treatment
24 hour profile	Islet function
Degree of complications	C-peptide levels
Peri-transplant documentation	Fasting
Islet preparation	Post-stimulation
Islet yield	Insulin requirement
Islet pretreatment	Glycosylated hemoglobin
Islet viability	24 hour profile
Islet sterility	Complications
Pancreas donor	*Experimental animal*
Islet treatment	Reliance on graft by its removal
Immuno-alteration methods	
Transplant method	
Transplant site	
Transplant technique	

need to be included. Post-transplant documentation requires the type and dosage of immunosuppression since prednisone, cyclosporin, and azathioprine have all been documented to adversely islet function. Diagnosis of rejection episodes is very difficult without biopsy and even then can be confused with auto-immune recurrence. The same studies obtained pre-transplant must be repeated post-transplantation. The effect of islet transplantation improves with time, especially soon after transplantation, and may gradually fail with increasing time, especially when marginal amounts of islet tissue are transplanted. Thus, these tests must be repeated at regular intervals in order to accurately represent the results of the transplant. In terms of animal islet transplantation, removal of the islet graft should be accomplished prior to the death of the animal in order to document return of the diabetic state to the recipient which confirms the observed functional results were indeed due to the graft. Histologic confirmation of the removed graft must be accomplished as well as confirmation of the recipients own islet status in the pancreas at time of sacrifice. If these criteria could be modified and accepted universally, then interpretation of results and sharing of knowledge would be much more efficient and effective in this area of transplanting insulin producing tissue.

The progress

Reviews of this concept are available [18, 20, 22]. As discussed above, the lack of standardized reporting of transplant results makes interpretation somewhat difficult and thus controversial. For example, a recent report by Warnock and Rajotte [40] begins to correlate the yield of islets to be transplanted with the clinical result in the dog model. The importance of this approach is emphasized when one considers the recent work also in dogs by Imamura [51] in which partially pancreatectomized dogs were presented with prolonged hyperglycemia or euglycemia. Those facing hyperglycemia lost beta cell mass and function compared with those which faced euglycemia, a point suggested long ago by Dohan and Lukens [53]. If one would perform islet transplants with marginal amounts of islet tissue, then one should expect those islets to be at risk to fail over time. If one then asks whether islet transplantation can prevent or stabilize the complications of diabetes without adequately documenting the degree of return to normal function following transplantation, then one may have a marginal islet transplant which may fail in time and thus not protect the recipient from the complications. One could incorrectly conclude that islet transplantation does not protect against the complications when one is actually observing that a marginal islet transplant does not last and thus would not protect the recipient from complications. This may be the basis of the current controversy regarding the effectiveness of islet transplantation.

Earlier work [18, 20, 22] suggested that islet transplantation into diabetic rats prevented or stabilized their complications. But, recent work by Orloff [53–55] comparing whole pancreas transplantation versus islet transplantation in rats suggests that only whole pancreas transplantation results in permanent reversal of the diabetic state and protection from the complications. It was also observed that longterm results of the islet recipients showed progressive loss of their function. This has also been observed by others [20]. In addition, the question of long term function of islet grafts has been raised in dog models [39]. However, the observation of marginally grafted dogs [56] and monkeys [35] losing their graft function with time when completely islet grafted animals did not [56, 20], again suggests that it is the amount of islets engrafted and surviving that is the critical factor. In fact, strict review of Orloff's islet transplanted rats reveal that they did not achieve the same degree of insulin responsi veness that the whole pancreas grafted animals achieved and were thus only marginally reversed from their diabetic state. Another report in rats suggests that marginally islet transplanted diabetic rats are not as protected from developing autonomic neuropathy as those that received twice as many islets with complete reversal of their diabetic state [57]. Thus, this controversy exists over the extent of islets needed to reverse the diabetic state, the duration of the transplant, and the ability to prevent or stabilize the complications of the diabetic recipient. Only by performing well documented studies, reporting the parameters suggested in Table 3, will the correct answer be learned by future investigations of this critically important concept.

The third concept:

The rejection of islet tissue can be prevented by one of three methods: a) immunosuppression, b) immuno-alteration, or c) immuno-isolation

The problems

Immunosuppression

Recipient toxicity. The use of immunosuppression as we know it today for preventing immune rejection of grafted organs results in too great a toxicity to be able to satisfy the objective for islet transplantation. Unlike the other organ transplants which are needed for life and thus, accept a relatively high degree of risk from potential treatment complications, islet transplantation represents a different kind of transplant. It essentially is a preventive organ transplant. It will be done as prophylaxis against the development of the secondary, micro-vascular complications of diabetes. As such, the risk-benefit ratio for using clinical immunosuppression for this purpose is unacceptable for the newly diagnosed diabetic when one considers that the average time from diagnosis of

Type 1, IDDM, to renal failure is 20 years in those patients who get it. The increased risks of infection and tumor production when proposed for such a long term prophylactic treatment are too great to consider for these patients when considering the use of the current triple and quadruple immunosuppressive therapies. In order to achieve acceptable recipient toxicity, there must either be a major, new change in immunosuppressive drugs or alternative measures employed with islets such as immuno-alteration or immuno-isolation techniques. It is only with these changes that islet transplantation can become considered as a practical alternative to insulin injections.

Islet toxicity. Not only are there important considerations for the recipient with immunosuppression, there appear to be significant risks to the transplanted islet as well from immunosuppression. For example, the diabetogeneic effects of prednisone are well known. Its use immediately post islet transplant may offer additional risks in causing an increased failure rate in islet autotransplanted dogs [58]. The islets are unique in organ transplantation in having to grow their own blood supply in the recipient in order to survive. This delicate situation immediately post transplant may be compounded by hyperglycemia that can occur [59]. Cyclosoporin has also been shown to cause decreased insulin biosynthesis and release in isolated islet cells [60]. Azathioprine has also been recently implicated as potentially beta cell toxic [61]. Thus, the three mainstays of modern immunosuppression all have evidence of islet toxicity. Their exact effect in early post-transplant islet failure is unknown.

The lack of specificity. The rather crude methods of immunosuppression in clinical use today are quite non-specific in their prevention of allograft rejection. The major reason for the lack of more specific immune suppressants is the lack of real understanding of the mechanisms of acute and chronic rejection of organ allografts. A description of the current understanding is located elsewhere is this book. With improvements in understanding, comes the opportunity to develop more specific immunosuppression. It is precisely this lack of specificity that makes the current immunosuppression approaches unrealistic for the prophylactic islet transplant.

Immuno-alteration

Documentation of the phenomenon. One of the most exciting potential developments for achieving the objective of transplanting islets without the use of immunosuppression in patients with diabetes is the demonstration in rodents of the ability to remove the immune, passenger, antigen presenting cells from the islets prior to transplantation resulting in their long term acceptance as an allograft or xenograft [21, 62–65]. Yet, this phenomenon has not been well documented in all the instances reported. Because the immunologic hypotheses of the phenomenon go against our previous understandings that suggest that antigen itself is the barrier to rejection [66, 67], universal acceptance of the phenomenon has not been achieved. Thus, documentation of the species, strain combinations, and in vitro reagents is imperative for the maximal information to be gained from all future studies.

Lack of specific reagents. The ideal immuno-alteration reagents would be 100% toxic to the immune cells while totally preserving islet cells. Most all the reagents employed to date have demonstrated some islet toxicity as well as immune cell toxicity. Thus, an investigator is trying to maximize the immune toxicity while minimizing islet toxicity in using these treatments. Some reagents are only available for usage in the mouse strains. Few reagents are available for large animal studies such as needed in the dog. While new, more specific reagents are being developed, documentation of their exact toxicity to both the immune and the islet cells must be determined. The effect of decreased islet mass resulting from exposure to these reagents must be clearly determined in order to interpret transplant results. This is especially true as regards the effects of transplanting marginal amounts of islet tissue, as was discussed above.

Combinations of reagents. It appears that as one moves out of the mouse model, it becomes more difficult to achieve success with single agents [65].

Table 4. Techniques for immuno-alteration.

In vitro approaches	In vivo approaches
Tissue culture techniques	Donor pre-treatment
7 day, 24° C culture	Fatty acid deficiency
High oxygen culture	Irradiation
In vitro treatment	Donor-recipient treatment
Antibodies and complement	Multiple donors
Polyclonal to Ia	Transient recipient treatment
Monoclonal to Ia	Immunosuppression
Monoclonal to dendritic cells	Cyclosporin alone
Monoclonal to interleukins	Anti-lymphocyte globulin
Ultraviolet light	Anti-oxygen free radical reagents
Islet processing	Recipient pre-treatment
Non-enzymatic	Low dose donor antigens
Very pure islets	
Single islet cells with reaggregation	
Cryopreservation	
	Combinations

Combinations of agents will most likely be required in approaching larger animals such as dogs or man. Since over a dozen single techniques have already been published (Table 4), it will take considerable time to evaluate these combinations as larger animal trials are initiated.

Large animal or human application. There is no conclusive proof that the phenomenon of immuno-alteration observed in rodents is observable in larger animals or man. While preliminary observations have been made [68, 69], they are really anecdotal reports at present. While there does not seem to be evidence to support either a positive or negative position in man for this phenomenon, these important observations await the development of effective clinical islet transplantation trials. Once a patient has been shown to be able to eliminate the exogenous insulin requirement after islet transplantation using immunosuppression, then this approach can be pursued more aggressively.

Immuno-isolation

Type of device. An important component of the hypothesis for initiating allograft rejection and for immuno-alteration is the required contact between the antigen presenting cell and the effector immune cell or cells. Thus, the concept of protecting engrafted tissue by a mechanical barrier is not a new one. Prehn, Weaver, and Algire [70–72] demonstrated the feasibility of this approach in the early 1950's. More recent reviews of this topic have been presented [73, 74]. The type of immuno-isolation device that would have the best potential clinical trials is not clear. Whether one considers using an extravascular diffusion device, an intravascular diffusion device, an intravascular ultrafiltration device or technique of microencapsulation, one must consider the major problems with each of these approaches. In some ways, the potential magnitude of these problems may be as major a consideration as the problems of circumventing rejection. Yet, the feasibility of each approach in animals has been shown.

Reagent biocompatibility. Each of the immuno-isolation approaches has its own set of problems. Both the extravascular diffusion device and the microencapsulated tissue would be implanted into the peritoneal cavity or the soft tissues. They therefore, need development of membranes that do not stimulate a fibroblastic response in the recipient. This is the primary problem which currently limits the effective diffusion capability of the device to a short time and also limits the survival of the enclosed graft. The intravascular devices need development of non-thrombogenic surfaces that also avoid protein deposition and an effective vascular interface if they are to became practical. While there are many other advantages and disadvantages to each of these approaches involved in their potential use in patients [74], these are the primary critical elements to be solved.

Functional documentation. Unfortunately, many reports of immuno-isolation devices provide little documentation of *in vitro* and *in vivo* function except in general terms such as recipient survival or fasting normoglycemia. The kinetics of glucose and insulin transfer both *in vitro* and *in vivo* need to be presented. Due to the predictable bioengineering principles involved in the design of an efficient insulin device, there have been many devices reported which one would predict would not be rapidly responsive but are reported to correct the animals glucose metabolism. Again, it is not known how responsive these devices need to be to prevent the complications of diabetes. But, adequate documentation of the items listed in Table 3 need to be the objective of future reports that describe the use of these devices.

The progress

Immunosuppression

The use of immunosuppressive agents in rodents for islet allografts has not been exceedingly effective [20]. Preliminary reports in dogs suggest cyclosporin A can be effective but at very high dosages that would not be tolerated in man without renal toxicity [75–77]. The use of standard triple therapy – prednisone, azothioprine, and cyclosporin, in the usual renal allograft dosages were not effective in our preliminary dog allograft studies. Our preliminary experience of islet transplantation in clinical trials with triple immunosuppression have so far not prevented rejection. As has been noted, toxicity of these agents has also been observed for islet tissue [58, 60, 61]. Thus, the role of immunosuppression in larger animals including man with freshly isolated islets remains to be determined in terms of both their permitting allograft acceptance and reducing islet toxicity.

Immuno-alteration

Snell [66] in 1957 suggested that passenger leukocytes transplanted from the donor with the graft may be responsible for initiating the mechanisms leading to graft rejection and that the parenchymal cells may not participate in this afferent reaction. Since that time, evidence has been recently increasing that the phenomenon of islet pretreatment which permits islet allograft and xenograft acceptance is a phenomenon [62–65]. Table 4 lists the different treatments that have resulted in graft acceptance. There are *in vitro* and *in vivo* approaches which have been used alone and in combination. In terms of tissue culture techniques, seven day culture of islets at 25° C [78, 79] and the use of high oxygen tension in culture [80] have resulted in prolongation of islet survival. In terms of *in vitro* treatment, a variety of antibodies against the passenger immune cells have been used for the same objective [65]. Islet treatment with ultraviolet light has also shown feasibility in partial selectivity for the passenger cells [81]. In terms of islet processing, there are several approaches that suggest purified islets or islet cells that are devoid of the passenger lympnoid cells as a result of the processing or purification can result in prolonged allograft acceptance [82–84]. Recently, it has been suggested that selection of proper freeze-thaw rates for islets can cause selective destruction of donor immune cells permitting prolonged islet survival as xenografts [85]. In terms of *in vivo* approaches, the use of donor pre-treatment has dramatically been recently demonstrated in terms of essential fatty acid deprivation of the donor permitting rat allograft survival without recipient immunosuppression [86]. While this is not a practical solution at present for clinical cadaver organ donors, understanding the mechanisms involved could certainly lead to practical approaches. The use of multiple donors using small amounts of islets from each donor apparently prevents an allograft response to any one of the donors [87, 88]. Transient immunosuppression to the recipient has usually been employed in combination with one or more of the other methods [65]. The recent use of anti-oxygen free radical reagents suggests more specific treatment of the cells involved in the rejection process [89]. Recipient pre-treatment to induce specific, donor unresponsiveness [90, 91] is another method that may lead to a tolerance that could lengthen islet graft survival. As one progresses from the mouse to larger organisms in considering human testing of this phenomenon, then one will most certainly need to consider conbinations of these various approaches.

Immuno-isolation

There has not been a great deal of progress published since the last review of this topic in 1984 [74]. Most recent effort has been focused on microencapsulation approaches. While Chang suggested this approach may be useful for islet transplants in 1972 [92], it was not demonstrated as feasible until Lim and Sun published their method of islet encapsulation in 1980 using an alginate-polylysine method [93]. While this technique has been shown to be effective in mice [94], many *in vitro* and *in vivo* details of this approach remain to be published. Table 5 presents a review of the four major approaches to immuno-isolation. While some of these points have been previously reviewed [74], the primary advantages and disadvantages of these approaches are presented.

A unique, and more natural approach to immuno-isolation are being explored by Selawry [95, 96] who is examining the immunoprivileged site of the testes and Tze [97, 98] who is examining the immunoprivileged site of the brain. While the feasibility of these sites are being demonstrated, additional studies are required to more completely define the mechanisms and practical problems of these approaches.

The fourth concept:

The prevention of auto-immune recurrences of type I, IDDM, can be accomplished by one of the methods used to prevent rejection

Table 5. Techniques for immuno-isolation.

Type of device	Advantages	Disadvantages

Extravascular Diffusion Chamber	Non-human islets
	Rejection protection
	Multiple sites
	No vascular interface
		Host fibroblastic response
		Diffusion limitations
		  Graft oxygenation
		  Graft nutrition
		  Islet function

Intravascular Diffusion Chamber	Non-human islets
	Rejection protection
	No host fibroblastic response
	Rapid difussion
	  Graft oxygenation
	  Graft nutrition
	  Islet function
		Host vascular access
		Anti-coagulation problems
		  Regional
		  Systemic
		Design limited function
		  Diffusion driven

Intravascular Ultrafiltration Chamber	Non-human islets
	Rejection protection
	No host fibroblastic response
	Eliminate diffusion restrictions
	Ultrafiltrate function
	  Graft oxygenation
	  Graft nutrition
	  Islet function
		Host vascular access
		Anti-coagulation problems
		  Regional
		  Systemic
		Protein deposition on membrane
		Ultrafiltrate limited function

Microencapsulation	Non-human islets
	Rejection protection
	Multiple sites
	No vascular access
		Host fibroblastic response
		Diffusion limitations
		  Graft oxygenation
		  Graft nutrition
		  Islet function
		Membrane stability

The problems

Understanding the nature of autoimmune diabetes

It seems to be accepted in most areas now that Type I, IDDM, is indeed an auto-immune disease [99]. Perhaps the most graphic example in man was Sutherland's documentation of auto-immune recurrence of diabetes in an identical twin who received a segmental pancreas transplant from her twin sister without immunosuppression [100]. However, the pathophysiologic mechanisms involved in the recurrence of human Type 1 diabetes are not well understood. There are two animal models of an autoimmune type of diabetes that are similar to that seen in man: the non-obese diabetic (NOD) mouse [101] and the biobreeding (BB) rat [102]. These two animal models have provided much to the understanding of Type 1, IDDM, in man. In terms of transplantation, they have provided interesting models to examine the question of autoimmune recurrence [103].

The progress

There is current controversy regarding the transplant results of normal islets into the BB rat and autoimmune recurrence. The first set of findings suggest that autoimmune recurrence of diabetes in this strain of rats is not MHC-restricted. Neonatal tolerance was induced in the BB rats prone for diabetes to different donor islet strains. While islets reversed the diabetic state post-transplant, diabetes recurred without regard to the donor strain [104, 105]. In other studies, again in neonatally tolerant BB recipients, the use of low temperature culture and ALS provided protection to the Lewis islets but still permitted rejection of the Wistar islets, suggesting MHC restriction [106]. Additional evidence also suggests MHC restriction such as the use of UV light in a donor pre-treatment regimen [107]. This is a very important concept to determine accurately in man. If correct, then the use of immuno-alteration techniques that can prevent rejection also have the potential of preventing the auto-immune recurrence of diabetes. Whether this concept is valid in man awaits effective clinical trials of islet transplantation.

The future

Each of the four concepts (Table 1) required to successfully achieve the objective of islet transplantation for patients with Type 1, IDDM, are developing to a critical point in animal studies that suggest the potential of establishing effective clinical trials in man. The mass isolation of islet tissue from the human pancreas seems close at hand. Animal studies of the function of islets in preventing the diabetic complications suggest the potential for similar protection in man. The rejection of islet transplants can be prevented by immuno-suppression, immuno-alteration, or by immuno-isolation. While the majority of these results have come from rodent studies, similar investigations are being initiated in larger animals. Current studies address the practical difficulties with each of these approaches and suggest directions for future clinical application. The final question of whether auto-immune recurrence of diabetes can be eliminated by immuno-alteration or immuno-isolation approaches remains to be determined.

Thus, 16 years after the demonstration of the first successful islet transplants in rodents, the stage appears to be set to determine the feasibility of islet transplantation in man. While unsuccessful islet trials have been accomplished in the past, the future seems both bright and challenging as this last critical step is approached that successful trials can be achieved. However, only by carefully designed and documented studies, will there be the potential of finding meaningful answers. The patients and the families who face the daily impact of this disease and its potential morbidity and mortality, depend upon the potential results of these future investigations. It is to their future, and to the future of achieving the objective of islet transplantation, that these continuing investigations are dedicated.

References

1. Diabetes in America, NIH Publication NO. 85–1468, 1985.
2. Williams PW: Notes on diabetes treated with extract and by grafts of sheep's pancreas. Br Med J 2: 1303, 1894.
3. Banting FG, Best CH: The internal secretion of the pancreas. J Lab Clin Med 7: 251, 1922.
4. Downing R: Historical review of pancreatic islet transplantation. World J Surg 8: 137–142, 1984.
5. Moskalewski S: Isolation and culture of the islets of Langerhans of the guinea pig. Gen Comp Endocrinol 5: 342–353, 1965.
6. Lacy PE, Kostianovsky M: Method for the isolation of intact islets of Langerhans from the rat pancreas. Diabetes 16: 35–39, 1967.
7. Lillehei RC, Ruiz JO, Acquino C, Goetz FC: Transplantation of the pancreas. Acta Endocrinol 83 (Suppl 205): 303, 1976.
8. Ricordi C, Lacy PE, Finke EH, Olack B, Scharp DW: An automated method for the isolation of human pancreatic islets. Diabetes 37: 413–420, 1988.
9. Scharp DW: The elusive human islet: variables involved in its effective recovery. In: van Schilfgaarde, Hardy M (eds) Transplantation of the endocrine pancreas in diabetes mellitus. Elsevier Science Publications, Amsterdam, 1988.
10. Corlett MP, Fonseca P, Scharp DW: Detrimental effect of warm ischemia on islet isolation in rats and dogs with protection by oxygen-free radical scavengers. J Surg Res, in press.
11. Scharp DW, Murphy JJ, Newton WT, Ballinger WF, Lacy PE: Transplantation of islets of Langerhans in diabetic Rhesus monkeys. Surgery 77: 100–105, 1975.

12. Scharp DW, Downing R, Merrell RC, Greider M: Isolating the elusive islet. Diabetes 29 (1): 19–30, 1980.
13. Scharp DW: Clinical feasibility of islet transplantation. Transplant Proc 16: 820–825, 1984.
14. Scharp DW, Alderson D, Kneteman NM: Optimization of islet preparations for clinical transplantation. Transplant Proc 18 (6): 1814–1816, 1986.
15. Scharp DW: Isolation and transplantation of islet tissue. World J Surg 8: 143–151, 1984.
16. Brown J, Danilovs JA, Clark WR, Mullen YS: Fetal pancreas as an organ donor. World J Surg 8: 152–157, 1984.
17. Mandel TE: Transplantation of organ cultured fetal pancreas. World J Surg 8: 158–168, 1984.
18. Federlin KF, Bretzel RG: The effect of islet transplantation on complications in experimental diabetes in rats. World J Surg 8: 168–178, 1984.
19. Rajotte RV, Warnock GL, Kneteman NM: Cryopreservation of insulin-producing tissue in rats and dogs. World J Surg 8: 179–186, 1984.
20. Gray DWR, Morris PJ: Developments in isolated pancreatic islet transplantation. Transplantation 43: 321–331, 1987.
21. Lacy PE, Scharp DW: Islet transplantation in treating diabetes. Ann Rev Med 37: 33–40, 1986.
22. Sutherland DER: Pancreas and islet transplantation I. experimental studies. Diabetologia 20: 161–185, 1981.
23. Sutherland DER: Pancreas and islet transplantation II. clinical trials. Diabetologia 20: 435–450, 1981.
24. Ballinger WF, Lacy PE: Transplantation of intact pancreatic islets in rats. Surgery 72: 175–186, 1972.
25. Reckard CR, Ziegler MM, Barker CF: Physiological and immunological consequences of transplanting isolated pancreatic islets. Surgery 74: 91–99, 1973.
26. Kemp CB, Knight MJ, Scharp DW, Ballinger WF, Lacy PE: Effects of transplantation site on the results of pancreatic islet isografts in diabetic rats. Diabetologia 9: 489–491, 1973.
27. Kolb E, Ruckert R, Largiader F: Intraportal and intrasplenic autotransplantation of pancreatic islets in the dog. Eur Surg Res 9: 419, 1977.
28. Kretschmer GJ, Sutherland DE, Matas AJ, Cain TL: Autotransplantation of pancreatic islets without separation of exocrine and endocrine tissue in totally pancreatectomized dogs. Surgery 82: 74–81, 1977.
29. Mehigan DG, Zuidema GD, Cameron JL: Pancreatic islet transplantation in dogs: critical factors in technique. Am J Surg 141: 208, 1981.
30. Alderson D, Farndon JR: The metabolic effects of islet transplantation in the diabetic dog. Transplant Proc 16: 831–833, 1984.
31. Alderson D, Walsh TN, Farndon JR: Islet cell transplantation in diabetic dogs: studies of graft function and storage. Br J Surg 71: 756–760, 1984.
32. Hesse, UJ, Sutherland DE, Gores PF, Sitges-Serra A, Najarian JS: Comparison of splenic and renal subcapsular islet autografting in dogs. Transplantation 41: 271–274, 1986.
33. Kretschmer GJ, Sutherland DE, Matas AJ, Payne WD, Najarian JS: Autotransplantation of pancreatic fragments of the portal vein and spleen of totally pancreatectomized dogs: a comparative evaluation. Ann Surg 187: 79, 1978.
34. Mehigan DG, Bell WR, Zuidema GD, Eggleston JC, Cameron JL: Disseminated intravascular coagulation and portal hypertension following pancreatic islet autotransplantation. Ann Surg 191: 287, 1980.
35. Gray DW, Warnock G, Sutton R, Peters M, McShane P, Morris PJ: Successful autotransplantation of isolated islets of Langerhans in the cynomolgus monkey. Br J Surg 73: 850, 1986.

36. Horaguchi A, Merrell RC: Preparation of viable islet cells from dogs by a new method. Diabetes 30: 445–458, 1981.

37. Warnock GL, Rajotte RV, Procshyn AW: Normoglycemia after reflux of islet-containing pancreatic fragments into the splenic vascular bed in dogs. Diabetes 32: 452, 1983.

38. Long JA, Britt LD, Olack BJ, Scharp DW: Autotransplantation of isolated canine pancreatic islet cells. Transplant Proc 15: 1332–1338, 1983.

39. Alejandro R, Cutfield RG, Scheinvold FL et al: Natural history of intrahepatic canine islet cell autografts. J Clin Invest 78: 1339–1348, 1986.

40. Warnock GL, Rajotte RV: Critical mass of purified islets that induce normoglycemia after implantation into dogs. Diabetes 37: 467–470, 1988.

41. Ricordi C, Finke E, Lacy PE: A method for the mass isolation of islets from the adult pig pancreas. Diabetes 35: 649–653, 1986.

42. Lacy PE, Lacy ET, Finke EH, Yasunami Y: An improved method for the isolation of islets from the beef pancreas. Diabetes 31: 109–111, 1982.

43. Gray DWR, McShane P, Grant A, Morris PJ: A method for isolation of islets of Langerhans from the human pancreas. Diabetes 33: 1055–1061, 1984.

44. Rajotte RV, Warnock GL, Evans M, Dawidson I: Isolation of viable islets of Langerhans from collagenase-perfused canine and human pancreata. Transplant Proc 19: 916, 1987.

45. Alderson D, Scharp DW, Kneteman NM: The isolation of purified islets of Langerhans. Transplant Proc 19: 916–917, 1987.

46. Alderson D, Kneteman NM, Olack BJ, Scharp DW: Isolation and quantification of canine islet tissue for transplantation. Transplantation 43 (4): 579–581, 1987.

47. Scharp DW, Lacy PE, Finke E, Olack BJ: Low-temperature culture of human islets isolated by the distension method and purified with Ficoll or Percoll gradients. Surgery 102: 869–879, 1987.

48. Scharp D, Lacy PL: Human islet isolation and transplantation. Diabetes 34 (1): 5A, 1985.

49. Alejandro R, Russell E, Jyriakides G, Miller J, Mintz DH: Islet cell transplantation in type I diabetes mellitus. Transplant Proc 19: 2359–2361, 1987.

50. Ramsay RC, Goetz FC, Sutherland DE, Mauer SM et al: Progression of diabetic retinopathy after pancreas transplantation for insulin dependent diabetes mellitus. NEJM 318: 208, 1988.

51. Imamura T, Koffler M, Helderman JH et al: Severe diabetes induced in subtotally pancreatectomized dogs by sustained hyperglycemia. Diabetes 37: 600–609, 1988.

52. Dohan RC, Lukens FEW: Lesions of the pancreatic islets produced in cats by administration of glucose. Science 105: 183, 1947.

53. Orloff MJ, Greenleaf GE, Urban P, Girard B: Lifelong reversal of the metabolic abnormalities of advanced diabetes in rats by whole-pancreas transplantation. Transplantation 41: 556–564, 1986.

54. Orloff MJ, Yamanaka N, Greenleaf GE, Huang Y, Hung D, Leng X: Reversal of mesangial enlargement in rats with long-standing diabetes by whole pancreas transplantation. Diabetes 35: 347–354, 1986.

55. Orloff MJ, Macedo A, Greenleaf GE, Girard B: Comparison of the metabolic control of diabetes achieved by whole pancreas transplantation in rats. Transplantation 45: 307–312, 1988.

56. Merrell RC, Maeda M, Basadonna G, Maricola F, Cobb L: Suppression, stress and accommodation of transplanted islets of Langerhans. Diabetes 34: 667–670, 1985.

57. Schmidt RE, Plurad SB, Olack BJ, Scharp DW: The effect of pancreatic islet transplantation and insulin therapy on experimental diabetic autonomic neuropathy. Diabetes 32: 532–540, 1983.

58. Scharp DW, Alderson D, Kneteman NM: The effect of immunosuppression on islet transplant function in the dog. Transplant Proc 12: 252–260, 1987.

476

59. Hayak A, Lopez AD, Beattie GM: Decrease in the number of neonatal islets required for successful transplantation by strict metabolic control of diabetic rats. Transplantation 45: 940–943, 1988.

60. Anderson A, Borg H, Hallberg A, Hellerstrom C, Sandler S, Schnell A: Long term effects of cyclosporin A on cultured mouse pancreatic islets. Diabetologia 27: 66, 1984.

61. Vivioni GL, Borgoglie MG, Fontana I, Leprini A, Valente V, Adezati L: Inhibition of islet insulin release by azathioprine. Presented at First International Congress on Pancreatic and Islet Transplantation, Stockholm, Sweden, 1988.

62. Lafferty KJ, Prowse SJ: Theory and practice of immuno regulation by tissue treatment prior to transplantation. World J Surg 8: 187–197, 1984.

63. Lacy PE: Experimental immuno-alteration. World J Surg 8: 198–203, 1984.

64. Bach FH, Morrow CE, Sutherland DER: Immunogenetic considerations in islet transplantation. The role of Ia antigen in graft rejection. World J Surg 8: 204–206, 1984.

65. Lacy PE: Islet transplantation. Clin Chem 32: 876, 1986.

66. Snell GD: The homograft rejection. Ann Rev Microbiol 2: 439, 1957.

67. Lafferty KJ, Prowse SJ, Simenovic C: Immunobiology of tissue transplantation: a return of the passenger leukocyte concept. Ann Rev Immol 1: 143, 1983.

68. Sollinger HW, Mack E, Cook K, Belzer FO: Allotransplantation of human parathyroid tissue without immunosuppression. Transplantation 36: 6, 1983.

69. Alejandro R, Latif Z, Noel J, Shienvold FL, Mintz DH: Effect of anti Ia antibodies, culture and cyclosporin on prolongation of canine islet allograft survival. Diabetes 36: 269–273, 1987.

70. Algire GH, Weaver JM, Prehn RT: Growth of cells in vivo in diffusion chambers. I. Survival of homografts in immunized mice. J Natl Canc Inst 15: 493, 1954.

71. Weaver JM, Algire GH, Prehn RT: The growth of cells in vivo in diffusion chambers. II. The role of cells in the destruction of homografts in mice. J Natl Canc Inst 15: 1737, 1955.

72. Algire GH: Diffusion chamber techniques for studies on cellular immunity. Ann N Y Acad Sci 69: 663, 1957.

73. Scharp DW, Mason NS, Sparks RE: The use of hybrid artificial organs to provide immunoisolation to endocrine grafts. In: Slavin S. (ed) Bone Marrow and Organ Transplantation; pp 601–618. Elsevier Science Publishers. Amsterdam, 1984.

74. Scharp DW, Mason NS, Sparks RE: Islet immunoisolation: the use of hybrid artificial organs to prevent islet tissue rejection. World J Surg 8: 221–229, 1984.

75. Alejandro R, Cutfield R, Sheivold FL, Latif Z, Mintz DH: Successful long-term survival of pancreatic islet allografts in spontaneous or pancreatectomy-induced diabetes in dogs. Cyclosporin induced unresponsiveness. Diabetes 34: 825–828, 1985.

76. Kneteman NM, Alderson D, Scharp DW: Cyclosporin A immuno-suppression of allotransplanted canine pancreatic islets. Transplant Proc 19: 950–951, 1987.

77. Kneteman NM, Alderson D, Scharp DW: Long-term normoglycemia in pancreatectomized dogs following islet allotransplantation and cyclosporin immunosuppression. Transplantation 44: 595–599, 1987.

78. Lacy PE, Davie JM, Finke EH: Prolongation of islet allograft survival following in vitro culture (24° C) and a single injection of ALS. Science 204: 312–313, 1979.

79. Lacy PE, Davie JM, Finke EH: Induction of rejection of successful allografts of rat islets by donor peritoneal exudate cells. Transplantation 28: 415–420, 1979.

80. Bowen KM, Andrus L, Lafferty K: Successful allotransplantation of mouse pancreatic islets to nonimmunosuppressed recipients. Diabetes 29: 98, 1980.

81. Lau H, Reemtsma K, Hardy MA: Prolongation of rat islet allograft survival by direct ultraviolet irradiation of the graft. Science 223: 607–608, 1984.

82. Pipeleers D, Pipeleers-Marichal M, Gepts W: Purified islet cell grafts are tolerated without

immunosuppressive treatment in allotransplanted diabetic rats. In abstracts, second assisi international symposium for advanced models for therapy of insulin dependent diabetes, Assisi, Italy, 1986.

83. Kakiaki K, Basadonna G, Merrell RC: Allotransplantation of islet endocrine aggregates. Diabetes 36: 315–319, 1987.

84. Serie JR, Hegre OD, Eide CR, Weinhaus AJ, Marshall SM: The successful allotransplantation of neonatal rat islets across multiple combined major and minor histocompatibility barriers. Transplantation 44: 739–741, 1987.

85. Coulombe MG, Warnock GL, Rajotte RV: Prolongation of islet xenograft survival by cryopreservation. Diabetes 36: 1086–1088, 1987.

86. Schreiner GF, Flye MW, Brunt E, Korber K, Lefkowith JB: Essential fatty acid depletion of renal allografts and prevention of rejection. Science 240: 1032–1033, 1988.

87. Gotah M, Maki T, Porter J, Nonaco AP: Pancreatic islet transplantation using H-2 incompatible multiple donors. Tansplant Proc 19: 957–959, 1987.

88. Goton M, Porter J, Kanai T, Munaco AP, Maki T: Multiple donor allotransplantation. A new approach to pancreatic islet transplantation. Transplantation 45: 1008–1011, 1988.

89. Mendola J, Wright JR, Lacy PE: The effect of oxygen free radical scavengers on immune destruction of murine islet in allograft rejection and in multiple low-dose Streptozotocin induced insulitis. Submitted, 1988.

90. Faustman D, Lacy PE, Davie JM, Hauptfeld V. Prevention of allograft rejection by immunization with donor blood depleted of Ia bearing cells. Science 217: 157–158, 1982.

91. Lau H, Reemtsma K, Hardy MA: Pancreatic islet allograft prolongation by donor specific blood transfusions treated with ultraviolet irradiation. Science 221: 754–756, 1983.

92. Chang TMS: Artificial cells. Springield, IL. Charles C. Thomas, 1972.

93. Lim F, Sun AM: Microencapsulated islets as bioartificial pancreas. Science 210: 908, 1980.

94. O'Chea CM, Cun AM: Encapsulation of rat islets of Langerhans prolongs xenograft survival in diabetic mice. Diabetes 35: 943–946, 1986.

95. Selawry HP, Whittington K: Extended allograft survival of islets grafted into intra-abdominally placed testis. Diabetes 33: 405–406, 1984.

96. Selawry HP, Fejaco R, Whittington K: Intratesticular islet allografts in the spontaneously diabetic BB/wmt. Diabetes 34: 1019–1024, 1985.

97. Tze WJ, Tai J: Successful intracerebral allotransplantation of purified pancreatic endocrine cells in diabetic rats. Diabetes 32: 1185–1187, 1983.

98. Tze WJ, Tai J: Allotransplantation of dispersed single pancreatic endocrine cells in diabetic rats. Diabetes 37: 383–392, 1988.

99. Eisenbarth GS: Type I diabetes mellitus, a chronic autoimmune disease. NEJM 314: 1360–1368, 1986.

100. Sibley RK, Sutherland DER, Goetz F, Michael AF: Recurrent diabetes mellitus in the pancreas iso and allograft. Lab Invest 53: 132, 1985.

101. Makino S, Muroaoka Y, Kishimoto Y, Hayashi Y: Genetic analysis in NOD mice. Exp Animals 34: 425–432, 1985.

102. Nakhooda AF, Like AA, Chappel GI, Wei CN, Marliss EB: The spontaneously diabetic Wistar rat (the 'BB' rat). Diabetologia 14: 199–207, 1978.

103. Naji A, Silvers WK, Bartlett ST, Francfort J, Barker CF: Immunologic factors in pathogenesis and treatment of human and animal diabetes. World J Surg 8: 214–220, 1984.

104. Weringer EJ, Like AA: Immune attach on pancreatic islet transplants in the spontaneously diabetic BB/w rat is not MHC restricted. J Immunol 134: 2382–2386, 1985.

105. Prowse SJ, Bellgrau D, Lafferty KJ: Islet allografts are destroyed by disease occurrence in the spontaneously diabetic BB rat. Diabetes 35: 110–114, 1986.

106. Woehrle M, Markmann JF, Silvers WK, Barker CF, Naji A: Transplantation of cultured pancreatic islets to BB rats. Surgery 100: 334–341, 1986.

107. Chabot JA, Lau H, Reemstma K, Hardy MA: Long term survival of islet allografts in spontaneously diabetic BB rats without chronic immunosuppression. Transplant Proc 18: 1851–1853, 1986.

17. The implantable artificial pancreas

J.L. SELAM

The pathogenesis of long-term complications associated with Insulin Dependent Diabetes Mellitus (IDDM) remains a contentious issue between two schools of thought: either accelerated macroangiopathy, microangiopathy, and neuropathy are genetically determined and independent of biochemical derangements; or they result from metabolic abnormalities. Although this issue is not yet decided, proponents of the 'metabolic' theory have gathered impressive clinical evidence [1–4], confirmatory data from animal models [5, 6], and demonstrable histologic changes [7–12] which correlate with metabolic abnormalities [13–18]. Conversely, there are other reports [19–24] either directly opposing or questioning this published evidence. Nevertheless, at present it is a reasonable assumption that long term diabetic abnormalities, with genetic factors play a modifying role.

Hyperglycemia is the most important, but not the only [25] metabolic abnormality potentially responsible for long-term complication. Even hypoglycemia might aggravate the complications of diabetes [26]. Conventional insulin therapy has been unable to normalize both blood glucose [27–29] and other metabolic and hormonal abnormalities [30]. In an ongoing National Survey in France, insulin-treated diabetics have been found to have a mean blood glucose of about 200 mg/dl and a normal Hemoglobin Alc in less than 10% of the cases [31].

Thus newer methods of intensified intermittent subcutaneous insulin injection (ISII) treatment have been used to achieve normal blood glucose levels in insulin-dependent or type 1 diabetes [32–35]. This treatment modality requires intensive patient and provider activity including multiple injections of insulin daily, multiple self blood glucose measurements daily and frequent clinic visits. Intensive subcutaneous insulin treatment includes multiple insulin delivery strategies, one of which is continuous subcutaneous insulin infusion (CSII), without continuous feed back control ('open loop' system).

The effectiveness of intensive ISII and CSII in studies using relatively smaller experimental groups of diabetic patients studied for a year or less

479

J.M. Dubernard and D.E.R. Sutherland (eds.), International Handbook of Pancreas Transplantation, 479–517.
© *1989 by Kluwer Academic Publishers.*

indicate that both intensive methods, i.e. ISII or CSII, can normalize glycosylated hemoglobin levels [35–39]. In larger nonresearch patients populations however, the long term safety and effectiveness of intensive ISII and CSII treatment appear unclear since glycosylated hemoglobin levels are not reduced into the normal range, and significant treatment-related complications are reported [40–50]. The frequency of severe hypoglycemic events using CSII has been reported to be higher [45, 48], equal [46–47] or lower [41, 51] when compared to ISII. Treatment with CSII however, has been associated with an increased frequency [2–17.5 fold] of ketoacidosis when compared to non-CSII treated patients [43–46, 53].

Two novel approaches to regulate blood glucose are under intensive evaluation; pancreatic transplantation and mechanical devices that control blood glucose concentration by means of feed back controlled ('closed loop') insulin delivery. The latter has been unproperly called 'artificial pancreas' [53].

Basically, a so-called artificial pancreas or artificial beta-cell consists of three basic components (Figure 1) a glucose sensor, insulin pump and a computer controller that regulates the administration of insulin based on a measured amount of glucose. Ideally, such a device should be small enough to offer the potential for implantatory. No such device is currently available. The present state of the art reviewed in terms of the individual components of the system and the recent progress and applications of these devices.

We exclude from the above definition the 'biological artificial pancreas' in which pancreatic cells are used in place of the sensor and delivery pump, inserted either within a chamber (extravascular bioartificial pancreas) [54, 55] or are just separated from the blood stream by a membrane (vascular bioartificial pancreas) [56–60]. We also exclude from the above definition the 'chemical artificial pancreas' in which insulin is fixed on a carrier and delivered according to the ambient blood glucose [61]. Both systems are at an early experimental plase and have to face specific problems different from those of a mechanical system.

From an historical point of view, the term and the concept artificial pancreas have been first employed in the early 70's by Albisser [53] and Pfeiffer [54]. However predecessors like Mirouze in 1962 for his pioneering work on blood glucose monitoring [62], Kadish in 1964 [63] for having described the first servo controlled insulin infusion system, Metcalf in 1934 [64] for having been the first to propose to administer insulin via a pump also deserved to be cited.

Glucose sensor

Blood glucose has been chosen as the parameter to regulate in the implantable artificial pancreas. However, it must be remembered that a) tissue glucose

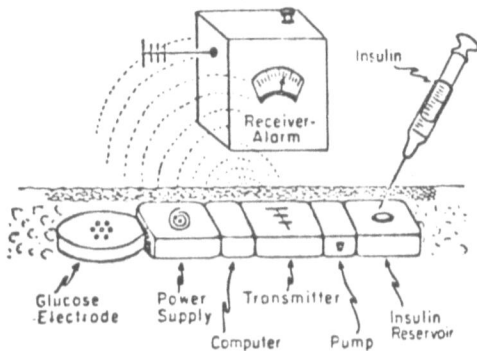

Figure 1. Schematic diagram of an ideal artificial pancreas (from Soeldner).

concentration – especially in the subcutaneous space – might be different from blood, and even might vary from one point to another of the body [64]. b) blood glucose is not physiologically only regulated by insulin along a single loop but by several hormones and – not of all – some insulin reaction are even totally independent from blood glucose, as the anticipatory insulin secretion triggered by meal ingestion before any glucose rise (cephalic phase) [65].

Although the development of glucose sensors has been tackled for more than 10 years, a sensor stable even for a few days only has not yet become available for wide clinical use.

The enzyme electrode sensor

Pioneers in the development of the enzyme electrode glucose sensor were Clark and Lyons [67]. Their sensor used a glucose oxidase solution sandwiched between semipermeable polymeric membranes to catalyze the reaction between glucose and oxygen to form gluconic acid and hydrogen peroxide. Initially, a pH electrode measured glucose concentration as a function of hydrogen ion concentration change which resulted from the formation of gluconic acid. Later versions used an oxygen electrode, also designed by Clark [68] to potentiometrically measure glucose concentration as a function of oxygen depletion.

In an attempt to refine the enzyme electrode design to make it suitable for use in an implantable artificial beta cell, Bessman and Schultz [69] (Figure 2) modified the original design of Clark by immobilizing and stabilizing the glucose oxidase by intra- and inter-molecular cross-linkages in a cloth matrix. Disks of the cloth matrix were cemented over the plastic membrane of a polarographic oxygen electrode.

The most advanced version of enzyme electrode glucose sensor is that developed by Miles Laboratories for their Biostator Glucose Controlled In-

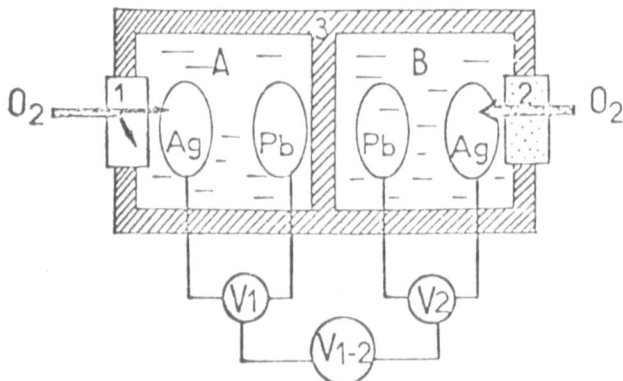

Figure 2. Enzymatic glucose electrode (from Bessman). (1) Glucose oxidase coated membrane. (2) Non-glucose oxidase coated membrane.

sulin Infusion System, and external version, version of the artificial pancreas. As described by Clarke and Santiago [70] this sensor consists of a membrane 1 cm in diameter, made up of solid phase glucose oxidase sandwiched between polyacrylamide and polycarbonate membranes. In contrast to previous versions that measured hydrogen perioxide polarographically. Double-layered protective membranes with differential pore sizes protect the hydrogen peroxide electrode from substances that might interface with the measurement.

Although designed for extracorporeal use the Biostator glucose sensor is relatively small (4 × 2.5 cm). It is accurate and stable with a useful operating range of 0 to 600 g/dl and has a response time of less than 1 min.

While this type of sensor obviously works well in an extracorporeal device, it has several drawbacks when considered for implantable uses. First, the length of time during which an enzyme electrode sensor retains its sensitivity and stability is short. Second, it shares the problem with other types of implantable sensors developed to date, namely of becoming encapsulated by fibrotic tissue and its communication with surrounding blood and body fluid disrupted shortly after implantation. With the sensors designed as needles and applied s.c. [71] services times of up to one week are reported [72] (Figure 3). The development is still in the laboratory stage with individually produced prototypes of electrodes. The problems of reproducible and cheap manufacture which, as experience with other sensors teaches, should represent the central problem, still oppose wide application, furthermore, the problems of storing the electrodes and their possible pretreatment before application must be solved. They must be in steady state when applied.

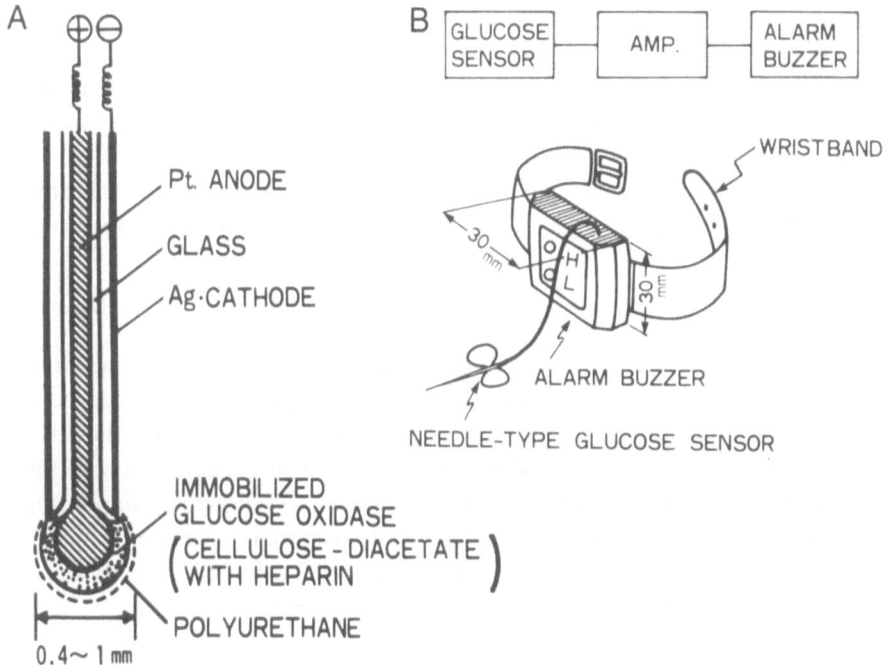

Figure 3. Needle-type glucose sensor (from Schichiri and Kawamori). (a) Principle. (b) Mounted on a watch-like system.

The electrochemical sensor

One way to avoid the problem of rapid degradation of enzyme electrodes is to design a sensor that can operate without enzymes. Noble metals such as platinum can be substituted for glucose oxidase to catalyze the oxidation of glucose. Several modes of operation are possible using this approach including fuel cell, polarographic, potentiometric, and potentiodynamic systems. Although the polarographic approach was taken by many other investigators in the field, Chang et al. [73] of Soeldner's group chose to use a fuel cell sensor in their initial experiments. The fuel cell consists of nonconsumable catalytic anode and cathode, an electrolyte, and a system of membranes to maintain the disparate anodic and cathodic environments. Since the fuel cell measures the electrical energy generated by the electrochemical oxidation of glucose, the system needs no applied current nor reference electrode, thereby reducing the problem of oxide formation and eliminating the problem of reference electrode degradation.

One difficulty with the electrochemical sensor is that it is relatively nonspecific, responding to a variety of endogenous substances such as ethanol, urea, monosaccharides other than glucose, and amino acids. In addition to affecting the accuracy of the response, these substances can cause deactivation of the platinum electrode. Selective membranes have been used to protect the electrode from these substances but these have not been entirely successful because of the small size of the interfering molecules. Additionally, these membranes increase the response time of the sensor.

Both the enzyme electrode and electrochemical sensors have yet to solve the problem of how to prevent the sensor from encapsulation once it is implanted.

The optical sensor

Laser absorption spectrometry is based on the fact that the glucose concentration in the aqueous humor of a human eye can be determined by the degree to which it causes rotation of the plane of a laser beam of light, and that there is a good correlation between blood glucose and glucose concentration in the anterior chamber. This method is a noninvasive technique for measuring glucose concentration [74]. Encouraging results in animals have been achieved recently by Rabinovitch et al. [75–77]. It remains to be seen whether this device can be miniaturized enough to make it practical.

Affinity sensors

These sensors are based on the affinity of glucose and a fluorescein-labeled analog for receptor sites specific to carbohydrate. They have only been tested in vitro so far. Concanavalin A is immobilized on the inner surface of a hollow fiber, which holds fluorescent dextran but allows diffusion of glucose into the fiber. Then an optical probe is inserted into the fiber to determine the quantity of dextran which remains unbound to the fiber walls. As glucose diffuses into the fiber, it displaces dextran, and the resulting change in fluid composition is detected and reported by the probe. Advantages of this system are that there is no membrane to create problems and that it can be tested with extremely small quantities of the mixture [78].

The computer controller

The function of the computer – controller is to regulate the administration of insulin based on measured amounts of glucose and using a special algorithm. An algorithm can be defined as a rule of procedure needed to solve a repetitious mathematical problem. Algorithms form the pattern by which a closed-loop insulin infusion system mimics the complex process of insulin secretion by a normal beta cell. It is based on glucose measurements alone rather than on the host of physiologic mediators of insulin release.

Glucose predictions with rising glucose concentrations

It was clear from early studies that a 5- or 10-min delay between blood withdrawal and glucose measurement introduced an inherent error or delay in closed-loop controls [79, 53]. Because of the delay in glucose measurement and insulin delivery, algorithms were developed so that insulin administration was based on an extrapolated or predicted glucose concentration. This prediction was a function of the actural glucose concentration and its rate of change over the previous few minutes.

Glucose predictions with declining glucose concentrations

The selection of projected glucose concentrations to control insulin delivery when blood glucose concentrations are declining rapidly have been designed so that insulin delivery can be blunted well before the onset of hypoglycemia. An alternate approach would be to activate a counter-regulatory system, such as a dextrose or glucagon infusion, as blood glucose concentrations fall below a given value. Both approaches were studied by the Toronto group [53, 80–82] although our experience was that activation of a glucose or glucagon infusion is seldom needed to avert hypoglycemia after meals when appropriate algorithms are selected [79, 83].

Selection of the glucose concentration-insulin infusion rate relationship

It became clear soon after development of the radioimmunoassay for insulin that the relationship between glucose concentrations and insulin secretory rates was not linear [84]. Foster developed a mathematical model that simulates an intravenous glucose tolerance test with a computer [85] to prod·ce acceptable glucose disappearance rates while it averts postprandial hypoglycemia during a simulated IVGTT. The algorithms selected contained elements of proportionate control that varied in sensitivity at different glucose levels and had a preselected limit to the insulin infusion rate. The term saturation control was used to describe these algorithms.

In 1973, the Toronto Group [86] proposed an algorithm for computer-controlled insulin delivery based on a hyperbolic tangent function. A dynamic control element was achieved through the calculation and use of a predicted glucose concentration, based on the average rate of change over the prior four minutes, applied to an exponential equation. The glucose-control algorithms were similar to those for insulin control except that they were proportionate to the measured rather than to the predicted glucose concentration.

A.H. Clemens and associates developed a series of control algorithms and control programs throughout the evolution of the Biostator GCIIS [82].

The Miles algorithms differed from those of the Toronto group in one aspect – they no longer used the hyperbolic tangent equation for the control of the static insulin release but introduced a biquadratic and, subsequently, a quadratic function, with the advantage that the new control constants could be selected in physiologically meaningful terms, such as the desired (basal) blood glucose level and the desired basal insulin infusion rate. The hyperbolic tangent function used inthe Toronto approach has the theoretic advantage of resembling more closely the sigmoidal pattern of insulin secretion at high glucose levels in the isolated rat pancreas perfused with glucose. While the Miles algorithm closely resembled the hyperbolic tangent control curve in the lower (physiologic) range, its maximal insulin release was limited by an operator-selected value. During the same period, we developed our own artificial pancreas (Figure 4) using several personal algorithms without [79] (Figure 5) then with projected functions [83]. Algorithms for subcutaneous [88] and intraperitoneal [89] insulin infusion have also been described. In both cases, the onset of hypoglycemic effect is delayed and the action is prolonged [90–93], which makes the feed back control difficult. For the IP route 'hybrid' control, including a preprogramed early infusion and a pure feed-back control infusion has been proposed, and shown to be infusion in a pure feed-back control algorithm. The preprogrammed infusion stimulates the important cephalic phase [65] and the time variant control characteristics provide the non linear biphasic response to a blood glucose in a normal pancreas [94]. We have shown that even with the IV route, this preprogrammed early injection may be beneficial [79].

Insulin pump

This is the most technically advanced part of the artificial pancreas. External pumps have been widely used in diabetes since the pioneering works of Slama, IV [95] and Pickup, SC [96]. The rate of the pump is usually adapted manually according to intermittent blood glucose testings ('open-loop', or better 'semi-closed-loop' system).

Externally portable devices

Approximately 30 different devices are commercially offered for insulin delivery alone. The majority are motor-driven syringes. The syringes are in part commercially available disposable plastic products with a volume of 1 to 3 ml (for one to three days supply), in part plungers or cylinders that are specially designed to achieve high accuracy or for reasons of pump drive design. With one model, the syringes are supplied pre-filled as cartridges (Nordisk-Infuser).

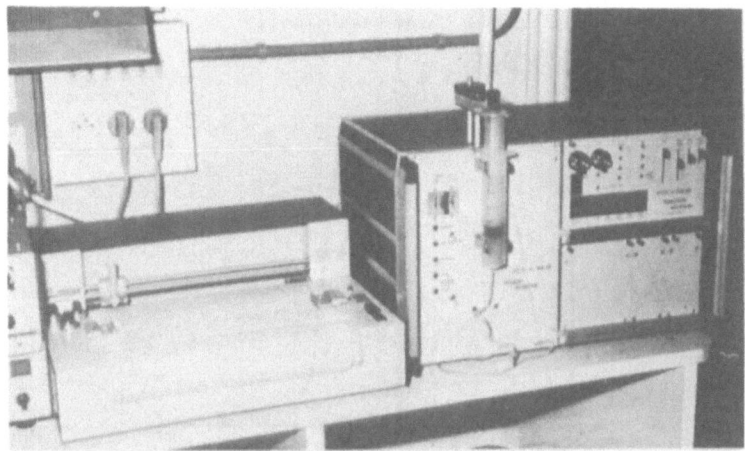

Figure 4. The external artifical pancreas used in Montpellier (Hyco-Aulas) with the glucose recorder (left) syringe pump (middle) and servo-computer (right).

The second pump principle to be encountered is the peristaltic or roller pump.

Pumps with electromagnetically driven pistons and two passive valves and a pre-filled plastic insulin reservoir have not yet reached the commercial stage. The technical data of the various types cannot be discussed here individually. Reference is made to what currently must be considered the most comprehensive survey on this topic [97].

With the general trend towards miniaturization of the devices, the reservoirs (syringes) are reduced more and more in size. Nearly all devices are suitable only for the s.c. route. The device shown in Figure 2 represents an example with a long-term reservoir (30 ml) for the central catheter route (currently mostly i.p.).

Implantable devices

Devices

With implantable devices, the number of active companies is clearly lower than with the external devices because of the greater technical complexity.

Devices with fixed rates

Only one company offers implants commercially for human use at present (Infusaid-Intermedics USA). This product is a purely mechanical pump. A titanium bellows is filled with the infusion liquid through a pierceable septum and is pressurized by means of an evaporating fluid (freon) [30] (Figure 6). The

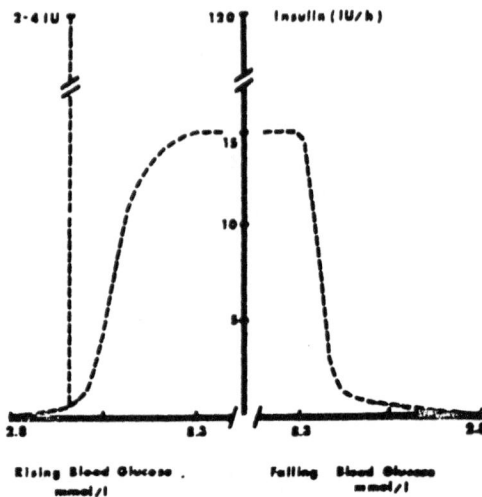

Figure 5. Original glucose/insulin algorithms used in the artifical pancreas shown in Figure 4.

fluid is driven out through a capillary flow resistor into a suitably placed catheter. According to the Hagen-Poisseuille law, the supply rate depends upon the differential pressure between the bellows interior and the catheter tip and viscosity of the fluid, in addition to the fixed dimensions of the capillary. The pressure in the bellows interior varies considerably with temperature and filling condition (because of the recoil force of the bellows). A change of 1° C induces a change of the internal pressure (and thus the rate) of approximately 4%, and temperature fluctuations of 5° C can be easily imagined to occur 1 cm below the skin. The variability of the rate as a function of the filling level, full compared with empty, amounts to approximately 7%. The pressure at the catheter tip fluctuates with the barometric pressure (height above sea-level), which is superimposed upon the psysiological pressure at the site of application (e.g. in the vein or in the peritoneum). The viscosity is a function of the temperature. The viscosity is selected as high as possible with insulin infusions in order to achieve the desired low flow rate with the largest possible capillary lumen (minimization of the risk of clogging because of possibly precipitated insulin). Apparently users of the devices can cope with these fluctuations by special precautionary measures when flying, mountaineering, in the sauna, with fever, etc.

The rates of these devices can only be changed on a long-term basis by replenishment and therefore are only conditionally suitable for diabetes therapy. This statement concerns the commercially available devices. Naturally, a rate control by valves is conceivable, and prototypes of this programmable infusaid pump are under clinical investigation for chemotherapy and insulin-therapy.

A

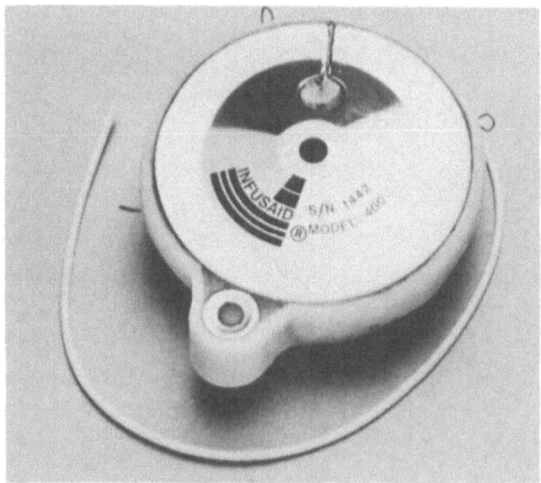

B

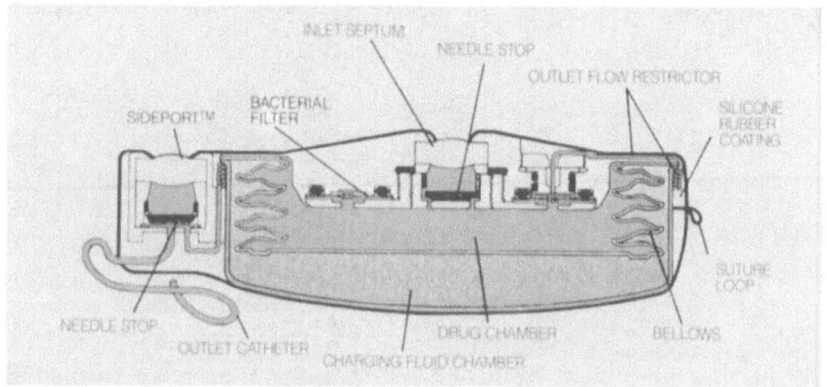

Figure 6. View (4) and diagram (b) of the Infusaid-Intermedics pump.

Devices with controllable variable rates

They are necessarily electromechanical. The information transfer from the external programming or control device takes place electromagnetically or magnetically; storage in the implant occurs electronically. The drug delivery itself is necessarily a mechanical process.

Sandia Laboratory pump – A prototype of the Sandia pump was first implanted by Schade et al. [99] in January 1981; it functioned for 5 months. The main difference between it and the Siemens pump is that the Sandia pump has its reservoir outside the pump capsule. To date, only Schade has implanted this pump, and no prototypes have been available for testing at other centers.

A

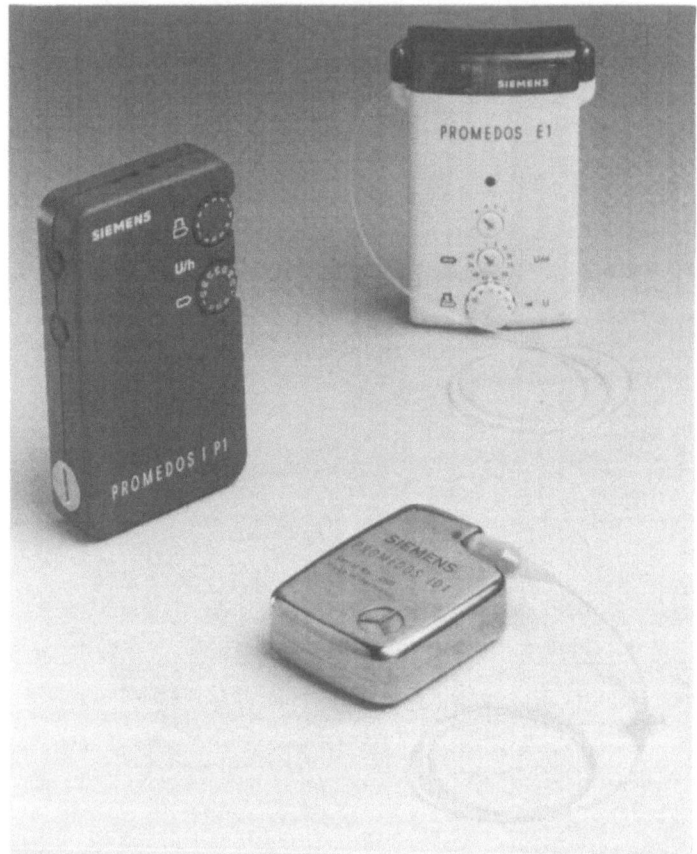

B

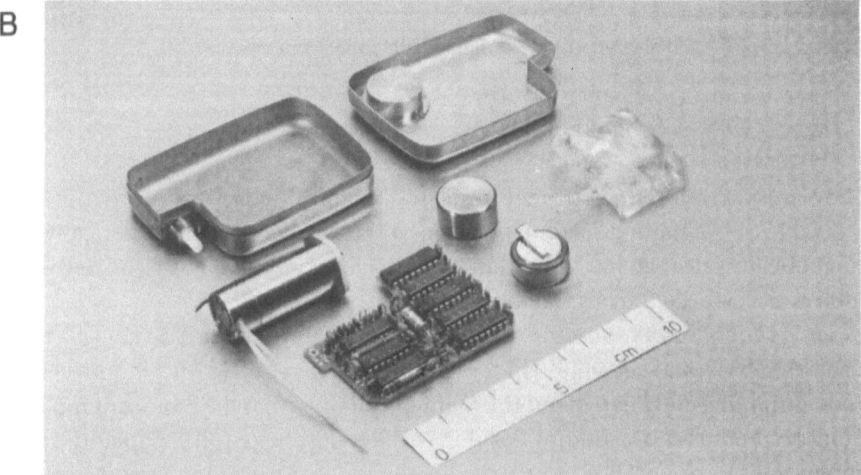

Figure 7. Siemens implantable pump (bottom A, B) with its remote controller (left A). Right A: portable peristaltic pump (Siemens, Promedos El).

Siemens pump (Figure 7). It was first implanted in 1981 in a human being by Irsigler et al. [100] at Vienna-Lainz by the Mehnert's group [101–103] in Munich and by Selam et al. [104] at Montpellier. Due to electronic defects the pump at Lainz was replaced 8 months later. After a further 4 months the second pump was explanted due to a catheter break. The other pumps functioned for about 12 months each. The continued problem of insulin instability seen in animal experimentation has prevented any further human implantation. The influence of mechanical shear forces on insulin used in roller pumps or the so-called diffusion forces present with synthetic reservoirs and tubing may have had additional effects upon insulin stability. There have been too few systematic studies to date to determine the real causes of the problem. In the meantime, the electronic switching system has been reworked. In Figure 7 we show the implantable pump and its programing unit. A second wave of human testings has been programmed for 1986.

Medtronic pump (Figure 8). It was first used in humans to deliver morphine, and has been implanted in dogs for insulin delivery [106]. Human implantation is planned as soon as problems with insulin aggregation are solved. The medtronic pump works on a peristaltic principle. A special feature is its programability by patient and physician using a computer terminal. Figure 8 shows the physician's programing unit (left and center), the pump (left foreground), the printer (right rear), and the patient's protable programing unit (right front).

Pacesetter pump (Figure 9). The Pacesetter pump was developed at Johns Hopkins University [107] and the prototype was built by Pacesetter Systems. Noteworthy is the use of the diaphragm. Freon gases used in the pump to create a negative pressure, so that there is no risk that insulin can leak out into the body. The pump is powered by a lithium battery. Reprograming of the pump over a telephone and computer modem has already been carried out with dogs. Individual pumps have functioned successfully in diabetic dogs for more than 3 years [108]. The insulin used in this system only comes in contact with metal, just as the Infusaid pump. This pump has recently been successfully clinically tested in the USA, by J. Hopkins and the UC Irvine Groups. A modified version (MIP, model 2000) using a full piston course in the ejection chamber, is presently tested for FDA premarket approval.

Other approaches

The valve-piston principle ranks among the earliest designs for drug delivery, with Bessman reporting on animal experiments as early as 1975 [109]. This

492

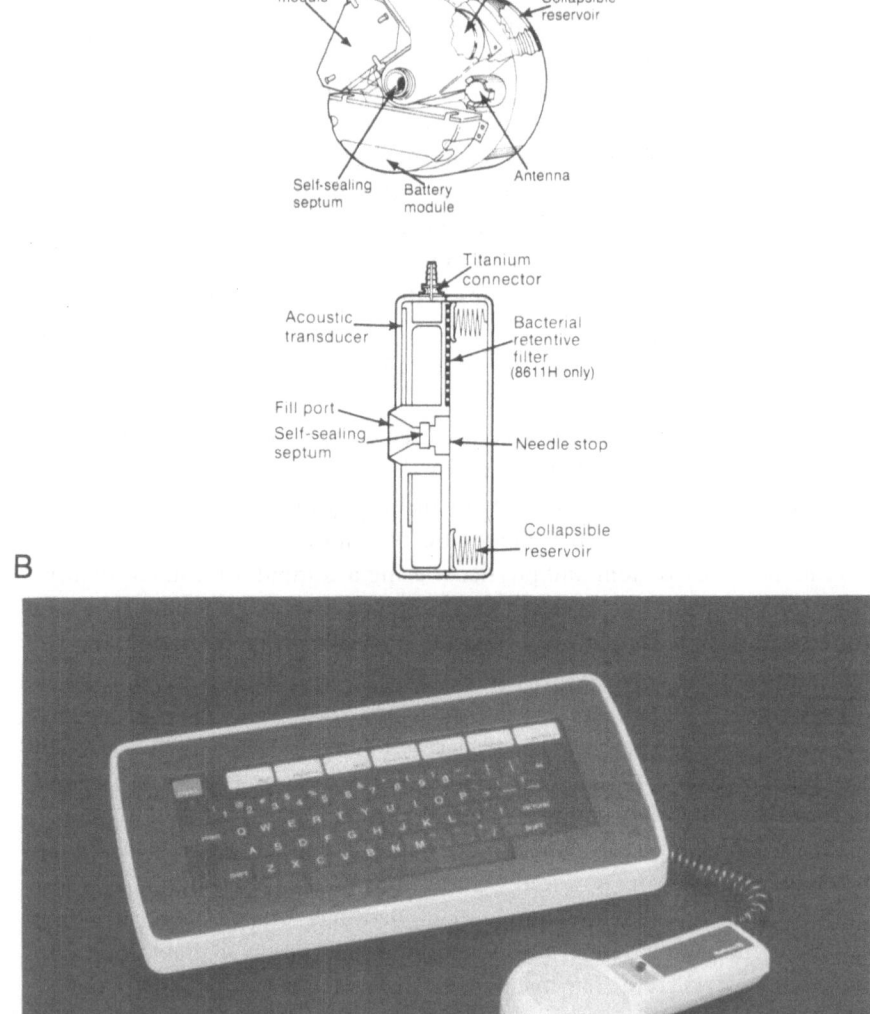

Figure 8. Medtronic Drug Administration System. The Medtronic Drug Administration System consists of an implantable infusion pump (DAD) (A) a variety of implantable catheters, an implantable access port, and a clinician's programmer. (B) The programmer can non-invasively program the implanted infusion pump to a specific prescription.

approach was discontinued. The same happened to another design described in [140] where the valve and piston were integrated in a plate of piezoelectric material. Already in the early 1970s and more recently, other groups were experimenting the pumps that operate according to the electro-osmotic principle [111–113] – nevertheless still in a very early development phase – and yet others with magnetic pellets [114]. The latter consist of implantable plastic matrices in which the drug is distributed as in depot preparations. Iron particles are embedded additionally. The administration rate can be influenced by applying an external magnetic alternating field.

Advantages and disadvantages of the different mechanisms.

Magnetic pellets. The rate control is not yet satisfactoryily solved. This technique is in the early development stage.

Electro-osmotic pump. The problem of the consumption of the electrodes as well as the replenishment of the reservoir are not satisfactorily solved.

Vapor-pressure pumps. Because of the simplicity of these bellow-capillary pumps they are well-proven for non-critical drugs that can be administered at predetermined rates with some variability as a result of varying external conditions.

For controlled drug delivery at variable rates, pumps of this type are not yet available, since the required totally leak proof valves are still lacking.

Syringe pumps. While in wide-spread use for external devices and s.c. infusion they are technically difficult to realize for implantable devices (plunger return, replenishment valve); this approach has apparently not yet been attempted.

Diaphragm pumps. The central problem is the susceptibility of the pumps to air bubbles located in or arising from the drug solution: gas in the pump chamber hampers the aspiration of further liquid because of its compressibility. The pulsated (non-physiological) delivery can also be a disadvantage with this principle when applied to the i.v. catheter route.

Peristaltic pumps (e.g. roller pumps). The quasi-continuous delivery that is also insensitive to bubbles and external influences permits a broad rate and application range. These pumps have been already used clinically as external devices; with implants only higher stability requirements for the insulin preparation prevent their wide-spread use.

494

A

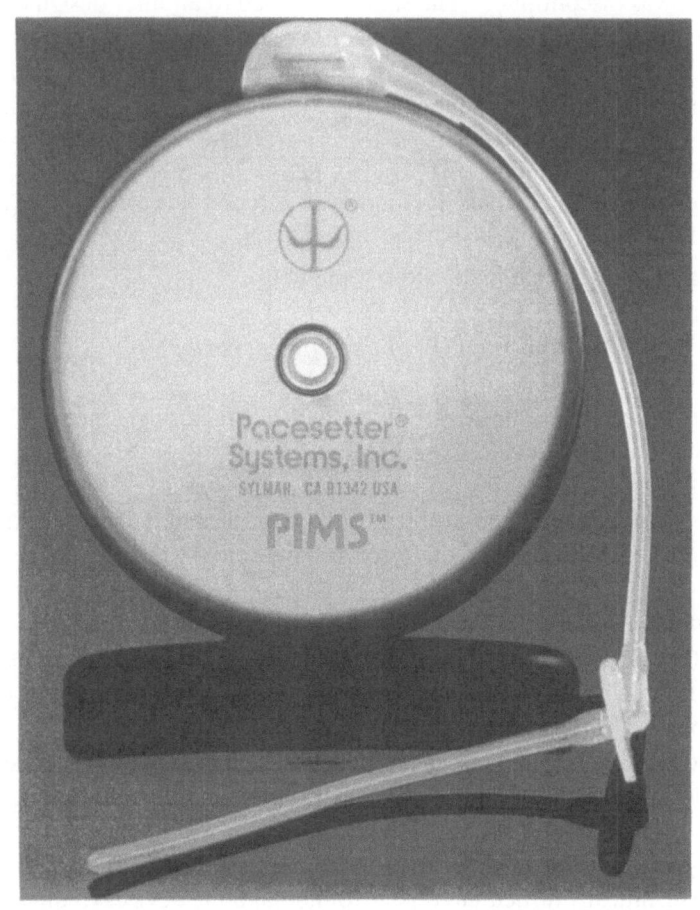

B

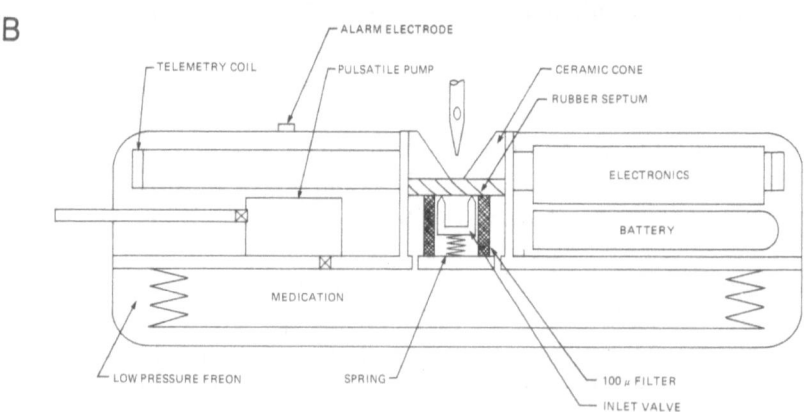

Figure 9. View (A) and diagram (B) of the Pacesetter (Minimed Technologies) Implantable pump.

Insulin

The physiochemical tendency of insulin to form macromolecular aggregates or fibrils seemed to cause no problem during the early years of insulin treatment but constitute a major problem for the development for insulin pumps.

Schade et al. [115] differentiate between the formation of macromolecular aggregates due to the association of insulin hexamers, and the association of multiple insulin fibrils with macromolecules arranged along a central axis. In contrast to crystals, insulin fibrils in an aqueous medium are extremely stable and biologically inactive.

Both the tendency toward aggregation and that toward fibril formation are aggravated by movement and body temperature, a fact which was not considered during bench tests for early pumps. The situation first became critical when pumps were worn by humans, and test groups were faced with catheter stoppage and aggregation in insulin reservoirs (Figure 15).

When the residual insulin is withdrawn from a pump reservoir prior to refill, high-pressure liquid chromatography (HPLC) shows that, in addition to aggregation, there are changes in the insulin monomer and the formation of dimers and plymers (Figure 16) [116, 117]. The monomer is the active form of insulin, so that biological effectiveness is reduced at polymerization.

Today, 6 years after the appearance of these problems, we have gained a bit more insight, but still have no definitive answers. Compromise solutions have been the changing of the milieu to an acidic pH or the addition of highly concentrated glycerol or other additives, which have made the further development of pump therapy possible. All the other trials were unsuccessful or unapplicable in vivo (Table 1).

Acidic insulin

When hydrochloric acid is used to change the pH level from 7.2 to the isoelectric point of 5.5 (where the number of positive and negative charges is equal), soluble zinc insulin rapidly crystallize [115]. Commercially available insulin solutions, therefore, have a pH value clearly above or below 5.5. In 1978 the only insulin which could pass a simple shake test without aggregation was the acid insulin from Hoechst AG. It has been used by our research team [92, 118–120] and by others [112–124] in portable externally worn devices ever since, for it has shown itself to be dependably more stable than any of its competitors to data [121]. Our group and Vienna-Lainz group has used acid insulin for more than 250 diabetics with portable external devices equipped with insulin reservoirs with a 3-week capacity. During a total of more than 200 patient years, both groups have not observed a single instance of catheter stoppage or aggregation in tubing or reservoir. However, this silution was rejected 'a priori' by the major companies, arguing that acidic insulin in pumps is transformed in an unacceptably high percentage of multiple derivatives [125]. We (Figure 10) were unable to demonstrate any transformation using an experimental acidic insulin (Organon), except desamidation [126] which has been shown to be inocuous [127] and almost as effective as he native insulin [128]. The risk of corrosion of metal parts of pumps due to acidity remains also to be demonstrated, as there were no corrosion reported with morphine, although acidic too.

Addition of surface-active substances

Hoechst south an additive for neutral insulin which would hinder aggregation, and chose the surface active product, Genapol, a pluronic polyol. (Pluronic polyols are poymers which can be chemically described as copolymers of polyoxypropylene and polyoxyethylene, with molecular weights between 1,000 and 15,000).

The first programable implants used in humans, the Siemens Promedos II, had a reservoir with a refill interval of 3 to 4 weeks, and used an insulin-Genapol solution. During a 2-year period in which four of these devices were used, not a single case of aggregation was observed.

Although this insulin-Genapol combination showed itself stable during intensive shake testing and in implanted pumps, when used in portable external devices massive aggregation was occasionally seen and led Hoechst to post-pone further implantations and to undergo additional intensive testing in dogs using implanted programmable pumps [129–131]. In addition to the Promedos II, developed especially for implantation by Siemens, the pumps from Medtronic and Pacesetter were also tested with Genapol-insulin [125]. The results led Hoechst to produce 2 different insulin, the original one for the non-peristaltic pumps, and a new, although still genapol-added, insulin for the peristaltic pumps.

Addition of glycerol

Buchwald et al. [132] and Rupp et al. [133] sought to solve the problem of insulin aggregation by adding highly concentrated glycerol (80 to 85%) to the insulin. The combination is continuously infused into the organism with a gas pressure Model 100 Infusion pump, which has a metal container and a silicone catheter.

Brange and Havelund [119] showed in 1981 that the addition of carbohydrates, such as fructose or glycerol, could prevent aggregation, but that when higher concentrations were used there was a lessening of chemical stability, and the growth of higher dimer and polymerization products.

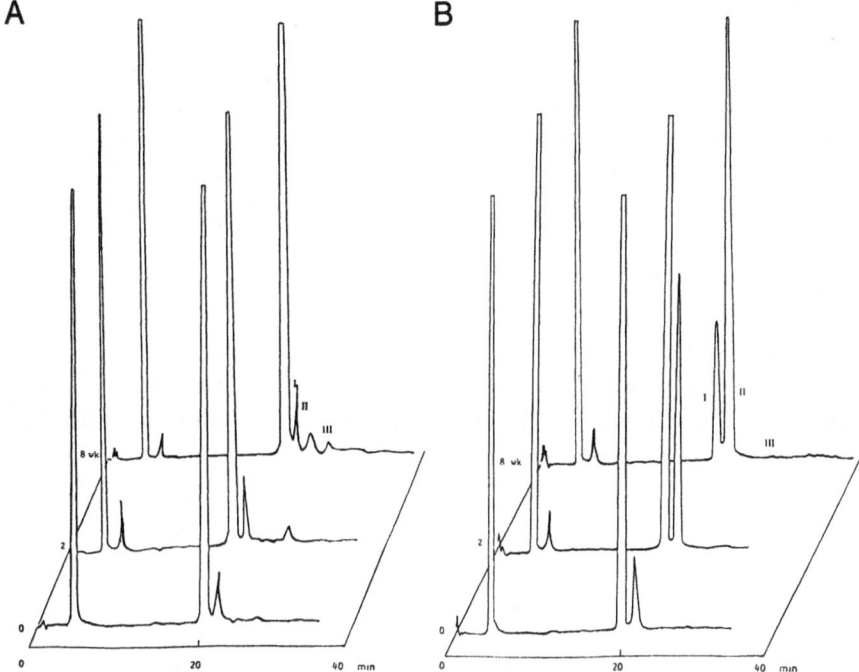

Figure 10. HPLC of neutral (4) and acidic (B) Organon insulin after 8 weeks of 37C agitation in pump. Peaks (from left to right) represent, preservative, insulin (at 20 min) desamido insulin and secondary peaks (dimers and polymers).

Using the two-dimensional HPLC method developed by Havelund and used by Brange, it was possible to determine polymerization products in the same analysis as degradation products. The glycerol-insulin mixture was examined at the time the pump was filled and again 3 weeks later when the reservoir was emptied prior to refill. It was discovered that, in addition to 8 to 12% insulin dimers and polymers, there were a considerable number of modified molecules in the monomer fraction. These monomers showed a diminution of biological activity in the mouse convulstion test, but surprisingly, no evidence of diminished biological activity had been observed in the metabolic control of the patients from whose pumps the insulin ad been withdrawn. In addition reduction of flow rate have been recently reported, leading to Buchwald's group to reduce their refill period to 1 week [133, 134] and to purpose methods or restoring correct flow [135].

Catheter

The catheter is probably the weakest part of the system. In addition to the risk of insulin deposition and catheter occlusion, they carry the risk of bioincompatibility, with, as a consequence, fibrin deposition (Figure 11), tissue growth (Figure 12) and, again occlusion (119, 120) (Figure 13). Therefore, factors like chemical comparison but also geometry are of a major importance.

Geometry

In an uncontrolled in vivo follow-up, we have noted that long (10–15 cm) catheters were better accepted than short ones (5–10 cm) [113, 136]. Diameter, sharpness of the extremity [137] and shape [138] of the catheters may also play a role.

Chemistry

Titanium

Titanium, is often used for the capsule of implantable pumps (e.g., Siemens, Infusaid, Medtronic, and Pacesetter) and for the insulin reservoir (e.g., infusaid and Pacesetter pumps). Titanium biocompatibility has already been demonstrated in the pacemaker field, where it has had long-term usage for human implantation. The optimum surface characteristics and the elimination of the diffusion problem help to explain its problem-free usage in the manufacture of insulin reservoirs.

Silicone rubber

Silicone rubber distinguishes itself by its high degree of elasticity and its limited thrombogenicity. The elasticity makes it an ideal material for the connective tubing between reservoir and catheter, particularly in peristaltic pumps, where this elasticity is exactly the characteristic desired.

Unfortunately, silicone has a tendency toward diffusion of both liquids and gases, so that special methods of pump encapsulation have had to be developed for use in implantable pumps [139].

The tissue biocompatibility of silicone rubber is almost as good as that of titanium, although Eaton et al. [140] and the research group at Vienna-Lainz [141] have seen peritoneal adhesions in individual cases.

A

B

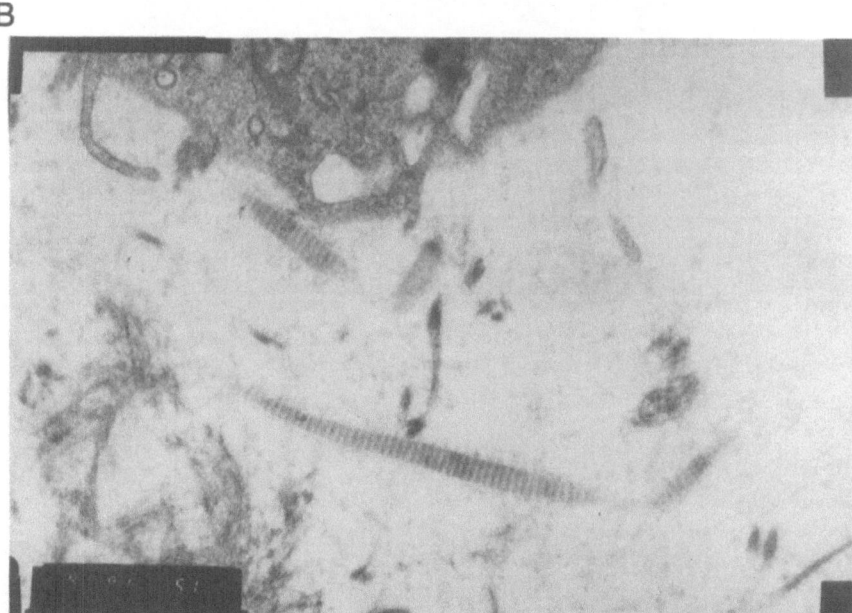

Figure 11. Scanning (A) and Transmission (B) electron microscopy of a chronic peritoneal insulin catheter obstructed by biological products. Note on B a giant cell (top) and collagen fibers.

A

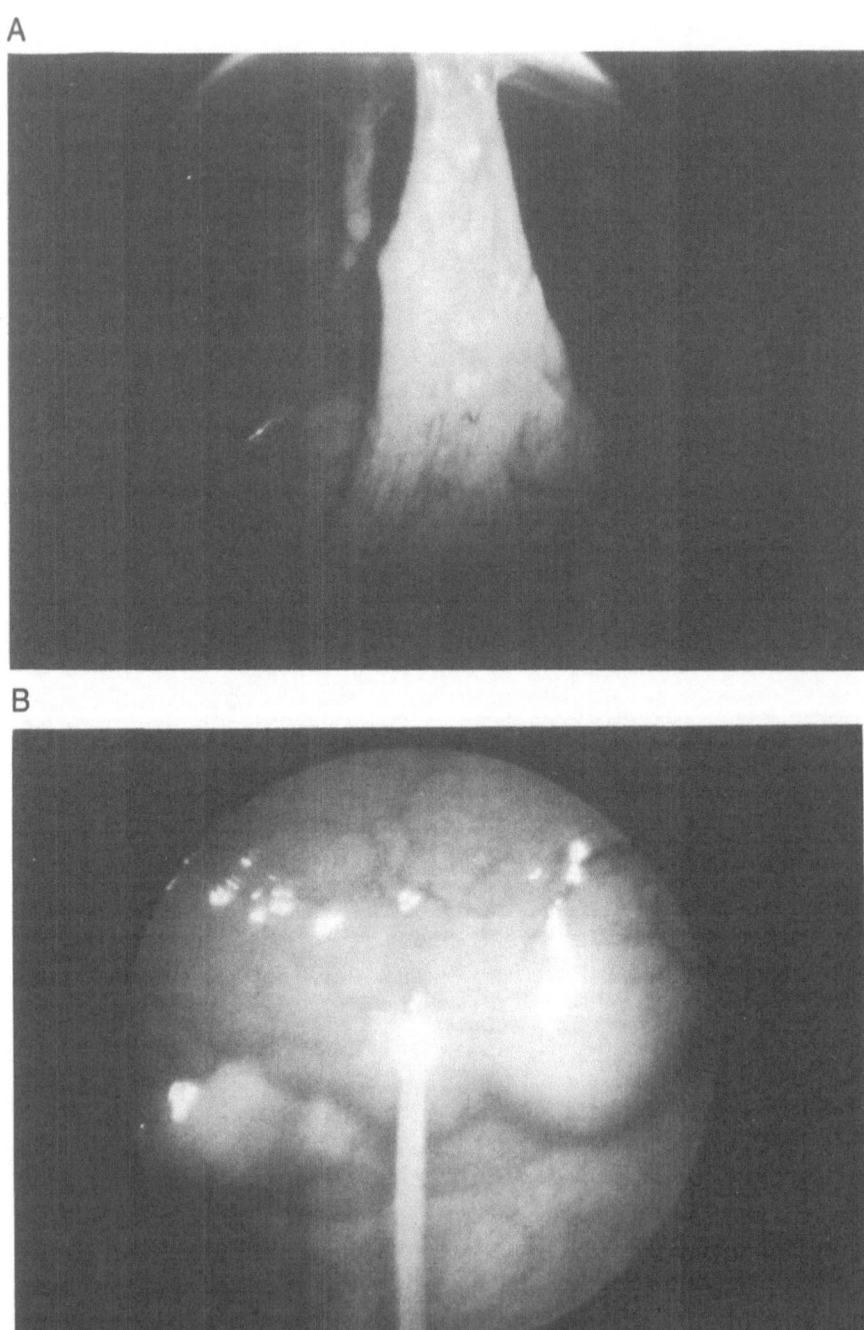

B

Figure 12. Laparoscopic view of chronic peritoneal catheters obstructed by omental adhesion (A) and fibrin olive-shaped deposition (B).

A

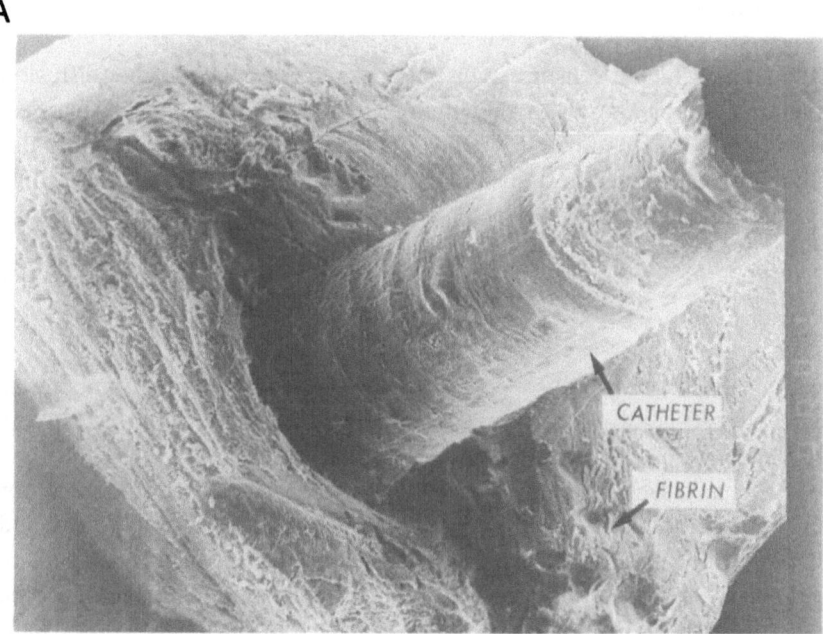

B

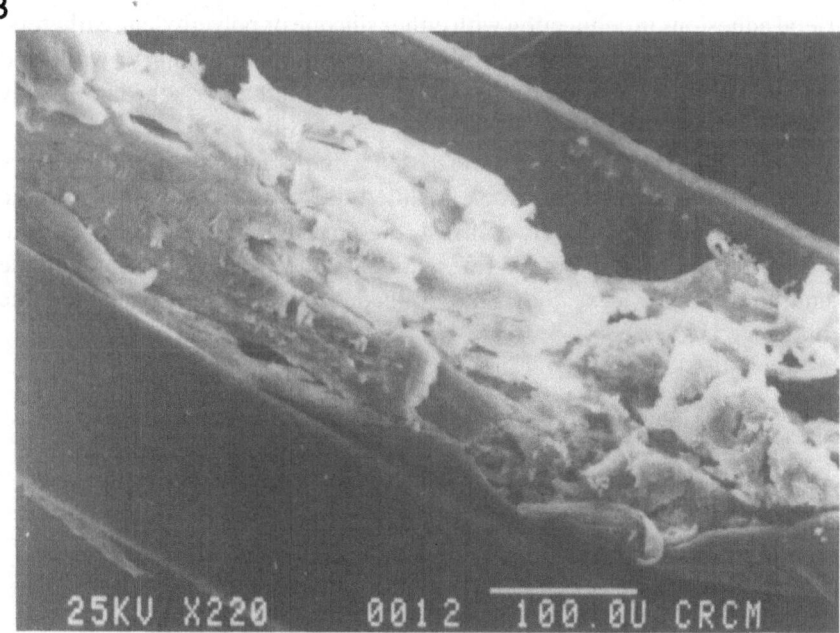

Figure 13. (A) Scanning electron microscopy of the tip of the catheter shown on Figure 12B. (B) Scanning electron microscopy of an obstructed IP catheter.

Polyurethane

Developers of glucose sensors favor polyurethane for its first-class diffusion characteristics, together with the minimal tissue reaction which it causes. However, it is this tendency toward diffusion that makes polyurethane unsuitable for the production of insulin catheters and reservoirs.

The thrombogenicity of polyurethane makes it a poor choice for i.v. use. To date, we have no reports of any i.p. applications.

Polyethylene

Polyethylene catheters have been generally regarded to be thrombogenic unless irrigated [142]. However, several researchers have reported success when they were used for insulin delivery.

We have used such catheters externally covered with Silastic (Siemens) for i.p. infusion without reaction at the point of entrance or in the skin tunnel, and without any thrombotic complications. Catheters examined endoscopically in the i.p. cavity appeared to be free-floating, although in individual cases some tissue growth had led to adhesions [119, 120, 136]. During laparoscopic examinations the Vienna Group found no difference in the number of omental or parietal adhesions in connection with either silicone or polyethylene catheters.

The greatest drawback of polyethylene is its limited ability to withstand stress and torque. Under mechanical stress, such a catheter can be irreversibly twisted out of shape or actually borken.

Where polyethylene catheters were used with implantable insulin delivery devices, several pumps had to be explanted due to catheter breakage some months after implantation. By contrast, there has not been a single report to the Registry sponsored by the International Study Group on Implantable Insulin Infusion Devices (ISGIID) of a silicone catheter being explanted due to breakage [143].

Routes of infusion

The subcutaneous route

Physiology

Although reduced when compared with conventional injections, local degradation of insulin persists after subcutaneous infusion, still variable and resulting in a 20–50% unpredictable loss of activity in certain individuals [144]. Moreover, the kinetics of resorption are not greatly different from those from subcutaneous injections. A mean delay of 136 min for the plasma insulin peak following a 1-h square wave of 6 U and a persistent hyperinsulinemia still 4 h after the bolus, under a 1-U/h basal infusion, were observed [120, 145]. The peak delay is shortened by 15–30 min [146, 147] if the bolus is given in a few minutes. However, the return to baseline is in any case sluggish, approximating 6–8 h.

Efficiency

The real superiority of continuous subcutaneous insulin infusion (CSII) over injections has been questioned [148]. In the authors opinion, the response is not ubiquitous. CSII is probably ineffective in brittle and insulin-resistant diabetes because it does not bypass the subcutaneous tissue, the poor resorption of which is probably involved in the mechanism of such forms of diabetes [149]. CSII is probably superior to injections in highly insulin-sensitive, low dose-requiring patients (pancreatectomized, hypophysectomized diabetics). In the average diabetic patient, it seems that CSII may be superior to twice-daily conventional insulin injections but not to multiple doses programs [152].

Feasibility

The technique of CSII is easy to handle and does not require sophisticated pumps or highly stable insulin because the reservoirs and catheters are changed frequently.

The risks and problems are limited to accidental under- or overdosage and local subcutaneous reactions. However, long-term acceptability is poorer than expected with a nonnegligible dropout rate [144, 150]. Unverifiable intermittent disconnections from pump must also be accounted for.

Finally, the authors recommend the subcutaneous route only for CSII in nonbrittle, insulin-dependent, but poorly controlled diabetes and only if the patients wish to avoid multiple injections or fixed mealtimes. This route is definitely not adapted to a feed-back controlled system.

The intravenous route

Physiology

The physiology of intravenously infused insulin was extensively investigated in the 1970s, as it was the route for insulin from the artificial pancreas. The intravenous infusion gives the fastest insulin response: Plasma insulin reaches its maximum and returns to baseline values in <30 min following a bolus [90]. However, this route invariably produces hyperinsulinemia [151, 152].

Efficiency

The efficiency of the intravenous route has been proven [151], even in the most severe forms of diabetes [145]. However, this advantage is balanced by the risk of rapid glucose rise in case of pump discontinuation [153] and rapid glucose fall during physical exercise [154].

Feasibility

The procedure for catheter insertion in a central vein is difficult and not innocuous. Technical requirements and patient constraints under portable intravenous pumps are as important as with the intraperitoneal route (see below). The risks of infection may be minimized by severe asepsy precautions, but not the risk of catheter obstruction by blood clotting, which was the mode of termination of the authors' only two chronic intravenous catheters after 8 and 6 months of constant infusion [92, 155]. However, results with totally implanted devices appear more encouraging [132, 133].

The intramuscular route

The intramuscular route has been proposed as an intermediate between the subcutaneous and intravenous routes, as it bypasses the subcutaneous barrier and has intermediate kinetics of absorption [156].

Encouraging results with the intramuscular route have been noted by some authors in insulin-resistant and brittle diabetes. However, the intramuscular route was rapidly abandoned because of very poor long-term feasibility: pain, muscle fibrosis, and abscesses were not infrequent.

The portal route

The portal route is theoretically the ideal route, as insulin is delivered primarily to the liver, thus reproducing the physiological portoperipheral insulin gradient [157].

So far, the portal route has been tested only in animals, with conflicting results [158–160, 152].

Owing to the potential risks of thrombosis and infection, it seems unlikely, at least with portable systems, that human testing will be ethically valid, unless the clear superiority and advantages of portal over peripheral infusion are definitely proven in long-term animal studies.

The intraperitoneal route

Physiology

Like the intravenous route, the intraperitoneal route bypasses the subcutaneous tissue and thus may be beneficial in patients with subcutaneously related problems (instability, insulin resistance), with the further advantage of a larger surface of resorption and no risk of catheter obstruction by clots.

The two major physiological advantages are a rapid insulin resorption [90, 93] and a partial portal uptake [161–162]. The plasma free insulin in 28 chronically pumped insulin-dependent diabetics (IDD) and 6 normal subjects were measured during 4 h after a standardized breakfast [93]. In the IDDs, insulin was infused as a 1-U/h basal rate and a 1-h superimposed meal dose intraperitoneally (n = 20) or subcutaneously (n = 8). The fasting plasma free insulin level was lower and bolus peaks occurred earlier in intraperitoneally than in subcutaneously treated patients (70 ± 6 vs 136 ± 28 min, respectively). Intraperitoneal values tended to return to baseline within the normal time (<3 h), whereas subcutaneous values were still elevated after 4 h (Figure 14). Many factors may affect the intraperitoneal insulin kinetics: High insulin concentrations [162] and instant boluses [162–163] instead of square waves seem to increase the rapidity of absorption. In the same way (Figure 15) higher bolus-induced peaks were observed when the intraperitoneal catheter was situated in the mid rather than the low abdomen [136] confirming for the first time that, as for the solutes, the peritoneum absorbs insulin better in the higher abdominal regions, probably owing to a lower pressure and more important venous and lymphatic circulations, specially in the diaphragmatic areas [164].

According to Schade et al. [162] up to 50% of intraperitoneally administered insulin is absorbed through the portal circulation, reproducing the normal portoperipheral insulin gradient. However, further experiments are needed to confirm those results and to demonstrate that the relative peripheral hypoinsulinemia also observed by the authors [93] is not due simply to partial in situ insulin degradation.

Efficiency

The efficiency of the intraperitoneal route appears for most [92, 165–167] but not all [168] of the authors superior to the subcutaneous and similar to the intravenous infusion of insulin. The authors' group conducted a short-term [92] and a long-term [119, 120] protocol for evaluation of the efficacy of intraperitoneal insulin. The short-term protocol consisted of three randomized 1 month periods of infusion in six brittle IDDs via a chronic catheter delivering insulin subcutaneously, intravenously, and intraperitoneally. The

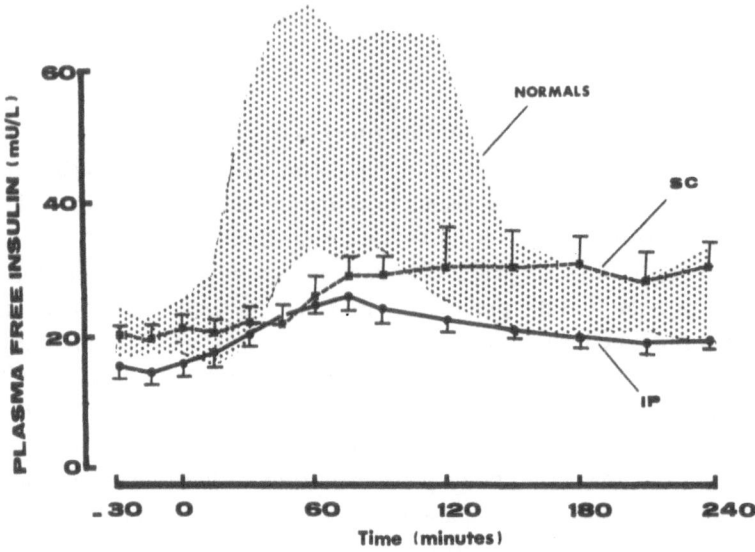

Figure 14. Plasma insulin kinetics following a bolus of insulin of 7 u at time 0 and a basal infusion of lu/h from −30 to +240 min. Solid line: IP infusion, dotted line SC infusion, shaded area: normal insulin response after a meal.

two last routes gave similar results, with significantly fewer hyperglycemic episodes and lower insulin requirements than observed with subcutaneous infusion. The long-term study was the follow-up of 40 chronically intraperitoneally pumped patients (present experience up to 1986, 80 patients). All patients had been poorly controlled by two to four daily subcutaneous injections. Mean CBG reached 127 ± 24 vs 192 ± 48 mg/ml before CPII and hemoglobin A_1 8.1 ± 1.1 vs $10.6 \pm 2.4\%$ before CPII. The results did not drift with time (1–27 months of continuous intraperitoneal infusion; mean 13 months). Daily insulin doses decreased from 63 ± 4 U/24 h before to 45 ± 3 U/24 h after 3 months of CPII. However it still remains to be demonstrated that the IP route is able to normalize the other metabolites and hormones abnormalities of diabetes [169].

Feasibility

The authors' experience [120] confirms that of Irsigler et al. [169], the only other group with a long-term wide experience with the intraperitoneal route through either portable or implantable pumps. In the present population treated with portable intraperitoneal pumps, the method was judged satisfactory by 90% of the patients, a result usually not attained by CSII [144].

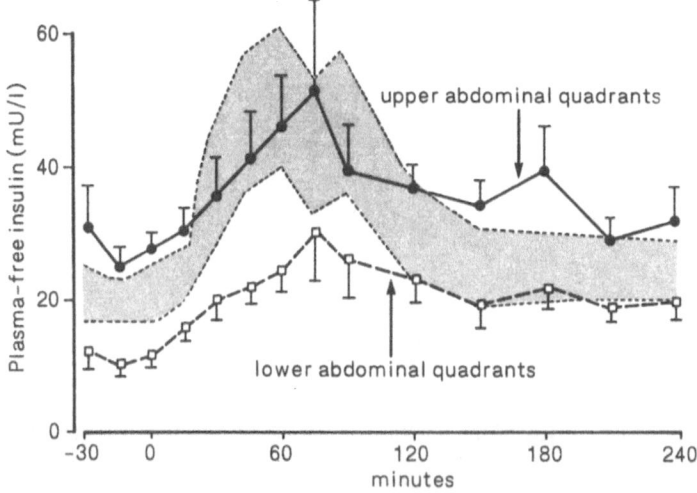

Figure 15. Plasma insulin kinetics following insulin infusion in different quadrants of the IP abdominal space. Legends as above.

The technical requirements for CPII via portable pumps include a reliable pump with long-duration insulin reservoir, to avoid too frequent manipulations and thus limit the risk of infection. The pump must be compact, robust, and of a sufficient impremeability at least for showers), as it cannot be removed on any occasion for safety reasons. The insulin must remain stable in the reservoir and must not precipitate in the permanently placed tubings. The authors are using preferentially the Promedos peristaltic pump (Siemens AG, Erlangen, F.R.G) equipped with a disposable polythetylene reservoir of 30 ml, filled with acidic U40 insulin (CS21; Hoechst AG, Frankfurt F.R.G.). Stabilized U100 neutral insulins (Hoechst, F.R.G. and Organon, France) have also been tested, with more variable results in Nordisk pumps. Technical requirements also include a robust, compatible, thin, chronic peritoneal catheter. A polyethylene catheter covered by silicon rubber (Siemens), was chosen by the authors. The technique of catheter insertion must be safe and simple. Thus, a non-surgical procedure using a blind needle technique was developed [92], which was used successfully for >80 catheter insertions.

The medical requirements include severe criteria for selection of the patients. Patients should be both poorly controlled (to provide a good biological advantages-to-constraints ratio) and reasonable motivated and reliable. Intensive education, severe asepsy instructions, free delivery of pumps and accessories, monthly consultation, 24 h/day technical and medical backup given by a specialized staff through an individualized unit are also of the utmost importance. In the authors' opinion, all the above precautions are a

508

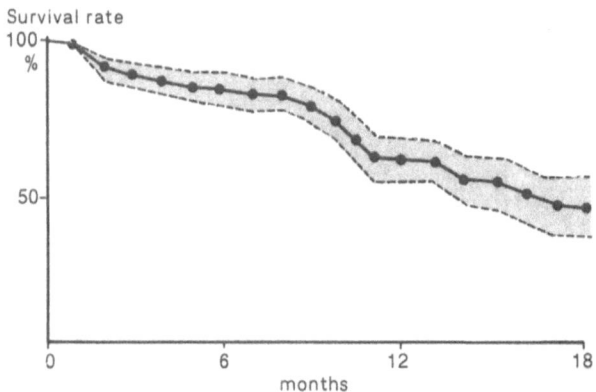

Figure 16. Actuarial analysis of the duration of chronic IP catheters. Personal study on 75 catheters.

sine qua non condition for the technique to be ethically acceptable.

Indeed, the most threatening clinical risk with intraperitoneal infusion is peritonitis. Only one case of local peritonitis, which was cured by antibiotics and surgical drainage, was observed by the authors. On the other hand, local infections at the skin exit were not rare: A mean of one infection every 35 patient-months, i.e., in 18 of the 71 catheters implanted, was obtained. Seven of the infected catheters had to be explanted because of persisting infection. Severe metabolic disorders were rare and never life threatening (one hypoglycemic coma and 1 severe ketoacidosis every 39 and 67 patient-months, respectively). Catheter-related problems were not rare, although breakages were usually repaired. Obstructions were usually irreversible, and led to six catheter explantations and a 50% survival rate of the catheters of 16 months (Figure 16). Intraluminal fibrin growth was noted in three cases, whereas enclosure of the catheter in a peritoneal adhesion was seen in the other three cases. In no case did precipitation of acidic insulin appear to be the primary cause of obstruction.

Finally, most of the problems and those constraints can be bypassed by implantable devices. The intraperitoneal route was used successfully by several groups [145] for insulin administration through totally implanted pumps. Peritoneal infections were never encountered, and the reasons for occasional premature termination of the experience were in most cases technical, i.e., pump or catheter related.

Conclusions

Contrarily to the optimistic previsions of the scientists in the 70s the implantable artificial pancreas is still not available.

However, bed-side and even wearable feed-back controlled devices are already in use, and the pumping part of the system has been already implanted in humans with success.

The remaining problem, before a complete and safe device can be envisaged, are the long term reliability of insulin, the reliability of the glucose sensor and the biocompatibility of the catheter for longer life duration (Figure 16).

It is wise to avoid previsions after the unexpected slowness of the progress in the 70's and 80's but we believe that it will probably taken some decades rather than some years before this technique will routinely replace the conventional injections – unless implantable pumps are satisfactory enough or transplantation progress go faster and win the competition?

Acknowledgments

Acknowledgments to G. Cavalie, M.A. Charles, P.A. Chaptal, D. Cavadore, P. Chanlat, M. Davies, M. Franetzki, J.P. Gagnol, P. Giraud, B. Hedon, C. Holleman, P. Humeau, K. Irsigler, H. Lapinski, M. Leguillette, P. Lord, J. Lozano, M. Mellet, P. Millet, J. Mirouze, A. Orsetti, T.C. Pham, M. Raymond, P. Remandet, R. Rouaud, S. Saeidi, A. Slingeneyer, D. Turner, P. Vic, K. Waxman and P. Zirinis for their precious help at different steps of the present work.

References

1. Johnson S: Retinopathy and nephropathy in diabetes mellitus. Comparison of the effects of two forms of treatment. Diabetes 9: 1–8, 1960.
2. Pirart J: Diabetes mellitus and its degenerative complications: a prospective study of 4,400 patients observed between 1947 and 1973. Diabetes Care 1: 168–188, 1978.
3. Job D, Eschwege E, Guyot-Argenton C et al: Effect of multiple daily insulin injections on the course of diabetic retinopathy. Diabetes 25: 463–469, 1976.
4. Eschwege E, Job D, Guyot-Argenton C et al: Delayed progression diabetic retionpathy by divided insulin administration: a further follow up. Diabetologia 16: 13–15, 1979.
5. Engerman R, Bloodworth JMB Jr, Nelson S: Relationship of microvascular disease in diabetes to metabolic control. Diabetes 26: 760–769, 1977.
6. Mauer SM, Stettes MW, Michael AF et al: Studies of diabetic nephropathy in animals and man. Diabetes 25 (2): 850–857, 1976.
7. Kilo C, Vogler N, Williamson JR: Muscle capillary basement membrane changes related to

aging and diabetes mellitus. Diabetes 21: 881–90, 1972.

8. Karam J, Rosenthal M, O'Donnell J et al: Discordance of diabetic microangiopathy in identical twins. Diabetes 25: 24–28, 1976.

9. Gander OP, Soeldner JS, Gleason RE et al: Monozygotic triplets with discordance for diabetes mellitus and diabetic microangiopathy. Diabetes 26: 469–479, 1977.

10. Osterby R: Early phases in the development of diabetic glomerulopathy. Acta Med Scand (Suppl) 574: 1–82, 1975.

11. Mauer SM, Barbosa J, Vernier RL et al: Development of diabetic vascular lesions in normal kidney transplants into patients with diabetes mellitus. N Engl J Med 295: 916–920, 1976.

12. Mauer SM, Miller K, Goetz FC et al: Immunopathology of renal extracellular membranes in kidneys transplanted into patients with diabetes mellitus. Diabetes 25: 709–712, 1976.

13. Beisswenger PJ, Spiro RG: Human glomerular basement membrane: chemical alteration in diabetes mellitus. Science 168: 596–598, 1970.

14. Gabbay KH: Hyperglycemia, polypol metabolism and complications of diabetes mellitus. Ann Rev Med 26: 521–536, 1975.

15. Spritz N: Nerve disease in diabetes mellitus. Med Clin North Am 62: 787–798, 1978.

16. Brownlee M, Cerami A: The biochemistry of the complications of diabetes mellitus. Ann Rev Biochem 50: 385–423, 1981.

17. Merimee TJ: A follow-up study of vascular disease in growth hormone deficient dwarfs with diabetes. N Engl J Med 298: 1217–1222, 1978.

18. Wolinsky H, Goldfischer S, Capron L et al: Hydrolase activities in the rat aorta. I. Effects of diabetes mellitus and insulin treatment. Circulation Res 42: 831, 1978.

19. Ashikaga T, Borodic G, Sims EA: Multiple daily insulin injections in the treatment of diabetic retinopathy. The Job study revisited. Diabetes 27: 592–596, 1978.

20. Knowles H: Long-term juvenile diabetes treated with unmeasured diet. Trans Assoc Am Physicians 84: 95–101, 1971.

21. Siperstein MC, Foster DW, Knowles HC Jr et al: Control of blood glucose and diabetic vascular disease. N Eng J Med 296: 1060–1063, 1977.

22. Siperstein MD, Unger RH, Madison LL: Studies of muscle capillary basement membranes in normal subjects, diabetic and prediabetic patients. J Clin Invest 47: 1973–1999, 1968.

23. Kalant N: Diabetic glomerulosclerosis. Current status. Can Med Assoc J 119: 146–153, 1978.

24. Clements RS Jr: Diabetic neuropathy-new concepts of its etiology. Diabetes 28: 604–611, 1979.

25. Pickup JC, Keen H, Parsons JA, Alberti KGMM: Continuous subcutaneous insulin infusion: improved blood glucose and intermediary metabolite control in diabetics. Lancet 2: 1255–1257, 1979.

26. Frier BM, Hilsted J: Does hypoglycemia aggrevate the complications of diabetes. The Lancer i: 1175–1177, 1985.

27. Service JS, Molnar GD, Rosevear JE et al: Mean amplitude of glycemic excursions, a measure of diabetic instability. Diabetes 29: 644–655, 1970.

28. Malone JI, Hellrung JM, Malphus EWK et al: Good diabetic control – a study in mass delusion. J Pediatr 88: 943–947, 1976.

29. Raskin R, Unger RH: Effect of insulin therapy on the profile of plasma immunoreactive glucagon in juvenile-type and adult-type diabetes. Diabetes 27: 411–419, 1978.

30. Anonymous: Effect of intensive treatment on substrate and hormonal abnormalities. In: Schade DS, Santiago JV, Skyler JS, Rizza RA (eds) Intensive insulin therapy; pp 71–87.

31. G.E.F.C.O.D.: Unpublished results.

32. Editorial: Evidence, implications, and corrolaries. Diabetes Care 4: 573–575, 1981.

33. Felig P, Bergman M: Intensive ambulatory treatment of insulin-dependent diabetes. Ann Intern Med 97: 225–230, 1982.

34. Rizza RA, Gerich JE, Haymond MW et al: Control of blood sugar in insulin-dependent diabetes: Comparison of an artificial endocrine pancreas, continuous subcutaneous insulin infusion, and intensified conventional insulin therapy. N Engl J Med 303: 1313–1318.

35. Tamborlane WV, Sherwin RS, Genel M, Felig P: Outpatient treatment of juvenile onset diabetes with a preprogrammed portable subcutaneous insulin infusion system. Am J Med 68: 190–196, 1980.

36. Champion MC, Shepherd GAA, Rodger NW, DuPrie J: Continuous subcutaneous infusion of insulin in the management of diabetes mellitus. Diabetes 29: 206–212, 1980.

37. Schiffrin A, Colle E, Belmonte M: Improved control in diabetes with continuous subcutaneous insulin infusion. Diabetes Care 3: 643–649, 1980.

38. Schiffrin A, Belmonte M: Combined continuous subcutaneous insulin infusion and multiple subcutaneous injections in type 1 diabeti patients. Diabetes Care 4: 595–600, 1981.

39. Home PD, Capaldo B, Burrin JM, Worth R, Alberti KGMM: A crossover comparison of continuous subcutaneous insulin infusion (CSII against multiple insulin injections in insulin-dependent diabetic subjects: improved control with CSII. Diabetes Care 5: 466–471, 1982.

40. Chiasson JL, Ducros F, Poliquin-Hamet M, Lopez D, Lecavalier L, Hameet P: Continuous subcutaneous insulin infusion versus multiple injections in the treatment of insulin dependent diabetes mellitus and the effect of metabolic control on microangiopathy. Diabetes Care 7: 331–337, 1984.

41. Muhlhauser I, Berger M, Sonnenberg G, Koch J et al: Incidence and management of servere hypoglycemia in 434 adults with insulin-dependent diabetes mellitus. Diabetes Care 8: 268–273, 1985.

42. Mecklenburg RS, Benson JW Jr, Becker NM et al: Clinical use of the insulin infusion pump in 100 patients with Type 1 diabetes. N Engl J Med 307: 513–518, 1982.

43. Peden NR, Bratten JT, McKendry JBR: Diabetic ketoacidosis during long-term treatment with continuous subcutaneous insulin infusion. Diabetes Care 7: 1–5, 1984.

44. Bending JJ, Pickup JC, Keen H: Frequency of diabetic ketoacidosis and hypoglycemic coma during treatment with continuous subcutaneous insulin infusion: an audit of medical care. Am J Med (In press), cited in letters, JAMA 253: No. 18, 1985.

45. Teutsch SM, Herman WH, Dwyer DM, Lane JM: Mortality among diabetic patients using continuous subcutaneous insulin infusion pumps. N Engl J Med 310: 361–368, 1984.

46. Mecklenburg RS, Benson EA, Benson JW Jr et al: Acute complications associated with insulin infusion pump therapy. Report of experience with 161 patients. JAMA 252: 3265–3269, 1984.

47. The Kroc Collaborative Study Group: Blood glucose control and the evolution of diabetic retinopathy and albuminuria. N Engl J Med 311: 365–372, 1984.

48. Unger RH: Special Comment. Meticulous control of diabetes: Benefits, risks, and precautions. Diabetes 31: 479–483, 1982.

49. White NH, Skor DA, Cryter PE, Levandoski LA, Brier DM, Santiago JV: Identification of type 1 diabetic patients at increased risk for hypoglycemia during intensive therapy. N Engl J Med 308: 485–491, 1983.

50. Hoeldtke RD, Boden G, Shuman CR, Owen OE: Reduced epinephrine secretion and hypoglycemia unawareness in diabetic autonomic neuropathy. Ann Int Med 96: 459–462, 1982.

51. Thorsteinsson B, Pramming S, Lauritzen T, Binder C: Frequency of biochemical hypoglycemia at different blood glucose levels in conventionally and pump-treated type 1 (insulin-dependent) diabetic patients. Diabetologia 27: 338A, 1984.

52. Eichner HL, Holleman C, Worcester B, Turner D, Woertz L, Selam JL, Charles MA: Reduction of severe hypoglycemic events in type I diabetic patients using CSII. Diabetes Research (in press).

53. Knight G, Boulton AJM, Ward JD: Success in reducing the rate of ketoacidosis in patients treated with continuous subcutaneous insulin infusion. European Association for the Study of Diabetes, London Abs. p. 297A, 1984.

53. Albisser AM, Leibel BS, Ewart TG, Davidovac Z, Botz CK, Wingg W, Schipper H, Gander R: Clinical control of diabetes by the artifical pancreas. Diabetes 23: 397–404, 1974.

54. Lim F, Sun A: Microencapsulated islets a bioartificial endocrine pancreas. Science 210: 908–910, 1980.

55. Altmann JJ, Houlbert D, Chollier A, Leduc A, McMillan P, Galletti PM: Encapsulated human islet transplants in diabetic rats. Trans Am Soc Artif Intern Organs 30: 3812–386, 1984.

56. Scharp DW, Mason NS, Sparks RE: Islet immuno-isolation: the use of hybrid artificial organs to present islet tissue rejection. World J Surg 8: 221–229, 1984.

57. Reach G, Poussier P, Sausse A, Assan R, Itoh M, Gerich JE; Functional evaluation of a bio-artificial pancreas using isolated islet perifused with blood ultrafiltrate. Diabetes 30: 296–301, 1981.

58. Reach G, Jaffrin MY, Vanhoutte C, Desjeux JF: Importance of convective transport in a model of bioartificial pancreas. Am Soc Artif Intern organs J 7: 85–90, 1984.

59. Reach G, Jaffrin MY, Desjeux JF: A U-shaped bioartificial pancreas with rapid glucose-insulin kinetics: in vitro evaluation and kinetic modelling. Diabetes 752: 761, 1984.

60. Orsetti A, Bouhaddioui N, Crespy S, Perez R: Analyse critique de la valeur fonctionnelle d'un pancreas bio-artificiel (modele a fibres creuses). C R Soc Biol 175: 228–234, 1981.

61. Browlee M, Cerami A: Glycosylated insulin complexed to concanavalin A: a biochemical basis for a closed-loop insulin delivery system. Diabetes 32: 499–504, 1983.

62. Mirouze J, Jaffiol C, Sany C: Enregistrement glycemique nycthemeral continu dans le diabete instable. Rev Fr Endocrinol Clin Metab 3: 337–353, 1962.

63. Kadish AH: Automation control of blood sugar I. A servomechanism for glucose monitoring and control. Am J Med Electron 3: 82, 1964.

64. Metcalf J: The administration of insulin by continuous injection. MB Thesis, university of Cambridge, 1934.

64. Kessler M, Hoper J, Volkhor HJ, Sailer D, Demling L: Tissue measurement of glucose with a new potential electrode in continuous insulin infusion therapy. KD Hepp and R Renner Ed, Schattauer, Stuttgart New York pp 19–26, 1985.

65. Woods SC, Porte D: Neural control of the endocrine pancreas. Phys Rev 54: 596–619, 1974.

66. Anonymous: Substrate and hormonal alteration in diabetes mellitus in intensive insulin therapy. Schade DS, Santiago JV, Styler JS and Rizza RA, Ed, Excerpta Medica, pp 36–70, 1983.

67. Clark LC Jr, Lyons C: Electrode systems for continuous monitoring in cardiovascular surgery. Ann N Y Acad Sci 102: 29, 1962.

68. Clark LC Jr: Monitor and control of blood and tissue oxygen tensions. Trans Am Soc Artif Intern Organs 2: 41, 1956.

69. Bessman SP, Schultz RD: Prototype glucose-oxydase sensor for the artificial pancreas. Trans Am Soc Artif Intern Organs 19: 361, 1973.

70. Clarke WL, Santiago JV: The characteristics of a new glucose sensor for use in artificial pancreatic beta cell. Artif Organs 1: 78, 1977.

71. Schichiri M, Kawamori R, Yamashki Y, Hakui N, Abe H: Wearable artificial pancreas with needle-type glucose sensor. Lancer 2: 1129, 1986.

72. Schichiri M, Kawamori R, Goriya Y, Yamasaki Y, Nomura Y: Diabetologia 24: 179–184, 1983.

73. Chang LW, Aisenberg S, Soeldner JS, Hiebert JM: Validation of bioengineering aspects of an implantable glucose sensor. Trans Am Soc Artif Intern Organs 352: 19, 1973.

74. March W, Engerman R, Rabinovitch B: Optical monitor of glucose. Trans Am Soc Artif Intern Organs 25: 28, 1979.

75. Kaiser N: Laser absorption spectroscopy with an ATR prism: noninvasive in vivo determination of glucose. Horm Metabl Res Suppl 7: 72, 1977.

76. Rabinovitch B, March W, Adams RL: Noninvasive glucose monitoring of the aqueous humor of the eye. I. Measurement of very small optical rotations. Diabetes Care 5: 254, 1982.

77. Rabinovitch B, March WF, Adams RL: Noninvasive glucose monitoring of the aqueous homor of the eye. II. Animal studies and the scleroal lens. Diabetes Care 5: 259.

78. Schultz J, Mansouri S, Goldstein I: Affinity sensors: a new technique for developing implantable sensors or glucose and other metabolities. Diabetes Care 5: 245, 1982.

79. Mirouze J, Selam JL, Pham TC, Cavadore D: Evaluation of exogenous insulin homeostasis by the artificial pancreas in insulin-dependent diabetes. Diabetologia 13: 273–278, 1977.

80. Botz CK: An improved control algorithm for an artificial B-cell. IEEE Trans Biomed Eng 23: 252–255, 1976.

81. Marliss EB, Murray FT, Stokes EF, Zinman B, Nakhooda AF, Denoga A, Leibel BS, Albisser AM: Normalization of glycemia in diabetics during meals with insulin and glucagon delivery by the artificial pancreas. Diabetes 26: 663–672, 1977.

82. Albisser AM, Leibel BS, Zinman B, Murray FT, Zingg W, Botz CK, Denoga A, Marliss EB: Studies with an artificial pancreas. Arch Intern Med 137: 639–649, 1977.

83. Soegijoko S, Selam SL, Ferrand D, Mirouze J: External artificial pancreas – 4th generation. 7th meeting of the Europ Soc Artif Org Geneva, 1980.

84. Curry DL, Bennett LL, Grodsky GM: Dynamics of insulin secretion by the perfused rat pancreas. Endocrinology 83: 572–584, 1968.

85. Foster RO: The dynamics of blood sugar regulation. M Sc Thesis, Massuchussett Institute of Technology, 1970.

86. Ewart TG, Albisser AM, Leibel BS, Davidovac Z, Zingg W: Computer analog of the endocrine pancreas. Int Symp on Dynamics Fluid Controls in Pysiological Systems. Iberall AS, Guyton AC. Editors Am Physiol Soc pp 509–511, 1973.

87. Clemens AH, Chang PH, Myers RW: The development of Biostator, a glucose controlled insulin infusion system (GCIIS). Horm Metabl Res Suppl 7: 22–33, 1977.

88. Schichiri M, Kawaviori R: Optimized algorithm for closed loop glycemic control in. Computer.

89. Piwernetz K, Renner R, Hepp KID. Attempt at glucose-controlled feed back regulatory of intraperitoneal insulin infusion.

90. Schade DA, Eaton RP, Friedman N, Spencer W: The intravenous, intraperitoneal, and subcutaneous routes of insulin delivery in diabetic man. Diabetes 28: 1068–1072, 1979.

91. Gyaram H, Bottermann P, Ehrhardt W, Blumel G: Pharmacokinetics of intraperitoneally injected insulin and the development of a cannula system to facilitate intraperitoneal injection. In: Brunetti P et al (eds): Artificial systems for insulin delivery. Raven Press, New York, 1983.

92. Selam JL, Slingeneyer A, Hedon B, Mares P, Beraud JJ, Mirouze J: Long-term ambulatory peritoneal insulin infusion of brittle diabetes with portable pumps: Comparison with intravenous and subcutaneous route. Diabetes Care 6: 105–111, 1983.

93. Selam JL, Raymond M, Jacquemin JL, Orsetti A, Richard JL, Mirouze J: Pharmacokinetics of insulin injected intraperitoneally via portable pumps. Diab Metab 11: 170–173, 1985.

94. Bergman RN, Bucolo RJ: Nonlinear metabolic dynamics of the pancreas and liver. J. Dynam Syst Trans ASME 95: 296–900, 1973.

95. Slama G, Hautecouverture M, Assan R, Tchobroutsky G: One to five days of continuous intravenous insulin infusion on seven diabetic patients. Diabetes 23: 732–738, 1974.

96. Pickup JC, Keen H, Parsons JA, Alberti KGMM: Continuous subcutaneous insulin infusion: an approach to achieving normoglycaemia. Br Med J 1: 204–207, 1978.
97. Novo Industry: Data on insulin infusion pumps, 1983.
98. Carlson GA, Bair REK, Goana JI Jr, Schidknecht HE, Love JT, Urenda R: An implantable, remotely programmable insulin infusion system. Med Prog Technol 9: 17, 1982.
99. Schade DS, Eaton RP, Edwards WS: A remotely programable insulin delivery system: successful short-term implantation in man. JAMA 247: 1848, 1982.
100. Irsigler K, Kritz H, Hagmuller G: Long-term continuous intraperitoneal insulin infusion with an implantable remote controlled insulin infusion device. Diabetes 30: 1072, 1981.
101. Hepp KD, Renner R, Funcke HJ, Mehnert H, Haerten R, Kresse H: Intravenous insulin therapy under conditions imitating physiological profiles. Diabetologia 11: 349, 1975.
102. Hepp KD, Renner R, Funcke HJ, Mehnert H, Haerten R, Kresse H: Glucose homeostasis under continuous intravenous insulin therapy in diabetics. Horm Metab Res Suppl 7: 72, 1977.
103. Hepp KD, Renner R, Piewernetz K, Mehnert H: Control of insulin-dependent diabetes with portable minaturized infusion systems. Diabetes Care 3: 309, 1980.
104. Walter H, Kemmler W, Kronski D, Franetzki M, Prestele K, Hepp KD, Renner R, Mehnert H: Implantation of a program-controlled device with intravenous insulin infusion in a patient with type I diabetes mellitus. In: Brunetti P et al (eds) Artificial systems for insulin delivery; p 313. Raven Press, New York, 1983.
105. Selam JL, Slingeneyer A, Chaptal PA: Total implantation of a remotely controlled insulin minipump in a human insulin dependent diabetic. Artif org 6: 315, 1982.
106. Elsberry D, Vadnais K, Bartelt K, VanKampen K: Abstr in artificial insulin-delivery systems. Workshop of the study group of EASD – Igls (Austria), 1984.
107. Fischell RE, Saudek C: A programmable implantable medication system: Application to diabetes – 6th Hawaii International Conference on system sciences, 1983.
108. Saudek C: Diabetes 35 (suppl): 82 (A), 1986.
109. Thomas LJ, Bessman SP: Trans Am Soc Artif in Organs 21: 516–522, 1975.
110. Schubert W, Baurschmidt P, Nagel J, Thull R, Schaldacl M: Med Biol Eng Comput 18: 527, 1980.
111. Kuhl D, Luft G: Deutsches Patent Nr 2626348, 1976.
112. Luft G, Kuhl D, Richter GJ: Med & Biol Eng Comput 16: 45–50, 1978.
113. Uhlig ELP, Graydon WF: Biomed Mater Res 1: 931–943, 1983.
114. Hsieh DST, Langer R, Folkman J: Proc Nat Acad Sci USA 78: 1863, 1981.
115. Schade D, Eaton R, DeLongo J, Saland L, Ladman A, Carlson G: Electron microscopy of insulin precipitates. Diabetes Care 5: 25, 1982.
116. Blackshear PJ, Rohde TD, Palmer JL, Wigness BD, Rupp WM, Buchwald H: Glycerol prevents insulin precipitation and interruption o flow in an implantable insulin infusion pump. Diabetes Care 6: 387, 1983.
117. Brang J, Havelund S: Properties of insulin solutions. In: Brunetti P et al (eds) Artificial systems for insulin delivery; p 89. Raven Press New York, 1983.
118. Selam JL, Slingeneyer A, Cahptal PA, Franetzki M, Prestele K, Mirouze J: One year continuous run with the totally-implantable Siemens pump in a human diabetic. In: Irsigler K, Kritz H, Lovett R (eds) Diabetes treatment with implantable insulin infusion systems; p 119. Urban & Schwarzenberg, Munich.
119. Selam JL, Giraud P, Mirouze J, Saeidi S: Continuous peritoneal insulin infusion with portable pumps: factors affecting the operating life of the chronic catheter. Diabetes Care 8: 34–38, 1985.
120. Selam JL, Slingeneyer A, Saeidi S, Mirouze J, Richard JL, Rodier M, Daynes B, Lapinski H: Experience with long-term peritoneal insulin infusion from external pumps. Diab Med 2: 41–44, 1985.

121. Selam JL, Mirouze J, Cavalie-Barthez G, Mellet M, Zirinis P, Gagnol JP, Humeau P: Insulin for portable pumps: influence of pH on in vitro stability in reservoirs. Diabetes 34: 200 (a) Artificial organs (in press), 1985.

122. Hepp KD, Renner R, vonFuncke HF: Glucose homestasis under continuous intravenous insulin therapy in diabetics. Horm Metabol Res Suppl 7: 72, 1977.

123. Irsigler K, Kritz H: Long-term continuous intravenous insulin therapy with a portable insulin dosage-regulating apparatus. Diabetes 28: 196, 1979.

124. Froesch ER, Blatter G, Morell B: Optimal blood sugar control in labile diabetics using a portable open-loop insulin infusion system with a flexible program. In: Hepp KRD, Kerner W, Pfeiffer EW (eds) Feedback-controlled and preprogramme insuline infusion in diabetes mellitus; p 198. Georg Thieme Verlag, Stuttgart, 1979.

125. Grau U: Chemical stability of insulin in a delivery system environment. Diabetologia 28: 458–463, 1985.

126. Selam JL, Zirinis P, Mellet M, Mirouze J: A stable insulin for implantable insulin delivery systems – in vitro studies with different containers and solvents. Diabetes Care, 1988.

127. Kritz H, Nagemnik C, Hagmuller G, Leddolter S, Olbert F, Mostbeck A, Denck H, Irsigler K: Long term results using different routes of infusion. In: Irsigler K et al (eds) Diabetes treatment with implantable insulin infusion systems; pp 81–102. Urban & Schwarzenberg, Munich, 1983.

128. Brange J, Langljaer L, Havelund S, Sorensen E: Chemical stability of insulin: neutral insulin solutions. Diabetologia 25: 143 (A), 1985.

129. Geisen K, Gerlach MH, Keil M: Morphological findings in pancreatectomized dogs with an implanted insulin dosing device: tissue reaction to the pump housing and to the vascular catheter. Horm Metab Res 15: 19??.

130. Geisen K, Jung S, Fiedler B: Result with a catheterless insulin delivery deice implanted in a pancreatectomized dog. Horm Metab Res 15: 111, 1983.

131. Geisen K, Jung S, Fiedler B: A remote programmable implantable insulin dosing device. II. Results of animal experiments. In: Federlin K, Pfeiffer EF, Raptis S (eds) Islet-pancreas transplantation and artificial pancreas; p 310. Georg Thieme Verlag, Stuttgart, 1982.

132. Buchwald H, Varco RL, Rupp WM: Treatment of a type II diabetic by a totally implantable insulin device. Lancet 6: 1233.

133. Rupp WM, Barbosa J, Blackshear PH, McCarthy HB, Rohde TD, Goldenberg F: Implantable insulin pump therapy in Type II diabetics. N Engl J Med 307: 265, 1982.

134. Rupp WH, Rohde TD, Wigness BD, Blackshear PH, Buchwald H: Clinical experiences with insulin-glycerol solution in an implantable pump. Transact Artif Org (in press).

135. Buchwald. Diabetes (Suppl 1). 35: 140 (A), 1986.

136. Selam JL, Giraud P, Hedon B, Saeidi S, Mirouze J, Orsetti A, Slingeneyer A: Factors affecting the operating life and efficiency of catheters for continuous intraperitoneal insulin infusion. In: Hepp, Renner (eds) Continuous insulin infusion therapy experience from one decade; pp 65–73. Shattauer, Stuttgart, 1985.

137. Selam JL: Personal unpublished results.

138. Lord P: Pacesetter unpublished results.

139. Franetzki M, Prestele K, Kresse H: Technological problems of miniaturized insulin dosing devices and some approaches to clinical trials. In: Hepp KO, Kerner W, Pfeiffer EF (eds) Feedback-controlled and preprogrammed insulin infusion in diabetes mellitus. Georg Thieme Verlag, Stuttgart, 1979.

140. Eaton RP, Schade DS, Pitcher L: Catheter encapsulation during prolonged intraperitoneal insulin infusion in a patient with a remote-controlled insulin delivery system. In: Irsigler R, Kritz H, Lovett R (eds) Diabetes treatment with implantable insulin infusion systems; Urban & Schwarzenberg, Munich, 1983.

516

141. Kritz H, Najemnik C, Hagmuller G, Leodolter S, Olbert F, Mostbeck A, Dench H, and Irsigler K: Long-term results using different routes of insulin infusion, in diabetes treatment with implantable insulin infusion systems, Irsigler K, Kritz H, Lovett R (eds) Urban & Schwarzenberg, Munich, 81, 1983.

142. Williams HF, Jarvis CW, Neal WA, Reynolds JW: Vascular thromboembolism complicating unbilical artery catheterization. Am J Roentgenol Radium Ther Nucl med 116: 475, 1972.

143. Knatterud G, Fisher M: Report from the international study group on implantable insulin delivery devices 8: 308–9, 1985.

144. Dupre J, Champion M, Rodger NW: Advances in insulin delivery in the management of diabetes mellitus. Clin Endocrinol Metabol 11: 525–549, 1982.

145. Selam JL, Mirouze J, Slingeneyer A, Hedon B, Millet P, Chaptal PA, Orsetti A: Two years experience of ambulatory peritoneal insulin infusion. In: Irsigler K, Kritz H, Lovett R (eds) Implantable delivery systems; pp 132–136 Urban & Schwartzenberg, Frankfurt, 1983.

146. Chisholm DJ, Kraegen EW: Pharmacokinetics of subcutaneous insulin with reference to pumps. Presented at the Toronto international workshop on insulin and portable delivery systems, June 9–11, Toronto, Canada.

147. Home PD, Pickup JC, Keen H, Alberti KGMM, Parson JA, Binder C: Continuous subcutaneous insulin infusion: comparison of plasma insulin profiles after infusion or bolus injection of the meal-time dose. Metabolism 30: 439–442, 1980.

148. Schiffrin A, Belmonte MM: Comparison between continuous subcutaneous insulin infusion and multiple injections of insulin, a one year prospective study. Diabetes 31: 255–264, 1982.

149. Pickup JC, Keen H, Viberti GC, White MC, Kohner EM, Parsons JA, Alberti KGMM: Continuous subcutaneous insulin infusion in the treatment of diabetes mellitus. Diabet Care 3: 290–300, 1980.

150. Who-study on CSII acceptability and efficiency. unpublished report.

151. Goriya Y, Bahoric A, Marliss EB, Zinman B, Albisser AM: Glycemic regulation using a programmed insulin delivery device. III: Long-term studies on diabetic dogs. Diabetes 28: 558–564, 1979.

152. Albisser AM, Nomura M, Greenberg GR, McPhedran NT: Metabolic control in diabetic dogs treated with autotransplants and insulin pumps. Diabetes 35: 97–100, 1986.

153. Miles JM, Rizza RA, Raymond MW, Gerich JD: Effects of acute insulin deficiency on glucose and ketone body turnover in man. Diabetes 29: 926–930, 1980.

154. Gooch BR, Abumrad NM, Robinson RP, Petrik M, Campbell D, Crofford OB: Exercise in insulin dependent diabetes mellitus: the effect of continuous infusion using the subcutaneous, intravenous and intraperitoneal sites. Diabet Care 6: 122–127, 1983.

155. Mirouze J, Selam JL: Clinical experience in human diabetics with portable and implantable insulin minipumps. Life Support Syst 1: 39–50, 1983.

156. Pickup JC, Home PD, Bilous RW, Alberti KGMM, Keen H: Management of severely brittle diabetes by continuous and intramuscular insulin infusion: evidence for a defect in subcutaneous insulin absorption. Br Med J 282: 347–350, 1981.

157. Field JB, Rojdmark S, Harding P, Ishida T, Chou MCY: Role of liver in insulin physiology. Diabet Care 3: 255, 1980.

158. Albisser AM, Botz CL, Leibel BS: Blood glucose regulation using an open-loop insulin delivery system in pancreatectomized dogs given glucose infusion. I: Portal square waves. Diabetologia 16: 129–133, 1979.

159. Rizza QA, Westland RE, Hall LD, Patton GS, Haymond MW, Clemens AH, Gerich JE, Service FJ: Effect of peripheral versus portal venous administration of insulin on postprandial hyperglycemia and glucose turn-over in alloxan, diabetic dogs. Mayo Clin Proc 56: 434–438, 1981.

160. Stevenson RW, Parsons JA, Alberti KGMM: Comparison of the metabolic responses to

portal and peripheral infusions of insulin in diabetic dogs. Metabolism 30: 745–752.

161. Nelson JA, Stephen R, Landau ST, Wilson DE, Tyler FH: Intraperitoneal insulin administration produces a positive portal-systemic blood insulin gradient in unanaesthetized unrestrained swine. Metabolism 31: 969–972, 1982.

162. Schade DS, Eaton RP, Davis T, Akiya F, Phinnem E, Kubica R. Vaughn EA, Day PW: The kinetics of peritoneal insulin absorption. Metabolism 30: 149–153, 1981.

163. Renner R, Piwernetz K, Hepp KD: Continuous intraperitoneal insulin treatment in type I diabetes: comparison between square wave infusion and bolus application. Diabetologia 25: 189A, 1983.

164. Kraft AR: Peritoneal electrolyte absorption, analysis of portal system, venous and lymphatic transport. Surgery 64: 148, 1968.

165. Irsigler K, Kritz H: Alternate routes of insulin delivery. Diabetes Care 3: 219–228, 1980.

166. Pozza G, Spotti D, Micossi P, Cristallo M, Melandri M, Piatti PM, Monti LD, Pontirolli AE: Long-term continuous intraperitoneal insulin treatment in brittle diabetes. Br Med J 286: 255–156, 1983.

167. Marshall SM, Husband DJ, Walford S, Wright PD, Alberti KGMM: Use of intraperitoneal insulin in birttle diabetes. Diabetologia 25: 179A, 1983.

168. Rizza RA, Service JF, Westland RE, Hall RD, Patton GS, Haymond MW, Gerich JE: Comparison of peripheral venous, portal, subcutaneous and intraperitoneal routes for insulin delivery in diabeti dogs. Presented at the workshop on artificial beta cells, September 19–290, Heviz, Hungary, 1979.

169. Irsigler K, Kritz H, Hagmuller G, Najemmik C, Leddolter S: Long-term safety of insulin infusion: the intravenous and intraperitoneal route for pump treatment. Diabetologia 25: 167A, 1983.

Note: since the preparation of the manuscript, the author has published recent reviews and data in the following articles:

(a) Selam JL: Development of implantable insulin pumps: long is the road. Diab. Medicine 5: 724–733, 1988.

(b) Selam JL: Peritoneum and intraperitoneal insulin administration. In: Bengmark S (ed) The peritoneum and peritoneal access; pp 179–191. Wright J and Sons Publ, London, 1989.

(c) Selam JL, Chaptal PA: The artificial pancreas. In: Kline J (ed) Handbook of medical bioengineering; pp 225–243. Acad Press Inc, San Diego, Calif, 1988.

(d) Selam JL: Towards the implantable artificial pancreas. In: Selam JL and Ensminger W (eds) Infusion systems; pp 55–98. Futura Publ Co, Mount Kisco, New York, 1987.

(e) Selam JL: Closed-loop pumps: update. In: Krall JP and Alberti KGMM (eds) World book of diabetes, Vol 3; pp 176–180. Elsevier Sci Publ, Amsterdam, December 28, 1988 Modification, The Netherlands, 1988.

18. Perspectives in pancreatic transplantation

J.M. DUBERNARD and D.E.R. SUTHERLAND

Although the ability of pancreatic transplants to establish a normoglycemic insulin-independent state in diabetic humans was shown by Lillehei and Kelly and associates in the late sixties [1, 2], technical and immunological problems limited its application for many years. During the past 10 years, however, the cumulative efforts of several international teams have elevated pancreatic transplantation from clinical experimentation to the edge of becoming a routine form of therapy method for selected patients with established or emerging complications of diabetes [3].

Several justifications for these efforts exist. First the degree of carbohydrate control achieved in patients with functioning pancreatic transplants [4, 5] exceeds that possible by any other therapy [6]. A successful graft completely eliminates the need for exogenous insulin, and previously diabetic patients maintain a virtually normal and constant blood glucose profile. The results of intravenous and oral glucose tolerance tests may show some mild abnormalities in some patients, but can be explained by the fact that the grafted pancreas is denervated and secretes the hormone into the systemic venous system rather than in the portal system (by most techniques). In addition, the recipients are on steroids for immunosuppression, and the beta cell mass may be reduced compared to normal from use of the segmental technique or loss from rejection episodes. Nevertheless, the metabolic abnormalities of diabetes are resolved, the patients are insulin-independent, they do not need a special diet, and they are usually rehabilitated [3].

The pancreas is a complex (dual) organ [7], composed almost entirely of exocrine tissue with only a small endocrine component in terms of mass. This arrangement lies at the heart of the surgical problems and the variety of techniques that have been devised for transplantation. The debate over technique is intertwined with the problem of early diagnosis of rejection. Both aspects are addressed in this book.

Data from the International Transplant Registry shows no differences in graft survival rates for whole versus segmental pancreas transplants [8]. Seg-

J.M. Dubernard and D.E.R. Sutherland (eds.), International Handbook of Pancreas Transplantation, 519–529.
© *1989 by Kluwer Academic Publishers.*

mental grafts can maintain normal glucose metabolism indefinitely, and normal glucose tolerance test results are also possible [4]. The patient with the currently longest functioning pancreas transplant (>10 years) received a segmental graft [9], and several others, transplanted when this technique was nearly exclusively applied, are more than 8 years with functioning grafts [8]. Theoretical advantages of whole pancreas grafts are a larger islet mass that may provide a greater reserve in case of rejection episodes, and increased blood flow, with perhaps, a lesser tendency to thrombose. Again the Registry shows no difference between whole and segmental grafts in regard to this complication [8], and the results with both approaches have improved as advances in immunosuppression have been applied and patient selection refined.

Both segmental and whole pancreas grafts can be procured from cadaver donors when a liver is also harvested. A longer and more complex operation is required when a whole pancreas is taken under these circumstances. However the fact that the complication rate is no higher when compared to the simple segmental technique, coupled with the theoretical advantages, indicates that a whole pancreas should be procured whenever possible.

Similarly, the Registry data shows equivalent graft survival rates for the duct management techniques used most frequently: duct obstruction, intestinal drainage, and bladder drainage. The three techniques are applicable to segmental as well as to whole pancreas transplantation. Duct obstruction is the simplest pancreas transplant method, requiring only 2 vascular and no other anastamoses. In the pre-cyclosporin era, this technique had the lowest surgical complication rate [10]. Duct obstruction transforms a dually functioning organ into a monofunctional graft, and basically should be regarded as a particular technique of islet transplantation. After a few months, only islets remain as parenchymal tissue in the graft [11]. Although not demonstrated in experimental animals [12] or in other clinical situations such as injection of autografts [13] or in situ remnants after a Whipple operation [14], a progression of fibrosis rather than chronic rejection, could be involved in the long-term deterioration of graft endocrine function observed in some patients. An adverse effect of duct-injection on function has yet to be proved, and if it does occur, its frequency is unknown; it is not inevitable, since normal glucose tolerance has been demonstrated in recipients of duct-injection segmental grafts followed for more than 8 years (personal observation). The duct obstruction technique, however, does not allow graft exocrine function to be monitored except in the immediate post-operative period of initial drainage when a delayed duct injection technique is employed [15]. Thus, long-term monitoring of function of a duct-obstructed grafts relies solely on endocrine parameters, and a marker for rejection independent of a decline in graft endocrine function does not exist except in cases of a simultaneously transplanted kidney from the same donor, where a rejection episode of the kidney, as indicated by an elevation of serum creatinine and finding on renal graft biopsy, may mirror events ongoing in the pancreas graft prior to deterioration in endocrine function as manifested by an increase in plasma glucose levels. Double transplants however, are only performed in recipients with end stage renal disease, and for the nonuremic, nonkidney transplant recipients of a pancreas transplant alone or for recipients of a pancreas after a kidney from a different donor, the graft survival rates have been significantly lower than in recipients of a kidney from the same donor (see chapter on Registry).

Enteric drainage is more physiological than the other technique, especially when pancreatic juice is diverted into the upper digestive tract. The architecturial integrity of the graft is preserved in most cases, and maintaining the exocrine-endocrine interactions could, theoretically, have a beneficial influence on overall graft function [7].

The most physiological technique used to date is paratopic transplantation [16], with gastric drainage of the pancreatic juice and portal venous drainage of the graft exocrine secretions. First passage of insulin through the liver, a major target organ of action, suppresses hepatic glucose production and theoretically should produce blood glucose and insulin levels that are lower or more normal than systemic drainage, with, also theoretically, a corresponding more salutary effect on microvascular complications. Studies in recipients with portal drained pancreas grafts have shown glucose levels (basal, postprandial, and during glucose tolerance tests to be slightly lower than in patients with systemic drained grafts, but the differences were not significant [17].

Monitoring of exocrine function in enteric drained cases is possible in the early postoperative period when a catheter draining the duct has been brought externally [16, 18]. For long term monitoring of graft function, however, the situation is the same as for duct injection, and only endocrine responses of the graft can be assessed. Again, the function of a simultaneously transplanted kidney from the same donor can give a clue to immunological events that may be ongoing in the pancreas graft, but in recipients of a pancreas transplant alone there are no parameters other than endocrine to monitor for rejection, and the graft survival rates are significantly lower in this group than in the doubly transplanted patients (see Registry chapter). Enteric drainage involves from two (segmental grafts invaginated into a Roux-en-Y-loop) to 5 (pancreatico-duodenal graft in a Roux-en-Y loop) intestinal closures or anastomoses, with the inherent risks of bacterial contamination, infection and fistula formation.

Urinary drainage of pancreatic graft exocrine secretions necessitates an anastomosis between the duct of segmental transplants or duodenum (or patch therof) of whole organ transplants and either the recipient's ureter [19] or bladder [20]. The latter is now prefered, but can also be complicated by local leakage, and microbial contamination from the donor duodenum with resultant infection is always a possibility. The major advantage of urinary drainage, however, is the ability to directly and permanently monitor exocrine function, a decrease preceding endocrine dysfunction during rejection episodes [20], thus leading to earlier treatment of rejection and higher graft survival rates than other techniques in nonuremic, nonkidney transplant patients and in those with end stage renal disease who have not received a kidney from the same donor (see Registry chapter).

To mimic as perfectly as possible the natural physiology of the pancreas, the ideal transplant procedure would be pancreatico-duodenal grafting, post-gastric diversion of the exocrine secretion and drainage of the venous effluent into the recipient portal vein, and retention of the donor spleen for hemodynamic reasons. Technical difficulties have prevented incorporation of all of these features into clinical transplantation. In addition, composite grafts that include the spleen produce the special problem of graft versus host disease due to the large amount of donor lymphatic tissue [22]. The results with the few pancreaticosplenic transplants reported in the literature have hot shown a convincing advantage over those without the spleen [23, 24], and the Registry data shows inclusion of the spleen to be detrimental (see Registry chapter).

The cause of the high rates of venous thrombosis for pancreas grafts reported is not entirely understood. The explanations usually given are low blood flow rates in the circulation from small to large pancreatic vessels, graft malposition with kinking and twisting; and graft pancreatitis. Although the efficacy of treatment has not been demonstrated, most centers administer anticoagulant or anti-platelet agents in the post-operative period, and accept the risk of bleeding which is already inherent in such a complex procedure. A distal splenic arteriovenous fistula, shown to reduce the thrombosis rate in animal experiments [25], has not been shown to prevent thrombosis in clinical cases. Theoretically, such a procedure could adversely affect function, by decreasing tissue perfusion and increasing graft venous pressure, and in non-human primates such a detrimental effect has been demonstrated [26].

It is essential that pancreas transplant teams objectively evaluate the numerous components and technical options of the procedure with objectivity. Comparison of two techniques applied by the same surgeons in the same center using the same immunosuppression is the only method of establishing parameters for a satisfactory answer to the many problems that remain unsolved. The number of transplants in each center are insufficient to address many issues and there is a need for cooperative studies. The most important issue is defining the indications for pancreatic transplantation particularly in the nonuremic, nonkidney transplant patients in whom immunosuppression would not otherwise be required.

At present, patients with end stage diabetic nephropathy (ESDN) are generally considered as acceptable candidates for a pancreas transplant, but in conjunction with a kidney. Kidney transplantation is the treatment of choice for uremic diabetic patients, and unlike other causes of renal failure, patient survival is significantly higher with renal transplantation than with hemodialysis [28]. Thus, for patients with ESDN, kidney transplantation should be performed, in which case immunosuppression is obligatory, and the addition of a pancreas entails only the surgical risk.

Microangiopathic complications are progressive, and cardiac and cardiovascular disease and infections account for the majority of deaths in diabetic patients [27], and is highest in those on hemodialysis. The need for anticoagulation during hemodialysis can cause hemorrhages and deterioration of vision in diabetic patients. Continuous ambulatory peritoneal dialysis (CAPD), with administration of insulin intraperitonealy, is better tolerated by some diabetic patients, but even this treatment is unsatisfactory for long-term management.

Renal transplantation does not solve all problems in the diabetic patient with ESDN, and cardiovascular disease, infection, difficulties in control of diabetes exacerbated by steroid administration are only some of the ones that persist or arise. Nevertheless, renal transplantation is the treatment of choice for ESDN [28]. The best results are obtained with living donors, but even with cadaveric organs, one year graft survival rates of over 80% have been reported [29]. Not all programs achieved such results by renal transplantation alone, and all aspects of diabetic care continue to require meticulous attention. Even though retinopathy and neuropathy may stabilize in some recipients with functioning renal allografts [30, 31], renal transplantation is no more than a palliative procedure. At long term, degenerative complications progress, and recurrence of diabetic nephropathy in the renal allograft has been clearly demonstrated [32]. Recurrence of diabetic nephropathy as a cause of loss of function has been rare, but only because no recipients of renal allografts done have long-term survival. With the increasing number of long-surviving diabetic recipients of kidney transplants [33], it may be predicted that graft failure from recurrence of disease will be seen more frequently.

Microscopic recurrence of diabetic nephropathy in a transplanted kidney is prevented by a simultaneous pancreas transplant [34] or a pancreas transplant soon after a kidney [35]. In diabetic patients with renal failure, pancreatic transplantation adds a potential source of morbidity. This risk has to be evaluated, taking into account the general condition of the patients, the technique of pancreatic transplantation and the timing of the procedures. The majority of pancreas transplant programs have preferred to perform renal and pancreas transplantation simultaneously. The largest experience with pancreas transplantation after a kidney is at the University of Minnesota, and the results with this approach have not been as good as with the simultaneous transplants. Both approaches are now used at the University of Minnesota [9].

The relative advantages and disadvantages of pancreas transplantation simultaneous or subsequent to a renal graft are not very apparent when a simple surgical technique (duct obstruction) is used, at least from a risk standpoint. However, no matter which technique is used, there may be an immunological advantage to the simultaneous procedure. According to the Registry, pancreas graft survival rates are higher in the patients who had simultaneous kidney transplants than when the pancreas was grafted alone or after the kidney [8]. One possible explanation is that recognition of rejection is easier and leads to earlier treatment in patients receiving a kidney from the same donor, with kidney rejection used as a marker for early diagnosis of pancreas rejection. A detailed analysis of Registry cases tends to support this hypothesis (see Registry chapter).

On the other hand, the patient survival rates are higher in recipients of pancreas transplants alone, and the number of patients in this category is gradually increasing as the results improve. It is in such patients that the potential benefit of pancreas transplantation is the greatest. To fulfill its promise, the indications for pancreatic transplantation in nonuremic, nonkidney transplant patients must be defined.

The degenerative complications of diabetes can evolve to a 'point of no return' beyond which the complication will be self-perpetuating without the possibility of being reversed by restoration of normal metabolism. The progression or proliferative retinopathy can be slowed by laser treatment but not stopped. A major question is whether earlier intervention by pancreas transplantation, at a time when microaneurysms and exsudates are appearing and progressing but without evidence of ischemia, could reverse or halt the progression of the lesions. Preliminary evidence suggests that even earlier intervention is required if pancreas transplantation alone is to have an effect [36]. In the short term, combined pancreas and kidney transplantation seems to have a stabilizing effect in uremic diabetic recipients [37].

Conversely, in patients with nephropathy, good metabolic control of diabetes can reduce glomerular hyperfiltration [38]. It is of the utmost importance to note that pancreatic transplantation in nonuremic, nonkidney transplant recipients has been associated with reversal of at least some of the microscopic lesions of diabetic nephropathy [39], even though the use of cyclosporin precluded detection of a saluatory effect on function [40].

Thus, pancreatic transplantation may be applicable to patients with early diabetic nephropathy with albuminuria, a situation in which progression is otherwise inevitable [41]. For retinopathy, an acute effect of pancreas transplant alone may not be apparent, although at long term a benefit may occur [36].

Clearly, the future of pancreatic transplantation lies in the application to diabetic patients with emerging microvascular complications. Pancreas transplantation should be performed at an early stage for a maximum therapeutic benefit. Because of the current need for generalized immunosuppression to prevent rejection of organ allografts, the selected patients must clearly be difficult to manage from the metabolic standpoint or be at high risk for secondary complications when treated by exogenous insulin. Methods to identify such patients are needed. High plasma levels of inactive renin are associated with microvascular complications in diabetic patients [42]. High levels of insulin-like growth factor I are also seen in patients who do have accelerated progression of diabetic retinopathy [43]. Diabetic children with stiff joints have a high incidence of subsequent microvascular complications [44]. Diabetic patients who have impaired counter-regulatory mechanisms are at high risk of having hypoglycemic reactions while on an insulin pump or other intensified insulin therapy regiment [45], and such patients can be identified by measurement of adrenergic responses to stress [46]. Individuals with such characteristics are the ones who are most likely to benefit.

The results of pancreas transplantation have to be improved for widespread application. Currently, one year graft function rates of more than 40% are being achieved world wide [8], and several institutions are reporting graft survival rates in selected patients of more than 70% [3]. Patient survival rates must also be improved, currently 80% at one year for all cases and 90% for patients without ESDN in the Registry [8]. Again several institutions have patient survival rates superior to 90% [3]. If these goals are achieved, pancreas transplantation has the potential to have the same impact on the treatment of diabetes as kidney transplantation has had on the treatment of end stage renal disease.

Pancreas transplantation, unlike heart or liver transplantation, is not an immediate life saving procedure. The objective of pancreas transplantation is to improve the quality of life and to favorably influence the secondary complications of diabetes that would otherwise arise several years hence. Pancreas transplantation is similar to kidney transplantation, in that if the kidney fails the patient can resume dialysis. Rejection, or other causes of pancreatic graft failure, should be followed by a return to exogenous insulin therapy and resumption of a life style no different than that achieved pretransplant.

When immunosuppressive therapy is improved to the point where side effects are minimal, and when results of transplantation are better, many more diabetic patients could be considered as candidates for pancreas transplantation and donor procurement will have to be increased. However, at this time, procurement should not be a problem. More than 7,000 kidney transplants are currently being done per year in the United States [47]. The yearly incidence of Type I diabetes in the United States is estimated at approximately 12,000 to 19,000 new cases per year, and less than half of the patients with the disease develop serious complications [27]. Thus, the current kidney transplant rate is

526

similar to the incidence of complicated Type I diabetes. Only a small proportion of the potential donors are currently used as a source of organs [48], but it should be possible to increase the procurement rate, and each donor could give the pancreas as well as other organs for transplantation.

Much enthusiasm has been generated for islet transplantation in recent years [49], but it is clearly only in the earliest investigative stages compared to clinical pancreas transplantation at this time. Human islet allografts have been unsuccessful in making diabetic recipients insulin independent [50, 51]. The manipulations associated with a relatively high success rate for islet transplantation in experimental animal models [52] have been difficult to reproduce [53], and even more difficult to employ for the human pancreas [54]. Islet preparation and transplantation are complex procedures for the transplant team. It is difficult to isolate a sufficient quantity of viable islets from a single human donor pancreas. It is uncertain whether the methods used in animals can be directly applied to the isolation and reduction in immunogenicity, and new approaches may be needed to develop islet transplantation into a clinical reality (see chapter on Islet Transplantation).

Pancreatic transplantation has contributed to the understanding of diabetes in several respects, including defining its autoimmune nature [55]. Recurrence of disease in pancreas transplants can be prevented by immunosuppression, and may be necessary no matter what strategies or circumstances are employed to prevent rejection [56]. Many other fundamental questions related to the nature of diabetes mellitus, such as etiology or its association with microvascular and other complications may also be forthcoming from observations in pancreas transplant recipients [57].

In conclusion, pancreas transplantation can effectively treat Type I diabetes in humans. Islet transplants have been successful in animals, and at this time pancreas transplantation is the only practical method of total endocrine replacement therapy in diabetic humans. Pancreas transplantation potential could be applied on a large scale as kidney transplantation. As future advances in immunosuppression occur, pancreas transplantation possibly could be routinely performed at a stage sufficiently early to prevent the development of diabetic nephropathy and other lesions, and supercede kidney transplants and other procedures in the management of complication-prone diabetic patients.

References

1. Kelly WD, Lillehei RC, Merkel FK et al: Allotransplantation of the pancreas and duodenum along with the kidney in diabetic nephropathy. Surgery 61: 827, 1967.
2. Lillehei RC, Simmons RL, Najarian JS et al: Pancreaticoduodenal allotransplantation: experimental and clinical experience. Ann Surg 172: 405–436, 1970.
3. Land W, Landgraff R: Clinical pancreas transplantation, the world experience. Proceedings

of the second international workshop on clinical pancreas transplantation. Transpl Proc 19 (Suppl No 4): 1–95, 1987.

4. Sutherland DER, Najarian JS, Greenberg BZ et al: Hormonal and metabolic effects of an endocrine graft. Vascularized segmental transplantation on the pancreas in insulin-independent patients. Ann Inter Med 95: 537, 1981.

5. Pozza G, Traeger J, Dubernard JM et al: Endocrine responses of type I (insulin-independent) diabetic patients following successful pancreas transplantation. Diabetologia 24: 244, 1983.

6. Malone JI, Hellrung JM, Malphus EW, Rosenbloom AL, Grgic A, Weber FT: Good diabetic control: a study in mass delusion. J Ped 88: 943–947, 1976.

7. Henderson JR, Daniel PM, Frasor PA: The pancreas as a single organ: the influence of the endocrine upon the exocrine part of the gland. Gut 22: 158, 1981.

8. Sutherland DER, Moudry KC: Pancreas transplant registry: history and analysis of cases 1966 to October 1986. Pancreas 2: 473–488, 1987.

9. Sutherland DER, Goetz FC, Moudry KC, Najarian JS: Pancreatic transplantation: a single institution's experience. Diabetes, Nutrition and Metabolism, in press.

10. Sutherland DER: Report of the international human pancreas and islet transplant registry cases through 1981. Diabetes 31 (Suppl 4): 112–116, 1982.

11. Blanc-Brunat N, Dubernard JM, Touraine JL, et al: Pathology of the pancreas after intraductal neoprene injection in dogs and diabetic patients treated by pancreatic transplantation. Diabetologia 25: 97, 1983.

12. Goozen HG, Bosman FT, van Schilfgaarde R: The effect of duct obliteration on histology and endocrine function of the canine pancreas. Transplantation 38: 13, 1984.

13. Rossi RL, Soeldner JS, Braasch JW, Heiss FW, Shea JA, Nugent FW, Watkins E, Silverman ML, Bolton J: Segmental pancreatic autotransplantation with pancreatic ductal occlusion after near total or total pancreatic resection for chronic pancreatitis. Ann Surg 203: 626–636, 1986.

14. Di Carlo V, Chiesa R, Pontiroli, AE, Pozza G, Carlucci M, Staudacher C, Secchi A, Cristallo M: Intraductal injection of neoprene to suppress native pancreatic exocrine secretion in humans: clinical and metabolic evaluation. Transpl Proc 16: 736–738, 1984.

15. Steiner E, Klima J, Niederwieser D et al: Monitoring of the pancreatic allograft by analysis of exocrine secretion. Transpl Proc 19: 2336–2338, 1987.

16. Calne RY: Paratopic segmental pancreas grafting: a technique with portal venous drainage. Lancet 1: 595–597, 1984.

17. Sutherland DER, Goetz FC, Moudry KC, Abouna GM, Najarian JS: Use of recipient mesenteric vessels for revascularization of segmental pancreas grafts: technical and metabolic considerations. Transpl Proc 19: 2300–2304, 1987.

18. Groth CG, Collste H, Lundgren G et al: Successful outcome of segmental human pancreatic transplantation with enteric exocrine diversion after modifications in technique. Lancet 2: 522–524, 1982.

19. Gil-Vernet JM, Fernandez-Cruz L, Andreu J, Figuerola D, Caralps A: Urinary tract diversion (UTD) in clinical pancreas transplantation. Transpl Proc 18: 1132–1133, 1986.

20. Sollinger H, Kalayoglu M, Hoffman RM et al: Experience with whole pancreas transplantation and pancreaticoduodenocystostomy. Transpl Proc 18: 1759–1761, 1986.

21. Prieto M, Sutherland DER, Fernandez-Cruz L et al: Experimental and clinical experience with urinary amylase monitoring for early diagnosis of rejection in pancreas transplantation. Transplantation 43: 71–79, 1987.

22. Deierhoi MH, Sollinger HW, Bozdec MJ et al: Lethal graft versus host disease in a recipient of pancreas-spleen transplant. Transplantation 41: 544–546, 1986.

23. Starzl TE, Iwatsuki S, Shaw BW: Pancreaticoduodenal transplantation in humans. Surg Gynecol Obstet 159: 265, 1984.

24. Koostra G, von Hooff JP, Jorning PJG et al: A new variant for whole pancreas grafting. Transpl Proc 19: 2314–2318, 1987.

25. Calne RY, McMaster P, Rolles K et al: Technical observations in segmental pancreas transplantation: observations on blood flow. Transpl Proc 12 (Suppl 2): 51–57, 1980.

26. du Toit DF, Heydenrych J, Smit B, Louw G, Zuurmond T, Laker L. Els D, Weideman A, Wolfe-Coote S, van der Merwe EA, Groenewald WA: Segmental pancreatic allograft survival in baboons treated with combined irradiation and cyclosporin: a preliminary report. Surgery, 97 (4): 447–453.

27. Harris MI, Hanaman RF: Diabetes in America. NIH Publication 85–1468, Bethesda, Maryland 1985.

28. Goetz FC, Elick B, Fryd D, Sutherland DER: Renal transplantation in diabetes. Clinics in endocrinology and metabolism 15: 807–821, 1986.

29. Sutherland DER, Fryd DS, Payne WD, Ascher N, Simmons RL, Najarian JS: Kidney transplantation in diabetic patients. Transpl Proc 19: 90–94, 1987.

30. Ramsay RC, Cantril HC, Knobloch WH, Goetz FC, Sutherland DER, Najarian JS: Visual parameters in diabetic patients following renal transplantation. Diabetic nephropathy 2(1): 26–29, 1983.

31. van der Vliet JA, Navarro X, Kennedy WR, Goetz FC, Najarian JS, Sutherland DER: The effect of pancreas transplantation on diabetic polyneuropathy. Transplantation 45: 368–370, 1988.

32. Mauer SM, Steffes MW, Connett J et al: Development of lesions in the glomerular basement membrane and mesangium after transplantation of normal kidneys to diabetic patients. Diabetes 32: 948–952, 1983.

33. Sutherland DER, Bentley FR, Mauer SM, Menth L, Nylander W, Goetz FC, Barbosa J, Ascher NL, Simmons RL, Najarian JS: A report of 26 diabetic renal allograft recipients alive with functioning grafts at 10 or more years after primary transplantation. Diabetic nephropathy 3: 39–43, 1984.

34. Bohman SO, Tyden G, Wilczek A: Prevention of kidney graft diabetic nephropathy by pancreas transplantation in man. Diabetes 34: 306, 1985.

35. Bilous RW, Mauer SM, Sutherland DER et al: The effects of pancreas transplantation on renal allograft glomerular structure in insulin-dependent (type I) diabetes mellitus. Diabetes 38 (Suppl 1): 262, 1989.

36. Ramsay RC, Goetz FC, Sutherland DER, Mauer SM, Robinson LL, Cantrill HL, Knobloch WH, Najarian JS: Progression of diabetic retinopathy after pancreas transplantation for insulin-dependent diabetes mellitus. New Engl J Med 318: 208–214, 1988.

37. Ulbig M, Kampik A, Landgraf R, Land W: The influence of combined pancreatic and renal transplantation on advanced diabetic retinopathy. Transpl Proc 19: 3554–3556, 1987.

38. Dahl-Jorgensen K, Brinchmann-Hansen O, Hanssen KF, Ganes T, Kierulf P, Smeland E, Sandvik L, Aagenaes O: Effect of near normoglycaemia for two years on progression of early diabetic retinopathy, nephropathy, and neuropathy: the Oslo study. Brit Med J 293: 1195–1199, 1986.

39. Bilous RW, Mauer SM, Sutherland DER, Steffes MW: Glomerular structure and function following successful pancreas transplantation for insulin-dependent diabetes. Diabetes 36: 43A, 1987.

40. DeFrancisco AM, Mauer SM, Steffes MW, Goetz FC, Najarian, JS, Sutherland DER: The effect of cyclosporin on native renal function in nonuremic diabetic recipients of pancreas transplants. J Diab Compl 1: 128–131, 1987.

41. Viberti GC, Hill RD, Jarre HRJ et al: Microalbuminuria as a predictor of clinical diabetic nephropathy. Lancet 1: 1430–1432, 1982.

42. Luetscher JA, Kraemer FS, Wilson DM et al: Increased plasma inactive renin: a marker to

microvascular disease. New Engl J Med 312–1412, 1985.

43. Merimee TJ, Zapf J, Froesch ER: Insulin-like growth factors: studies in diabetes with and without retinopathy. New Engl J Med 309: 527, 1983.
44. Rosenbloom AL, Silverstein JH, Lezotte DC et al: Limited joint mobility in childhood diabetes mellitus indicates increased risk for microvascular disease. New Engl J Med 305: 191, 1981.
45. Ungar RH: Meticulous control of diabetes: Benefits, risks and precautions. Diabetes 31: 479, 1982.
46. White N, Skor DA, Cryer PE et al: Identification for type I diabetic patients at increased risk for hypoglycemia during intensive therapy. New Engl J Med 308: 485, 1983.
47. Health Care Financing Administration (HCFA) office of special programs: End-stage renal disease program medical information system, facility survey tables, department of health and human services, USA, HCFA, January 1–December 31, 1986.
48. Bart KJ, Macon EJ, Whittier FC et al: Cadaveric kidneys for transplantation. A paradox of shortage in the face of plenty. Transplantation 31: 374, 1981.
49. Lacy PE: Islet transplantation. Diabetes annual 3, pp 189–200, 1987.
50. Sutherland DER, Matas AJ, Goetz FC et al: Transplantation of dispersed pancreatic islet tissue in humans: autografts and allografts. Diabetes 29 (Suppl 1): 34, 1980.
51. Scharp DW, Lacy PE: Human islet isolation and transplantation. Diabetes 34 (Suppl 1): 5A, 1985.
52. Faustman D, Hauptfeld V, Lacy P, Davie J: Prolongation of murine islet allograft survival by pretreatment of islets with antibody directed to Ia determinants. Proc Natl Acad Sci USA 78: 5156.
53. Gores PF, Sutherland DER, Platt JL, Bach FH: Depletion of donor Ia+ cells before transplantation does not prolong islet allograft survival. J Immunol 137: 1482–1485, 1986.
54. Scharp DW, Lacy PE, Finke E et al: Low temperature culture of human islets isolated by the distention method and purified with ficoll or percoll gradients. Surgery 102: 869–879, 1987.
55. Sibley RK, Sutherland DER, Goetz FC, et al: Recurrent diabetes mellitus in the pancreas iso- and allograft. A light and electron microscope and immunohistochemical analysis of four cases. Lab Invest 53: 132–144, 1985.
56. Sutherland DER, Goetz FC, Sibley RK: Recurrence of disease in pancreas transplants. Diabetes 38 (Suppl 1): 85–87, 1989.
57. Barker CF, Naji A, Perloff LJ et al: Invited commentary: An overview of pancreas transplantation. Biologic aspects. Surgery 92: 113, 1982.

Index of subjects

532

538

540